Mental Disorders Around the World

Mental Disorders Around the World

Facts and Figures from the WHO World Mental Health Surveys

Edited by

Kate M. Scott
University of Otago

Peter de Jonge
University of Groningen

Dan J. Stein
University of Cape Town

Ronald C. Kessler
Harvard University

CAMBRIDGE UNIVERSITY PRESS

CAMBRIDGE
UNIVERSITY PRESS

University Printing House, Cambridge CB2 8BS, United Kingdom

One Liberty Plaza, 20th Floor, New York, NY 10006, USA

477 Williamstown Road, Port Melbourne, VIC 3207, Australia

314-321, 3rd Floor, Plot 3, Splendor Forum, Jasola District Centre, New Delhi - 110025, India

79 Anson Road, #06-04/06, Singapore 079906

Cambridge University Press is part of the University of Cambridge.

It furthers the University's mission by disseminating knowledge in the pursuit of education, learning and research at the highest international levels of excellence.

www.cambridge.org
Information on this title: www.cambridge.org/9781107115705
DOI: 10.1017/9781316336168

First published 2018

A catalogue record for this publication is available from the British Library

Library of Congress Cataloging in Publication data

Names: Scott, Kate M. (Kate Margaret), 1960- editor. | Jonge, Peter de, 1969- editor. | Stein, Dan J., editor. | Kessler, Ronald C., editor.
Title: Mental disorders around the world : facts and figures from the WHO World Mental Health surveys / edited by Kate M Scott, Peter de Jonge, Dan J Stein, Ronald C Kessler.
Description: Cambridge ; New York, NY : Cambridge University Press, 2017. | Includes bibliographical references and index.
Identifiers: LCCN 2017051828 (print) | LCCN 2017053203 (ebook) | ISBN 9781107115705 (Hardback) | ISBN 9781107115705 (hardback)
Subjects: | MESH: Mental Disorders—epidemiology | Health Surveys | Global Health—statistics & numerical data | Statistics
Classification: LCC RA790.5 (ebook) | LCC RA790.5 (print) | NLM WM 140 | DDC 362.2—dc23
LC record available at https://lccn.loc.gov/2017051828

ISBN 978-1-107-11570-5 Hardback

Contents

Section III – Overview

Acknowledgements

We are grateful to the many thousands of World Mental Health (WMH) survey respondents around the world who gave of their time so generously; in so doing they have added immeasurably to our understanding of the epidemiology of mental disorders. For this volume, the editors would like to acknowledge the contributions of all the researchers who have been part of the WMH Surveys Initiative, only a proportion of whom are represented as authors on chapters included in this volume. We are particularly indebted to Carmen Lim, University of Otago, Dunedin, who carried out most of the statistical analyses for this book. Additional statistical analyses for specific chapters were conducted by Hisateru Tachimori (Chapter 21), Maria Petukhova (Chapter 11), and Klaas Wardenaar (Chapter 20). We would also like to acknowledge the contribution of the analysts and staff of the WMH Data Collection and Data Analysis Centre at the Department of Health Care Policy, Harvard Medical School, whose foundational data management and analytical work underpins the statistical analyses undertaken for this volume. We thank Teresa Gorman, Department of Health Care Policy, Harvard Medical School, for her administrative assistance. Finally, we greatly appreciate the funding provided for the statistical analyses undertaken by Carmen Lim through grants to Kate Scott in 2015 and 2016 from the James Hume Family Bequest, Dunedin, New Zealand.

This project was carried out in conjunction with the World Health Organization WMH Surveys Initiative. We thank the WMH staff for assistance with instrumentation, fieldwork, and consultation on data analysis. These activities were supported by the United States National Institute of Mental Health (NIMH; R01 MH070884), the John D. and Catherine T. MacArthur Foundation, the Pfizer Foundation, the United States Public Health Service (R13-MH066849, R01-MH069864, and R01 DA016558), the Fogarty International Center (FIRCA R03-TW006481), the Pan American Health Organization, Eli Lilly and Company, Ortho-McNeil Pharmaceutical Inc., GlaxoSmithKline, and Bristol-Myers Squibb. A complete list of WMH publications can be found at www.hcp.med.harvard.edu/wmh.

The 2007 Australian National Survey of Mental Health and Wellbeing is funded by the Australian Government Department of Health and Ageing. The São Paulo Megacity Mental Health Survey is supported by the State of São Paulo Research Foundation (FAPESP) Thematic Project Grant 03/00204-3. The Bulgarian Epidemiological Study of common mental disorders EPIBUL is supported by the Ministry of Health and the National Center for Public Health Protection. The Chinese WMH Survey Initiative is supported by the Pfizer Foundation. The Shenzhen Mental Health Survey is supported by the Shenzhen Bureau of Health and the Shenzhen Bureau of Science, Technology, and Information. The Colombian National Study of Mental Health (NSMH) is supported by the Ministry of Social Protection. The Mental Health Study Medellín – Colombia was carried out and supported jointly by the Center for Excellence on Research in Mental Health (CES University) and the Secretary of Health of Medellín. The ESEMeD project is funded by the European Commission (Contracts QLG5-1999-01042, SANCO 2004123, and EAHC 20081308), the Piedmont Region (Italy); Fondo de Investigación Sanitaria, Instituto de Salud Carlos III, Spain (FIS 00/0028); Ministerio de Ciencia y Tecnología, Spain (SAF 2000-158-CE); Departament de Salut, Generalitat de Catalunya, Spain; Instituto de Salud Carlos III (CIBER CB06/02/0046, RETICS RD06/0011 REM-TAP); and other local agencies and by an unrestricted educational grant from GlaxoSmithKline. Implementation of the Iraq Mental Health Survey (IMHS) and data entry were carried out by the staff of the Iraqi Ministry of Health and Ministry of Planning with direct support from the Iraqi IMHS team with funding from both the Japanese and European Funds through United Nations Development Group Iraq Trust Fund (UNDG ITF). The Israel National Health Survey is funded by the Ministry of Health with support from the Israel National Institute for Health Policy and Health Services Research and the National Insurance Institute of Israel. The World Mental Health Japan (WMHJ) Survey is supported by the Grant for Research on Psychiatric and Neurological Diseases and Mental Health (H13-SHOGAI-023, H14-TOKUBETSU-026, H16-KOKORO-013) from the Japan Ministry of Health, Labour and Welfare. The Lebanese Evaluation of the Burden of Ailments and Needs Of the Nation (L.E.B.A.N.O.N.) is supported by the Lebanese Ministry of Public Health, the WHO (Lebanon), National Institute of Health/Fogarty International Center (R03 TW006481-01), anonymous private donations to IDRAAC, Lebanon, and unrestricted grants from, Algorithm, AstraZeneca, Benta, Bella Pharma, Eli Lilly, Glaxo Smith Kline, Lundbeck, Novartis, OmniPharma, Phenicia, Pfizer, Servier, and UPO. The Mexican National Comorbidity Survey (MNCS) is supported by The National Institute of Psychiatry Ramon de la Fuente (INPRFMDIES 4280) and by the National Council on Science and Technology (CONACyT-G30544-H), with supplemental support from the PanAmerican Health Organization (PAHO). Te Rau Hinengaro: The New Zealand Mental Health Survey (NZMHS) is supported by the New Zealand Ministry of Health, Alcohol Advisory Council, and the Health Research Council. The Nigerian Survey of Mental Health and Wellbeing (NSMHW) is supported by the WHO (Geneva), the WHO (Nigeria), and the Federal Ministry of Health, Abuja, Nigeria. The Northern Ireland Study of Mental Health was funded by the Health and Social Care Research and Development Division of the Public Health Agency. The Peruvian WMH Study was funded by the National Institute of Health of the Ministry of Health of Peru. The Polish project Epidemiology of Mental Health and Access to Care–EZOP Project (PL 0256) was supported by Iceland, Liechtenstein, and Norway through funding from the EEA Financial Mechanism and the Norwegian Financial Mechanism. EZOP project was co-financed by the Polish Ministry of Health. The Portuguese Mental Health Study was carried out by the Department of Mental Health, Faculty of Medical Sciences, NOVA University of Lisbon, with collaboration of the Portuguese Catholic University, and was funded by Champalimaud Foundation, Gulbenkian Foundation, Foundation for Science and Technology (FCT), and Ministry of Health. The Romania WMH study projects 'Policies in Mental Health Area' and 'National Study regarding Mental Health and Services Use' were carried out by National School of Public Health and Health Services Management (former National Institute for Research and Development in Health), with technical support of Metro Media Transilvania, the National Institute of Statistics-National Centre for Training in Statistics, SC Cheyenne Services SRL, Statistics Netherlands and were funded by Ministry of Public Health (former Ministry of Health) with supplemental support from Eli Lilly Romania SRL. The South Africa Stress and Health Study (SASH) is supported by the US National Institute of Mental Health (R01-MH059575) and National Institute of Drug Abuse with supplemental funding from the South African Department of Health and the University of Michigan. The Psychiatric Enquiry to General Population in Southeast Spain – Murcia (PEGASUS-Murcia) Project has been financed by the Regional Health Authorities of Murcia (Servicio Murciano de Salud and Consejería de Sanidad y Política Social) and Fundación para la Formación e Investigación Sanitarias (FFIS) of Murcia. The Ukraine Comorbid Mental Disorders during Periods of Social Disruption (CMDPSD) study is funded by the US National Institute of Mental Health (RO1-MH61905). The US National Comorbidity Survey Replication (NCS-R) is supported by the National Institute of Mental Health (NIMH; U01-MH60220) with supplemental support from the National Institute of Drug Abuse (NIDA), the Substance Abuse and Mental Health Services Administration (SAMHSA), the Robert Wood Johnson Foundation (RWJF; Grant 044708), and the John W. Alden Trust.

The views and opinions expressed in this book are those of the authors and should not be construed to represent the views of the WHO, other sponsoring organizations, agencies, or governments.

Contributors

Sergio Aguilar-Gaxiola, MD, PhD
Center for Reducing Health Disparities
University of California Davis School of Medicine
Davis, CA, USA

Ali Al-Hamzawi, MBCh.B, MD, FICMS
College of Medicine
Al-Qadisiya University
Diwaniya governorate, Iraq

Jordi Alonso, MD, PhD
Health Services Research Unit, IMIM-Hospital del Mar Medical Research Institute
Pompeu Fabra University (UPF)
CIBER en Epidemiología y Salud Pública (CIBERESP)
Barcelona, Spain

Laura Helena Andrade, MD, PhD
Section of Psychiatric Epidemiology – LIM 23
Institute of Psychiatry, University of São Paulo Medical School
São Paulo, Brazil

Corina Benjet, PhD
Department of Epidemiologic and Psychosocial Research
National Institute of Psychiatry Ramón de la Fuente Muñiz
Mexico City, Mexico

Evelyn J. Bromet, PhD
Department of Psychiatry
Stony Brook University
Stony Brook, NY, USA

Ronny Bruffaerts, PhD
Universitair Psychiatrisch Centrum – Katholieke Universiteit Leuven (UPC-KUL)
Campus Gasthuisberg
University of Leuven, Belgium

Brendan Bunting, PhD
School of Psychology
Ulster University
Londonderry, United Kingdom

José Miguel Caldas-de-Almeida, MD, PhD
Department of Mental Health,
Faculdades de Ciências Médicas
Universidade Nova de Lisboa
Lisbon, Portugal

Graça Cardoso, MD, PhD
Department of Mental Health,
Faculdades de Ciências Médicas
Universidade Nova de Lisboa
Lisbon, Portugal

Somnath Chatterji, MD
Department of Information, Evidence and Research
World Health Organization
Geneva, Switzerland

Louisa Degenhardt, PhD
National Drug and Alcohol Research Centre
University of New South Wales
Sydney, Australia

Koen Demyttenaere, MD, PhD
Department of Psychiatry, University Hospital Gasthuisberg
Katholieke Universiteit Leuven (KUL)
Leuven, Belgium

Sara Evans-Lacko, PhD
Institute of Psychiatry, Psychology and Neuroscience, King's College London
PSSRU, London School of Economics and Political Science
London, United Kingdom

John Fayyad, MD
Institute for Development, Research, Advocacy and Applied Care (IDRAAC)
Beirut, Lebanon

Marina Piazza Ferrand, ScD, MPH
Universidad Cayetano Heredia
National Institute of Health
Lima, Peru

Silvia Florescu, MD, PhD
National School of Public Health, Management and Development
Bucharest, Romania

Giovanni de Girolamo, MD
Istituti di Ricovero e Cura a Carattere Scientifico (IRCCS)
St. John of God Clinical Research Centre
Brescia, Italy

Meyer D. Glantz, PhD
Department of Epidemiology, Services, and Prevention Research (DESPR)
National Institute on Drug Abuse (NIDA)
National Institute of Health (NIH)
Bethesda, MD, USA

Oye Gureje, MD, PhD, FRCPsych
Department of Psychiatry
University of Ibadan
Ibadan, Nigeria

Lauren S. Hallion, PhD
Department of Psychology
University of Pittsburgh
Pittsburgh, PA, USA

Josep Maria Haro, MD, PhD
Parc Sanitari Sant Joan de Déu
Universitat de Barcelona
CIBERSAM
Barcelona, Spain

Yanling He, MD
Shanghai Mental Health Center
Shanghai Jiao Tong University, School of Medicine
Shanghai, People's Republic of China

Steven G. Heeringa, PhD
Survey Research Center, Institute for Social Research
University of Michigan
Ann Arbor, MI, USA

Hristo Hinkov, MD, PhD
National Center for Public Health and Analyses
Sofia, Bulgaria

Chiyi Hu, MD, PhD
Shenzhen Institute of Mental Health
Shenzhen Kangning Hospital
Shenzhen, People's Republic of China

Yueqin Huang, MD, MPH, PhD
Institute of Mental Health
Peking University
Beijing, People's Republic of China

James I. Hudson, MD, ScD
Biological Psychiatry Laboratory, McLean Hospital
Belmont, MA, USA
Department of Psychiatry, Harvard Medical School
Boston, MA, USA

Peter de Jonge, PhD
Developmental Psychology, Department of Psychology, Rijksuniversiteit Groningen
Interdisciplinary Center Psychopathology and Emotion Regulation
Department of Psychiatry, University Medical Center Groningen
Groningen, The Netherlands

Elie G. Karam, MD
Department of Psychiatry and Clinical Psychology, St George Hospital University Medical Center, Balamand University, Faculty of Medicine
Institute for Development, Research, Advocacy and Applied Care (IDRAAC)
Beirut, Lebanon

Norito Kawakami, MD, DMSc
Department of Mental Health
School of Public Health
The University of Tokyo
Tokyo, Japan

Ronald C. Kessler, PhD
Department of Health Care Policy
Harvard Medical School
Boston, MA, USA

Andrzej Kiejna, PhD, MD
Wroclaw Medical University
University of Lower Silesia
Wroclaw, Poland

Karestan C. Koenen, PhD
Department of Epidemiology
Harvard T. H. Chan School of Public Health
Boston, MA, USA

Viviane Kovess-Masféty, MD, PhD
Ecole des Hautes Etudes en Santé
Publique (EHESP), EA 4057
Paris Descartes University
Paris, France

Sing Lee, MB, BS
Department of Psychiatry
Chinese University of Hong Kong
Tai Po, Hong Kong

Jean-Pierre Lépine, MD
Hôpital Lariboisière Fernand Widal,
Assistance Publique Hôpitaux de Paris
Universités Paris Descartes-Paris Diderot
INSERM UMR-S 1144
Paris, France

Daphna Levinson, PhD
Mental Health Services,
Ministry of Health
Jerusalem, Israel

Carmen C. W. Lim, MSc
Department of Psychological
Medicine, University of Otago
Dunedin, New Zealand
Queensland Brain Institute, University of
Queensland, St. Lucia Queensland
Centre for Mental Health Research,
The Park Centre for Mental Health,
Brisbane, Australia

John J. McGrath, MD, PhD
Queensland Brain Institute, University
of Queensland, St.Lucia
Queensland Centre for Mental Health Research,
The Park Centre for Mental Health,
Brisbane, Australia

Maria Elena Medina-Mora, DrPH
National Institute of Psychiatry
Ramón de la Fuente Muñiz
Mexico City, Mexico

Jacek Moskalewicz, PhD
Institute of Psychiatry and Neurology
Warsaw, Poland

Fernando Navarro-Mateu, PhD, MD
UDIF-SM, Subdirección General de
Planificación, Innovación y Cronicidad,
Servicio Murciano de Salud
IMIB-Arrixaca
CIBERESP-Murcia
Murcia, Spain

Lauren C. Ng, PhD
Department of Psychiatry
Boston University School of Medicine
and Boston Medical Center
Boston, MA, USA

Andrew A. Nierenberg, MD
Department of Psychiatry, Harvard Medical School
Bipolar Clinic and Research Program,
Massachusetts General Hospital
Boston, MA, USA

Matthew K. Nock, PhD
Department of Psychology
Harvard University
Cambridge, MA, USA

Beth-Ellen Pennell, MA
Survey Research Center, Institute for Social Research
University of Michigan
Ann Arbor, MI, USA

José Posada-Villa, MD
Faculty of Social Sciences
Colegio Mayor de Cundinamarca University
Bogota, Colombia

Andrew Ratanatharathorn, MA
Department of Epidemiology
Mailman School of Public Health
Columbia University
New York, NY, USA

Annelieke Roest, PhD
Interdisciplinary Center Psychopathology
and Emotion Regulation
Department of Psychiatry, University
Medical Center Groningen
Groningen, The Netherlands

Ayelet Meron Ruscio, PhD
Department of Psychology
University of Pennsylvania
Philadelphia, PA, USA

Sukanta Saha, PhD
Queensland Brain Institute,
University of Queensland,
St. Lucia Queensland Centre for Mental
Health Research, The Park Centre
for Mental Health,
Brisbane, Australia

Nancy A. Sampson
Department of Health Care Policy
Harvard Medical School
Boston, MA, USA

Kate M. Scott, PhD
Department of Psychological Medicine
Dunedin School of Medicine
University of Otago
Dunedin, New Zealand

Victoria Shahly, PhD
Department of Health Care Policy
Harvard Medical School
Boston, MA, USA

Derrick Silove, MB ChB, FRANZCP, MD
School of Psychiatry, University of New South Wales
Academic Mental Health Unit and Psychiatry
Research and Teaching Unit, South
Western Sydney Local Health District
Sydney, NSW, Australia

Dan J. Stein, FRCPC, PhD
Department of Psychiatry and Mental Health
University of Cape Town
Cape Town, Republic of South Africa

Hisateru Tachimori, PhD
National Institute of Mental Health
National Center of Neurology and Psychiatry
Tokyo, Japan

Margreet ten Have, PhD
Trimbos-Instituut, Netherlands Institute
of Mental Health and Addiction
Utrecht, The Netherlands

Graham Thornicroft, PhD
Centre for Global Mental Health
Institute of Psychiatry, Psychology and Neuroscience
King's College London
London, United Kingdom

Yolanda Torres, MPH, Dra.HC
Center for Excellence on Research in Mental Health
CES University
Medellin, Colombia

Brianna Turner, PhD
Department of Psychology, University of Victoria
Victoria, BC, Canada
Department of Psychology, Harvard University
Cambridge, MA, USA

Maria Carmen Viana, PhD, MD
Department of Social Medicine
Federal University of Espirito Santo
Vitoria, Brazil

Klaas J. Wardenaar, PhD
Interdisciplinary Center Psychopathology
and Emotion Regulation
Department of Psychiatry, University
Medical Center Groningen
Groningen, The Netherlands

David R. Williams, MPH, PhD
Department of Society, Human
Development and Health
Harvard T. H. Chan School of Public Health
Boston, MA, USA

Alan M. Zaslavsky, PhD
Department of Health Care Policy
Harvard Medical School
Boston, MA, USA

Chapter 1 Introduction

Kate M. Scott, Peter de Jonge, Dan J. Stein, Ronald C. Kessler

The study of the epidemiology of mental disorders in the World Health Organization (WHO) World Mental Health (WMH) surveys provides information on the prevalence and distribution of mental disorders in general populations around the world, together with much additional information on age-of-onset, severity, role impairment, treatment, and risk factors. This information is critically important for the improvement of population mental health. It provides foundational data for a wide array of interventions and policies ranging from the broad public health approaches of mental health promotion and prevention through to specialist mental health treatment and service delivery planning.

This volume is the fifth in the series of books on the WMH Surveys Initiative. The first volume, based on the first 17 countries to complete surveys, presented the epidemiology of mental disorders by country, allowing a country-specific description of methods and discussion of findings (Kessler and Üstün 2008). The next three volumes focused on specific topics within the broad field of psychiatric epidemiology: mental–physical comorbidity (Volume 2; Von Korff *et al.* 2009); suicide (Volume 3; Nock *et al.* 2012); and the disability and societal costs associated with mental disorders (Volume 4; Alonso *et al.* 2013). The current volume, based on 29 surveys conducted in 26 countries, takes a disorder-specific approach, presenting descriptive epidemiological data on a wide range of mental disorders as defined by the *Diagnostic and Statistical Manual of Mental Disorders*, fourth edition (DSM-IV). A key feature of this volume is that a common set of statistical analyses devised specifically for this volume was used for all disorders, with just a few exceptions resulting from data constraints. Some of the findings have been published in journal articles and many are published here for the first time. This consistent approach to data analysis, building on the consistent, rigorous approach to survey methodology that is one of the great strengths of the WMH surveys, allows readers to make comparisons of epidemiological estimates across disorders and across countries.

The book is organized in three sections. The next chapter in this introductory section, Chapter 2, places the WMH surveys in historical context by outlining the development of psychiatric epidemiology, as well as the struggles of the field to reach consensus on how to define and measure mental ill-health. This chapter also provides a discussion of some of the methodological criticisms levelled at the WMH surveys and other studies using similar methods. Chapter 3 finishes the section with a detailed description of WMH methods, covering the many aspects of survey design and implementation, questionnaire development, and analytical approach. Methods chapters are often skipped as boring or too technical: we urge readers not to do so as this chapter offers a fascinating insight into the challenge and complexity of cross-national survey design and implementation.

Chapters 4–19 that comprise Section II of this book focus on specific disorders. Each chapter begins with an overview of the known epidemiology of the disorder and then presents and discusses the WMH findings on disorder prevalence, onset distributions, lifetime risk, impairment, socio-demographic correlates, comorbidity with other mental disorders, and service use. The tables provide results at increasing levels of aggregation: country-specific, aggregated across country income groups and WHO regions, and aggregated across all countries combined. Although the disorders are based on DSM-IV diagnoses, where changes in diagnostic criteria from DSM-IV to DSM-5 have occurred these are outlined and their implications discussed. As noted above, a core set of analyses was undertaken for all disorders, data permitting. But the chapters are nonetheless diverse, over and above their differing results. Additional analyses were undertaken for specific disorders where there were strong research imperatives to do so. Findings from earlier WMH analyses are also presented or discussed where relevant. A further factor contributing to variation across chapters is that they are written by a wide range of experts, who have used their knowledge of the specific disorders to select which findings to present and highlight.

Some comment on disorder omissions and inclusions in Section II is in order. The WMH surveys assessed most of the major DSM-IV mental disorders, but not all. Schizophrenia and related psychotic disorders were not included in the surveys because they cannot be accurately assessed using fully structured lay-administered interviews in non-institutionalized populations. The neurodegenerative disorders of ageing were not assessed, nor were some of the rarer disorders, such as somatoform and dissociative disorders. Of the disorders that were assessed in the WMH surveys almost all have been included in this volume, with two exceptions. One omission is obsessive compulsive disorder, which was not measured by the WMH diagnostic interview with sufficient accuracy in all surveys. The other omission is anorexia nervosa, which was not included due to insufficient case numbers. The one chapter in Section II that is not focused on a DSM mental disorder is Chapter 19. We include this chapter because psychotic-like symptoms, occurring outside the context of a psychotic disorder, are a topic of increasing interest to the mental health research community.

The third section of the book moves from the disorder-specific perspective to a broader view encompassing all disorders in three chapters. Chapter 20 on comorbidity uses the WMH data to investigate what the observed patterns of comorbidity among mental disorders might signify in terms of underlying constructs or 'latent structure'. Although this topic has been extensively studied previously, this chapter is novel in the inclusion of such a wide range of mental disorders and in its examination of the cross-national stability of comorbidity patterns. Chapter 21 on service use examines how treatment seeking for mental health problems varies across disorders, across levels of disorder severity, and across socio-demographic groups. The findings of this chapter are an important testament to the gap between clinical need and treatment access, especially among those with lower education and income who are encountering barriers to accessing specialist mental health care, even when their mental disorders are severe. The cross-national perspective highlights that this gap between need and treatment uptake is particularly glaring in low-income countries.

Finally, Chapter 22 integrates and discusses the findings of the volume as a whole, presenting summary statistics for each disorder to allow a comparison across disorders and across countries. This chapter highlights the consistent patterns across countries emerging from the WMH data in when and in whom mental disorders present. The chapter also documents and discusses some provocative patterns of cross-national variation in disorder prevalence and impairment, although there are constraints on the interpretation of these patterns due to the difficulty of ensuring methodological consistency in a large cross-national study. The chapter closes with a discussion of the policy implications of the findings and future research directions.

Our hope is that this book will be of interest to a wide readership. It is likely to be of particular value to researchers, clinicians, students, and policy-makers in the fields of mental health and public health who want the most up-to-date information on the epidemiology of mental disorders cross-nationally. It is a unique resource for those with an interest in a specific mental disorder in its provision of detailed disorder-specific WMH findings that are discussed in the context of other published research on the disorder. The book also offers a mine of information for those who have more general questions, such as what the prevalence of mental disorders is and how prevalence varies across countries; at what age mental disorders tend to develop and who is at most risk; which mental disorders are most persistent and which are most disabling; and how treatment varies across individuals, disorders, service settings, and countries. Collectively, this body of information is an essential empirical foundation for policy and treatment initiatives in global mental health. Conducting cross-national comparative studies of mental disorders is immensely challenging but we believe that the wealth of findings presented in this volume is testament to the great value of doing so.

References

Alonso J., Chatterji S., He Y. (eds) (2013) *The Burdens of Mental Disorders: Global Perspectives from the WHO World Mental Health Surveys*. Cambridge University Press, New York.

Kessler R.C., Üstün T.B. (eds) (2008) *The WHO World Mental Health Surveys: Global Perspectives on the Epidemiology of Mental Disorders*. Cambridge University Press, New York.

Nock M.K., Borges G., Ono Y. (eds) (2012) *Suicide: Global Perspectives from the WHO World Mental Health Surveys*. Cambridge University Press, New York.

Von Korff M., Scott K.M., Gureje O. (eds) (2009) *Global Perspectives on Mental–Physical Comorbidity in the WHO World Mental Health Surveys*. Cambridge University Press, New York.

Chapter 2

The Cross-National Epidemiology of Mental Disorders

Dan J. Stein, Peter de Jonge, Ronald C. Kessler, Kate M. Scott

Introduction

Successive advances have been made in our understanding of the epidemiology of mental disorders over the past several decades. These gradual advances in our understanding in turn rest on a foundation of incremental progress in various areas, including conceptualization of mental disorders, community survey methodology and data analysis, and global collaborative research networks. The World Mental Health (WMH) Surveys Initiative, comprising the largest and most sophisticated coordinated set of community surveys on mental disorders to date, exemplifies the progress that has been made and provides a state-of-the-art portrayal of the epidemiology of mental disorders around the world. In this background chapter, we provide some relevant historical and theoretical context in order to outline the scope and value of the WMH surveys, and to address some key criticisms of the work.

Operationalization of Mental Disorders

Mental disorders have been recognized and described by clinicians for millennia (Kendler 2009). Hippocrates and many other physicians of the ancient world provided detailed descriptions of depression and alcohol dependence; conditions which we now include under the rubric of 'common mental disorders'. In the nineteenth century, Kraepelin and others working in mental hospital settings delineated psychotic disorders such as schizophrenia and bipolar disorder: entities that are now often termed 'serious mental disorders'. Freud, Janet, Westphal, and others working in outpatient settings described a range of anxiety and impulse-control disorders. Mental disorders were classified and categorized in early editions of the *Diagnostic and Statistical Manual of Mental Disorders* (DSM), and of the *International Statistical Classification of Diseases* (ICD).

At the same time, by the middle of the twentieth century, a number of problems in psychiatric classifications were readily apparent (Spitzer *et al.* 1980). A particularly important issue that came to light was disagreement between clinicians in different countries about the diagnosis of schizophrenia; in the United Kingdom there was a comparatively high threshold for diagnosis of this condition, while in the United States there was a much lower threshold (Cooper *et al.* 1969). Critics reported that healthy individuals who feigned mental illness could readily be admitted to a psychiatric hospital (Rosenhan 1973). In order to address these problems, researchers began to develop diagnostic criteria to operationalize psychiatric disorders; for example, the Feighner criteria were developed by Robins and colleagues and the Research Diagnostic Criteria were developed by Spitzer and colleagues (Kendler *et al.* 2010).

This work in turn provided the basis for the third edition of the DSM, published by the American Psychiatric Association in 1980. This volume, led by Spitzer, provided diagnostic criteria for a range of mental disorders and so enabled clinicians across the United States to more reliably determine the presence of diagnostic entities. The manual was translated into a range of languages and within a few years became the dominant nosology for psychiatric research across the globe. The diagnostic criteria were incorporated into clinician-administered diagnostic interviews, they formed the basis for inclusion criteria into clinical trials of pharmacotherapy and psychotherapy for mental disorders, and they provided a foundation for community and clinical surveys of mental disorders in a range of different settings.

Subsequent decades saw the publication of DSM-IV and DSM-5, as well as further revisions of the ICD. Whereas DSM-III broke new ground by providing a novel approach to the operationalization of mental disorders, DSM-IV and DSM-5 made incremental progress, with changes to the diagnostic criteria based on accumulating research (Frances *et al.* 1989). Thus, for example, high thresholds for the introduction of new disorders in DSM-IV and DSM-5 were set, and the focus was on evidence-based refinement of the diagnostic criteria of existing mental disorders. DSM is produced by the American Psychiatric Association, and recent revisions have emphasized the importance of diagnostic validity (that is, going beyond the earlier emphasis on reliability of operational criteria to focus on evidence supporting the relevant construct) (Kupfer & Regier 2011). ICD is produced by the World Health Organization (WHO), and recent efforts at revision have emphasized the importance of clinical utility and of global applicability (Reed & Ayuso-Mateos 2011). Nevertheless, DSM-IV and the research version of ICD-10 have a good deal of overlap, and there are ongoing attempts to harmonize DSM-5 and ICD-11 (Regier *et al.* 2013).

Community Surveys Methodology

A range of advances in the methodology of community surveys have been crucial for contemporary epidemiology of mental disorders. Once diagnostic criteria had been developed for psychiatric disorders, an immediate question was whether they could feasibly be administered in the community, for example, by master's level clinicians (Weissman *et al.* 1978). A key advance was the development of a fully structured lay interview based on the Feighner criteria, the Research Diagnostic Criteria, and the DSM-III diagnostic criteria: the Diagnostic Interview Schedule (DIS) (Robins *et al.* 1984). Work on the DIS was supported by the National Institute of Mental Health Center for Epidemiological Studies, which funded the Epidemiological Catchment Area study in the United States; the first large multi-site community survey of mental disorders to be based on the new approach to the operationalization of mental disorders. Comparison of data from lay-administered interviews with independent clinician-administrated interviews indicated acceptable reliability and validity.

Subsequent work on a new diagnostic instrument was undertaken by the WHO in collaboration with the US Alcohol, Drug, and Mental Health Administration in order to include criteria from the ICD, and to translate the instrument into a range of different languages (Kessler 2000b). This first version of the Composite International Diagnostic Interview (CIDI) was made available in 1990, and included both DSM-III and ICD-10 criteria, with subsequent versions incorporating DSM-III-R and DSM-IV diagnostic criteria. The CIDI has a range of features designed to improve the reliability and validity of the data obtained from lay-administered interview, including efforts to increase respondent understanding, motivation, and ability to provide accurate survey responses (Kessler and Üstün 2004). Such features, and the concordance of the CIDI with clinical diagnosis, are discussed in more detail in the next chapter.

Prior to the DIS and CIDI, psychiatric epidemiology lagged behind work done in other areas of health. The DIS and CIDI allowed a new generation of psychiatric epidemiology research (Dohrenwend and Dohrenwend 1982), which employed operational definitions of mental disorders, and so provided rigorous data on their prevalence and correlates. A number of key lessons emerged from this new generation of studies, which include a range of surveys focusing on particular mental disorders, such as the National Vietnam Veterans Readjustment Study (Schlenger *et al.* 2007) and the National Epidemiological Survey on Alcohol and Related Conditions (Hasin & Grant 2015). First, depression, anxiety disorders, and substance-use disorders are highly prevalent conditions in the United States. Second, these disorders have an early age-of-onset, protracted course, and high comorbidity. Third, mental disorders are associated with significant impairment, as well as high costs to society. Finally, mental disorders are significantly under-diagnosed and under-treated.

The new generation of epidemiological research on mental disorders has also provided a series of lessons about particular mental disorders. Consider, for example, some key findings on anxiety disorders (Kessler *et al.* 2010). First, data on prevalence of different psychiatric disorders has emphasized that anxiety disorders are the most common class of psychiatric disorders, perhaps speaking to the adaptive value of fear responses (Stein & Nesse 2011). Second, data on onset and course have emphasized that many anxiety disorders precede mood and substance-use disorders, so emphasizing the potential clinical value of early recognition and robust treatment (Goodwin & Gorman 2002). Third, data on comorbidity have emphasized that depression and generalized anxiety disorder (GAD) have similarly high levels of comorbidity and of associated impairment; such work has contributed to the conceptualization of GAD as an independent diagnostic entity (Kessler 2000a). Fourth, work on the treatment gap in anxiety disorders has given impetus to the emergence of consumer advocacy organizations that work to promote awareness of these conditions (Stein *et al.* 2001). Analogous lessons have emerged for a range of psychiatric conditions.

Global Collaborative Research Networks

Soon after the development of the DIS, studies were undertaken with this instrument in a number of different countries (Weissman *et al.* 1994, 1996). The CIDI, based on a newer version of the DSM, and including ICD diagnostic criteria, was developed with the explicit aim of being translated into a range of different languages and being used in different regions of the globe, with modifications being made to ensure cross-cultural compatibility – including a range of work to address cross-national variations in the vocabulary of distress (see also Chapter 3). Comparison of data from across countries allows an initial approach to the question of how the prevalence and correlates of mental disorders differ across different contexts. However, in order to fully exploit the richness of data from different contexts and countries, international consortia that gather and pool such data are needed. Fortunately, such work has advanced in the past two decades.

Surveys using the DIS and DSM-III criteria in a limited number of countries suggested that although there were some differences in prevalence of mental disorders across different contexts, the conditions assessed (mood, anxiety, and substance-use disorders) were common, and individuals with these conditions had substantial unmet treatment needs (Weissman *et al.* 1994, 1996). Given that the WHO focuses on the ICD for its work on data gathering and policy formulation, this organization created a cross-national network of researchers using the CIDI in different countries, the WHO International Consortium in Psychiatric Epidemiology (ICPE) (2000). Data from the ICPE emphasized the high prevalence, early onset, substantial persistence, and high comorbidity of mental disorders in a range of different settings. In addition, however, ICPE investigators were able to pool epidemiological data to provide input on questions about risk of disorders; thus for example an ICPE analysis of predictors of onset and persistence of GAD found that history of specific phobia may be a risk marker for GAD onset (Kessler *et al.* 2002).

A revision of the CIDI in the late 1990s provided the impetus for the WHO to establish the WMH Surveys Initiative, and to encourage countries around the world to use the revised CIDI to undertake nationally representative surveys. Grants from a number of agencies, including the National Institutes of Health in the United States allowed the creation of a core infrastructure for the Initiative, so leveraging expertise and allowing cost-saving for participating countries. Many low and middle-income countries, which had not previously participated in psychiatric epidemiological research and which lacked both financial and human resources to undertake such work, were now able to conduct high-quality and large-scale community surveys, and to build capacity in psychiatric epidemiology. The WMH Surveys Initiative now comprises over 30 countries, and includes more than 150,000 respondents (see Chapter 3).

The WMH surveys have brought enormous scope and value to psychiatric epidemiology, providing, for the first time, rigorous data on the prevalence and correlates of a range of mental disorders in a wide range of low, middle, and high-income countries. Notably, coincident with the collection, analysis, and publication of this new body of data, we have witnessed the emergence of the new field of global mental health (Patel 2012; Becker & Kleinman 2013). Indeed, just as epidemiology can be conceptualized as a key pillar of public health, so work such as that of the WMH surveys and the Global Burden of Disease study (GBD Collaborators, Murray *et al.* 2015) has provided a foundation for global mental health, which in turn has emphasized the high disability due to mental disorders, and the large treatment gap associated with these conditions. The WMH Surveys Initiative has provided a key evidence base for the clarion call of global mental health for 'no health without mental health' (Prince *et al.* 2007).

Criticisms of Contemporary Psychiatric Nosology and Epidemiology

The operationalization of mental disorders provided by DSM and ICD, advances in survey methodology outlined earlier, and the development of global collaborative research networks such as the WMH surveys all lay the foundation for remaining chapters of this volume to describe the cross-national epidemiology of a wide range of mood, anxiety, substance-use, and disruptive behaviour/impulse-control disorders. At the same time, it is relevant to consider a number of the key criticisms of these foundations, and so of the work described in this volume. We consider in turn, some related criticisms of contemporary psychiatric nosology, of the approach of the WMH surveys, and of the employment of the CIDI across different regions of the world.

Criticisms of current psychiatric nosology include those emphasizing the reification of mental disorders, artefactual comorbidity, and vested interests. Some argue that psychiatrists now use checklists to make diagnoses; they are unaware of symptoms not listed in DSM, and they fail to appreciate that diagnostic criteria are merely an hypothesis about how a disorder most commonly presents – for any particular patient current diagnostic constructs may not serve well (Hyman 2010; Kendler 2016). Patients often have more than one DSM diagnosis, which suggests that some of this comorbidity is artefactual in nature (Maj 2005). Neuroscientifically minded critics have argued that some of these flaws reflect the fact that diagnostic operationalizations are not sufficiently based on biological discoveries; neurocircuitry-based constructs, it has been suggested, may ultimately provide a more valid and useful foundation for assessment and treatment (Insel *et al.* 2010). More sceptical critics have argued that more disorders translate into increased sales, and that psychiatry has colluded with the pharmaceutical industry to inappropriately apply Western diagnostic constructs in non-Western contexts, ignoring the issue of fundamental differences in the structure of distress and psychopathology across the globe, and instead medicalizing non-pathological distress and deviance (Moynihan *et al.* 2002; Stein 2015).

Certainly, the diagnostic operationalization embedded in contemporary psychiatric nosology reflects the status of our current knowledge of mental disorders. At the same time, considerable effort has been made to establish and to improve the diagnostic validity and clinical utility of modern diagnostic constructs (Reed & Ayuso-Mateos 2011; Regier *et al.* 2013). Such efforts avoid reification by focusing on the evidence in support of contrasting diagnostic conceptualizations and operationalizations, fully accepting that symptoms lie on dimensions and that disorders have fuzzy boundaries with non-disorder and with one another. Conflicts of interest are rigorously addressed, and participation of a broad range of stakeholders is vigorously encouraged (Stein & Phillips 2013). While new biologically based conceptual frameworks such as the Research Domain Criteria (RDoC) may well be useful in informing future research (Cuthbert & Insel 2010), it is by no means clear that superior diagnostic constructs for clinical work will easily be found (Stein 2014). Indeed it is unlikely that the next editions of DSM and ICD will represent a paradigm shift; it is much more likely that they will represent iterative improvement (Kendler & First 2010).

Related criticisms have been made of both the WMH surveys and of global mental health; emphasizing that psychiatric epidemiology and public mental health are flawed insofar as they rely on DSM and ICD operationalizations (Summerfield 2012). On the one hand, some critics have argued that given that we already know that mental disorders are highly prevalent and under-diagnosed and under-treated, the WMH surveys add little that is new (Weich & Araya 2004). On the other hand, others argue that WMH and global mental health have inflated the prevalence of mental disorders and their associated disability; the argument is that policymakers should not be misled by such data, and should be careful not to conflate psychological distress with medical disorder (Summerfield 2012). Those who are less sceptical of contemporary psychiatric nosology and epidemiology still have a range of other criticisms. These include that the CIDI takes insufficient account of cultural idioms of distress, that the reliance on recall biases age-of-onset and lifetime prevalence estimations, and that the cross-sectional design of the WMH surveys makes it difficult for causal factors underlying mental disorders to be delineated.

While it is important to be aware of the limitations of any scientific research and consequent efforts at advocacy, the sophistication of the WMH surveys and of efforts in global mental health should not be underestimated. Although it is true that WMH surveys have relied on DSM and ICD diagnostic conceptualizations and operationalizations, they have also made important contributions to psychiatric nosology by rigorously comparing different diagnostic constructs (Ruscio *et al.* 2007; Lee *et al.* 2009; Karam *et al.* 2010; Stein *et al.* 2010, 2013; McLaughlin *et al.* 2015). Relatedly, WMH surveys have documented how the symptoms of common mental disorders lie on dimensions, and have contributed to psychiatric nosology by evaluating the impact of choosing different cut-points and thresholds for determining the presence of disorders. Finally, the WMH surveys have expended significant energy on addressing cross-national variations in the vocabulary of distress, in optimizing recall of symptoms, and in improving analyses of risk and resilience factors (see Chapter 3). Similarly, the discipline of global mental health has emphasized the importance for public health of appreciating the range that spans serious mental disorders, psychological distress, and well-being, and of addressing the specific social and cultural context within which psychiatric symptoms emerge.

Indeed, we would argue that in a number of respects there has been significant convergence between nosological advances, clinical neuroscience, psychiatric epidemiology, and global mental health; this convergence has helped address critiques of contemporary psychiatric theory, and has contributed to strengthening clinical practice and mental health policy. Thus, for example, the question of how to define a case has long been debated in each of these arenas. The WMH surveys have made an important contribution to this issue by measuring symptom severity of specific mental disorders, by paying particular attention to the question of how best to delineate subthreshold from clinical symptomatology, and by providing an evidence base for proposals to improve the operationalization of diagnostic entities in DSM and ICD. Relatedly, an emphasis on the dimensional nature of psychiatric symptomology has been a key issue in psychiatric nosology, clinical neuroscience, psychiatric epidemiology, and global mental health. Thus DSM-5 introduced new chapters on related psychiatric conditions, emphasized that psychiatric symptoms lie on dimensions of severity and are present across disorders, and provided a range of trans-diagnostic symptom measures. RDoC has emphasized that symptoms lie on dimensions and cut across different disorders; and WMH analyses have investigated different cut-points and thresholds for determining mental disorder.

Conclusion

The subsequent chapters of this volume provide data on the cross-national descriptive epidemiology of a wide range of mental disorders. Certainly our epidemiological data are only as good as our current study instruments, as the memory of survey respondents permits, and as their willingness to participate fully in the interview process allows. Still, notwithstanding the limitations of current diagnostic operationalizations, survey methodology, and global research collaborative networks, these data provide the most comprehensive available perspective on the prevalence and distribution of mental disorders around the world. Taken together, they provide a compelling picture of the burden of mental disorders and of the treatment gap; information that is crucial for those working to improve mental health policies and services. At the same time, the data are an important bridge across the classical divide between psychiatric epidemiology and clinical practice, asking and answering a range of important questions about the prevalence and correlates of mental disorders, and providing clinicians with key facts and figures about the most important conditions seen in everyday work. We believe that the wealth of analyses provided in this volume comprise an important step in the evolution of epidemiological research on mental disorders. Our hope is that they also provide a foundation from which to evaluate future policy and clinical interventions aimed at increasing access to and effectiveness of mental disorder treatments.

References

Becker, A.E. and Kleinman, A. (2013). Mental health and the global agenda. *New England Journal of Medicine*, 369, 1380–1.

Cooper, J.E., Kendell, R.E., Gurland, B.J., *et al.* (1969). Cross-national study of diagnosis of the mental disorders: some results from the first comparative investigation. *American Journal of Psychiatry*, 10 Suppl, 21–9.

Cuthbert, B. and Insel, T. (2010). The data of diagnosis: new approaches to psychiatric classification. *Psychiatry*, 73, 311–4.

Dohrenwend, B.P. and Dohrenwend, B.S. (1982). Perspectives on the past and future of psychiatric epidemiology. The 1981 Rema Lapouse Lecture. *American Journal of Public Health*, 72, 1271–9.

Frances, A.J., Widiger, T.A., and Pincus, H.A. (1989). The development of DSM-IV. *Archives of General Psychiatry*, 46, 373–5.

GBD Collaborators, Murray, C.J., Barber, R.M., *et al.* (2015). Global, regional, and national disability-adjusted life years (DALYs) for 306 diseases and injuries and healthy life expectancy (HALE) for 188 countries, 1990–2013: quantifying the epidemiological transition. *Lancet*, 386, 2145–91

Goodwin, R.D. and Gorman, J.M. (2002). Psychopharmacologic treatment of generalized anxiety disorder and the risk of major depression. *American Journal of Psychiatry*, 159, 1935–7.

Hasin, D.S. and Grant, B.F. (2015). The National Epidemiologic Survey on Alcohol and Related Conditions (NESARC) Waves 1 and 2: review and summary of findings. *Social Psychiatry and Psychiatric Epidemiology*, 50, 1609–40.

Hyman, S.E. (2010). The diagnosis of mental disorders: the problem of reification. *Annual Review of Clinical Psychology*, 6, 155–79.

Insel, T., Cuthbert, B., Garvey, M., *et al.* (2010). Research domain criteria (RDoC): toward a new classification framework for research on mental disorders. *American Journal of Psychiatry*, 167, 748–51.

Karam, E.G., Andrews, G., Bromet, E., *et al.* (2010). The role of criterion A2 in the DSM-IV diagnosis of posttraumatic stress disorder. *Biological Psychiatry*, 68, 465–73.

Kendler, K.S. (2009). An historical framework for psychiatric nosology. *Psychological Medicine*, 39, 1935–41.

(2016). The phenomenology of major depression and the representativeness and nature of DSM criteria. *American Journal of Psychiatry*, 173, 771–80.
Kendler, K.S. and First, M.B. (2010). Alternative futures for the DSM revision process: iteration v. paradigm shift. *British Journal of Psychiatry*, 197, 263–5.
Kendler, K.S., Munoz, R.A., and Murphy, G. (2010). The development of the Feighner criteria: a historical perspective. *American Journal of Psychiatry*, 167, 134–42.
Kessler, R.C. (2000a). The epidemiology of pure and comorbid generalized anxiety disorder: a review and evaluation of recent research. *Acta Psychiatrica Scandinavica Supplementum*, 7–13.
(2000b). Psychiatric epidemiology: selected recent advances and future directions. *Bulletin of the World Health Organization*, 78, 464–74.
Kessler, R.C., Andrade, L.H., Bijl, R.V., *et al.* (2002). The effects of co-morbidity on the onset and persistence of generalized anxiety disorder in the ICPE surveys. International Consortium in Psychiatric Epidemiology. *Psychological Medicine*, 32, 1213–25.
Kessler, R.C., Ruscio, A.M., Shear, K., *et al.* (2010). Epidemiology of anxiety disorders. *Current Topics in Behavioral Neurosciences*, 2, 21–35.
Kessler, R.C. and Üstün, T.B. (2004). The World Mental Health (WMH) Survey Initiative Version of the World Health Organization (WHO) Composite International Diagnostic Interview (CIDI). *International Journal of Methods in Psychiatric Research*, 13, 93–121.
Kupfer, D.J. and Regier, D.A. (2011). Neuroscience, clinical evidence, and the future of psychiatric classification in DSM-5. *American Journal of Psychiatry*, 168, 672–4.
Lee, S., Tsang, A., Ruscio, A.M., *et al.* (2009). Implications of modifying the duration requirement of generalized anxiety disorder in developed and developing countries. *Psychological Medicine*, 39, 1163–76.
Maj, M. (2005). "Psychiatric comorbidity": an artefact of current diagnostic systems? *British Journal of Psychiatry*, 186, 182–4.
McLaughlin, K.A., Koenen, K.C., Friedman, M.J., *et al.* (2015). Subthreshold posttraumatic stress disorder in the World Health Organization World Mental Health Surveys. *Biological Psychiatry*, 77, 375–84.
Moynihan, R., Heath, I., and Henry, D. (2002). Selling sickness: the pharmaceutical industry and disease mongering. *British Medical Journal*, 324, 886–91.
Patel, V. (2012). Global mental health: from science to action. *Harvard Review of Psychiatry*, 20, 6–12.
Prince, M., Patel, V., Saxena, S., *et al.* (2007). No health without mental health. *Lancet*, 370, 859–77.
Reed, G.M. and Ayuso-Mateos, J.L. (2011). Towards a more clinically useful International World Health Organisation classification of mental disorders. *Revista Psiquiatria Salud Mental*, 4, 113–6.
Regier, D.A., Kuhl, E.A., and Kupfer, D.J. (2013). The DSM-5: classification and criteria changes. *Official Journal of the World Psychiatric Association*, 12, 92–8.
Robins, L.N., Helzer, J.E., Weissman, M.M., *et al.* (1984). Lifetime prevalence of specific psychiatric disorders in three sites. *Archives of General Psychiatry*, 41, 949–58.
Rosenhan, D.L. (1973). On being sane in insane places. *Science*, 179, 250–8.
Ruscio, A.M., Chiu, W.T., Roy-Byrne, P., *et al.* (2007). Broadening the definition of generalized anxiety disorder: effects on prevalence and associations with other disorders in the National Comorbidity Survey Replication. *Journal of Anxiety Disorders*, 21, 662–76.
Schlenger, W.E., Kulka, R.A., Fairbank, J.A., *et al.* (2007). The psychological risks of Vietnam: the NVVRS perspective. *Journal of Traumatic Stress*, 20, 467–79.
Spitzer, R.L., Williams, J.B., and Skodol, A.E. (1980). DSM-III: the major achievements and an overview. *American Journal of Psychiatry*, 137, 151–64.
Stein, D.J. (2014). An integrative approach to psychiatric diagnosis and research. *World Psychiatry*, 13, 51–3.
(2015). Disorder versus deviance: where to draw the boundary? *Philosophy, Psychiatry and Psychology*, 21, 262–5.
Stein, D.J., Koenen, K.C., Friedman, M.J., *et al.* (2013). Dissociation in Posttraumatic Stress Disorder: evidence from the World Mental Health Surveys. *Biological Psychiatry*, 73, 302–12.
Stein, D.J. and Nesse, R.M. (2011). Threat detection, precautionary responses, and anxiety disorders. *Neuroscience and Biobehavioral Reviews*, 35, 1075–9.
Stein, D.J. and Phillips, K.A. (2013). Patient advocacy and DSM-5. *BMC Medicine*, 11, 133.
Stein, D.J., Ruscio, A.M., Lee, S., *et al.* (2010). Subtyping social anxiety disorder in developed and developing countries. *Depression and Anxiety*, 27, 390–403.
Stein, D.J., Wessels, C., Zungu-Dirwayi, N., *et al.* (2001). Value and effectiveness of consumer advocacy groups: a survey of the anxiety disorders support group in South Africa. *Depression and Anxiety*, 13, 105–7.
Summerfield, D. (2012). Afterword: against "global mental health". *Transcultural Psychiatry*, 49, 519–30.
Weich, S. and Araya, R. (2004). International and regional variation in the prevalence of common mental disorders: do we need more surveys? *British Journal of Psychiatry*, 184, 289–90.
Weissman, M.M., Bland, R.C., Canino, G.J., *et al.* (1994). The cross national epidemiology of obsessive compulsive disorder. The Cross National Collaborative Group. *Journal of Clinical Psychiatry*, 55 Suppl, 5–10.
(1996). The cross-national epidemiology of social phobia: a preliminary report. *International Clinical Psychopharmacology*, 11 Suppl 3, 9–14.
Weissman, M.M., Myers, J.K., and Harding, P.S. (1978). Psychiatric disorders in a U.S. urban community: 1975–1976. *American Journal of Psychiatry*, 135, 459–62.
WHO International Consortium in Psychiatric Epidemiology (2000). Cross-national comparisons of the prevalences and correlates of mental disorders. WHO International Consortium in Psychiatric Epidemiology. *Bulletin of the World Health Organization*, 78, 413–26.

Chapter 3

Methods of the World Mental Health Surveys

Ronald C. Kessler, Steven G. Heeringa, Beth-Ellen Pennell, Nancy A. Sampson, Alan M. Zaslavsky

Introduction

The World Mental Health (WMH) Surveys Initiative is a World Health Organization (WHO) initiative designed to help countries carry out and analyse epidemiological surveys of the burden of mental disorders in their populations (www.hcp.med.harvard.edu/wmh). This chapter provides a broad overview of the methods used in the surveys. Throughout the chapter we emphasize the consistent aspects of sampling, data collection, measurement, and analysis that were used across all WMH surveys. The core of the standardized procedures used in all these areas was the use of the same diagnostic interview, the WHO Composite International Diagnostic Interview (CIDI) version 3.0 (Kessler & Üstün 2004). The CIDI is a fully structured research diagnostic interview designed for use by trained lay interviewers who do not have clinical experience. The version of the CIDI used in the surveys reported here generates diagnoses of mental disorders according to the definitions and criteria of both the 10th edition of the *International Statistical Classification of Diseases and Related Health Problems* (ICD-10) and 4th edition of the *Diagnostic and Statistical Manual of Mental Disorders* (DSM-IV) systems, although only DSM-IV criteria are used here. Consistent WHO translation, back-translation, and harmonization procedures were used to modify the CIDI for use in each WMH country (Harkness *et al.* 2008). The same interviewer training materials, training programmes, and quality control monitoring procedures were also used across WMH surveys to guarantee cross-survey comparability of data (Pennell *et al.* 2008).

The use of these standardized procedures has been critical for WMH success, as a core mission of WMH is to allow countries that might not otherwise be able to implement mental health needs assessment surveys to do so by building on the existing WMH infrastructure. The use of standardized materials reduces costs for each country and makes it easier to implement high-quality surveys by building on tried and true procedures. This applies not only to instrumentation and data collection but also to analysis, as WMH uses a centralized data processing and cross-national peer consultation model to allow less experienced collaborators to work with world-class statisticians and psychiatric epidemiologists to analyse, interpret, and write scientific reports about their data.

The WMH Samples

The sampling procedures used in the WMH surveys are closely related to those originally developed for the World Fertility Survey (WFS) programme, one of the first and largest efforts to coordinate a global gathering of survey data (Verma, Scott & O'Muircheartaigh 1980). The decisions made in developing sample designs for the WMH surveys drew heavily on the lessons of the WFS experience. Like the WFS and more recent successful international programmes of community survey research, the WMH surveys required collaborating countries to employ probability sample designs to select nationally or regionally representative samples of adults for the survey interview. The aim of sampling in the WMH surveys was to obtain a representative sample of the household population in the country or region under study. This usually involved drawing a multi-stage clustered area probability sample of households in the population and then selecting one, or in some cases two, respondents from each sampled household using probability methods without replacement. These sample designs were standardized across countries based on the principles of probability sampling, but with less emphasis placed on the specific probability sample design features employed across countries in recognition of the fact that countries varied widely in the information available to develop a sample frame from which the WMH sample could be selected.

In order to achieve the level of coordination in sampling required across countries, we established a WMH Data Collection Coordination Centre at the Institute for Social Research (ISR) at the University of Michigan in the United States. The Survey Research Center (SRC) at ISR is one of the leading academic survey research organizations in the world, with a long history of leadership in the development and implementation of large community surveys (www.src.isr.umich.edu). The Survey Sampling group at SRC, under the direction of Steve Heeringa, supervised WMH sampling, while the Survey Implementation group, under the supervision of Beth-Ellen Pennell, supervised WMH interviewer training and field implementation.

Focusing first on sampling, the SRC group began by developing a list containing a common set of requirements and performance standards that the probability sample design in each WMH survey was required to meet. Unique opportunities available in individual countries were then used to develop a sampling plan that achieved these requirements and to meet the WMH standards. The staff of the WMH Data Collection Coordination Centre worked closely with local collaborators to develop these sample design plans. The plans were reviewed by a panel of technical experts and then revised based on feedback from this panel. Once the design was finalized, day-to-day oversight of implementation was the responsibility of the local research team.

Most WMH countries developed a similar sampling plan that featured multistage area probability sampling. Several countries, though, adopted alternative probability sampling procedures, such as the use of a national registry or combined uses of area probability methods and registry sampling to achieve the required probability sampling of the designated target population. All these samples, though, were probability samples. No WMH survey used a convenience sample, an interviewer-managed quota sample, or any other non-probability method of sample selection.

The Target Populations

Probability sample surveys are designed to describe a *target population* of elements that spans a specific geographic space during a specific window of time. Although it might seem obvious how to do this, a number of important considerations arise as soon as one begins to consider the possibilities. Should persons who were temporary residents, guest workers, or those who had legal claim to medical treatment or services be included in the sample? What about people who were incapable of participating in the survey because they were institutionalized, or cognitively or physically impaired, and what about people living in remote places that would require disproportionate amounts of survey resources to sample and interview? In the end, a decision was made to allow the answers to these questions to vary across countries within a range of options described below.

The *survey population* is defined as the subset of the target population that is truly eligible for sampling under the survey design (Groves *et al.* 2004). A decision was needed to decide what restrictions would apply in each participating WMH country to establish a survey population definition that would conform to the survey's scientific objectives, available sample frames, and budget limitations. Multiple dimensions were included here. One of these involved the age range of the sample. WMH was designed to focus on adults. However, the age that defines adulthood (commonly referred to as the 'age of majority') varies across countries (most typically either 18 or 21). In addition, some countries decided to impose an upper age limit on the sample (usually 65). Other dimensions that defined the survey population involved geographic scope limitations (most typically excluding otherwise eligible people who lived in remote areas of the country), language restrictions, citizenship requirements, and whether to include special populations such as persons living in military barracks and group quarters or persons who were institutionalized at the time of the survey (e.g., hospital patients, prison inmates). These varied somewhat across countries.

Table 3.1 provides a summary of the survey populations for the 29 WMH surveys included in this volume. Starting with the different age limits, the vast majority of the surveys had a minimum age of 18 years. The lowest minimum age was age 16 (New Zealand, although analysis of the New Zealand data is restricted to respondents 18 and above in cross-national reports for comparability with other countries) and the oldest was 21 (Israel). For maximum age requirements, Colombia, Mexico, and the regional surveys carried out in Beijing and Shanghai mandated that respondents be no older than 65 or 70. Turning to the geographic scope of the survey population, 19 of the 29 surveys defined the geographic scope of their survey population as the entire country, whereas the Nigerian survey was restricted to specific regions and the national surveys in Colombia and Mexico were restricted to urban places above a specified population size (e.g., more than 2,500 persons in Mexico). A few surveys, finally, were restricted to specific metropolitan areas. These included the

Table 3.1 WMH sample characteristics by World Bank income categories[a]

Country by income category	Survey[b]	Sample characteristics[c]	Field dates	Age range	Sample size: Part I	Part II	Part II and age ≤ 44[d]	Response rate[e]
Low/lower-middle-income-countries								
Colombia	NSMH	All urban areas of the country (approximately 73% of the total national population)	2003	18–65	4,426	2,381	1,731	87.7
Iraq	IMHS	Nationally representative	2006–7	18–96	4,332	4,332	–	95.2
Nigeria	NSMHW	21 of the 36 states in the country, representing 57% of the national population. The surveys were conducted in Yoruba, Igbo, Hausa, and Efik languages	2002–4	18–100	6,752	2,143	1,203	79.3
PRC[f] (Beijing/Shanghai)	B-WMH/S-WMH	Beijing and Shanghai metropolitan areas	2001–3	18–70	5,201	1,628	570	74.7
PRC[f] (Shenzhen)[g]	Shenzhen	Shenzhen metropolitan area. Included temporary residents as well as household residents	2005–7	18–88	7,132	2,475	–	80.0
Peru	EMSMP	All urban areas of the country	2004–5	18–65	3,930	1,801	1,287	90.2
Ukraine	CMDPSD	Nationally representative	2002	18–91	4,725	1,720	541	78.3
TOTAL					(36,498)	(16,480)	(5,332)	82.2
Upper-middle-income countries								
Brazil (São Paulo)	São Paulo Megacity	São Paulo metropolitan area	2005–8	18–93	5,037	2,942	–	81.3
Bulgaria	NSHS	Nationally representative	2002–6	18–98	5,318	2,233	741	72.0
Colombia (Medellin)[h]	MMHHS	Medellin metropolitan area	2011–12	19–65	3,261	1,673		97.2
Lebanon	LEBANON	Nationally representative	2002–3	18–94	2,857	1,031	595	70.0
Mexico	M-NCS	All urban areas of the country (approximately 75% of the total national population)	2001–2	18–65	5,782	2,362	1,736	76.6
Romania	RMHS	Nationally representative	2005–6	18–96	2,357	2,357	–	70.9
South Africa[g]	SASH	Nationally representative	2002–4	18–92	4,315	4,315	–	87.1
TOTAL					(28,927)	(16,913)	(3,072)	78.5
High-income countries								
Australia[g]	NSMHWB	Nationally representative	2007	18–85	8,463	8,463	–	60
Belgium	ESEMeD	Nationally representative. The sample was selected from a national register of Belgium residents	2001–2	18–95	2,419	1,043	486	50.6
France	ESEMeD	Nationally representative. The sample was selected from a national list of households with listed telephone numbers	2001–2	18–97	2,894	1,436	727	45.9
Germany	ESEMeD	Nationally representative	2002–3	19–95	3,555	1,323	621	57.8

(cont.)

Table 3.1 *(cont.)*

Country by income category	Survey[b]	Sample characteristics[c]	Field dates	Age range	Sample size			Response rate[e]
					Part I	Part II	Part II and age ≤ 44[d]	
Israel	NHS	Nationally representative	2003–4	21–98	4,859	4,859	–	72.6
Italy	ESEMeD	Nationally representative. The sample was selected from municipality resident registries	2001–2	18–100	4,712	1,779	853	71.3
Japan	WMHJ 2002–6	11 metropolitan areas	2002–6	20–98	4,129	1,682	–	55.1
Netherlands	ESEMeD	Nationally representative. The sample was selected from municipal postal registries	2002–3	18–95	2,372	1,094	516	56.4
New Zealand[g]	NZMHS	Nationally representative	2003–4	18–98	12,790	7,312	–	73.3
Northern Ireland	NISHS	Nationally representative	2005–8	18–97	4,340	1,986	–	68.4
Poland	EZOP	Nationally representative	2010–11	18–65	10,081	4,000	2,276	50.4
Portugal	NMHS	Nationally representative	2008–9	18–81	3,849	2,060	1,070	57.3
Spain	ESEMeD	Nationally representative	2001–2	18–98	5,473	2,121	960	78.6
Spain (Murcia)	PEGASUS–Murcia	Murcia region	2010–12	18–96	2,621	1,459	–	67.4
United States	NCS-R	Nationally representative	2001–3	18–99	9,282	5,692	3,197	70.9
TOTAL					(81,839)	(46,309)	(10,706)	62.6
IV TOTAL					(147,264)	(79,702)	(19,110)	69.5

[a]The World Bank (2012) Data and Statistics. Accessed 12 May 2012 at: http://data.worldbank.org/country. Some of the WMH countries have moved into new income categories since the surveys were conducted. The income groupings above reflect the status of each country at the time of data collection. The current income category of each country is available at the preceding URL.

[b]NSMH (The Colombian National Study of Mental Health); IMHS (Iraq Mental Health Survey); NSMHW (The Nigerian Survey of Mental Health and Wellbeing); B-WMH (The Beijing World Mental Health Survey); S-WMH (The Shanghai World Mental Health Survey); EMSMP (La Encuesta Mundial de Salud Mental en el Peru); CMDPSD (Comorbid Mental Disorders during Periods of Social Disruption); NSHS (Bulgaria National Survey of Health and Stress); MMHHS (Medellín Mental Health Household Study); LEBANON (Lebanese Evaluation of the Burden of Ailments and Needs of the Nation); M-NCS (The Mexico National Comorbidity Survey); RMHS (Romania Mental Health Survey); SASH (South Africa Health Survey); NSMHWB (National Survey of Mental Health and Wellbeing); ESEMeD (The European Study of the Epidemiology of Mental Disorders); NHS (Israel National Health Survey); WMHJ 2002–6 (World Mental Health Japan Survey); NZMHS (New Zealand Mental Health Survey); NISHS (Northern Ireland Study of Health and Stress); EZOP (Epidemiology of Mental Disorders and Access to Care Survey); NMHS (Portugal National Mental Health Survey); PEGASUS-Murcia (Psychiatric Enquiry to General Population in Southeast Spain-Murcia); NCS-R (The US National Comorbidity Survey Replication).

[c]Most WMH surveys are based on stratified multistage clustered area probability household samples in which samples of areas equivalent to counties or municipalities in the United States were selected in the first stage followed by one or more subsequent stages of geographic sampling (e.g., towns within counties, blocks within towns, households within blocks) to arrive at a sample of households, in each of which a listing of household members was created and one or two people were selected from this listing to be interviewed. No substitution was allowed when the originally sampled household resident could not be interviewed. These household samples were selected from census area data in all countries other than France (where telephone directories were used to select households) and the Netherlands (where postal registries were used to select households). Several WMH surveys (Belgium, Germany, Italy, Poland) used municipal or country resident registries to select respondents without listing households. The Japanese sample is the only totally un-clustered sample, with households randomly selected in each of the 11 metropolitan areas and one random respondent selected in each sample household. 19 of the 29 surveys are based on nationally representative household samples.

[d]Australia, Brazil, Colombia (Medellin), Iraq, Israel, Japan, New Zealand, Northern Ireland, PRC (Shenzhen), Romania, South Africa and Spain (Murcia) did not have an age restricted Part II sample. All other countries, with the exception of Nigeria, PRC (Beijing WMH; Shanghai WMH), and Ukraine (which were age restricted to ≤39), were age restricted to ≤44.

[e]The response rate is calculated as the ratio of the number of households in which an interview was completed to the number of households originally sampled, excluding from the denominator households known not to be eligible either because of being vacant at the time of initial contact or because the residents were unable to speak the designated languages of the survey. The weighted average response rate is 69.5%.

[f]People's Republic of China.

[g]For the purposes of cross-national comparisons we limit the sample to those 18+.

[h]Colombia moved from the 'low/lower-middle-income' to the 'upper-middle-income' category between 2003 (when the Colombian National Study of Mental Health was conducted) and 2010 (when the Medellin Mental Health Household Study was conducted), hence Colombia's appearance in both income categories. For more information, please see footnote a.

surveys in Beijing, Shanghai, and Shenzhen in the People's Republic of China (PRC), São Paulo in Brazil, Peru, Medellin in Colombia (distinct from the earlier national Colombian survey), Murcia in Spain (distinct from the earlier national Spanish survey), and a series of large cities in Japan.

Sampling Frames

Probability sampling requires a sampling frame that provides a high level of coverage for the defined survey population. The sampling frame is defined as the list or equivalent enumeration procedure that identifies all population elements and enables the sampler to assign nonzero selection probabilities to each element (Kish 1965). We carefully reviewed the available choices of sample frames with the collaborators in each WMH country before deciding on a final frame. Options could have included population registries, new or existing area probability sampling frames, postal address lists, voter registration lists, and telephone subscriber lists. The final choice of the frame for each country was determined by a number of factors, including the extent of coverage and statistical efficiency of available frame alternatives, the cost of developing and using the frame for sample selection, and the experience of the data collection organization in the use of the sample frame. These final sampling frames were generally of three types: (1) a database of individual contact information provided in the form of national population registries, voter registration lists, postal address lists, or household telephone directories; (2) a multistage area probability sample frame (Kish 1965); or (3) a hybrid multistage frame that combined area probability methods in the initial stages and a registry or population list in the penultimate and/or final stages of sample selection. Table 3.1 identifies the sample frame type chosen in each of the participating surveys.

Complex Sample Designs for the WMH Surveys

The goal of all survey sample designs is either to minimize sampling variance and bias for a fixed total cost or to minimize total cost while meeting predetermined analysis objectives. The analysis objectives are typically formulated as fixed targets for the variance and bias components of the total survey error for key survey estimates or the parameter estimates for important population models. In the WMH survey programme, there was no single path to this goal. The surveys shared a set of common analysis objectives, primarily centred on the estimation of the population prevalence and correlates of mental disorders. Survey cost structures were highly variable from one country to another, depending on factors such as availability and accessibility of survey infrastructure (government or commercial survey organizations), availability and costs for databases and map materials required to develop sample frames, labour rates for field interviewers and team leaders, and transportation costs for getting trained interviewers to distributed samples of households. Total funding for the surveys also varied widely across countries. In many cases funding restrictions not only limited the total size of the interviewed sample but also limited the scope of the survey populations or the use of costly sample design options.

The individual WMH sample designs employed the full range of probability sampling techniques that survey statisticians can use to improve sample precision and reduce costs. Stratification of the samples by geographic regions and demographic characteristics was used to increase sample precision and control sample allocation. Multistage designs with modest clustering in the initial stages of sampling were used to control travel time and expenses. A version of the 'double sampling' technique (Cochran 1977) was used in the vast majority of surveys to determine the subsample of initial Part I CIDI screening interview respondents who would complete the more intensive Part II CIDI diagnostic questionnaire. This two-part approach is discussed in more detail in the next section of this chapter.

The variety of designs used in different WMH surveys is a reflection of the differences in the essential survey conditions faced by the collaborators. With the exception of a small number of studies that sampled adults directly from high-quality population registries, the great majority of WMH surveys used a multistage area probability sampling method. The population registry approach is very attractive when this option is available because it avoids within-household selection and weighting. A few other countries chose a first-stage probability sample of households directly from national postal lists (e.g., the Netherlands) or telephone directories (e.g., France) and then chose random respondents within the selected households. Germany used a two-stage design that involved a first-stage sampling of municipalities and a second-stage sampling of adults from population registries available within each of the selected municipalities. A number of other countries used a similar design but added an intermediate second-stage sampling of electoral or postal districts before selecting eligible adults from a district registry (e.g., Italy) or an enumerated list of residents within selected districts (e.g., Ukraine).

The vast majority of WMH surveys, though, used three-stage or four-stage area probability designs. The three-stage designs began with a primary stage sample of a probability sample of census enumeration districts or neighbourhood units selected with probabilities proportional to size, followed by a second-stage sampling of households within the first-stage units, and a third-stage random selection of an eligible adult within a sampled household. Countries that used four-stage designs expanded this same basic approach by beginning with the selection of large county or municipal units and then progressing to the selection of area segment blocks, then to households, and then to respondents within households. All WMH surveys that used within-household selection of respondents did so with an objective household selection table method developed by Kish (1949). In a probability subsample of households in some countries, the spouses of selected respondents also selected to take part in the survey.

It is important to note that considerable effort was required to construct the frames for the WMH samples in countries where preexisting survey frames did not already exist. In Lebanon, for example, area probability methods were used to build the frame and select a multistage sample due to the fact that only limited population data existed in Lebanon. The primary stage of sampling consequently selected area segments (sectors) from a comprehensive list developed by the WMH collaborators stratified by region and urbanicity. From this list, 342 area segments were selected with probabilities proportional to size. Prior to the second stage of sampling, the Lebanese team sent trained field staff to each selected area segment to create a comprehensive list of all housing units in the segment. Once this enumerative list was completed for each area segment, a second-stage sample was selected of housing units and then of respondents within households.

The WMH guidelines specified a target response rate target of 65% based on a precise method required to calculate the response rate (the American Association for Public Opinion Research RR4 definition; American Association for Public Opinion Research 2000; www.aapor.org). This target response rate was achieved by 21 of the 29 surveys, with five having response rates in the range 70–75%, five in the range 75–80%, and six over 80%. The eight surveys that failed to meet the target had response rates in the range 45.9–57.8%. It is noteworthy that all of these eight surveys were carried out in high-income countries (Australia, Belgium, France, Germany, Japan, Netherlands, Poland, Portugal). This is consistent with other evidence that difficulties contacting respondents because they are away from the household are greatest in high-income countries, where people have a higher probability than elsewhere of being away from home in the evening and on weekends, and also that marketing surveys have become so common in high-income countries that the willingness of people to participate in surveys has declined substantially over time (Couper & de Leeuw 2003). Surveys remain sufficiently novel in lower-income countries, though, that response rates are generally higher than in high-income countries. Survey response rates are, of course, also influenced by many other factors, including government privacy rules, population resistance to survey participation, the experience and norms of the chosen data collection organization, and availability of financial resources to invest in incentives or other refusal aversion efforts.

The Two-Part Interview Design

As noted above, in the vast majority of WMH surveys (the exceptions being Iraq, Israel, Romania, and South Africa, where all respondents were administered the full interview), the interview was divided into two parts, with the questions in Part I administered to all respondents and the questions in Part II administered to a probability subsample of respondents based on responses to the Part I questions. The reason for doing this was that the total interview was quite long and sometimes required the interviewer to return to the respondent's household a second or even third time to complete the entire interview. As many respondents did not have any mental disorders, though, we did not need all of these *non-cases* to achieve maximum statistical power in comparing to cases. This meant that we could realize considerable cost saving by terminating the interview for a probability subsample of non-cases as soon as we learned that they did not meet criteria for any mental disorder. This was accomplished with the two-part interview design. The interview began with a series of basic descriptive warm-up questions and then evaluated lifetime presence of a wide range of core mental disorders. All (100%) of the respondents who met criteria for any of these disorders were continued into Part II, which included questions about a wide range of correlates of the core disorders and also assessed mental disorders of secondary interest. In addition, a probability subsample of other Part I respondents (i.e., those who did not meet criteria for any core disorder) were also selected to complete Part II, while interviews with the remaining non-cases were ended after the completion of the Part I questions.

There has been a good deal of confusion on the part of some journal article reviewers about this two-part design, the most common concern being that the Part II sample over-estimates prevalence because it does not include all non-cases. This concern is unwarranted due to the fact that the Part II data were weighted to adjust for the under-sampling of Part II cases. For example, if we included only a random one-fourth (0.25) of all Part I non-cases in the Part II sample in a given country, each of those Part II non-cases would be assigned a weight of 4.0 (1.0/0.25) to compensate for their under-sampling. This means that if the estimated prevalence of a given lifetime mental disorder was 10% in the Part I sample it would still be 10% in the weighted Part II sample. In a similar way, estimates of the correlates of disorder would be expected to be unbiased in the Part II sample compared to the Part I sample.

However, the *precision* of these estimates might be lower in the Part II sample due to the fact that the denominator sample size on which estimates were based would be smaller. Four observations are relevant with regard to precision. First, the precision of estimates increases at a decreasing rate as the number of non-cases increases relative to cases, with the optimal allocation being 1:1 (Schlesselman 1982). The number of non-cases selected for the Part II sample was generally in the range 15–33%, yielding more non-cases than cases of every single disorder in every survey. Second, the Part II sample was poststratified (a term described later in this chapter) in order to adjust for any discrepancies that existed between the measured characteristics of the non-cases selected into Part II and those not selected into Part II. Third, the certainty selections into Part II included 100% of not only respondents with any lifetime core disorder but also of any subthreshold manifestation of the core disorders, increasing power to distinguish cases from near-cases. Fourth, probability of selection into Part II among other non-cases was made proportion to the number of eligible respondents in the sample household in all surveys that used household sampling. This is a subtle point that edges into the discussion of weighting later in this chapter. Briefly, though, the precision of estimate is inversely related to the variance of sample weights. Both the probability of selection into Part I and the conditional probability of selection into Part II among Part I respondents contributed to this total weight. The Part I weight is *inversely* proportional to the number of eligible respondents in each household due to the fact that we selected only one respondent per household (with the exception of the small couples sample) no matter how many eligible people resided in the household. This led to an over-sampling of people living alone and an under-sampling of people living in married couples and even more so of people living in households with three or more eligible respondents. The Part I weight corrects for this differential representation. By sampling non-cases into Part II with probabilities *proportional* to number of eligible household members we were able partially to cancel out the variance in Part I weights for non-cases. So, for example, while people living alone were over-represented in the Part I sample (due to having a 100% chance of selection as the household respondent versus a 50% chance for people living with a spouse, a 33% chance for people living with a spouse and one other adult household resident, etc.), they were under-sampled in the selection of non-cases into the Part II sample, making their proportion in the unweighted Part II sample closer to their true population proportion than it was in the unweighted Part I sample.

Nonresponse Surveys

Collaborators in all countries were encouraged to carry out systematic nonresponse surveys in an effort to evaluate and, to the extent possible, correct for the effects of systematic survey nonresponse. The basic design of the nonresponse survey was to select a stratified probability subsample of initial survey non respondents who were approached one last time and asked to participate in a *brief* (typically 10–20 minutes of interview time) interview that would provide the investigators with basic information about people who were not able to participate in the full survey. Respondents were typically offered a financial incentive to participate in this brief survey. The survey was typically carried out either by telephone or face-to-face. The questions in the survey included a small number of basic socio-demographics (e.g., age, gender, education, marital status) and diagnostic stem questions for diagnoses of core mental and substance disorders. Importantly, identical questions were asked in the main survey. Comparison of responses to these questions in the main sample and the nonrespondent sample was used to make inferences about nonresponse bias, while weighting adjustments described below were used to adjust the main sample for these biases.

Weighting

Person-level analysis weights that incorporated factors for sample selection, nonresponse, and poststratification (i.e., weighting the sample distributions on one or more variables or multivariate profiles to equal the distribution known to exist in the population, with the population targets typically coming from government census data) were constructed for each WMH survey dataset. In a number of cases these weights were developed by survey statisticians on the individual country research teams, while weights were constructed in other cases by the staff of the WMH Data Analysis Coordination Centre at Harvard Medical School (HMS) using sample design and population control data supplied by the local project teams. The case-specific analysis weights were used in computing estimates of descriptive statistics for the survey population and for estimating the descriptive statistics reported in this volume.

Construction of Analysis Weights

In general, the final analysis weight for each WMH survey respondent was computed as the product of the three weight components:

$$W_{final,i} = W_{sel,i} \cdot W_{nr,i} \cdot W_{psc,i}$$

where:

$W_{sel,i}$ = the selection weight factor for respondent $i = 1, \ldots, n$;

$W_{nr,i}$ = the nonresponse weight adjustment factor for respondent $i = 1, \ldots, n$; and

$W_{psc,i}$ = the poststratification factor for respondent $i = 1, \ldots, n$.

The exact sequence of weight calculation steps differed slightly across surveys. In some countries, a separate nonresponse adjustment step was skipped and the final weight was derived as the product of the sample selection factor and a final, all-encompassing, poststratification to external population controls.

The sample selection weight was designed to compensate for the differing sampling probabilities for selecting individuals as WMH respondents. The selection weight factor, W_{sel}, was generally the product of the reciprocals of three probabilities: $W_{sel,hh}$, the reciprocal of the multistage probability of selecting the respondent's housing unit selection from the sample frame; $W_{sel,resp}$, the reciprocal of the conditional probability of selecting the WMH respondent at random within the eligible household (Kish 1965); and W_{sel}, *Part II*, the reciprocal of the probability that an eligible WMH survey respondent was subsampled to complete the in-depth Part II diagnostic section of the WMH interview.

The nonresponse adjustment weight, W_{nr}, could be computed to account for differential patterns of response across categories of eligible respondents for a country-specific survey. When this weight was applied, nonresponse adjustments to survey weights were based on endogenous data; that is, on data from the sample frame that was known for both sample respondents and nonrespondents. In baseline or cross-sectional surveys such as the WMH studies described here, the data available to develop nonresponse adjustments is often limited to geographic and possibly demographic information available for respondents and nonrespondents in the sample frame, such as population census data collected by the government.

In cases where nonresponse adjustment was implemented, a nonrespondent survey of the sort described above was used to generate this weight. The nonresponse sample was first weighted to be representative of all nonrespondents using within-household probability of selections weights (see below) and then this weighted subsample was compared to the similarly weighted main sample in an effort to determine if the two samples differed meaningfully on the variables assessed. When differences of this sort were found, either a weighting class method or a propensity modelling approach (Little & Rubin 2002) was used to develop the adjustment factors.

The weight calculations for most of the WMH survey datasets, however, did not include a separate nonresponse adjustment. Instead, an adjustment for differential nonresponse and sample noncoverage of the survey population was integrated into one consolidated adjustment in the poststratification weighting step, which is described below. In such cases, the factor W_{nr} can be viewed as taking a value of 1.0 in the final composite weight calculation. Readers who are interested in detailed case studies of nonresponse adjustment weighting for selected WMH data sets are referred to Alonso *et al.* (2004) and Kessler & Üstün (2004).

The final component in the WMH individual analysis weight is a poststratification factor, W_{ps}. The poststratification weighting adjustment differs from the nonresponse adjustment factors in that poststratification weighting uses data that are exogenous to the survey design to calibrate the weights for survey estimation. The WMH poststratification used estimates of population values from external sources such as a recent national census or demographic population estimation programme to standardize the sampling weights to known population distribution values, such as the distribution of the population of the cross-classification of age (in categories), gender, and education. The logic of the general procedure used in each country involved forming a matrix of adjustment cells by cross-classifying age, gender, and major geographic regions (data permitting) of the survey population. Within each cell of this matrix, the poststratification weight factors were computed as the ratio of the external population count for each cell to the sum of computed sample selection weights for the WMH survey cases assigned to that cell:

$$W_{pstrat,c,i} = \frac{\hat{N}_c}{\sum_{i \in c}^{n_c} W_{sel,i} \cdot W_{nr,i}}$$

where:

$W_{pstrat,c,i}$ = the poststratification factor for all cases in cell c;
$\hat{N}_c$ = the WMH country population estimate for cell c;
n_c = WMH country sample size in cell c;
$W_{sel,i}$ = the composite sample selection weight for case $i = 1, \ldots, n_c$;
$W_{nr,i}$ = the nonresponse adjustment for case $i = 1, \ldots, n_c$.

In some countries, it was possible to include much more information than a few socio-demographic and geographic variables due to the availability of much more detailed population data on a wide range of social and demographic variables that were also assessed in the WMH survey. In cases of this sort, data analyses were carried out to compare the WMH survey data, with other weights imposed on the data, to the population data in an effort to pinpoint any variables that were meaningfully discrepant between the two. When the number of such variables was small, a modified poststratification table of the sort described in the last paragraph could have been carried out that constructed poststratification tables from only those variables. However, this procedure would run the risk of creating discrepancies between the weighted sample and the population on other variables that were originally non-discrepant. In order to guard against this possibility, propensity score adjustment was used whenever a large number of poststratification variables were present (Rosenbaum & Rubin 1983). In this approach, logistic regression analysis was used to develop a multivariate prediction equation from the poststratification variables that discriminated between the WMH sample and the population, where a dichotomous outcome variable was used to distinguish the sample from the population in an analysis that combined both data files. This prediction equation allowed for interactions among the poststratification variables and sequentially evaluated a wide range of predictors, arriving at a final model that included core variables (i.e., age, gender, education, geography) and significant discriminating variables. Appropriately weighted predicted probabilities generated from this final equation were used to adjust the final WMH sample to approximate the multivariate distribution of the population on these variables.

Although poststratification can potentially reduce sampling variances for survey estimates, the primary purpose of weighting is to eliminate potential sources of bias that would be present in an unweighted analysis. Those biases could arise due to differences in the original selection probabilities for respondents, differential nonresponse (probabilities of observation), and differential sample noncoverage for elements of the target population. However, the pursuit of 'unbiasedness' can have a price in the form of increased variance of survey estimates compared to an unweighted estimate based on the same sample size. Weighting effects on standard errors arise due to several factors, including the association between the distributions of the weights and the variables of interest and variance of the weight values assigned to the individual cases. In the process of developing the final analysis weights for the WMH data sets, sensitivity analyses were conducted to determine the effect of extreme weight values on the estimated sampling errors and potential bias of key survey estimates. If sampling variances proved highly sensitive to the most extreme weight values, the computed weights in the extreme lower and upper ranges were trimmed using methods that retained the sum of weights but distributed those weights across cases at each tail of the distribution. This trimming was typically carried out for respondents with the highest and lowest 1–2% of weights and in extreme cases for those in the highest and lowest 5% of weights. For a detailed example of how this was done in one WMH survey, see Kessler *et al.* (2004).

Sampling Error and Inference from the WMH Survey Data

The WMH surveys are based on a variety of probability sample designs – each design adapted to the resources, experiences, and cost structures that are unique to the collaborating countries. Despite the variations in probability sample design forms, each survey is designed to support robust, design-based estimation of population statistics, such as prevalence of mental health in a chosen survey population.

The survey literature refers to designs like the ones used in the WMH surveys as *complex designs*, a loosely used term meant to denote the fact that the sample incorporates special design features such as stratification, clustering, and differential selection probabilities (i.e., weighting) that analysts must consider in computing sampling errors and confidence intervals for sample estimates of descriptive statistics and model parameters. Standard programmes in statistical analysis software packages assume simple random sampling (SRS) or independence of observations in computing standard errors for sample estimates. In general, the SRS assumption results in the underestimation of variances of survey estimates of descriptive statistics and model parameters. This means that the confidence intervals based on computed variances that assume independence of observations will be biased (generally too narrow) and design-based inferences will be affected accordingly. This section focuses on sampling error estimation and construction of confidence intervals for WMH survey estimates of descriptive statistics, such as means, proportions, ratios, and coefficients for linear and logistic regression models.

Over the past 50 years, advances in survey sampling theory have guided the development of a number of methods for estimating variances from complex sample data sets correctly. Several sampling error programmes that implement these complex sample variance estimation methods were available to WMH data analysts. The two most common approaches were the Taylor series linearization method (and corresponding approximation to its variance) and resampling variance estimation methods such as the Balanced Repeated Replication method and the Jackknife Repeated Replication (JRR) method (Rust 1985). The sampling error estimates presented in the substantive chapters of this volume were for the most part estimated in SUDAAN Version 9 (Research Triangle Institute 2002) using the Taylor series linearization method, although some of the more complex estimates required the use of the JRR method, which we implemented in special SAS macros (SAS Institute Inc. 2011) written by staff of the WMH Data Collection Coordination Centre.

As noted earlier in this chapter in the discussion of the WMH sample designs, the WMH surveys, like most other sample designs in health-related surveys, use stratification and clustering. Stratification is introduced to increase the statistical and administrative efficiency of the sample. Sample elements are selected as clusters in multistage designs to reduce travel costs and improve interviewing efficiency. Disproportionate sampling of population elements may be used to increase the sample sizes for subpopulations of special interest, resulting in the need to employ weighting in the estimation of population prevalence or other descriptive statistics. Relative to SRS, each of these complex sample design features influences the size of standard errors for survey estimates. Figure 3.1 illustrates the effects of these design features on standard errors of estimates. The curve plotted in this figure represents the SRS standard error of an estimate as a function of sample size. At any chosen sample size, the effect of sample stratification is generally a reduction in standard errors relative to SRS. Clustering of sample elements and designs that require weighting for unbiased estimation generally produce larger standard errors than an SRS sample of equal size (Kish 1965).

The combined effects of stratification, clustering and weighting on the standard errors of estimates are termed the *design effect* (D^2) and are measured by the ratio:

$$D^2 = \frac{SE(p)^2_{complex}}{SE(p)^2_{srs}} = \frac{Var(p)_{complex}}{Var(p)_{srs}}$$

where:

D^2 = the design effect;
$Var(p)_{complex}$ = the complex sample design variance of the sample statistic p; and
$Var(p)_{srs}$ = the simple random variance of p.

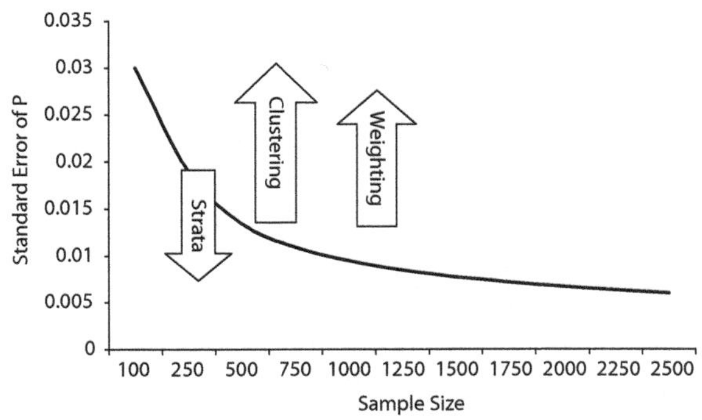

Figure 3.1 Complex sample design effects on standard errors of prevalence estimates (illustration for P = 0.10)

Table 3.2 presents the design effects for estimates of lifetime, 12-month, 30-day, 12-month/lifetime, 30-day/12-month prevalence of two illustrative DSM-IV disorders considered in this volume; one of them the most prevalent of the disorders assessed in the WMH surveys (specific phobia) and the other a relatively uncommon disorder (bipolar disorder). With only a small number of exceptions, design effects are greater than 1.0 but relatively modest in elevation, with a median in the range 1.5–1.8 across time frames for specific phobia and 1.2–1.6 for bipolar disorder. It is noteworthy that design effects are generally larger for the higher-prevalence disorder and, within disorders, higher for the time frames with higher than lower prevalence. This is because frequency of multiple cases occurring within sample clusters decreases, and with it the design effect due to clustering, as prevalence decreases. Design effects are for the most part somewhat larger when results are pooled across countries compared to when they are estimated within countries for the same reason. It needs to be remembered, though, that the sample size increases dramatically when data are combined across countries, resulting in substantial decreases in standard errors of estimates despite the relatively small increases in design effects.

Measures

Mental Disorders

As noted earlier in this chapter, mental disorders were assessed with the WHO CIDI version 3.0 (Kessler & Üstün 2004), a fully structured lay-administered research diagnostic interview. DSM-IV criteria were used in making diagnoses. A wide range of anxiety, mood, disruptive behaviour, and substance-use disorders were included in the assessment, along with questions about psychotic experiences. In each case, the CIDI assessed lifetime prevalence of the disorder and then obtained retrospective data about age-of-onset (AOO), prevalence of the disorder at any time in the 12 months before interview and, among those with 12-month recency, presence in the 30 days before interview. While we reserve discussion of specific disorder-specific measurement characteristics for the disorder-specific chapters, we discuss more general issues about measurement here.

As retrospective reports of lifetime occurrence of mental disorders play a central part in the analyses presented in this volume, it is important to recognize that previous research suggests that these reports can be inaccurate due to recall error (Giuffra & Risch 1994; Simon & VonKorff 1995; Patten 2003; Moffitt *et al.* 2010). This problem is not unique to interviews about mental disorders but has been recognized in many other areas of investigation by survey methodologists for years. A considerable amount of methodological research has been carried out by survey methodologists to address the problem (e.g., Turner & Martin 1985; Tanur 1992; Sudman *et al.* 1996). This research has advanced considerably in recent years as cognitive psychologists have become interested in the survey interview as a natural laboratory for studying cognitive processes (Schwarz & Sudman 1994, 1996; Sirken *et al.* 1999). A number of important insights have emerged from these studies about practical ways to improve the accuracy of retrospective reports. These insights and methods were used in the modified version of the CIDI developed for use in the WMH surveys (Kessler & Üstün 2004, 2008). We also used the results of survey methodologist research to address two other challenges in evaluating mental disorders: that mental disorders are embarrassing and, like other embarrassing behaviours, tend to be under-reported (Tourangeau & Yan 2007); and that some of the survey questions used to assess symptoms of mental disorders are necessarily rather complex, leading to the risk of comprehension errors (Schober *et al.* 2004).

We review the aspects of the interview modifications we made to address the above challenges that are most relevant to the current volume. Before doing so, though, we note that methodological analyses of the WMH data provide compelling evidence for the success of these improvements. This is true in three ways. First, a 10-year follow-up survey of the respondents in the WMH survey carried out in the United States did

Table 3.2 Design effects of prevalence estimates of two selected disorders (SP, specific phobia; BPD, broadly defined bipolar disorder) in the WMH surveys

	Time frame of prevalence estimates									
	Lifetime (LT)		12-month		30-day		12-month/LT		30-day/12-month	
	SP	BPD	SP	BPD	SP	BPD	SP	BPD	SP	BPD
Low/lower-middle-income-countries										
Colombia	2.8	1.7	3.1	1.6	2.4	2.3	1.8	1.4	1.7	1.9
Iraq	2.1	2.0	2.1	3.3	1.9	–	2.5	1.8	2.0	–
Nigeria	2.6	1.6	1.8	1.8	1.4	1.3	1.9	1.0	1.6	1.5
Peru	1.1	1.2	1.0	1.3	1.0	0.4	2.7	0.8	0.9	0.5
PRC (Beijing/Shanghai)[a]	2.3	2.3	2.3	2.7	1.8	1.1	0.8	1.1	2.6	1.4
PRC (Shenzhen)	1.9	1.8	2.3	1.7	1.5	1.8	3.0	1.3	1.0	1.5
Upper-middle-income countries										
Brazil	1.5	1.2	1.5	1.5	1.4	1.4	1.4	1.7	2.7	1.6
Bulgaria	0.8	2.3	1.6	2.5	1.3	–	1.7	1.6	1.1	–
Colombia (Medellin)	2.4	2.0	2.3	1.7	2.1	1.2	2.1	1.5	1.4	1.0
Lebanon	1.3	1.6	1.4	2.0	1.5	2.0	0.9	1.0	1.4	1.3
Mexico	2.2	1.6	1.7	1.2	1.2	1.0	1.4	1.2	1.9	1.3
Romania	1.7	1.2	1.8	0.9	2.1	1.2	1.9	1.3	1.7	1.1
High-income countries										
Australia	–	2.0	–	1.8	–	1.4	–	1.6	–	1.9
Belgium	3.9	–	2.3	–	1.9	–	1.0	–	1.6	–
France	1.2	–	1.7	–	1.5	–	2.2	–	1.4	–
Germany	2.1	–	1.7	–	0.9	–	1.1	–	1.5	–
Israel	–	1.3	–	1.4	–	1.2	–	1.1	–	1.1
Italy	2.0	–	1.6	–	1.3	–	0.6	–	0.7	–
Japan	0.9	1.4	1.0	1.2	1.1	1.0	1.3	1.2	1.2	1.0
Netherlands	1.9	–	1.8	–	1.8	–	1.0	–	1.3	–
New Zealand	1.7	2.0	1.6	1.7	1.6	1.4	1.5	1.4	2.2	1.9
Northern Ireland	1.6	1.2	1.5	0.8	1.3	0.4	1.0	1.2	1.2	0.9
Poland	1.3	1.0	1.2	0.8	1.2	0.6	1.4	0.8	1.0	0.5
Portugal	1.5	1.3	1.3	1.3	1.5	1.0	0.9	1.1	1.0	1.0
Spain	1.7	–	2.1	–	2.0	–	1.8	–	1.1	–
Spain (Murcia)	1.1	3.5	1.0	2.0	0.7	1.5	0.8	1.2	0.9	1.5
United States	1.4	1.4	1.7	1.3	2.1	1.2	3.0	1.2	1.4	1.9
Cross-national combinations of countries										
Low/lower-middle-income	2.3	1.8	2.2	1.8	1.8	1.8	2.2	1.2	1.6	1.6
Upper-middle-income	1.7	1.5	1.7	1.5	1.5	1.4	1.5	1.5	2.0	1.4
High-income	1.8	1.7	1.7	1.5	1.6	1.2	1.7	1.3	1.5	1.6

[a]People's Republic of China

not find the problem found in previous longitudinal psychiatric epidemiological surveys of a large number of respondents in the follow-up who reported pre-baseline lifetime disorders that were not reported in the baseline interview (Borges *et al.* 2008). This is an important finding because it indicates that the approach we used for assessment was successful in reducing the most extreme problems of long-term recall failure. Second, the problem found in previous psychiatric epidemiological surveys of AOO reports being substantially over-represented in the five years before interview do not occur in the WMH surveys (Kessler *et al.* 2007b, 2008), as shown by the fact that the distributions of AOO reports are much more substantively plausible. Again, this finding suggests that our approach to assessment addressed the problem of long-term recall failure. Third, as detailed in disorder-specific chapters of the volume, blinded clinical reappraisal interviews carried out in conjunction with a number of WMH surveys documented good concordance between diagnoses of the disorders considered here and independent clinical diagnoses made by training research diagnostic clinical interviewers (Haro *et al.* 2006).

These improvements were achieved by beginning with evaluations of problems in earlier versions of the CIDI made by survey methodologists in preparation for an earlier US survey that was the foundation for the WMH surveys (Kessler *et al.* 1998, 1999, 2000). Four main methodological challenges highlighted in those evaluations became the focus of CIDI 3.0 revision efforts: (1) that respondents might not understand some of the CIDI questions about lifetime prevalence, a number of which include multiple clauses and vaguely defined terms; (2) that some respondents might not understand the task implied by the lifetime prevalence questions, which requires careful memory search that is unlikely to be carried out unless respondents are clearly instructed to do so; (3) that respondents might not be motivated to put in the hard work required to think back over their entire lives and answer lifetime recall questions accurately, especially in light of the fact that many CIDI questions deal with potentially embarrassing and stigmatizing experiences; and (4) that respondents might not be able to answer some CIDI questions accurately, especially those that ask about characteristics of mental disorders that are difficult to remember. AOO comes in as especially important as part of this fourth challenge, as previous research has shown that AOO is often difficult to recall accurately even when respondents are motivated to do so (Belli 1998; Prohaska *et al.* 1998). The strategies used in CIDI 3.0 to address these four challenges are discussed in detail elsewhere (Kessler & Üstün 2004, 2008) and will only be briefly reviewed here.

Question Comprehension

It is obvious that ambiguous questions are likely to be misconstrued, but it's perhaps less obvious just how ambiguous most structured surveys questions are and how often respondents must 'read between the lines' to make sense of them. Debriefing studies of earlier versions of the CIDI found that a great many respondents misunderstood important aspects of key diagnostic questions. The reason for this lies partly in the fact that many terms in surveys are vaguely defined. But beyond this is the more fundamental fact that the survey interview situation is a special kind of interaction in which the standard rules of conversation – rules that help fill in the gaps in meaning that exist in most speech – do not apply. Unlike the situation in normal conversational practice, the respondent in the survey interview often has only a vague notion of the person to whom he is talking or the purpose of the conversation (Cannell *et al.* 1968). The person who asks the questions (the interviewer) is not the person who formulated the questions (the researcher), and the questioner is often unable to clarify the respondent's uncertainties about the intent of the questions. Furthermore, the flow of questions in the survey interview is established prior to the beginning of the conversation, which means that normal conversational rules of give and take in question and answer sequences do not apply. This leads to more misreading than in normal conversations even when questions are seemingly straightforward (Clark & Schober 1992), a problem that is compounded when the topic of the interview is one that involves emotional experiences that are in many cases difficult to describe with clarity.

In an effort to investigate this problem debriefing interviews were carried out with community respondents who were administered sections of the CIDI; they were asked to explain what they thought the questions meant and why they answered the way they did (Kessler *et al.* 1998; Kessler 1999). Four discriminating features were found among questions that had high versus low levels of misunderstanding. First, some questions were too complex. Second, some questions involved vaguely defined terms. Third, some questions asked about odd experiences that could plausibly be interpreted in more than one way, such as questions about seeing and hearing things that others do not. Many respondents were found to have a tendency to normalize these questions and to respond positively when the correct answer was actually negative. Fourth, some questions were misunderstood because of *contextual* misunderstanding; that is, a misunderstanding that derived more from the position of the question in the flow of the interview than from lack of clarity in the question.

Based on these results, we carried out detailed CIDI debriefing interviews with volunteer respondents in methodological studies to support the development of CIDI 3.0 by pinpointing questions with each of the above four types of comprehension problems. Misunderstandings based on complex questions were addressed by breaking down the original CIDI questions into less complex subquestions. Especially complex questions were presented in a Respondent Booklet (RB) that provided a visual aid to respondents as the questions were being read by the interviewer. Misunderstandings based on the vagueness of terms were addressed by introducing clarifications and examples. Misunderstandings based on normalization of questions about odd experiences were addressed by prefacing the questions with clarification that we were actually asking about odd experiences and informing respondents that it was important for us to learn how often these experiences occur. Contextual misunderstandings were resolved by reordering questions to remove the contextual effects and by adding clarifying clauses in questions where residual confusion might exist. Although the number of modifications of this sort was so large that each one cannot be reviewed here, examples of each of the main types of modifications are presented elsewhere (Kessler *et al.* 2000).

Task Comprehension

Respondents also sometimes misunderstand the fundamental task they are being asked to carry out. Debriefing studies showed this was especially common with the diagnostic stem questions in the CIDI (Kessler *et al.* 2000). These stem questions are the first questions asked in each diagnostic section. They are used to determine whether a lifetime syndrome of a particular sort might have ever occurred. These questions provide what are, in effect, brief vignettes and ask the respondent whether they have ever had an experience of this sort. If a diagnostic stem question is endorsed, additional questions are asked to assess the specifics of the syndrome. If all diagnostic stem questions for a particular disorder are denied, the remaining questions about this syndrome are skipped.

Our methodological studies found that substantial confusion arises from respondent failure to understand the purpose of diagnostic stem questions. In particular, only about half of pilot respondents in our studies of the earlier version of CIDI interpreted these questions as they were intended; namely, as a request to engage in active memory search and to report the lifetime occurrence of episodes of the sort in the question. The other respondents interpreted the question as a request to report whether a memory of such an episode was readily accessible. These latter respondents did not believe that they were being asked to engage in active memory search and did not do so. Not surprisingly, the latter respondents were much less likely than those who understood the intent of the question to remember lifetime episodes.

Why did so many respondents misinterpret the intent of these lifetime recall questions? As Marquis and Cannell (1969) discovered in their early research on standard interview practice, respondents are generally ill informed about the purposes of the research and poorly motivated to participate actively. Furthermore, cues from interviewers often reinforce the inclination of respondents to participate in a halfhearted way. For example, when an interviewer asks a question that requires considerable thought, the respondent is likely to assume in the absence of instructions to the contrary that the interviewer is operating under normal conversational rules and, as such, is really asking for an immediate and appropriate answer. Cannell and colleagues (1981) showed that this conversational convention can be minimized by explicitly instructing respondents to answer completely and accurately; the use of such instruction can substantially improve the quality of data obtained in surveys. Based on this result, we built in clarifying statements throughout CIDI 3.0 aimed at informing respondents that accuracy was important. See (Kessler *et al.* 2000) for examples of statements.

Motivation

One problem with emphasizing to respondents the need to work hard at a series of demanding and potentially embarrassing recall tasks is that more respondents than otherwise may refuse to engage in the task. Recognition of this problem among survey methodologists has led to the development of motivational techniques intended to increase the chances that respondents will accept the job of answering completely and accurately. Two techniques that have proven to be particularly useful in this regard were used in CIDI 3.0. The first is the use of motivational components in instructions; that is, introductory remarks at the beginning of a survey that clarify the research aims in order to motivate respondents to provide a more complete and accurate report than they would otherwise. Respondents are known to be willing to undertake laborious and possibly painful memory searches if they recognize some altruistic benefit of doing so (Cannell *et al.* 1981). Based on this evidence, we developed and presented a statement containing a clear rationale for administering the interview and emphasized the importance of the survey for social policy purposes.

The second technique is contingent reinforcement embedded in the interviewer feedback probes. Consistent with research on behavioural modification of verbal productions through reinforcement (e.g., Centers 1963), several survey researchers have demonstrated that verbal reinforcers such as 'thanks' and 'that's useful' can significantly affect the behaviour of survey respondents (Marquis & Cannell 1969). Based on this observation, Cannell and his associates developed a method for training interviewers to use systematic feedback – both positive and negative – to reinforce respondent effort in reporting (Oksenberg *et al.* 1979). The central feature of this method is the use of structured feedback statements coordinated with the content and timing of instructions aimed at reinforcing respondent performance. It is important to recognize that it is performance that is being reinforced rather than the content of particular answers. For example, a difficult recall question may be prefaced with the instruction: 'This next question may be difficult, so please take your time before answering'. In contingent feedback instruction, interviewers issue some expression of gratitude whenever the respondent seems to consider his or her answer carefully, whether they remember anything or not. Alternatively, the interviewer might instruct the precipitous respondent: 'You answered that awfully quickly. Was there anything (else), even something small?' Such invitations to reconsider would occur whenever the respondent gives an immediate answer whether or not anything was reported. Experiments document clearly that the combined use of these contingent reinforcement probes with instructions explaining the importance of careful and accurate reporting leads to substantial improvement in recall of health-related events in general population surveys, including validated dates of medical events (Miller & Cannell 1977; Vinokur *et al.* 1979). Importantly, their results also showed that self-enhancing response biases are reduced when these strategies are used, as indicated by both a decreased tendency to underreport potentially embarrassing conditions and behaviours (e.g., gynaecological problems, seeing an X-rated movie) and a decreased tendency to over-report self-enhancing behaviours (e.g., number of books read in the last three months, having read the editorial page of the newspaper the previous day). Based on these results, the contingent feedback approach was included as a fundamental part of the interviewer training materials developed for CIDI 3.0.

The Ability to Answer Accurately

Research on basic cognitive processes has shown that memories are organized and stored in structured sets of information packages commonly called schemas (Markus & Zajonc 1985). When the respondent has a history of many instances of the same experience that cannot be discriminated, the separate instances tend to blend together in memory to form a special kind of memory schema called a 'semantic memory', a general memory for a prototypical experience (Jobe *et al.* 1990; Means & Loftus 1991). For example, the person may have a semantic memory of what panic attacks are like but, due to the fact that he has had many such attacks in his lifetime, cannot specify details of any particular panic attack. In comparison, when a respondent has had only a small number of lifetime experiences of a certain sort or when one instance stands out in memory as much different from the others, a memory can likely be recovered for that particular episode. This is called an 'episodic memory'.

In the case of memories of illness experiences, memory schemas tend to include not only semantic memories of prototypic symptoms but also personal theories about causes, course, and cure (Leventhal *et al.* 1984; Skelton & Croyle 1991). Some of these theories will conceptualize the experience in illness terms, while other theories will conceptualize the experience as a moral failing, a punishment from God, or a normal reaction to stress (Gilman 1988). These interpretations can influence the extent to which different memory cues are capable of triggering the schemas. The effects of memory schemas and the difference between semantic and episodic memories are central themes in research on autobiographical memory. In the survey context, a critical issue related to this research is whether the respondent is able to recover episodic memories in answering a particular survey question or if the respondent is answering the question by drawing inferences of what the past must have been like on the basis of more general semantic memories.

Research shows that people are more likely to recover episodic memories for experiences that are recent, distinctive, and unique, while people are more likely to rely on semantic memories for experiences that are frequent, typical, and regular (Brewer 1986; Belli 1988; Menon 1994). When a survey question is designed to ask about a particular instance of an experience, it must be posed in such a way that the respondent knows he is being asked to recover an episodic memory. Furthermore, the researcher must have some basis for assuming that an episodic memory can be recovered for this experience. If it cannot, a question that asks for such a memory implicitly invites the respondent to guess rather than to remember and this can have adverse effects on quality of reporting later in the interview (Pearson *et al.* 1992). In comparison, when a question is designed to recover a semantic memory or to use semantic memories to arrive at an answer by estimation, that should be made clear.

One difficulty with these injunctions in the case of retrospective recall questions about lifetime mental disorders is uncertainty about what level of recall accuracy to expect. Therefore, as part of the CIDI pilot work in preparation for the WMH surveys, we debriefed pilot respondents with an explicit eye towards pinpointing questions that were difficult to answer on the basis of episodic memory. When questions of this sort were discovered, an attempt was made to revise the questions to reduce the memory problem, either by allowing explicitly for estimation (e.g., explicitly asking respondents to provide a rough estimate), by providing categorical responses that reduce the complexity of the task, or by decomposing the question into subquestions that mimic effective memory search processes.

AOO questions are of special importance in this regard, as our pilot data showed that some people had quite a vivid memory of their first (and often only) episode of some mental disorders, especially when these disorders had rapid onsets, as in the case of panic attacks, whereas other people had only a vague memory of their first onset. The latter cases tended to involve accretion disorders (i.e., disorders that come on slowly) that occurred to people who subsequently had a great many other episodes. Based on a good deal of exploratory pilot work we finally developed an approach to this problem that proved to be simple and very effective: to ask people at the beginning of the AOO sequence if they had a *clear* memory of their first episode. As it turned out, the vast majority of people are able to answer this meta-question with no difficulty. We then varied subsequent questions depending on the answer to that first question. Respondents who reported having a clear memory were asked a follow-up question that simply asked them for their age when that first episode occurred. Respondents who reported not having a clear memory, in comparison, were asked a more complex set of question about the earliest age they could clearly remember a particular episode and their best estimate of *about* how old they were when they had their first episode. We carried out an experimental study to evaluate the effects of these questions by randomly assigning a group of community respondents to receive either a standard AOO question or our more complex series of AOO probes. The results were dramatic in showing that our new AOO probes resulted in much more substantially plausible AOO reports than those obtained in response to standard AOO questions (Knäuper *et al.* 1999). In particular, the implausible pattern found in earlier studies of AOO reported clustered in the five years before interview was not found in responses to our AOO questions.

Combining Strategies

We also used some additional strategies to deal with two or more of the above problems at once. The most important of these is a life review section that we developed for use in CIDI 3.0 near the beginning of the interview in an effort both to motivate and to facilitate active memory search in answering diagnostic stem questions. This section starts out with an introduction that explains to respondents that the next questions might be difficult to answer because they require respondents to review their entire lives. The introduction then goes on to say that despite this difficulty it is very important for the research that these questions are answered accurately. The introduction ends with the injunction to 'please take your time and think carefully before answering'.

The diagnostic stem questions for all core CIDI diagnoses are then administered directly following this commitment question. The questions are all included in the RB with a written instruction to 'take your time and think carefully before answering'. Interviewers are instructed to read the diagnostic stem questions slowly in an effort to emphasize their importance and to use motivational probes to encourage active memory search. Our intent in developing this section was both to explain the serious and difficult nature of the task and to motivate respondents to engage in the active memory search we hoped to stimulate by combining all the stem questions after a fairly detailed motivational introduction. We also recognized, based on our debriefing studies, that CIDI respondents quickly learn the logic of the stem-branch structure after a few sections and recognize that they can shorten the interview considerably by saying no to the stem questions. This problem is removed by asking all the stem questions near the beginning of the interview before the logic of the stem-branch structure becomes clear. Another important reason for including the section near the beginning of the interview is that pilot study respondents told us in debriefing interviews that their energy flagged as the interview progressed, making it much more difficult to carry out a serious memory search later in the interview than at the beginning.

We carried out an experiment to evaluate the effects of using this lifetime review section in conjunction with motivational probes. A random sample of 200 community respondents was randomized either to an earlier version of CIDI or to a version that was identical except that it included the life review section at the beginning of the interview. As reported in more detail elsewhere (Kessler *et al.* 1998), this experiment documented that the life review section led to a significant increase in the proportion of respondents who endorsed diagnostic stem questions. For example, while 26.7% of respondents in the standard CIDI condition endorsed a diagnostic stem question for major depression, a significantly higher 40.6% did so in the life review condition. Importantly, a clinical validity study documented that this increased prevalence of stem endorsement was not accompanied by a reduction in sensitivity with regard to clinical diagnoses, documenting that additional true cases were discovered by the use of the life review section and the accompanying commitment and motivation probes. These results were the basis of adopting the lifetime review section in CIDI 3.0.

Socio-demographics

We consider seven socio-demographic variables in this volume: cohort (i.e., year of birth, approximately with a measure of age-at-interview), age at onset of the disorder (which, as noted above, was based on retrospective reports), gender, employment status at the time of interview, marital status at the time of interview, educational level, and household income in the year before interview. These variables were selected based on the fact that they are the most commonly considered socio-demographic characteristics in previous descriptive epidemiological studies of mental disorders. It is important to appreciate that we do not conceptualize these variables as causes of mental disorders but merely as descriptive correlates that are useful in locating the segments of the population most likely to experience these disorders.

Cohort is discretized into quartiles for purposes of our descriptive analyses to distinguish respondents who are in the age ranges 18–29, 30–44, 45–59, and 60+. AOO, in comparison, is divided into quartiles that are specific to each disorder in light of the fact that AOO distributions differ markedly across disorders. The 25% of lifetime cases with the earliest AOO for a given disorder are described as early-onset cases, the next 25% early-average, the next 25% late-average, and the 25% with latest onsets as late-onset cases. In regression analyses predicting course of illness, we also subtract current age from AOO to compute a continuous measure of time-since-onset (TSO). The logic of doing this is discussed below in the subsection on analysis methods for predicting course of illness.

Employment status was assessed in the WMH surveys using a nonexclusive coding scheme that allowed us to capture information about individuals in multiple roles (e.g., part-time female workers who considered themselves homemakers; retirees who were also students). We used a hierarchical coding scheme to simplify these codes in the current volume by classifying each respondent into only one of five categories using a hierarchical scheme. The hierarchy coded everyone who reported being employed as employed no matter what other categories they reported, others as retired no matter what other categories they reported, others as homemakers no matter what other categories they employed, and remainder as 'others', where the latter category was made up largely of individuals who reported being unemployed and/or disabled.

Marital status was classified into three categories of being either never married, currently married, or previously married, where the latter category included separated as well as widowed and divorced people. Respondents who reported that they were currently cohabiting in a marriage-like relationship were classified as married. Educational status was coded using a seven-category scheme that was more complex than we would have liked but was necessary because of the wide variation in educational attainment across countries. The categories were no education, some primary, finished primary, some secondary, finished secondary, some college, and finished a BA-level college education. The number of respondents with more than a college education was too small for consideration as a separate category. Given that the number of years required for primary, secondary, and college degrees differed across countries, we used the standards in each country to develop codes rather than requiring the same number of years of education for a given designation across countries.

Household income, finally, posed a special challenge because of the many different currencies used across countries. There is also the question of whether we wanted to think of income in terms of cross-national comparisons, in which case we might have transformed all incomes into a constant metric, such as one that describes purchasing power (Taylor 2003). However, as discussed in more detail below in the section on analysis methods, this was not our intent. Instead, we were interested in pooled within-country comparisons. And as a result, we used a cross-national scoring system that is common in international research on welfare economics (Solow 1967): to classify families in terms of percentile of pretax household per family member income using the local currency with values less than 50% of the median as having low income, those with higher incomes up to the median as having low-average income, those above the median up to two times the median as having high-average income, and those greater than two times the median as having high-income. Note that even though this is a within-country classification scheme, the proportions of the population in each category can vary across countries.

Role Impairment

An earlier WMH volume focused on the burdens of mental disorders (Alonso *et al.* 2013). One of the aspects of disease burden considered in that volume was disorder-specific role impairment (Ormel *et al.* 2013). This is an aspect of disease burden that is of special importance from a societal perspective (Murray & Lopez 2013) and is the one element of disease burden considered in this volume. Role impairment was assessed with a modified version of the Sheehan Disability Scales (SDS; Sheehan *et al.* 1996), a widely used self-report measure of condition-specific disability. Our modified version of the SDS consists of four questions, each asking the respondent to rate on a 0–10 visual analogue scale the extent to which a particular disorder 'interfered with' activities in one of four role domains during the month in the past year when the disorder was most severe. The four domains include: (i) 'your home management, like cleaning, shopping, and taking care of the (house/apartment)' (home); (ii) 'your ability to work' (work); (iii) 'your social life' (social); and (iv) 'your ability to form and maintain close relationships with other people' (close relationships). The 0–10 response options were presented in a visual analogue format with labels for the response options of None (0), Mild (1–3), Moderate (4–6), and Severe (7–10). A global SDS disability score was also created by assigning each respondent the highest SDS domain score reported across the four domains.

Previous methodological studies have documented good internal consistency reliability across the SDS domains (Leon *et al.* 1997; Hambrick *et al.* 2004; Leu *et al.* 2015; Horberg *et al.* 2016), a result that we replicated in the WMH data by finding Cronbach's alpha (a measure of internal consistency reliability) in the range 0.82–0.97 across countries. Importantly, reliability was consistently high in low/lower-middle-income (0.91), upper-middle (0.91), and high-income (0.88) countries (Ormel *et al.* 2008). Previous methodological studies have also documented good discrimination between role functioning of cases and controls based on SDS scores in studies of major depression (Leu *et al.* 2015), social phobia (Hambrick *et al.* 2004), posttraumatic stress disorder (PTSD) (Connor & Davidson 2001), panic disorder (Leon *et al.* 1997), and substance abuse (Pallanti *et al.* 2006). Similar results were found in the WMH surveys based on responses to a question asked after the SDS about: 'How many days out of 365 in the past year were you totally unable to work or carry out you normal activities because of (the illness)?' We examined the strength of SDS scores predicting variation in this relatively objective measure of disability. If the SDS measures genuine disability, we would expect correlations to be significant and comparable for physical and mental disorders. This is, in fact, what we found although the correlations varied across national income level. In high-income countries, the multiple correlations of the four SDS domain scores predicting days-out-of-role were 0.56 for mental disorders and 0.50 for physical conditions, while the comparable correlations in upper-middle-income countries were 0.42 for mental disorders and 0.37 for physical conditions, and in low and lower-middle-income countries were 0.38 for mental disorders and 0.34 for physical conditions (Ormel *et al.* 2008).

It is important to recognize that the SDS scales are *condition-specific*. That is, respondents were asked to rate the interference in role functioning caused by a particular disorder rather than the interference caused by all their health problems. This focused approach to questioning allows SDS scores to be compared across disorders without adjusting for comorbidity. However, this requires respondents with multiple health problems to sort out the relative effects of their various conditions on their overall functioning. An indication that respondents are able to do this comes from controlled treatment studies that have documented significant improvements in SDS measures of condition-specific role functioning with treatment for generalized anxiety disorder (GAD) (Davidson *et al.* 2004), panic disorder (Bertani *et al.* 2004), and major depression (Hudson *et al.* 2007). Because they are condition-specific, the SDS scales were administered separately for each of the disorders considered in this volume.

Treatment/Service Use

The WMH surveys include considerable information about patterns of service use and treatment, including information on both prevalence of lifetime treatment (Wang *et al.* 2007b), treatment adequacy (Wang *et al.* 2007a), barriers to treatment (Andrade *et al.* 2014), and treatment dropout (Wells *et al.* 2013). The investigation of all these issues is beyond the scope of this volume, but we nonetheless present data on past-year treatment among respondents with each of the disorders considered here. This information comes from questions that asked all Part II WMH respondents if they ever saw any one of a wide range of professionals or attended a self-help group because of 'problems with your emotions, nerves, or your use of alcohol or drugs'. The list of professionals varied across countries depending on local options, but in each case the list included the full range of commonly available local treatment providers in each of four broad treatment sectors. The first was the *mental health specialist sector*. Included here were visits to a psychiatrist, psychologist, psychiatric social worker, psychiatric nurse, and mental health or substance abuse counsellor, along with use of a mental health helpline, as well as overnight admissions for a mental health or drug or alcohol problem to any treatment setting. The second sector was the *general medical sector*, which included visits to a general practitioner, other medical doctor, nurse, occupational therapist, or any other healthcare professional exclusive of those in a specialty mental health treatment setting. The third sector was the *human services sector*, which included visits to any religious or spiritual advisor or to a social worker or counsellor in any setting other than a specialty mental health setting. The final sector was the *complementary-alternative medical (CAM) sector*, which included any other type of healer such as an herbalist or homeopath, or participation in a self-help or support group.

Respondents who reported lifetime use of any of these types of services were then probed to ask about treatment in the 12 months before interview. We focus in this volume on treatment at any time in the 12 months before interview. It is noteworthy that prior WMH studies (e.g., Wang *et al.* 2007a; Thornicroft *et al.* 2016) have also made a distinction between receiving any treatment and receiving a type of treatment that would be considered sufficiently intense to be considered potentially helpful or adequate. We did not do that here, as controversy exists about the threshold for defining minimally adequate treatment in different parts of the world. Instead, we merely report the proportion of people with a 12-month disorder who received any 12-month treatment. We also consider treatment for any self-defined problem with emotions, nerves, or alcohol-drug problems even though the analyses focus on particular disorders, as the WMH surveys did not enquire about disorder-specific 12-month treatments. As a result, the estimates of the treatment rates of 12-month disorders should be considered upper bound estimates.

Translation

CIDI 3.0 was developed initially in English. One of the fundamental challenges in an undertaking such as the WMH Survey Initiative is to achieve both equivalence in meaning and consistency in measurement across surveys and have multiple languages. This is a special challenge in studying mental disorders, as the symptoms of these are described and interpreted differently in different cultures (Prince & Tcheng-Laroche 1987; Cheng 2001), making it necessary in some cases to use substantially different terms or even questions in different countries to assess the presence versus absence of these symptoms. Another complexity is that the CIDI source language, English, has a larger lexicon (stock of vocabulary) than any other known language. This can mean that distinctions made in English cannot be matched in one or more target languages. The opposite can also be true with respect to certain areas of lexical or grammatical distinctions, in which the source language may not specify enough detail necessary for translation into a given target language.

WMH collaborators were given guidelines for translation and adaptation of the CIDI aimed at achieving both equivalence in meaning and consistency in measurement across surveys. A detailed discussion of these guidelines is presented elsewhere (Harkness *et al.* 2008) and will not be repeated here. We merely note that these guidelines were modifications of longstanding WHO guidelines for translation, back-translations, and harmonization that were updated by the staff of the WHO Data Collection Coordination Centre under the direction of BE Pennell in collaboration with the WMH Co-Principal Investigators.

Countries were instructed that the central aim of the translation process was to achieve target language versions of the English questionnaire that were *conceptually equivalent* in each of the countries/cultures rather than literal equivalence in terms of word-for-word translation. It was emphasized that the translation should sound natural in each language (in as far as that is possible in standardized instruments) and to perform in comparable fashion across the populations and languages. Independent assessors who were experts on cross-national translation reviewed the CIDI translations and found that these aims were generally achieved, but that some of the translations were at times too close to the English questionnaire language formulation and structure to sound 'natural'.

Countries were required to follow a six-step process in achieving these aims. These steps included: (1) forward translation; (2) expert panel review; (3) independent back-translation; (4) harmonization of vocabulary and formulation across different country versions of a shared language (if appropriate); (5) pretesting and cognitive interviewing; and (6) final revision, creation, and documentation of a final version of the translated questionnaire. A detailed description of each of these steps is presented elsewhere (Harkness *et al.* 2008).

Pretesting

Consistent with best-practices recommendations (Sheatsley 1983; Converse & Presser 1986; Groves *et al.* 2004; Harkness *et al.* 2004; Smith 2004), pretests of the instrument and procedures were carried out in each WMH survey prior to main study implementation. This should not be confused with the pretesting phase of translation that was described in the last subsection, as the latter focused only on translation, whereas the larger subsequent pretesting phase evaluated not only the instrument but all survey procedures. The pretests were designed to mirror the main study in most aspects, except in some cases using experienced interviewer supervisors for pretest data collection rather than the interviewers who carried out the main survey. Pretest interviews were evaluated by debriefing interviewers to identify potential problem areas with the instrument and survey procedures, checking the distributions of items for high rates of missing data and out-of-range values, and using behaviour coding of audio-taped pretest interviews to pinpoint questions that were often misread or often elicited respondent requests for clarification.

Pretesting is especially important in cross-national studies (Smith 2004) because of the challenges associated with working in many different languages and social contexts (Smith 2004). A separate series of pretests was consequently required in each WMH country. Initial pretests focused on evaluating the translations. Later pretests evaluated the interview schedule and field procedures. The number of the latter pretest rounds varied from one to three, with approximately two-thirds of the countries conducting just one round of pretests and most others two rounds. The pretest debriefing sessions identified country-specific difficulties with questionnaire wording and response categories that were modified prior to the beginning of production interviewing. These sessions, along with quantitative analyses of responses, also detected skip pattern errors in the paper and pencil interview (PAPI) version and programming errors in the computer-assisted personal interview (CAPI) version that were corrected prior to the beginning of production interviewing. The pretests also allowed the investigators to evaluate the adequacy of survey procedures and sample management systems.

Interviewer Training and Quality Control Monitoring

Although large-scale cross-national surveys have been undertaken for decades (Heath *et al.* 2005 provide a concise history), there is surprisingly little written research on the practical aspects of training and supervising interviewers to achieve high-quality survey data. Cultural adaptation of survey methods is widely recognized to be necessary to achieve equivalence in measurement across countries (Bulmer 1998; Jowell 1998; Kuechler 1998; Lynn 2001). However, few details are provided in the literature as to how to achieve this equivalence across the many phases of a project's development. In the absence of such standards of practice, many cross-national projects have been left to accept the research traditions of individual countries, which vary widely in methodological rigour. An approach at the other extreme is to implement a 'one-size-fits-all' methodology that naively imposes the same procedure and protocols across all countries and cultures based on the assumption that good practices in one culture will be good practice in other cultures (Harkness *et al.* 2002).

The WMH Survey Initiative sought to implement an approach between these two extremes by establishing guidelines that set minimum standards for each phase of project implementation but allowed for country-specific adaptations. We saw this earlier in the chapter in the discussion of probability sampling methods that allowed for country-specific variations. The difficulty for the staff of the WMH Data Collection Coordination Centre was determining when variations in approach were necessary and appropriate rather than simply expedient. Staying with the above sampling example, survey organizations in some parts of the world have a tradition of quota sampling and respondent substitution that violates the WMH requirement of probability sampling. This kind of potential conflict between local practice and best practices was found in every phase of the WMH survey implementation.

A detailed description of the WMH data quality control standards established by the WMH Data Collection Coordination Centre and the ways in which these standards were implemented in the individual WMH countries is presented elsewhere (Pennell *et al.* 2008). These standards were subsequently used by the senior members of the WMH Data Collection Coordination Centre to take the lead in developing internationally recognized guidelines for best practices in cross-national comparative survey research more generally (www.ccsg.isr.umich.edu). Issues of interviewer recruitment and training, research ethics, field structure, data collection procedures and quality control, and data preparation are all included in these guidelines. We will not discuss here the main practical decisions made in establishing WMH field procedures, such as the decision to have interviews carried out face-to-face rather than by telephone and the decision to use both paper and pencil and computer-assisted versions of the survey and to allow individual countries to choose which of the two modes they were able to use, but refer the reader to a detailed discussion of these decisions elsewhere (Pennell *et al.* 2008).

Interviewer Hiring and Training

The previous section made it clear that CIDI 3.0 is a complex instrument. Successful implementation of such an instrument requires interviewers to be highly trained. We consequently placed high importance on careful interviewer training and quality assurance monitoring. In some countries, the research team was responsible for interviewer recruitment and management, while in other countries the interviewing component was subcontracted to an external survey organization. Before starting the interviewer recruitment and training process, each country sent at least two interviewer supervisors to a 'train-the-trainer' session presented by the WMH Data Collection Coordination Centre at the University of Michigan in the United States. These sessions lasted an average of six days and were designed to prepare the interviewer supervisors to train and monitor interviewer performance, as well as to manage data collection and data processing in their country. Through these sessions, research teams obtained all of the information and materials necessary to train their own interviewing staff using consistent procedures. These trainers, who in almost all countries came from a pool of experienced interviewers, then trained a team of supervisors to help in interviewer recruitment, training, and field quality control monitoring. Many countries were required to recruit and hire new interviewers for the WMH survey, while others were able to use existing field staff from ongoing survey organizations. In most countries where new interviewers were recruited, recruitment was carried out in the general population. In a few countries, though, interviewers were recruited exclusively from among college students. Careful centralized screening procedures were used in this hiring process.

Interviewer training was divided into two parts: general interviewing techniques and CIDI-specific training. General interviewing training (GIT) was designed to introduce interviewers to the basic components of standardized questionnaire administration (e.g., question reading, appropriate techniques for probing and seeking clarification, providing feedback, and accurate data recording). GIT sessions ranged from two to three days in most countries. In addition, countries that used computer-assisted interviewing had a GIT component focused on computer hardware and software use. Some countries added other country-specific topics in their GIT session, such as New Zealand's inclusion of cultural empathy to Maori and Pacific Islander households and Colombia's special training on interacting with governmental authorities and armed guerrilla and paramilitary groups. All interviewers were required to demonstrate competence with GIT concepts and procedures through a variety of tests before moving on to study-specific training.

Study-specific training averaged 30 hours across countries. The content was presented as a mix of lecture and round-robin practice sessions focused on general project background and importance, rules for obtaining informed consent, definitions of eligibility and respondent selection procedures, specifics of the precise interview procedures, and discussion of production requirements. Hands-on practice was stressed throughout. Trainers assessed the skill level of each interviewer in small group exercises and often held tailored 'after-hours' special sessions to address areas where interviewers needed additional assistance and practice. Most countries included in the training team a clinical consultant, typically a psychiatric social worker or clinical psychologist, who provided interviewers with background information about the kinds of symptoms of emotional problems they would encounter during production interviewing. This clinical contact person (CCP) was also a resource person for both interviewers and respondents during data collection to address the needs of respondents who might require a referral for follow-up and interviewers who might need to debrief after a particularly difficult interview. In most cases, the CCP was available to interviewers 24 hours a day, seven days a week. Many countries developed protocols that allowed interviewers to contact their CCP privately, without first going through a supervisor to provide interviewers a unique opportunity to speak freely about their own and their respondents' experiences.

Quality Control Monitoring

Importantly, all countries required interviewers to pass a certification test before being approved for production work. Interviewers who did not pass the certification process were either terminated from the project or received additional retraining and another opportunity to obtain certification. Interviewer training often continued during the production phase of the project through such means as periodic in-person seminars, telephone conference calls, and bulletins or newsletters.

Special procedures were also developed to monitor interviewer performance during production. Systematic monitoring is critical to survey data quality assurance (Billiet & Loosveldt 1988; Fowler & Mangione 1990). Consistent with best-practices guidelines for survey implementation (Biemer & Lyberg 2003), four areas of performance were the main targets of quality assurance monitoring: detection and prevention of falsified information, compliance with the interviewing rules and guidelines set forth in the training manual, performance of noninterview tasks, and identification of interviewer-questionnaire interface problems.

These areas were evaluated by a number of methods including supervisor reinterview of selected cases, supervisor verification of key survey elements through spot recontact of respondents, direct observation of interviews, audio-recording, questionnaire review, analysis of performance and production measures, keystroke/trace file analysis (files that record keystrokes and movement of the interviewer through the computerized instrument), and mock interviews/tests of knowledge and practice. Interviewers were terminated from production interviewing if they were found through these methods not to be able to perform up to required standards. The recommended supervisor-to-interviewer ratio of one supervisor for every 8–10 interviewers was used in the majority of countries that used paper and pencil data collection, while lower ratios were used in countries with computer administration based on the greater control over the data collection process afforded by computerized interviewing (Williams 1986; Lavrakas 1993).

Statistical Analysis Methods

Prevalence of the Outcome Variables

The main focus of this volume is on prevalence and basic descriptive predictors of mental disorders. We look at prevalence in several time frames. *Lifetime prevalence* represents the proportion of people in the population who, to date, have ever met criteria for the disorder. This is the first outcome measure we report for each mental disorder. It is important to recognize that some unknown number of respondents will develop these disorders in the future, which means that lifetime risk of the disorders is generally higher than lifetime prevalence. It is possible to estimate the proportion of the population who are likely to experience the disorder at some time in their life, which is known as *morbid risk*, by making assumptions about the stability of AOO distributions across birth cohorts. We do not emphasize morbid risk in this volume due to concerns about the implausibility of this assumption. Instead, we focus on lifetime prevalence as a conservative estimate of the proportion of the population ever affected by each disorder considered, although we also report morbid risk. It is important for the reader to recognize that estimates of lifetime prevalence represent *lower bound* estimates of the proportions of the population who will ever experience the disorders, while estimates of morbid risk probably over-estimate the proportion of people in a survey cohort who will ever experience the disorders considered here because of the likelihood that transition probabilities of onset risk vary over cohorts in ways that have probably led to increased risk in more recent cohorts, although sample bias (e.g., prior mortality among people in the original population cohorts from which the sample was selected and low response rates among especially ill living members of these cohorts) could introduce conservative bias even in estimates of morbid risk.

We also report *12-month prevalence* of each disorder, the proportion of the population who are in an active episode of the disorder as some time in the past 12 months. Estimates of 12-month prevalence are in many ways of more practical policy importance than estimates of lifetime prevalence, as many health care organizations update their plans for service delivery needs on an annual basis. And we report *30-day prevalence*, the proportion of the population who are in an active episode of the disorder in the month of interview, as 30-day prevalence is the best estimate we have in WMH of the current direct burden of each disorder. It is noteworthy, though, that 30-day prevalence might be under estimated for some disorders due to the fact that respondents are given latitude in when to schedule their interviews, leading to likely under-representation of times when they are severely impaired.

The ratio of 12-month prevalence to lifetime prevalence provides a rough estimate of long-term disorder persistence, whereas the ratio of 30-day prevalence to 12-month prevalence provides a rough estimate of episode or symptom persistence, although both of these estimates have to be considered only approximations. We present both of these ratios in an effort to disaggregate our estimates of 30-day prevalence into components due to lifetime prevalence, long-term persistence, and episode persistence. As we will see at numerous places in the volume, the predictors of 30-day prevalence are often due to associations of the significant predictors with only one of these components. And in some rare cases we even find significantly positive associations of a given predictor with one component but negative associations with other components. This disaggregated information is important because it has implications both for theory development and for intervention targeting. Based on this fact, in each chapter we present integrated information on patterns and predictors of lifetime, 12-month, and 30-day prevalence in the total sample, along with parallel information about 12-month prevalence among lifetime cases and 30-day prevalence among 12-month cases.

Estimating Cumulative Lifetime Probability Distributions

Some insight into the difference between lifetime prevalence and morbid risk can be obtained by looking at *cumulative lifetime probability curves*. These curves are graphic depictions of the increase in the proportion of people in the population who experience a given disorder as they age. For example, if 1% of the population first experiences a given disorder at age 12, 1% of the remainder at age 13, 1% of that remainder at age 14, and so on, then the *cumulative* proportion of the population that experiences the disorder as of given ages will be 1% at age 12, 1% + 1% × (100% – 1%) at age 13, and, more generally, the age *t* cumulative proportion + 1% × (100% – the age *t* cumulative proportion) at age *t*+1. We used the actuarial method (Halli *et al.* 1992) to make these calculations. The actuarial method is somewhat different from and preferable to the more conventional Kaplan-Meier method (Lee & Go 1997) in the way it handles ties. This curve gives us information about when in the life course each disorder typically begins. Given that we generated these curves separately for each survey, we felt that it would be more intuitive for readers for us to report ages at fixed percentiles of the distribution in tabular form than to show actual curves. As a result, we prepared a table for each disorder listing the age at which an estimated 5%, 10%, 25%, 50%, 75%,

90%, 95%, and 99% of all the people who will ever have an onset of the disorder in their lifetime had their first onset. These ages are reported separately for each survey as a way to let readers how stable estimates across the surveys. We arbitrarily defined lifetime risk as ending at age 75, given that the numbers of respondents in the survey older than this age were small.

As we noted in the previous subsection of this chapter, it is possible to make a projection of the proportion of the population that is likely to experience a given disorder at some time in their life using cumulative lifetime probability curves, which is known as morbid risk. We did this in order to define the denominator for calculating the percentiles noted in the previous paragraph. In conjunction with reporting ages of selected percentiles of the age-of-onset distributions of the disorders for each survey, we also reported projected morbid risk and we recorded for comparison purposes lifetime prevalence (i.e., the proportion of survey respondents that had an onset of the disorder as of the time of interview). In cases where the great majority of people have onsets early in life, as with attention-deficit/hyperactivity disorder, lifetime prevalence and projected morbid rick are virtually identical. In cases where a substantial proportion of people develop the disorder later in life, in comparison, lifetime prevalence is considerably lower than projected morbid risk.

Socio-demographic Correlates of Lifetime Disorders

As noted above, we think of the socio-demographic variables examined in this volume as descriptive correlates, not causes. As a result, we use information about a number of time-varying socio-demographics assessed at the time of interview (employment status, marital status, education, family income) as 'predictors' of first onset and course of disorders, even though these socio-demographic variables in many cases first occurred many years after the onset of the disorders. We do this because we are using the statistical analyses of these associations in order to describe associations rather than to examine the predictive associations of temporally primary socio-demographic variables with the subsequent first onset or course of mental disorders.

For the same reason (i.e., our focus on description rather that prediction), the associations of each time-varying socio-demographic variable reported in this volume are adjusted only for age, gender, and survey. The associations are not adjusted for the overlap of time-varying socio-demographic variables with each other (e.g., for the fact that people with high education generally have higher incomes than people with low education; or for the fact that married women are more likely to be homemakers than unmarried women). We look at unadjusted (for other time-varying socio-demographics) associations because we want to present clear descriptions of the distributions of mental disorders across individual socio-demographic variables rather than to partition the joint importance of multiple socio-demographic variables in predicting mental disorders.

We control for gender and age, though, in 'predicting' lifetime disorders for the following reasons. We control for gender because there are well-known gender differences in many mental disorders (Frank 2002). We control for age because people who have lived longer have more time-at-risk to develop disorders and would be expected, all else equal, to have higher lifetime prevalence of disorders. This is not always the case, though, because there can be changes in prevalence over time, as when the proportion of young adults who ever had an illicit drug use disorder might be higher than the proportion of older adults with that disorder due to an increase in the use of drugs among children, adolescents, and young adults in more recent cohorts in the country. In addition to cohort effects, though, recall of childhood disorders becomes lower with age. Another possibility is that embarrassment about having had one or more disorders can be greater among older people, leading to an increase in conscious nondisclosure with age. A final noteworthy possibility is that some mental disorders are associated with increased risk of early mortality not only because of suicide (Whiteford *et al.* 2013) but also elevated risk of all-cause mortality (Charlson *et al.* 2016), leading to increasing attrition bias against lifetime history of mental disorder mental with increasing age.

We also control for survey in 'predicting' lifetime disorders. We do this by including a series of dummy predictor variables in each equation to represent individual surveys. When all 29 surveys are included in the analysis, we use 28 dummy control variables in this way. It is important to appreciate our rationale for doing this: that we are explicitly focusing on pooled within-survey associations and consciously deciding not to examine between-survey variation in prevalence of mental disorders. It would have been possible to use information about between-survey differences in central tendencies and/or distributions of predictors to predict between-survey variation in prevalence of mental disorders. Indeed, some other researchers have done exactly that by putting together published WMH country-level results (Duckers *et al.* 2016).

We chose not to examine cross-national differences in prevalence because the WMH surveys were optimized to search for patterns of central tendency and to highlight the most stable of such patterns across countries rather than to optimize examination of the reasons for cross-national differences. A serious effort to study cross-national differences would have led us to modify the sample designs of the WMH surveys to make them representative not only of countries but also of major regions within countries to increase the sample of spatial units. We would also have collected extensive data on both contemporary and short-term historical contextual factors for each country, as well as regions within countries that might explain the time–space variation in prevalence we observed in the data. Indeed, this examination of time–space variation has been the approach we have taken in the rare occasions we have studied cross-national differences in the WMH data (Seedat *et al.* 2009). And even there we carried out the analysis to study variation in associations (i.e., gender differences in lifetime prevalence of individual disorders as of age 25) rather than prevalence in order to capitalize on the fact that these associations are less sensitive to the influence of relatively arbitrary diagnostic thresholds on estimates of cross-national differences than are prevalence estimates.

More general comparisons of cross-national differences in predictors of prevalence, in comparison, are faced with the daunting task of making sense of differences across only about two dozen data points (i.e., surveys) by selecting from the literally hundreds of plausible potentially causal variables that might account for this variation. With such a small sample it is virtually impossible to draw unequivocal conclusions about important predictors. For example, an association of country-level economic development with prevalence might actually be due to between-country differences in methodological variables (e.g., response rate, which, as noted in Table 3.1, is considerably lower for surveys in high-income than lower-income countries).

As we focus on pooled within-survey associations, a question can be raised whether we should weight our data by population size or survey sample size. We chose the latter due to the fact that the countries included in WMH are not in any way representative of all countries in the world, making it impossible to estimate world-wide prevalence or correlates of mental disorders from our pooled data. Instead, we consider each survey as having a level of importance equivalent to its sample size in generating estimates of central tendency, leading us to use weights that represent sample size rather than population size.

Discrete-time survival analysis with person-year used as the unit of analysis (Efron 1988) was used to study the predictors of first onset of each disorder. The discrete-time approach was chosen over the more traditional Cox proportional hazards analysis approach because our information about timing of onsets was available only for discrete intervals of time (i.e., years of age). The discrete-time models were operationalized as logistic regression models with person-year the unit of analysis and first onset of the focal disorder as outcomes. This approach treats each year of each respondent's life as a separate observational record, building a dataset containing $n \times t$ person-year records for a sample of n respondents with an average of t years of life at the time of interview. Each record is coded for the year of life it represents and is assigned a score of either 0 or 1 on the outcome (i.e., first lifetime onset of the disorder) depending on whether or not the disorder had a first onset in that year. Years of life after first onset of the disorder are excluded from analysis. By pooling years in this way and controlling for person-year, as we do in the analysis, we estimate a series of within-year models for the predictors of first onset of the disorder in year t among respondents who never had the disorder as of year t-1 that are combined to obtain a single parameter estimate for each predictor across all years.

Survival coefficients and their standard errors were exponentiated and are reported here as odds-ratios (ORs) with 95% confidence intervals. Confidence intervals were estimated using the design-based Taylor series linearization method (Wolter 1985) implemented in the SAS software system (SAS Institute Inc. 2011) to adjust for the weighting and clustering of the WMH data. Multivariate significance tests for sets of dummy variables to characterize a single socio-demographic characteristic (e.g., a two-degree of freedom test for the three categories of marital status) were carried out using Wald χ^2 tests based on Taylor series coefficient variance-covariance matrices. Statistical significance was consistently evaluated using 0.05-level two-sided tests.

An issue of note in discussing the person-year models is that the nearly 80,000 respondents in the pooled Part II sample across all surveys considered here typically generated well over 2 million person-years in the dataset for each discrete-time survival model. This made it computationally intensive to estimate these models. This problem was addressed by using *case-control sampling* to reduce the number of observations used in estimating the models. In this approach, 100% of the person-years with first onsets of the outcome disorder were compared to a probability sample of 10 times as many control person-years selected with stratification from the full set of person-years prior to first onset of the disorder and weighted to have a sum of weights equal to the sum of weights in the full set of control person-years in the pooled cross-national sample. As the logistic link function is used in these models, the coefficients are not biased by selecting a subsample of controls (Schlesselman 1982). Furthermore, the ratio of 10 controls for every one case is large enough that any increase in statistical power achieved by adding more controls would be trivial.

The initial models included predictors for gender, age-at-interview (i.e., cohort), and survey. These ORs can be interpreted as the relative-odds of lifetime prevalence for women versus men or for respondents of certain ages at interview versus those of other ages, compared to other respondents in the same survey averaged over all person-years of risk and across surveys, with these averages taking into consideration time–space variation in number of new cases of the disorders in the cross-national dataset. The latter means that any existing variation in ORs associated with a given predictor is weighted in favour of observations in the age ranges and in the surveys with highest concentrations of cases. Subsequent models added one and only one time-varying socio-demographic variable. These ORs can be interpreted as the relative-odds of lifetime prevalence for respondents with given values on the time-varying predictor *as of the time of interview* compared to other individuals of the same age-at-interview and gender averaged over all person-years of risk and across surveys.

Decomposing Socio-demographic Correlates of 30-day Prevalence

We noted above that data are reported for each disorder on lifetime, 12-month, and 30-day prevalence as well as for 12-month prevalence among lifetime cases and 30-day prevalence among 12-month cases. We also noted that we are especially interested in 30-day prevalence because this is our most direct estimate of the burden of the disorder in the population (i.e., an estimate of the proportion of population in an episode of the disorder at a given point in time). When we looked at socio-demographic correlates, we consequently began with a consideration of associations with 30-day prevalence and then we decomposed this association into its component parts of associations with lifetime prevalence in the total population, associations with 12-month prevalence among lifetime cases, and associations with 30-day prevalence among 12-month cases. It sometimes occurs that a socio-demographic variable is significantly associated with 30-day prevalence due to only one of those three component associations. The distinction among the three is potentially important for policy planning purposes, as the primary preventive interventions designed to reduce high lifetime risk of a given disorder in a particular segment of the population would be quite different from the secondary interventions designed to reduce persistence of the disorder or clinical interventions to treat active episodes.

Unlike the person-year models used to predict lifetime prevalence, the models to predict 30-day prevalence were person-level models estimated in the total sample with a logistic link function using the same design-based Taylor series linearization method as in the person-year survival models. The same predictors were also used in the model for 30-day prevalence as the model for lifetime prevalence. The models for 12-month prevalence among lifetime cases and 30-day prevalence among 12-month cases, in comparison, while also based on person-level data arrays, were estimated in subgroups rather than in the total sample and included among the predictors two separate predictors representing components of age-at-interview: AOO of the disorder and TSO. AOO and TSO sum to equal age-at-interview. We considered these two components separately because previous research has shown that they often have opposite signs in predicting the course of a disorder, with early AOO often associated with a more persistent course of illness but TSO inversely associated with 12-month and 30-day prevalence among lifetime cases (McLaughlin *et al.* 2010). It is only when both components are included as predictors in the same model that these opposite-sign associations can be seen clearly.

Comorbidity among Disorders

Even though this volume focuses on disorder-specific analyses, it is important to recognize that common mental disorders are highly comorbid (Kessler *et al.* 2011) and that comorbidity is associated with persistence (Wardenaar *et al.* 2014), severity (Ormel *et al.* 2008), and treatment (Wang *et al.* 2007a) of individual disorders. While a thorough analysis of comorbidity is beyond the scope of this volume, we present basic information on comorbidity in each disorder-specific chapter and we also present a special chapter that provides associations between lifetime disorders, and findings from analyses examining the structure of comorbidity (Chapter 20). In each disorder-specific chapter, we present information on the proportions of lifetime and 12-month cases that also meet criteria over the same time periods for any mood, anxiety, disruptive behaviour/impulse-control, and substance-use disorder, as well as for any of these disorders. In addition, we present information on the typical AOO sequence between each focal disorder and the disorders with which it is comorbid. Simple cross-tabulation methods were used to generate these results. The more complex methods used in the chapter on comorbidity are described in that chapter.

Treatment of 12-month Disorders

As noted above in the section on measures, our condition-specific investigation of treatment in this volume focuses on treatment for problems with emotions, nerves, or substance-use problems in the 12 months before interview among respondents with each of the disorders considered here. We consider separately treatment in the mental health specialty, general medical, human services, and CAM sectors along with any type of treatment across these sectors. We present only basic information on the proportion of respondents with each 12-month disorder that received each of these types of treatment at any time in the 12 months before interview. We also examined these same associations in subsamples of respondents based on level of role impairment based on previous evidence that the treatment rate is considerably higher among people with seriously impairing mental disorders (Mojtabai *et al.* 2011). Simple cross-tabulation methods were used to generate these results. In the separate chapter on treatment across disorders (Chapter 21) we also examine socio-demographic correlates of treatment seeking.

Disorder-Specific Analyses

Some chapters contain analyses that expand on the cross-disorder analyses described above, but the rationale for and logic of those analyses are described in the chapters in which they are used. Included here are both methods for addressing more complex research questions than the basic research questions assessed in parallel across all chapters and also methods for dealing with special missing data problems. Item-level missing data were uncommon in the WMH surveys due to the fact that skip errors were minimized by the fact that we used computer-assisted interviewing for most surveys and implemented a rigorous post-interview data checking protocol in the surveys that used paper and pencil administration so that missing data could be filled in quickly in brief phone calls to respondents shortly after their interview was completed. However, in some cases there were structural problems involving a skip error in early surveys that was fixed in later surveys or the use of only a screening assessment in the main survey that was only validated later in clinical reappraisal interviews, requiring us to use regression-based imputation to estimate individual scores. In the vast majority of cases, where a variable had a very small amount of missing data, we imputed the missing values using a single regression-based imputation with an error term. The PROC MI procedure with a single imputation in SAS 9.3 (SAS Institute Inc. 2011) was used for this purpose. The method of multiple imputation (MI; Rubin 1987) was used for more complex imputations, in which case we generated 10 imputations for each missing value and used standard procedures to adjust estimates of standard errors of parameter estimates to take into consideration the fact that many (or all) values were imputed rather than observed. These methods are discussed in more detail in the chapters in which they were used.

Acknowledgements

Portions of this chapter appeared previously in: Heeringa, S. G., Wells, J. E., Hubbard, F., Mneimneh, Z. N., Chiu, W. T., Sampson, N. A., & Berglund, P. A. (2008). Sample designs and sampling procedures. In *The WHO World Mental Health Surveys: Global Perspectives on the Epidemiology of Mental Disorders*, eds. R. C. Kessler & T. B. Üstün, pp. 14–32. New York: Cambridge University Press; Kessler, R. C. & Üstün, T. B. (2008). The World Health Organization Composite International Diagnostic Interview. In *The WHO World Mental Health Surveys: Global Perspectives on the Epidemiology of Mental Disorders*, eds. R. C. Kessler & T. B. Üstün, pp. 58–90. New York: Cambridge University Press; Pennell, B. E., Mneimneh, Z., Bowers, A., Chardoul, S., Wells, J. E., Viana, M. C., Dinkelmann, K., Gebler, N.,

Florescu, S., He, Y., Huang, Y., Tomov, T., & Vilagut, G. (2008). Implementation of the World Mental Health surveys. In *The WHO World Mental Health Surveys: Global Perspectives on the Epidemiology of Mental Disorders*, eds. R. C. Kessler & T. B. Üstün, pp. 33–57. New York: Cambridge University Press; Harkness, J., Pennell, B. E., Villar, A., Gebler, N., Aguilar-Gaxiola, S., & Bilgen, I. (2008). Translation procedures and translation assessment in the World Mental Health Survey Initiative. In *The WHO World Mental Health Surveys: Global Perspectives on the Epidemiology of Mental Disorders*, eds. R. C. Kessler & T. B. Üstün, pp. 91–113. New York: Cambridge University Press; Haro, J. M., Arbabzadeh-Bouchez, S., Brugha, T. S., de Girolamo, G., Guyer, M. E., Jin, R., Lepine, J. P., Mazzi, F., Reneses, B., Vilagut Saiz, G., Sampson, N. A., & Kessler, R. C. (2008). Concordance of the Composite International Diagnostic Interview Version 3.0 (CIDI 3.0) with standardized clinical assessments in the WHO World Mental Health surveys. In *The WHO World Mental Health Surveys: Global Perspectives on the Epidemiology of Mental Disorders*, eds. R. C. Kessler & T. B. Üstün, pp. 114–30. New York: Cambridge University Press. All © 2008, World Health Organization, used with permission.

References

Andrade, L. H., Alonso, J., Mneimneh, Z., *et al.* (2014). Barriers to mental health treatment: results from the WHO World Mental Health surveys. *Psychological Medicine* 44, 1303–17.

Alonso, J., Angermeyer, M. C., Bernert, S., *et al.* (2004). Sampling and methods of the European Study of the Epidemiology of Mental Disorders (ESEMeD) project. *Acta Psychiatrica Scandinavica Supplement* 109, 8–20.

Alonso, J., Chatterji, S., & He, Y. (2013) (eds.) *The Burdens of Mental Disorders: Global Perspectives From the WHO World Mental Health Surveys*. New York: Cambridge University Press.

American Association for Public Opinion Research. (2000). Standard definitions: final dispositions of case codes and outcome rates for surveys. www.aapor.org. Accessed 17 April 2011.

Belli, R. F. (1988). Color blend retrievals: compromise memories or deliberate compromise responses? *Memory and Cognition* 16, 314–26.

(1998). The structure of autobiographical memory and the event history calendar: potential improvements in the quality of retrospective reports in surveys. *Memory* 6, 383–406.

Bertani, A., Perna, G., Migliarese, G., *et al.* (2004). Comparison of the treatment with paroxetine and reboxetine in panic disorder: a randomized, single-blind study. *Pharmacopsychiatry* 37, 206–10.

Biemer, P., & Lyberg, L. (2003). *Introduction to Survey Quality*. New York: John Wiley & Sons.

Billiet, J., & Loosveldt, G. (1988). Interviewer training and quality of responses. *Public Opinion Quarterly* 52, 190–211.

Borges, G., Angst, J., Nock, M. K., Ruscio, A. M., & Kessler, R. C. (2008). Risk factors for the incidence and persistence of suicide-related outcomes: a 10-year follow-up study using the National Comorbidity Surveys. *Journal of Affective Disorders* 105, 25–33.

Brewer, W. F. (1986). What is autobiographical memory? In D. C. Rubin, ed., *Autobiographical Memory*. New York: Cambridge University Press, pp. 25–49.

Bulmer, M. (1998). The problem of exporting social survey research. *American Behavioral Scientist* 42, 153–67.

Cannell, C. F., Fowler, F. J., & Marquis, K. H. (1968). The influence of interviewer and respondent psychological and behavioral variables on the reporting in household interviews. *Vital and Health Statistics* 2, 1–65.

Cannell, C. F., Miller, P. V., & Oksenberg, L. (1981). Research on interviewing techniques. In S. Leinhardt, ed., *Sociological Methodology*. San Francisco, CA: Jossey-Bass Publishers, pp. 389–487.

Centers, R. (1963). A laboratory adaptation of the conversational procedure for the conditioning of verbal operants. *Journal of Abnormal Psychology* 67, 334–9.

Charlson, F. J., Baxter, A. J., Dua, T., *et al.* (2016). Excess mortality from mental, neurological, and substance use disorders in the Global Burden of Disease Study 2010. In V. Patel, D. Chisholm, T. Dua, R. Laxminarayan, & M. E. Medina-Mora, eds., *Mental, Neurological, and Substance Use Disorders: Disease Control Priorities, Third Edition (Volume 4)*. Washington, DC: The World Bank Publications, pp. 41–66.

Cheng, A. T. (2001). Case definition and culture: are people all the same? *British Journal of Psychiatry* 179, 1–3.

Clark, H. H., & Schober, M. F. (1992). Asking questions and influencing answers. In J. M. Tanur, ed., *Questions about Questions: Inquiries into the Cognitive Bases of Surveys*. New York: Russell Sage Foundation, pp. 15–48.

Cochran, W. G. (1977). *Sampling Techniques*. New York: John Wiley & Sons.

Converse, J., & Presser, S. (1986). *Survey Questions: Handcrafting the Standardized Questionnaire*, Sage Series No. 63. Thousand Oaks, CA: Sage Publications.

Connor, K. M., & Davidson, J. R. T. (2001). SPRINT: a brief global assessment of post-traumatic stress disorder. *International Clinical Psychopharmacology* 16, 279–84.

Couper, M. P., & de Leeuw, E. D. (2003). Nonresponse in cross-cultural and cross-national surveys. In J. A. Harkness, F. J. R. Van de Vijver, & P. P. Mohler, eds., *Cross-Cultural Survey Methods*. Hoboken, NJ: John Wiley & Sons, pp. 155–77.

Davidson, J. R., Bose, A., Korotzer, A., & Zheng, H. (2004). Escitalopram in the treatment of generalized anxiety disorder: double-blind, placebo controlled, flexible-dose study. *Depression and Anxiety* 19, 234–40.

Duckers, M. L., Alisic, E., & Brewin, C. R. (2016). A vulnerability paradox in the cross-national prevalence of post-traumatic stress disorder. *British Journal of Psychiatry* 209, 300–5.

Efron, B. (1988). Logistic regression, survival analysis, and the Kaplan-Meier curve. *Journal of the American Statistical Association* 83, 414–25.

Fowler, F., & Mangione, T. (1990). *Standardized Survey Interviewing: Minimizing Interviewer-Related Error.* Newbury Park, CA: Sage Publications, Inc.

Frank, E. ed. (2002). *Gender and Its Effects on Psychopathology*. Washington, DC: American Psychiatric Association.

Gilman, S. (1988). *Disease and Depresentation: Images of Illness from Madness to AIDS.* Ithaca, NY: Cornell University Press.

Giuffra, L. A., & Risch, N. (1994). Diminished recall and the cohort effect of major depression: a simulation study. *Psychological Medicine* 24, 375–83.

Groves, R. M., Fowler, F. J., Couper, M. P., *et al.* (2004). *Survey Methodology.* Hoboken, NJ: John Wiley & Sons.

Halli, S. S., Rao, K. V., & Halli, S. S. (1992). *Advanced Techniques of Population Analysis.* New York: Plenum.

Hambrick, J. P., Turk, C. L., Heimberg, R. G., Schneier, F. R., & Liebowitz, M.R. (2004). Psychometric properties of disability measures among patients with social anxiety disorder. *Journal of Anxiety Disorders* 18, 825–39.

Harkness, J. A., Pennell, B. E., & Schoua-Glusberg, A. (2004). Survey questionnaire translation and assessment. In S. Presser, J. Rothgeb, M. P. Couper, *et al.*, eds., *Methods for Testing and Evaluating Survey Questionnaires.* Hoboken, NJ: John Wiley & Sons, pp. 453–74.

Harkness, J., Pennell, B. E., Villar, A., *et al.* (2008). Translation procedures and translation assessment in the World Mental Health Survey Initiative. In R. C. Kessler, & T. B. Üstün, eds., *The WHO World Mental Health Surveys: Global Perspectives on the Epidemiology of Mental Disorders.* New York: Cambridge University Press, pp. 91–113.

Harkness, J. A., Van de Vijver, J. R., & Mohler, P. P. (2002). *Cross-Cultural Survey Methods.* New York: John Wiley & Sons.

Haro, J. M., Arbabzadeh-Bouchez, S., Brugha, T. S., *et al.* (2006). Concordance of the Composite International Diagnostic Interview Version 3.0 (CIDI 3.0) with standardized clinical assessments in the WHO World Mental Health Surveys. *International Journal of Methods in Psychiatric Research* 15, 167–80.

Heath, A., Fisher, S., & Smith, S. (2005). The globalization of public opinion research. *Annual Review of Political Science* 8, 297–333.

Horberg, N., Kouros, I., Ekselius, L., & Ramklint, M. (2016). The Swedish version of the Sheehan Disability Scale-a valid and brief measure of functioning. *European Journal for Person Centered Healthcare* 4, 208–14.

Hudson, J. I., Perahia, D. G., Gilaberte, I., *et al.* (2007). Duloxetine in the treatment of major depressive disorder: an open-label study. *BMC Psychiatry* 7, 43.

Jobe, J. B., White, A. A., Kelley, C. L., *et al.* (1990). Recall strategies and memory for health-care visits. *Milbank Quarterly* 68, 171–89.

Jowell, R. (1998). How comparative is comparative research? *American Behavioral Scientist* 42, 168–77.

Kessler, R. C. (1999). The World Health Organization International Consortium in Psychiatric Epidemiology (ICPE): initial work and future directions – the NAPE Lecture 1998. Nordic Association for Psychiatric Epidemiology. *Acta Psychiatrica Scandinavica* 99, 2–9.

Kessler, R. C., Aguilar-Gaxiola, S., Alonso, J., *et al.* (2008). Lifetime prevalence and age of onset distributions of mental disorders in the World Mental Health Survey Initiative. In R. C. Kessler & T. B. Üstün, eds., *The WHO World Mental Health Surveys: Global Perspectives on the Epidemiology of Mental Disorders.* New York: Cambridge University Press, pp. 511–21.

Kessler, R. C., Amminger, G. P., Aguilar-Gaxiola, S., *et al.* (2007a). Age of onset of mental disorders: a review of recent literature. *Current Opinion in Psychiatry* 20, 359–64.

Kessler, R. C., Angermeyer, M., Anthony, J. C., *et al.* (2007b). Lifetime prevalence and age-of-onset distributions of mental disorders in the World Health Organization's World Mental Health Survey Initiative. *World Psychiatry* 6, 168–76.

Kessler, R. C., Berglund, P., Chiu, W. T., *et al.* (2004). The US National Comorbidity Survey Replication (NCS-R): design and field procedures. *International Journal of Methods in Psychiatric Research* 13, 69–92.

Kessler, R. C., Mroczek, D. K., & Belli, R. F. (1999). Retrospective adult assessment of childhood psychopathology. In D. Shaffer, C. P. Lucas, & J. E. Richters, eds., *Diagnostic Assessment in Child and Adolescent Psychopathology.* New York: Guilford Press, pp. 256–84.

Kessler, R. C., Ormel, J., Petukhova, M., *et al.* (2011). Development of lifetime comorbidity in the World Health Organization World Mental Health Surveys. *Archives of General Psychiatry* 68, 90–100.

Kessler, R. C., & Üstün, T. B. (2004). The World Mental Health (WMH) Survey Initiative version of the World Health Organization (WHO) Composite International Diagnostic Interview (CIDI). *International Journal of Methods in Psychiatric Research* 13, 93–121.

Kessler, R. C., & Üstün, T. B. (2008). The World Health Organization Composite International Diagnostic Interview. In R. C. Kessler & T. B. Üstün, eds., *The WHO World Mental Health Surveys: Global Perspectives on the Epidemiology of Mental Disorders*. New York: Cambridge University Press, pp. 58–90.

Kessler, R. C., Wittchen, H. U., Abelson, J. M., *et al.* (1998). Methodological studies of the Composite International Diagnostic Interview (CIDI) in the US National Comorbidity Survey. *International Journal of Methods in Psychiatric Research* 7, 33–55.

Kessler, R. C., Wittchen, H. U., Abelson, J. M., & Zhao, S. (2000). Methodological issues in assessing psychiatric disorder with self-reports. In A. A. Stone, J. S. Turrkan, C. A. Bachrach, *et al.*, eds., *The Science of Self-Report: Implications for Research and Practice*. Mahwah, NJ: Lawrence Erlbaum Associates, pp. 229–55.

Kish, L. (1949). A procedure for objective respondent selection within the household. *Journal of the American Statistical Association* 44, 380–7.

(1965). *Survey Sampling*. New York: John Wiley & Sons.

Knäuper, B., Cannell, C. F., Schwarz, N., Bruce, M. L., & Kessler, R. C. (1999). Improving accuracy of major depression age-of-onset reports in the US National Comorbidity Survey. *International Journal of Methods in Psychiatric Research* 8, 39–48.

Kuechler, M. (1998). The survey method: an indispensable tool for social science research everywhere? *American Behavioral Scientist* 42, 178–200.

Lavrakas, P. J. (1993). *Telephone Survey Methods: Sampling, Selection, and Supervision*. Thousand Oaks, CA: Sage Publications.

Lee, E. T., & Go, O. T. (1997). Survival analysis in public health research. *Annual Review of Public Health* 18, 105–34.

Leon, A. C., Olfson, M., Portera, L., Farber, L., & Sheehan, D. V. (1997). Assessing psychiatric impairment in primary care with the Sheehan Disability Scale. *The International Journal of Psychiatry in Medicine* 27, 93–105.

Leu, S. H., Chou, J. Y., Lee, P. C., *et al.* (2015). Validity and reliability of the Chinese version of the Sheehan Disability Scale (SDS-C). *Asia-Pacific Psychiatry* 7, 215–22.

Leventhal, H., Nerenz, D., & Steele, D. J. (1984). Illness representations and coping with health threats. In A. Baum, S. E. Taylor, & J. E. Singer, eds., *Handbook of Psychology and Health*. Hillsdale, NJ: Erlbaum Associates, pp. 219–52.

Little, R. J. A., & Rubin, D. B. (2002). *Statistical Analysis with Missing Data, Second Edition*. New York: John Wiley & Sons.

Lynn, P. (2001). Developing quality standards for cross-national survey research: five approaches. *International Journal of Social Research Methodology* 6, 323–36.

Markus, H., & Zajonc, R. B. (1985). The cognitive perspective in social psychology. In G. Lindzey & E. Aronson, eds., *The Handbook of Social Psychology*. New York: Random House, pp. 137–230.

Marquis, K. H., & Cannell, C. F. (1969). *A Study of Interviewer–Respondent Interaction in the Urban Employment*. Ann Arbor, MI: Survey Research Center, University of Michigan.

McLaughlin, K. A., Green, J., Gruber, M. J., *et al.* (2010). Childhood adversities and adult psychiatric disorders in the National Comorbidity Survey Replication II: associations with persistence of DSM-IV disorders. *Archives of General Psychiatry* 67, 124–32.

Means, B., & Loftus, E. F. (1991). When personal history repeats itself: decomposing memories for recurring events. *Applied Cognitive Psychology* 5, 297–318.

Menon, A. (1994). Judgements of behavioral frequencies: Memory search and retrieval strategies. In N. Schwartz & S. Sudman, eds., *Autobiographical Memory and the Validity of Retrospective Reports*. New York: Springer-Verlag, pp. 161–72.

Miller, P. V., & Cannell, C. F. (1977). Communicating measurement objectives in the survey interview. In D. M. Hirsch, P. V. Miller, & F. G. Kline, eds., *Strategies for Communication Research*. Beverly Hills, CA: Sage Publications, pp. 127–51.

Moffitt, T. E., Caspi, A., Taylor, A., *et al.* (2010). How common are common mental disorders? Evidence that lifetime prevalence rates are doubled by prospective versus retrospective ascertainment. *Psychological Medicine* 40, 899–909.

Mojtabai, R., Olfson, M., Sampson, N. A., *et al.* (2011). Barriers to mental health treatment: results from the National Comorbidity Survey replication. *Psychological Medicine* 41, 1751–61.

Murray, C. J. L., & Lopez, A. D. (2013). Measuring the global burden of disease. *New England Journal of Medicine* 369, 448–57.

Oksenberg, L., Vinokur, A., & Cannell, C. F. (1979). The effects of instructions, commitment and feedback on reporting in personal interviews. In C. F. Cannell, L. Oksenberg, & J. M. Converse, eds., *Experiments in Interviewing Techniques. DHEW Publication No. (HRA) 78-3204*. Washington, DC: Department of Health, Education, and Welfare, pp. 133–99.

Ormel, J., Petukhova, M., Chatterji, S., *et al.* (2008). Disability and treatment of specific mental and physical disorders across the world. *British Journal of Psychiatry* 192, 368–75.

Ormel, J., Petukhova, M. V., Chatterji, S., *et al.* (2013). Disorder-specific disability and treatment of common mental and physical disorders. In J. Alonso, S. Chatterji, & Y. He, eds., *The Burdens of Mental Disorders: Global Perspectives from the WHO World Mental Health Surveys*. New York: Cambridge University Press, pp. 171–85.

Pallanti, S., Bernardi, S., & Quercioli, L. (2006). The shorter PROMIS questionnaire and the internet addiction scale in the assessment of multiple addictions in a

high-school population: prevalence and related disability. *CNS Spectrums* 11, 966–74.
Patten, S. B. (2003). Recall bias and major depression lifetime prevalence. *Social Psychiatry and Psychiatric Epidemiology* 38, 290–6.
Pearson, R. W., Ross, M., & Dawes, R. M. (1992). Personal recall and the limits of retrospective questions in surveys. In J. M. Tanur, ed., *Questions about Questions: Inquiries into the Cognitive Bases of Surveys*. New York: Russell Sage Foundation, pp. 65–94.
Pennell, B. E., Mneimneh, Z., Bowers, A., *et al.* (2008). Implementation of the World Mental Health Surveys. In R. C. Kessler & T. B. Üstün, eds., *The WHO World Mental Health Surveys: Global Perspectives on the Epidemiology of Mental Disorders*. New York: Cambridge University Press, pp. 33–57.
Prince, R., & Tcheng-Laroche, F. (1987). Culture-bound syndromes and international disease classifications. *Cultural Medical Psychiatry* 11, 3–52.
Prohaska, V., Brown, N. R., & Belli, R. F. (1998). Forward telescoping: the question matters. *Memory* 6, 455–65.
Research Triangle Institute (2002). *SUDAAN: Professional Software for Survey Data Analysis, Version 8.0.1.* Research Triangle Park, NC: Research Triangle Institute.
Rosenbaum, P. R., & Rubin, D. B. (1983). The central role of the propensity score in observational studies for causal effects. *Biometrika* 70, 41–55.
Rubin, D.B. (1987). *Multiple Imputation for Nonresponse in Surveys*. New York: Wiley.
Rust, K. (1985). Variance estimation for complex estimators in sample surveys. *Journal of Official Statistics* 1, 381–97.
SAS Institute Inc. (2011). *SAS/STAT® Software, Version 9.3 for Windows*. Cary, NC: SAS Institute Inc.
Schlesselman, J. J. (1982). *Case–Control Studies: Design, Conduct, Analysis*. New York: Oxford University Press.
Schober, M. F., Conrad, F. G., & Fricker, S. S. (2004). Misunderstanding standardized language in research interviews. *Applied Cognitive Psychology* 18, 169–88.
Schwarz, N., & Sudman, S., eds. (1994). *Autobiographical Memory and the Validity of Retrospective Reports*. New York: Springer-Verlag.
eds. (1996). *Answering Questions: Methodology for Determining Cognitive and Communicative Processes in Survey Research*. San Francisco, CA: Jossey-Bass Publishers.
Seedat, S., Scott, K., Angermeyer, M. C., *et al.* (2009). Cross-national associations between gender and mental disorders in the World Health Organization World Mental Health Surveys. *Archives of General Psychiatry*, 66, 785–95.
Sheatsley, P. B. (1983). Questionnaire construction and item writing. In P. H. Rossi, J. D. Wright, & A. B. Anderson, eds., *Handbook of Survey Research: Quantitative Studies in Social Relations*. New York: Academy Press, pp. 195–230.
Sheehan, D. V., Harnett-Sheehan, K., & Raj, B. A. (1996). The measurement of disability. *International Clinical Psychopharmacology* 11 (Suppl 3), 89–95.
Simon, G. E., & VonKorff, M. (1995). Recall of psychiatric history in cross-sectional surveys: implications for epidemiologic research. *Epidemiologic Reviews* 17, 221–7.
Sirken, M. G., Herrmann, D. J., Schechter, S., *et al.*, eds. (1999). *Cognition and Survey Research*. New York: John Wiley & Sons.
Skelton, J. A., & Croyle, R. T. (1991). *Mental Representation in Health and Illness*. New York: Springer-Verlag.
Smith, T. W. (2004). Developing and evaluating cross-national survey instruments. In S. Presser, J. M. Rothgeb, M. P. Couper, *et al.*, eds., *Methods for Testing and Evaluating Survey Questionnaires*. New York: John Wiley & Sons, pp. 431–52.
Solow, R. (1967). *Inequality and Poverty*. New York: W.W. Norton and Company.
Sudman, S., Bradburn, N., & Schwarz, N. (1996). *Thinking about Answers: The Application of Cognitive Processes to Survey Methodology*. San Francisco, CA: Jossey-Bass Publishers.
Tanur, J. M. (1992). *Questions about Questions: Inquiries into the Cognitive Bases of Surveys*. New York: Russell Sage Foundation.
Taylor, M. P. (2003). Purchasing power parity. *Review of International Economics* 11, 436–52.
Thornicroft, G., Chatterji, S., Evans-Lacko, S., *et al.* (2017). Under-treatment of people with major depressive disorder in 21 countries. *British Journal of Psychiatry* 210, 119–24.
Tourangeau, R., & Yan, T. (2007). Sensitive questions in surveys. *Psychological Bulletin* 133, 859–83.
Turner, C., & Martin, E. (1985). *Surveying Subjective Phenomena*. New York: Russell Sage Foundation.
Verma, V., Scott, C., & O'Muircheartaigh, C. (1980). Sample designs and sampling errors for the World Fertility Survey. *Journal of the Royal Statistical Society* 143, 431–73.
Vinokur, A., Oksenberg, L., & Cannell, C. F. (1979). Effects of feedback and reinforcement on the report of health information. In C. F. Cannell, L. Oksenberg, & J. M. Converse, eds., *Experiments in Interviewing Techniques*. Ann Arbor, MI: Survey Research Center, University of Michigan.
Wang, P. S., Aguilar-Gaxiola, S., Alonso, J., *et al.* (2007a). Use of mental health services for anxiety, mood, and substance disorders in 17 countries in the WHO World Mental Health Surveys. *Lancet* 370, 841–50.
Wang, P. S., Angermeyer, M., Borges, G., *et al.* (2007b). Delay and failure in treatment seeking after first onset of mental disorders in the World Health Organization's World Mental Health Survey Initiative. *World Psychiatry* 6, 177–85.
Wardenaar, K. J., van Loo, H. M., Cai, T., *et al.* (2014). The effects of co-morbidity in defining major depression

subtypes associated with long-term course and severity. *Psychological Medicine* 44, 3289–302.

Wells, J. E., Browne, M. O., Aguilar-Gaxiola, S., *et al.* (2013). Drop out from out-patient mental healthcare in the World Health Organization's World Mental Health Survey Initiative. *The British Journal of Psychiatry* 202, 42–9.

Whiteford, H. A., Degenhardt, L., Rehm, J., *et al.* (2013). Global burden of disease attributable to mental and substance use disorders: findings from the Global Burden of Disease Study 2010. *Lancet* 382, 1575–86.

Williams, B. J. (1986). Suggestions for the application of advanced technology in Canadian collection operations. *Journal of Official Statistics* 2, 555–60.

Wolter, K. M. (1985). *Introduction to Variance Estimation.* New York: Springer.

World Bank (2012). Data and Statistics. http://data.worldbank.org/country. Accessed 12 May 2012.

Chapter 4

Major Depressive Disorder

Evelyn J. Bromet, Laura Helena Andrade, Ronny Bruffaerts, David R. Williams

Introduction

Major depression is a serious, recurrent disorder linked to diminished role functioning, medical morbidity, and mortality (Üstün *et al.* 2004). The magnitude and consequences of depression are underscored by a recent Global Burden of Disease (GBD) report that ranks depression as the second leading cause of 'years lived with disability', or YLDs, in the world (GBD Collaborators, Vos *et al.* 2015).

Prior to the National Comorbidity Survey (NCS) in the United States (Kessler *et al.* 1994), direct information on the prevalence of clinical depression based on structured diagnostic assessments came from a small, non-representative number of geographic areas. The first community surveys administered the Diagnostic Interview Schedule for DSM-III (Robins *et al.* 1981) in specific catchment areas and cities in the United States, Canada, Puerto Rico, France, West Germany, Italy, Lebanon, Taiwan, Korea, and New Zealand. The lifetime prevalence of major depressive disorder (MDD) ranged from 1.5% (Taiwan) to 19.0% (Lebanon), with midpoints of 9.2% (West Germany) and 9.6% (Canada) (Weissman *et al.* 1996). The 12-month prevalence ranged from 0.8% (Taiwan) to 5.8% (New Zealand), with midpoints of 3.0% (United States) and 4.5% (France). In the 1990s, the Composite International Diagnostic Interview (CIDI) for DSM-III-R and DSM-IV (Kessler *et al.* 1998) was administered in both national and regional surveys in the United States, Canada, Brazil, Chile, Mexico, the Czech Republic, Germany, the Netherlands, Turkey, and Japan. The prevalence rates were broadly consistent with rates reported for the prior surveys (Andrade *et al.* 2003). That is, lifetime rates ranged from 1.0% (Czech Republic) to 16.9% (United States), with midpoints of 8.3% (Canada) and 9.0% (Chile); and 12-month rates ranged from 0.3% (Czech Republic) to 10% (United States), with midpoints of 4.5% (Mexico) and 5.2% (West Germany).

This body of research broke new ground by focusing on clinical depression (MDD) rather than depressive symptom severity, but the surveys were not designed as replications. Thus, they did not use standardised protocols for sample selection, instrument translation, interviewer training, quality control, or risk factor measurement. Indeed, the variability in the prevalence estimates was difficult to interpret because of these substantial differences in methodology. As noted in Chapter 3, the WHO World Mental Health (WMH) Surveys Initiative was established as an attempt to control these methodological factors in order to better assess the cross-national prevalence of disorders along with their risk factors. We previously reported that in 18 WMH countries, the lifetime prevalence of DSM-IV major depressive episodes (i.e., all depressive episodes independent of DSM diagnostic hierarchy rules) ranged from 6.5% (Japan) to 19.2% (United States), with a midpoint across all countries of 13% (Bromet *et al.* 2011). The 12-month prevalence ranged from 2.2% (Japan) to 10.4% (São Paulo, Brazil) with a midpoint of 5%, similar to that found in previous surveys. In this chapter, we report the rates of MDD (depressive episodes that are not part of other disorders, such as bipolar disorder) in a larger number of sites.

In almost every previous survey, gender and marital status were significantly associated with the prevalence of depression. Women had an approximately two fold increased risk compared to men, and previously married respondents had a significantly higher rate than currently married respondents. The relationship of age to depression varied by country income level. In higher-income countries, depression declined with age, while in poor countries, depression increased with age. Other socio-economic factors, e.g., education and income, had less consistent relationships with depression in the different countries. Moreover, comorbidity was the rule rather than the exception (Richards 2011; Kessler & Bromet 2013). Another disturbing finding across these surveys was that only a small percentage reported receiving care during their depressive episodes. Those who sought help often received services from the general medical sector (Regier *et al.* 1993). Few studies, however, examined the degree to which seeking care from different types of providers was linked to the level of impairment of the depressive episodes.

This chapter provides descriptive data on the epidemiology of MDD in 29 WMH surveys. Country-specific findings are presented on the prevalence, persistence, and age-of-onset (AOO) of MDD. Comorbidity, impairment, use of services, and sociodemographic correlates are also presented for the entire sample and for countries grouped into World Bank income-level strata.

Method

MDD was assessed in all 29 of the WMH surveys included in this volume (see Chapter 3 and Table 4.1 for listing). The Sheehan impairment data were not collected for The European Study of the Epidemiology of Mental Disorders (ESEMED) countries, so these six European countries are excluded from Table 4.3.

DSM-IV MDD requires the presence of five of the nine cardinal symptoms of depression listed in the DSM. The nine symptoms are: depressed mood and markedly diminished interest or pleasure (one of these must be present to meet diagnostic criteria for MDD), clinically significant weight gain/loss or appetite disturbance, insomnia or hypersomnia, psychomotor agitation or retardation, fatigue or loss of energy, feelings of worthlessness or excessive guilt, diminished ability to concentrate or think clearly, and recurrent thoughts of death or suicide. To meet DSM-IV criteria for MDD, symptoms must persist for two weeks or longer, be present for most of the day nearly every day and cause significant distress or impairment. In addition, episodes must occur outside the context of other conditions, such as bipolar disorder. Clinical reappraisal studies conducted in several countries found good agreement between CIDI-MDD and clinician diagnoses from blinded reappraisal interviews (Haro *et al.* 2006). Previous research also found that the latent structure of the symptoms of depression was consistent across countries (Simon *et al.* 2002).

Results

Prevalence and Persistence

The average lifetime prevalence of MDD in the 29 countries combined is 10.6% (Table 4.1). The average rate is highest in the high-income countries (12.6%; range 6.1% [Japan] to 21.0% [France]), intermediate in the upper-middle-income countries (9.2%; range 2.9% [Romania] to 16.9% [São Paulo, Brazil]), and lowest in the poorest countries (7.1%; range 3.1% [Nigeria] to 14.6% [Ukraine]). We also show the country-specific lifetime rates for men and women separately (Appendix Tables 4A.1 and 4A.2). The average lifetime rate is 13.5% for women and 7.5% for men. Among women, the average rate is highest in the high-income countries (16.0%; range 4.0% [Poland] to 26.6% [France]), intermediate in the upper-middle-income countries (12.2%; 3.3% [Romania] to 23.0% [São Paulo, Brazil]), and lowest in the poorest countries (8.8%; 3.2% [Shenzhen, PRC] to 19.5% [Ukraine]). Among men, the average rate is also highest in the high-income countries (9.0%; range 1.9% [Poland] to 14.8% [France]), but similar in the upper-middle (5.9%; 2.5% [Romania] to 10.0% [São Paulo]) and poor countries (5.4%; 2.8% [Nigeria] to 8.6% [Ukraine]). It is also interesting to note that in six high-income countries (the United States, the Netherlands, Portugal, Northern Ireland, New Zealand, and France), more than one in five women has a lifetime history of MDD. In eight high-income countries (the same six plus Belgium and Australia), more than one in ten men has a lifetime history of MDD.

The average 12-month rate (4.5%) is approximately half that of the lifetime rate. However, although the differences are statistically significant, the overall rates among high, middle, and poorer-income countries, 4.8%, 4.6%, and 3.6%, respectively, are less discrepant than the lifetime rates. None of the country-specific rates exceeds 10%. Among women (Appendix Table 4A.1), however, while the average 12-month rate is 5.8%, the country-specific rates exceed 10% in Northern Ireland, São Paulo, and Ukraine. Exceptionally low female rates (<2%) are found in Nigeria, Beijing/Shanghai, Romania, and Poland. Among men (Appendix Table 4A.2), the average 12-month rate is 3.0%. Relatively higher rates of MDD (~5%) are found in Ukraine, São Paulo, Northern Ireland, and the US, while exceptionally low male rates (<1.5%) are found in Nigeria, Bulgaria, Romania, Japan, and Poland.

While current burden (30-day prevalence) of MDD is low in all countries combined (1.7% on average), both the lowest (0.2%, Nigeria) and the highest (4.8%, Ukraine) current rates of MDD are found in low/lower-middle-income countries. The average rate for women is 2.3%, and consistent with the overall rate, both the lowest and highest rates are found in Nigeria (0.1%)

Table 4.1 Prevalence of DSM-IV major depressive disorder (MDD) in the World Mental Health surveys

Country	Lifetime prevalence		12-month prevalence		30-day prevalence		12-month prevalence of MDD among lifetime cases		30-day prevalence of MDD among 12-month cases		Sample size used
	%	SE	%	SE	%	SE	%	SE	%	SE	
Low/lower-middle-income countries	**7.1**	**0.2**	**3.6**	**0.1**	**1.5**	**0.1**	**50.7**	**1.2**	**40.5**	**1.8**	**36,498**
Colombia	12.0	0.7	5.3	0.4	1.6	0.2	44.7	2.7	30.2	4.0	4,426
Iraq	7.2	0.6	3.9	0.4	1.5	0.3	54.0	4.3	38.1	5.3	4,332
Nigeria	3.1	0.3	1.1	0.1	0.2	0.1	34.3	3.9	18.6	5.3	6,752
Peru	6.4	0.4	2.7	0.2	0.7	0.1	42.0	3.0	25.9	4.8	3,930
PRC (Beijing/Shanghai)	3.5	0.4	1.8	0.3	0.6	0.1	51.5	5.2	32.3	6.8	5,201
PRC (Shenzhen)	6.1	0.4	3.5	0.3	1.4	0.2	56.9	2.5	41.3	4.2	7,132
Ukraine	14.6	0.7	8.4	0.6	4.8	0.4	57.8	2.2	57.0	2.8	4,725
Upper-middle-income countries	**9.2**	**0.3**	**4.6**	**0.2**	**2.0**	**0.1**	**49.5**	**1.1**	**43.0**	**1.5**	**28,927**
Brazil	16.9	0.9	9.4	0.6	4.2	0.3	56.0	1.7	44.8	2.4	5,037
Bulgaria	5.6	0.4	2.5	0.3	1.5	0.2	44.7	3.8	59.8	3.4	5,318
Colombia (Medellin)	9.9	0.8	3.8	0.4	1.4	0.3	37.9	2.9	36.9	5.1	3,261
Lebanon	9.9	0.9	4.8	0.6	2.0	0.3	48.5	3.1	41.1	4.9	2,857
Mexico	7.3	0.5	3.6	0.3	1.6	0.2	49.2	2.8	44.9	3.7	5,782
Romania	2.9	0.4	1.5	0.3	0.4	0.2	49.8	5.9	29.2	8.2	2,357
South Africa	9.8	0.7	4.9	0.4	1.6	0.3	50.0	2.7	33.3	4.8	4,315
High-income countries	**12.6**	**0.2**	**4.8**	**0.1**	**1.7**	**0.1**	**38.0**	**0.6**	**35.4**	**0.9**	**81,839**
Australia	13.5	0.5	5.0	0.3	2.0	0.2	36.8	1.9	40.9	2.8	8,463
Belgium	14.1	1.0	5.0	0.5	1.9	0.4	35.2	2.8	39.0	6.9	2,419
France	21.0	1.1	5.9	0.6	1.5	0.4	27.9	2.6	26.1	5.4	2,894
Germany	9.9	0.6	3.0	0.3	1.0	0.2	30.1	2.1	34.4	4.8	3,555
Israel	9.8	0.5	5.9	0.4	1.7	0.2	59.7	2.3	28.8	2.9	4,859
Italy	9.9	0.5	3.0	0.2	1.4	0.2	30.2	1.9	45.4	5.4	4,712
Japan	6.1	0.4	2.2	0.3	0.3	0.1	35.2	3.4	14.9	3.9	4,129
New Zealand	16.3	0.4	5.8	0.3	1.7	0.1	35.2	1.6	29.1	1.9	12,790
Northern Ireland	16.3	0.8	7.9	0.5	3.2	0.3	48.2	2.0	40.9	2.9	4,340
Poland	3.0	0.2	1.3	0.1	0.4	0.1	41.9	2.3	33.1	4.5	10,081
Portugal	16.7	0.7	6.8	0.5	2.8	0.3	40.5	2.1	41.1	3.1	3,849
Spain	10.6	0.5	4.0	0.3	1.7	0.2	37.5	1.9	42.9	4.5	5,473
Spain (Murcia)	13.8	0.8	6.0	0.4	2.6	0.4	43.4	2.0	43.6	3.7	2,621
Netherlands	17.9	1.0	4.9	0.5	1.4	0.4	27.3	2.6	28.6	6.9	2,372
United States	16.9	0.5	6.8	0.3	2.5	0.2	40.5	1.3	36.6	1.7	9,282
All countries combined	**10.6**	**0.1**	**4.5**	**0.1**	**1.7**	**0.0**	**42.1**	**0.5**	**38.0**	**0.7**	**147,264**

(cont.)

Table 4.1 (*cont.*)

Country	Lifetime prevalence		12-month prevalence		30-day prevalence		12-month prevalence of MDD among lifetime cases		30-day prevalence of MDD among 12-month cases		Sample size used
	%	SE	%	SE	%	SE	%	SE	%	SE	
WHO regions[a]											
Region of the Americas	12.4	0.3	5.6	0.2	2.2	0.1	45.2	0.9	38.3	1.2	31,718
African region	5.7	0.3	2.6	0.2	0.8	0.1	44.8	2.3	29.5	4.0	11,067
Western Pacific region	10.9	0.2	4.2	0.1	1.4	0.1	38.7	1.1	33.5	1.5	37,715
Eastern Mediterranean region	8.9	0.3	4.9	0.3	1.7	0.1	55.1	1.8	34.3	2.3	12,048
Western European region	13.9	0.2	5.1	0.1	2.0	0.1	36.3	0.8	38.9	1.5	32,235
Eastern European region	6.0	0.2	3.1	0.1	1.6	0.1	51.0	1.6	51.8	2.0	22,481
Comparison between countries[b]	$F_{28,v} = 97.1^*$, $P < 0.001$		$F_{28,v} = 49.7^*$, $P < 0.001$		$F_{28,v} = 30.7^*$, $P < 0.001$		$F_{28,v} = 13.4^*$, $P < 0.001$		$F_{28,v} = 5.7^*$, $P < 0.001$		
Comparison between low-, middle-, and high-income country groups[b]	$F_{2,v} = 259.6^*$, $P < 0.001$		$F_{2,v} = 27.0^*$, $P < 0.001$		$F_{2,v} = 8.0^*$, $P < 0.001$		$F_{2,v} = 72.3^*$, $P < 0.001$		$F_{2,v} = 10.7^*$, $P < 0.001$		
Comparison between WHO regions[b]	$F_{5,v} = 177.6^*$, $P < 0.001$		$F_{5,v} = 48.9^*$, $P < 0.001$		$F_{5,v} = 21.0^*$, $P < 0.001$		$F_{5,v} = 31.1^*$, $P < 0.001$		$F_{5,v} = 10.9^*$, $P < 0.001$		

*Significant at the 0.05 level, two-sided test.

[a]**Region of the Americas** (Colombia, Mexico, Brazil, Peru, United States, Colombia (Medellin)); **African region** (South Africa, Nigeria); **Western Pacific region** (PRC (Shenzhen), PRC (Beijing and Shanghai), Japan, Australia, New Zealand); **Eastern Mediterranean region** (Israel, Iraq, Lebanon); **Western European region** (Belgium, France, Germany, Italy, Netherlands, Spain, Northern Ireland, Portugal, Spain (Murcia)); **Eastern European region** (Romania, Poland, Bulgaria, Ukraine).

[b]Wald design-corrected F-tests were used to determine if there is variation in prevalence estimates across countries. The denominator degree of freedom, v, is 5429.

PRC: People's Republic of China

Table 4.2 Comorbidity of major depressive disorder (MDD) with other DSM-IV disorders, all countries combined

	MDD cases with comorbid disorders							
	Anxiety disorder[a]		Disruptive behaviour/impulse-control disorder[b]		Substance-use disorder[c]		Any mental disorder[d]	
	%	SE	%	SE	%	SE	%	SE
Lifetime comorbidity[e]								
Lifetime	**48.6**	0.6	**12.3**	0.4	**17.2**	0.5	**57.9**	0.5
12-month	**54.6**	0.9	**15.0**	0.6	**18.0**	0.7	**63.3**	0.9
12-month comorbidity[f]								
12-month	**45.0**	0.8	**8.7**	0.5	**6.8**	0.5	**50.5**	0.9
Temporal priority of MDD[g]								
Lifetime	**15.7**	0.6	**19.5**	1.3	**38.5**	1.4	**15.8**	0.5
12-month	**18.1**	0.8	**21.7**	1.8	**42.7**	2.1	**17.4**	0.8

[a]Respondents with panic disorder, generalized anxiety disorder, social phobia, specific phobia, agoraphobia, post-traumatic stress disorder or separation anxiety disorder.
[b]Respondents with intermittent explosive disorder, conduct disorder, attention-deficit disorder, oppositional defiant disorder, binge-eating disorder or bulimia nervosa.
[c]Respondents with alcohol abuse with or without dependence or drug abuse with or without dependence.
[d]Respondents with any disorder listed above.
[e]Percentage of respondents with either lifetime or 12-month MDD who also meet lifetime criteria for at least one of the other DSM-IV disorders.
[f]Percentage of respondents with 12-month MDD who also meet 12-month criteria for at least one of the other disorders.
[g]Percentage of respondents with either lifetime or 12-month MDD and at least one of the other disorders, whose age-of-onset of MDD is reported to be younger than the age-of-onset of all comorbid disorders under consideration.

and Ukraine (6.6%). Among men, the average across all countries combined is 1.0%. The highest current rate is found in Ukraine (2.6%), and the lowest is found in Poland (0.1%), a World Bank high-income country (Appendix Tables 4A.1 and 4A.2).

Column 4 of Table 4.1 shows the indirect indicator of persistence of MDD (12-month prevalence among lifetime cases). At 42.1% for all countries combined, this value indicates that MDD is one of the less persistent disorders relative to other disorders featured in this volume, confirming its episodic nature. It is also interesting to note that the pattern for country income levels is reversed, with the highest rates of persistence occurring in the poorest (50.7%) and upper-middle (49.5%) income countries and the lowest (38.5%) found in high-income countries. Seven sites have persistence rates ≥50%: Israel, South Africa, São Paulo, Ukraine, PRC Shenzhen, PRC Beijing/Shanghai, and Iraq. Similar country income patterns are found for women and men. Among both women and men, the average 12-month persistence rate was 43.0%. Among women, eight sites have rates that exceeded 50% (Israel, Northern Ireland, South Africa, São Paulo, Lebanon, Ukraine, Shenzhen, and Iraq). Among men, seven sites have rates ≥50% (Israel, Romania, São Paulo, Ukraine, Shenzhen, Beijing/Shanghai, and Iraq).

The last column of Table 4.1 shows the indirect indicator of symptom persistence of MDD (30-day prevalence among 12-month cases). Of note, the combined average symptom persistence rate (38.0%) is only four points lower than the combined average disorder persistence rate (42.1%), but the variability among countries both within and across income level is very high. The two countries with highest symptom persistence are Bulgaria (59.8%) and Ukraine (57.0%), while the two lowest are Nigeria (18.6%) and Japan (14.9%). The average cross-national rates are slightly higher for women (39.7%) than for men (34.5%). Among women, three countries have rates exceeding 50% (Shenzhen, Ukraine, and Bulgaria), and three have rates lower than 20% (Nigeria, France, and Japan). Among men, only Ukraine's rate exceeds 50%, while the Netherlands, Japan, and Poland have rates under 20%.

Age-of-Onset

Appendix Figure 4A.1 shows the AOO curves for the three country income groups. The median (interquartile range; IQR) AOO across all countries is 38 (24–53). The average AOO is youngest in the high-income countries (38; 24–53), intermediate in the upper-middle-income countries (40; 26–55), and oldest in the poorest countries (42; 26–57).

The average projected risk of MDD at age 75 is 19.6%, suggesting that nearly 20% of WMH respondents will have a depressive episode at some point in their lives. The average lifetime risk is 21.1% in high-income countries, 18.3% in middle-income countries, and 17.6% in the poorest countries. Of note, the lifetime risk exceeds 30% in São Paulo and France, but is under 10% in Nigeria, Beijing/Shanghai, Romania, and Poland.

Comorbidity

Table 4.2 shows the comorbidity of MDD with anxiety, disruptive behaviour/impulse-control, and substance-use disorders for all countries combined. Half of respondents with lifetime MDD also have a lifetime anxiety disorder, though fewer met criteria for impulse-control or substance-use disorders. Similar proportions are found in the comparison of 12-month MDD with other 12-month disorders. Most importantly, fewer than 20% of respondents have had their first episode of depression prior to the onset of anxiety disorder, consistent with the earlier AOO of anxiety disorders described in Chapters 6–12. About one-fifth of cases of MDD began prior to onset of a disruptive behaviour/impulse-control disorder, and about one-third began prior to onset a substance-use disorder. Overall, MDD temporally precedes other disorders only 15–17% of the time.

Role Impairment

Table 4.3 provides country-specific data on severe role impairment for respondents with 12-month MDD in the 23 countries that administered the Sheehan Disability Scale (SDS) in the CIDI depression module. The four subscales (home, work, relationship, social) and 'any' impairment (one or more subscales with a score of 7+ out of 10) are included. It is important to note that the findings reported here are based solely on self-reports. Three findings are especially noteworthy. First, about half of respondents (57.0%) report severe impairment in at least one domain. Second, rates of severe impairment are highest in the high-income (63.9%), intermediate in the upper-middle-income (53.7%), and lowest in the poor (43.9%) countries. The highest rates of any severe impairment are found in Northern Ireland (73.2%) and Australia (70.8%), while

Table 4.3 Severity of role impairment (Sheehan Disability Scale: (SDS)) associated with 12-month major depressive disorder, by country

Country	Proportion with severe role impairment (SDS score: 7–10)										Number of 12-month cases
	Home		Work		Relationship		Social		Any[a]		
	%	SE	%	SE	%	SE	%	SE	%	SE	
Low/lower-middle-income countries	**26.3**	**1.6**	**21.8**	**1.5**	**22.7**	**1.6**	**24.0**	**1.6**	**43.9**	**1.7**	**1,355**
Colombia	23.9	3.4	23.5	3.4	31.8	4.5	27.2	4.1	50.0	4.6	246
Iraq	53.0	6.2	46.7	5.8	38.6	6.8	39.2	5.9	64.3	5.6	182
Nigeria	18.2	7.3	9.8	4.1	4.7	3.2	8.4	4.3	22.3	7.8	75
Peru	22.3	5.3	18.3	5.6	25.4	4.3	33.0	5.5	48.3	6.4	103
PRC (Beijing/Shanghai)	27.1	7.2	13.9	4.7	11.0	3.7	12.8	3.8	38.9	8.5	87
PRC (Shenzhen)	5.2	1.8	7.3	2.3	14.4	3.6	16.7	3.3	26.3	3.5	230
Ukraine	34.7	2.1	26.8	2.8	21.8	1.9	24.1	2.7	47.8	1.9	432
Upper-middle-income countries	**33.9**	**1.7**	**35.1**	**1.9**	**33.6**	**1.7**	**36.2**	**1.7**	**53.7**	**1.9**	**1,422**
Brazil	33.7	3.1	34.9	3.9	32.4	2.8	36.7	2.9	50.6	3.8	491
Bulgaria	31.9	4.6	38.6	5.1	34.6	4.3	37.8	5.1	49.7	4.7	145
Colombia (Medellin)	32.4	4.9	33.0	5.4	30.6	4.8	33.3	4.8	54.6	5.5	151
Lebanon	43.5	7.5	39.6	8.4	41.7	4.8	48.5	5.3	66.8	5.6	127
Mexico	29.5	4.2	31.9	3.8	31.2	3.9	30.8	4.0	48.5	3.9	242
Romania	33.7	7.8	39.8	8.1	30.1	8.1	25.3	7.8	44.0	8.6	40
South Africa	36.1	3.5	35.1	3.5	34.9	5.1	34.3	3.8	60.6	3.4	226
High-income countries	**37.4**	**1.2**	**38.7**	**1.1**	**36.4**	**1.1**	**45.9**	**1.1**	**63.9**	**1.1**	**3,160**
Australia	38.4	3.8	45.0	3.8	41.9	3.6	57.2	3.8	70.8	3.1	438
Israel	45.6	3.2	43.3	3.3	32.7	3.1	33.7	3.2	59.5	3.2	280
Japan	28.0	6.0	36.1	7.5	35.5	5.6	24.9	7.1	54.0	7.7	83
New Zealand	32.4	2.1	42.2	2.2	36.6	2.2	48.3	2.2	66.9	2.1	742
Northern Ireland	47.3	4.0	47.2	3.0	39.0	3.2	56.0	3.5	73.2	3.5	375
Poland	43.3	4.6	36.4	5.1	37.1	4.3	46.4	5.7	58.9	5.5	125
Portugal	28.6	3.3	29.3	2.9	27.2	3.2	30.5	3.6	56.3	3.8	293
Spain (Murcia)	37.6	7.6	38.2	7.4	40.5	6.9	40.7	6.9	48.1	6.7	154
United States	37.8	2.5	29.5	2.1	35.6	1.6	45.8	1.9	62.1	2.3	670
All countries combined	**34.1**	**0.8**	**34.0**	**0.8**	**32.7**	**0.8**	**39.0**	**0.8**	**57.0**	**0.9**	**5,937**

(cont.)

Table 4.3 (*cont.*)

Country	Proportion with severe role impairment (SDS score: 7–10)										Number of 12-month cases
	Home		Work		Relationship		Social		Any[a]		
	%	SE	%	SE	%	SE	%	SE	%	SE	
WHO regions											
Region of the Americas	32.8	1.5	30.0	1.5	32.9	1.3	37.7	1.3	54.7	1.6	1,903
African region	31.9	3.3	28.8	3.1	27.9	4.1	28.2	3.2	51.6	3.5	301
Western Pacific region	29.0	1.6	35.1	1.6	33.1	1.6	42.5	1.6	59.3	1.6	1,580
Eastern Mediterranean region	47.1	2.8	43.6	2.8	36.4	2.6	38.9	2.6	62.6	2.6	589
Western European region	38.6	2.6	38.8	2.3	35.0	2.2	43.6	2.5	62.1	2.6	822
Eastern European region	35.5	1.8	31.6	2.1	27.3	1.6	31.9	2.2	49.8	1.8	742
Comparison between countries[b]	$F_{22,v} = 6.6^*$, $P < 0.001$		$F_{22,v} = 8.0^*$, $P < 0.001$		$F_{22,v} = 5.3^*$, $P < 0.001$		$F_{22,v} = 10.1^*$, $P < 0.001$		$F_{22,v} = 8.9^*$, $P < 0.001$		
Comparison between low-, middle-, and high-income countries[b]	$F_{2,v} = 16.0^*$, $P < 0.001$		$F_{2,v} = 38.0^*$, $P < 0.001$		$F_{2,v} = 25.7^*$, $P < 0.001$		$F_{2,v} = 58.0^*$, $P < 0.001$		$F_{2,v} = 49.1^*$, $P < 0.0001$		
Comparison between WHO regions[b]	$F_{5,v} = 6.7^*$, $P < 0.001$		$F_{5,v} = 5.5^*$, $P < 0.001$		$F_{5,v} = 3.0^*$, $P = 0.012$		$F_{5,v} = 5.6^*$, $P < 0.001$		$F_{5,v} = 6.0^*$, $P < 0.001$		

*Significant at the 0.05 level, two-sided test.
[a]Highest severity category across four SDS role domains.
[b]Wald design-corrected F-tests were used to determine if there is variation in impairment severity across countries. The denominator degree of freedom, v, is 5429.
PRC: People's Republic of China

the lowest are found in Beijing/Shanghai (26.3%) and Nigeria (22.3%). Third, across the four impairment domains, social impairment is most strongly impacted in the wealthier countries, while impairment in the home domain edges out the social domain in low-income sites.

Treatment

The last column of Table 4.4 shows the percent of 12-month MDD cases, across all countries combined, who report treatment seeking in the year prior to interview. Overall, 54.5% of respondents in high, 29.5% in upper-middle, and 18.0% in low/lower-middle-income countries report treatment of any kind. Consistent with the previous population-based studies starting with the Epidemiological Catchment Area Study (ECA), the largest percent of individuals with MDD seek care from general medical providers. In high-income countries, where mental health specialty services are more available, close to one-third of respondents with 12-month MDD seek care from a mental health specialist. In each sector, high-income country respondents have the largest and low/lower-middle-income country respondents the lowest percent seeking services. Overall, few respondents seek care in the human services or CAM sectors.

Table 4.4 also shows that help-seeking from the mental health specialty sector is associated with level of impairment. In high-income countries, the percent seeking this type of care increases from 19.1% (mild), to 22.0% (moderate), to 35.0% (high impairment). This pattern is repeated for general medical providers in high-income countries. It is difficult to interpret the results for the upper-middle and low/lower-middle-income countries without information on the types and accessibility of services available when the surveys were implemented.

Socio-demographic Correlates

Table 4.5 shows the associations of demographic variables with current burden (30-day prevalence) of MDD, lifetime history of MDD, disorder persistence (12-month/lifetime) and symptom persistence (30-day/12-month) for all countries combined. With regard to current burden of MDD, there are no marked differences across the age-cohorts, with only respondents aged 45–59 having a significantly elevated prevalence compared to respondents ages 60+. It is important to note, however, that this apparent lack of difference masks quite different age-related patterns found in analyses by country income stratum. In low/lower-middle- and upper-middle-income countries, current burden is highest in the oldest (60+) cohort. But in high-income countries, the pattern is reversed, with current burden being higher among the three younger cohorts relative to the oldest cohort (data not shown).

The female:male ratio for MDD prevalence is 2:1 in most countries and 3:1 in the upper-middle-income countries. Regarding employment status, in all countries combined and in high-income countries, homemakers and respondents in the 'other category' (unemployed or disabled) are twice as likely to have MDD as employed respondents. In upper-middle- and low/lower-middle-income countries, the 'other' category also carries a significantly higher likelihood of MDD. In low/lower-middle-income countries only, being retired is associated with two fold increased odds of MDD compared to being employed, independent of age and gender.

Consistent with prior literature, in all sites, respondents who were previously married and those who have not graduated from college are significantly more likely to have current MDD compared to married respondents and to college graduates. Higher household income is a protective factor in all except low/lower-middle-income countries, where there is no association with current MDD.

The demographic associations found for current MDD are for the most part similar for lifetime MDD. There are a couple of notable differences, however. For age, after adjusting for gender, person-years, and country, odds of MDD decrease in a linear fashion from younger to older cohorts. This pattern is consistent across the three country income groups. This may reflect a true cohort effect such that rates of depression are higher among younger cohorts; or it may reflect age-related recall bias whereby older respondents are less likely to recall episodes of MDD earlier in their lives, or other methodological factors such as differential mortality. The fact that the age-related pattern in lifetime prevalence is consistent across country income groups while the age-related pattern in current burden differs substantially across country income groups is because current burden reflects both lifetime history and persistence of disorder. As noted above, disorder persistence is higher in the lower-income countries. A further noteworthy difference is that household income is not associated with the risk of developing depression in all countries combined or in separate analyses of

Table 4.4 Among those with 12-month major depressive disorder, percent reporting treatment in the past 12 months by Sheehan impairment severity

Sector of treatment	Sheehan Disability Scale category[a]											
	Mild impairment (score: 1–3)			Moderate impairment (score: 4–6)			Severe impairment (score: 7–10)			Any impairment		
	%	SE	Comparison between country income groups[b]	%	SE	Comparison between country income groups[b]	%	SE	Comparison between country income groups[b]	%	SE	Comparison between country income groups[b]
Specialty mental health[c]												
Low/lower-middle-income countries	–	–	$F_{2,v} = 12.5^*$,	**3.8**	0.9	$F_{2,v} = 31.9^*$,	**9.4**	1.8	$F_{2,v} = 58.4^*$,	**6.5**	0.9	$F_{2,v} = 131.1^*$,
Upper-middle-income countries	**8.1**	2.5	$P < 0.001$	**14.0**	2.3	$P < 0.001$	**19.9**	1.7	$P < 0.001$	**15.3**	1.2	$P < 0.001$
High-income countries	**19.1**	2.8		**22.0**	1.9		**35.0**	1.3		**28.9**	0.8	
All countries combined	**10.7**	1.5		**15.5**	1.2		**27.2**	1.0		**21.7**	0.6	
General medical[d]												
Low/lower-middle-income countries	**6.0**	2.3	$F_{2,v} = 10.6^*$,	**10.6**	2.2	$F_{2,v} = 36.6^*$,	**9.7**	1.4	$F_{2,v} = 127.7^*$,	**8.4**	1.0	$F_{2,v} = 228.8^*$,
Upper-middle-income countries	**23.2**	5.6	$P < 0.001$	**9.5**	1.5	$P < 0.001$	**16.2**	1.6	$P < 0.001$	**14.5**	1.1	$P < 0.001$
High-income countries	**23.8**	3.5		**32.3**	2.1		**43.4**	1.4		**37.8**	0.9	
All countries combined	**17.3**	2.1		**21.3**	1.3		**31.6**	1.0		**27.2**	0.6	
Any health care[e]												
Low/lower-middle-income countries	**6.4**	2.3	$F_{2,v} = 22.8^*$,	**13.7**	2.1	$F_{2,v} = 44.5^*$,	**17.5**	2.1	$F_{2,v} = 124.4^*$,	**13.8**	1.2	$F_{2,v} = 249.2^*$,
Upper-middle-income countries	**29.5**	6.3	$P < 0.001$	**22.0**	2.4	$P < 0.001$	**29.7**	2.1	$P < 0.001$	**26.0**	1.2	$P < 0.001$
High-income countries	**35.8**	3.7		**44.9**	2.2		**59.3**	1.4		**51.7**	1.0	
All countries combined	**24.0**	2.3		**31.5**	1.5		**45.6**	1.1		**38.9**	0.7	
Human services[f]												
Low/lower-middle-income countries	–	–	–	**2.1**	0.8	$F_{2,v} = 2.3$,	**5.5**	1.4	$F_{2,v} = 4.0^*$,	**3.4**	0.7	$F_{2,v} = 2.7$,
Upper-middle-income countries	–	–		**2.2**	0.9	$P = 0.10$	**4.2**	0.8	$P = 0.02$	**3.9**	0.8	$P = 0.07$
High-income countries	**5.1**	1.7		**4.1**	0.7		**7.3**	0.8		**5.1**	0.4	
All countries combined	**3.7**	1.1		**3.1**	0.5		**6.3**	0.6		**4.5**	0.3	
CAM[g]												
Low/lower-middle-income countries	–	–	$F_{2,v} = 2.3$,	**3.7**	1.2	$F_{2,v} = 1.7$,	**2.1**	0.8	$F_{2,v} = 21.9^*$,	**2.3**	0.5	$F_{2,v} = 20.5^*$,
Upper-middle-income countries	**5.3**	2.5	$P = 0.10$	**2.6**	0.9	$P = 0.18$	**4.2**	0.9	$P < 0.001$	**3.2**	0.6	$P < 0.001$
High-income countries	**4.3**	1.5		**5.0**	0.9		**10.1**	0.9		**6.6**	0.5	
All countries combined	**3.5**	0.9		**4.1**	0.6		**7.4**	0.6		**5.1**	0.3	

Table 4.4 (*cont.*)

Sector of treatment	Sheehan Disability Scale category[a]											
	Mild impairment (score: 1–3)			Moderate impairment (score: 4–6)			Severe impairment (score: 7–10)			Any impairment		
	%	SE	Comparison between country income groups[b]	%	SE	Comparison between country income groups[b]	%	SE	Comparison between country income groups[b]	%	SE	Comparison between country income groups[b]
Any non-health care[h]												
Low/lower-middle-income countries	**3.6**	1.9	$F_{2,v} = 1.7$, $P = 0.19$	**5.8**	1.4	$F_{2,v} = 2.8$, $P = 0.06$	**7.5**	1.6	$F_{2,v} = 16.2^*$, $P < 0.001$	**5.6**	0.8	$F_{2,v} = 13.4^*$, $P < 0.001$
Upper-middle-income countries	**6.4**	2.7		**4.5**	1.3		**7.2**	1.0		**6.3**	0.9	
High-income countries	**8.8**	2.2		**8.5**	1.2		**15.2**	1.1		**10.4**	0.6	
All countries combined	**6.4**	1.3		**6.8**	0.8		**12.1**	0.7		**8.6**	0.4	
Any treatment[i]												
Low/lower-middle-income countries	**9.4**	2.9	$F_{2,v} = 20.9^*$, $P < 0.001$	**18.4**	2.3	$F_{2,v} = 37.9^*$, $P < 0.001$	**22.8**	2.4	$F_{2,v} = 110.4^*$, $P < 0.001$	**18.0**	1.4	$F_{2,v} = 211.3^*$, $P < 0.001$
Upper-middle-income countries	**35.3**	6.5		**24.9**	2.6		**33.3**	2.1		**29.5**	1.4	
High-income countries	**40.9**	3.8		**47.2**	2.2		**62.9**	1.4		**54.5**	1.0	
All countries combined	**28.5**	2.5		**34.6**	1.5		**49.5**	1.1		**42.1**	0.8	

*Significant at the 0.05 level, two-sided test.
A dash indicates low cell counts (<5 cases).
[a]Highest severity category across four SDS role domains.
[b]Wald design-corrected F-tests were used to determine if there is variation in prevalence estimates across country income groups. The denominator degree of freedom, v, is 5429; only generated where there is more than one stable cell (≥5 cases) for each combination of treatment sector and Sheehan impairment.
[c]The mental health specialist sector, which includes psychiatrist and non-psychiatrist mental health specialists (psychiatrist, psychologist, or other non-psychiatrist mental health professional; social worker or counsellor in a mental health specialty setting; use of a mental health helpline; or overnight admissions for a mental health or drug or alcohol problems, with a presumption of daily contact with a psychiatrist).
[d]The general medical sector (general practitioner, other medical doctor, nurse, occupational therapist, or any healthcare professional).
[e]The mental health specialist sector or the general medical sector.
[f]The human services sector (religious or spiritual advisor or social worker or counsellor in any setting other than a specialty mental health setting).
[g]The CAM (complementary and alternative medicine) sector (any other type of healer such as herbalist or homeopath, participation in an internet support group, or participation in a self-help group).
[h]The human services sector or CAM.
[i]Any treatment listed above.

Table 4.5 Bivariate associations between socio-demographic correlates and DSM-IV major depressive disorder (MDD), all countries combined

Correlates	30-day MDD[a]		Lifetime MDD[b]		12-month MDD among lifetime cases[c]		30-day MDD among 12-month cases[c]	
	OR	(95% CI)	OR	(95% CI)	OR	(95% CI)	OR	(95% CI)
Age-cohort								
18–29	**0.9**	(0.8–1.1)	**11.6***	(10.6–12.7)				
30–44	**1.1**	(1.0–1.3)	**6.4***	(5.9–6.9)				
45–59	**1.2***	(1.0–1.4)	**3.4***	(3.2–3.6)				
60+	**1.0**		**1.0**					
Age-cohort difference[d]	$\chi^2_3 = 18.3^*, P < 0.001$		$\chi^2_3 = 2{,}918.4^*, P < 0.001$					
Age-of-onset								
Early					**1.9***	(1.7–2.2)	**0.6***	(0.5–0.7)
Early-average					**1.1**	(1.0–1.2)	**0.6***	(0.5–0.8)
Late-average					**1.0**	(0.9–1.1)	**0.7***	(0.6–0.9)
Late					**1.0**		**1.0**	
Age-of-onset difference[d]					$\chi^2_3 = 169.1^*, P < 0.001$		$\chi^2_3 = 34.2^*, P < 0.001$	
Time since onset (continuous)					**0.98***	(0.98–0.99)	**1.02***	(1.01–1.02)
Gender								
Female	**2.2***	(2.0–2.5)	**1.9***	(1.8–1.9)	**1.1***	(1.0–1.3)	**1.2***	(1.0–1.3)
Male	**1.0**		**1.0**		**1.0**		**1.0**	
Gender difference[d]	$\chi^2_1 = 216.4^*, P < 0.001$		$\chi^2_1 = 931.0^*, P < 0.001$		$\chi^2_1 = 7.9^*, P = 0.005$		$\chi^2_1 = 4.8^*, P = 0.028$	
Employment status								
Student	**0.9**	(0.7–1.3)	**1.2***	(1.1–1.4)	**1.6***	(1.3–2.1)	**0.7**	(0.5–1.1)
Homemaker	**1.4***	(1.2–1.6)	**0.9**	(0.9–1.0)	**1.3***	(1.2–1.5)	**1.3***	(1.1–1.6)
Retired	**1.1**	(0.9–1.3)	**0.8***	(0.7–0.9)	**1.4***	(1.2–1.6)	**1.1**	(0.9–1.4)
Other	**2.6***	(2.3–3.0)	**1.4***	(1.3–1.5)	**1.9***	(1.7–2.2)	**1.6***	(1.3–1.9)
Employed	**1.0**		**1.0**		**1.0**		**1.0**	

Table 4.5 ***(cont.)***

Correlates	30-day MDD[a]		Lifetime MDD[b]		12-month MDD among lifetime cases[c]		30-day MDD among 12-month cases[c]	
	OR	(95% CI)	OR	(95% CI)	OR	(95% CI)	OR	(95% CI)
Employment status difference[d]	$\chi^2_4 = 188.8^*$, $P < 0.001$		$\chi^2_4 = 173.6^*$, $P < 0.001$		$\chi^2_4 = 122.2^*$, $P < 0.001$		$\chi^2_4 = 33.2^*$, $P < 0.001$	
Marital status								
Never married	**1.0**	(0.9–1.2)	**1.3***	(1.2–1.4)	**1.3***	(1.2–1.5)	**0.9**	(0.7–1.0)
Divorced/separated/widowed	**1.9***	(1.7–2.1)	**1.7***	(1.6–1.8)	**1.2***	(1.1–1.3)	**1.0**	(0.8–1.1)
Currently married	**1.0**		**1.0**		**1.0**		**1.0**	
Marital status difference[d]	$\chi^2_2 = 102.8^*$, $P < 0.001$		$\chi^2_2 = 415.3^*$, $P < 0.001$		$\chi^2_2 = 32.8^*$, $P < 0.001$		$\chi^2_2 = 2.9$, $P = 0.239$	
Education level								
No education	**2.3***	(1.7–3.2)	**1.5***	(1.3–1.8)	**1.7***	(1.3–2.4)	**1.1**	(0.7–1.7)
Some primary	**2.2***	(1.8–2.8)	**1.3***	(1.2–1.4)	**1.9***	(1.6–2.3)	**1.4***	(1.1–1.8)
Finished primary	**2.0***	(1.6–2.6)	**1.3***	(1.2–1.4)	**1.5***	(1.2–1.8)	**1.3***	(1.0–1.7)
Some secondary	**2.0***	(1.6–2.4)	**1.2***	(1.1–1.3)	**1.4***	(1.2–1.6)	**1.6***	(1.3–2.0)
Finished secondary	**1.5***	(1.3–1.8)	**1.2***	(1.1–1.3)	**1.1**	(1.0–1.3)	**1.3***	(1.0–1.5)
Some college	**1.4***	(1.2–1.7)	**1.2***	(1.1–1.3)	**1.3***	(1.1–1.5)	**1.1**	(0.9–1.3)
Finished college	**1.0**		**1.0**		**1.0**		**1.0**	
Education level difference[d]	$\chi^2_6 = 73.4^*$, $P < 0.001$		$\chi^2_6 = 62.7^*$, $P < 0.001$		$\chi^2_6 = 63.4^*$, $P < 0.001$		$\chi^2_6 = 23.0^*$, $P = 0.001$	
Household income								
Low	**1.4***	(1.2–1.6)	**1.0**	(1.0–1.1)	**1.7***	(1.5–1.9)	**1.1**	(0.9–1.3)
Low-average	**1.3***	(1.1–1.5)	**1.0**	(1.0–1.1)	**1.4***	(1.3–1.6)	**1.1**	(0.9–1.3)
High-average	**1.1**	(0.9–1.2)	**1.0**	(1.0–1.1)	**1.1***	(1.0–1.3)	**0.9**	(0.8–1.2)
High	**1.0**		**1.0**		**1.0**		**1.0**	
Household income difference[d]	$\chi^2_3 = 29.9^*$, $P < 0.001$		$\chi^2_3 = 1.4$, $P = 0.701$		$\chi^2_3 = 97.2^*$, $P < 0.001$		$\chi^2_3 = 2.3$, $P = 0.503$	
N[e]	**147,264**		**6,221,577**		**16,339**		**6,842**	

*Significant at the 0.05 level, two-sided test.
[a]These estimates are based on logistic regression models adjusted for age, gender, and country.
[b]These estimates are based on survival models adjusted for age-cohorts, gender, person-years, and country.
[c]These estimates are based on logistic regression models adjusted for time since MDD onset, age of MDD onset, gender, and country.
[d]Chi-square test of significant differences between blocks of socio-demographic variables.
[e]Denominator N: 147,264 = total sample; 6,221,577 = number of person-years in the survival models; 16,339 = number of lifetime MDD cases; 6,842 = number of 12-month MDD cases.

high-, upper-middle-, and low/lower-middle-income countries.

There are two further findings of note in relation to disorder persistence. First, early AOO is associated with a two fold increased likelihood of MDD persistence. Second, the gender ratio is less pronounced (relative to lifetime risk) in all countries combined and in high- and upper-middle-income countries (ORs ~1.1) and is non-significant in low/lower-middle-income countries (OR = 1.0). Overall, being employed, better educated, currently married, and having a higher household income are protective factors against persistence of disorder in all countries combined and in high- and upper-middle-income countries. In poor countries, lower household income is significantly associated with persistence, although as noted above, it is not significantly associated with current or lifetime prevalence.

The factors associated with persistence of symptoms (30-day/12-month) are older AOO, female gender, homemaker or 'other' occupation, and lower education. Given the reduced sample size, few associations are statistically significant in the country income group-specific analyses.

Discussion

Consistent with previous cross-national reports, the WMH prevalence estimates of MDD varied considerably among countries, but the highest prevalence estimates were found in some of the wealthiest countries in the world. Many of our findings are consistent with prior studies; others shed new light on the epidemiology of depression around the globe. Before discussing the findings, however, it is important to clarify the methodological factors that potentially influence the prevalence and risk factors for depression. One basic issue reported in Chapter 3 is the variability in response rates across countries, which in some cases were quite low. In a previous paper, we examined whether there was an obvious association between the response rates for the WMH surveys and the prevalence of depression, and no clear association was observed (Bromet *et al.* 2011). Another limitation for studying depression is that in settings where treatment was unavailable, the most depressed people might have been unable to participate. This might have contributed to the lower prevalence rates found in low compared to high-income countries, although it does not explain their higher 12-month and current persistence rates. A third limitation for understanding the epidemiology of depression is that the WMH Surveys Initiative involved household surveys, and people in jails, prisons, hospitals, or living on military bases were not part of the sampling frame. The WMH surveys also did not interview people who were highly intoxicated or had severe cognitive or physical disabilities. Thus, the rates of MDD presented here should be regarded as conservative. Yet another limitation that impacts potential comparisons of prevalence rates among the WMH sites is the 10–15-year gap in life expectancy in WMH poor compared to wealthy countries (Riley 2005). Thus, the WMH cross-sectional samples reflect survivor bias, which could be of considerable importance for understanding differences in the rates and correlates of depression in high-, upper-middle-, and low/lower-middle-income countries. Lastly, there may have been cross-national differences in the willingness to disclose personal information about depression, in the extent to which MDD was stigmatized, and in the recall of lifetime episodes, especially episodes that occurred more than a year before the interview. This too may help to explain the unusually low rates of MDD found in some of the WMH countries.

Despite these limitations, the current findings shed important light on the prevalence, and demographic, comorbidity, and service use patterns in countries around the globe, including settings like Ukraine, that had no previous population-based data on depression. Regarding prevalence, it is noteworthy that while the lifetime and 12-month rates were significantly higher in wealthier countries, persistence of MDD was significantly higher in the low/lower-middle-income WMH countries. Although differential recall of distal compared to recent episodes of depression by country income level could have contributed to this result, it is also likely that the higher persistence is related to environmental conditions, particularly the combination of a lack of treatment resources coupled with extremely adverse socio-economic conditions. The latter would also explain why in low-income countries, household income was not related to prevalence but was associated with persistence of MDD.

Consistent with prior population studies, MDD was strongly comorbid with other disorders. Because the average AOO for MDD was older than was the case for anxiety, impulse-control, and substance-disorders, MDD rarely preceded the onset of these disorders. As noted in many WMH publications, the cross-sectional nature of the surveys impedes our ability to confirm AOO. It is also possible that error in recall of previous lifetime episodes varied by country, by income level, or by geographic location. Longitudinal data collection is required to best document the time of onset so that the causes and consequences of MDD can be disentangled (Wells & Horwood 2004; Patten 2009). Differential recall, however, should not have affected the findings on current prevalence of MDD and associated risk factors.

In this regard, three socio-demographic patterns merit special comment. First, consistent with prior epidemiologic research, women had twice the odds of MDD compared to men (as was true for other internalizing disorders, like anxiety), but gender was not a particularly strong correlate of persistence. Indeed, with minor exceptions, the percentages of women and men with persistent MDD (12-month/lifetime and 30-day/12-month) differed by only a few points. Thus, women have a greater likelihood of developing disorder, but once present, the persistence rates appear similar. Most prior research on gender differences in depression has focused on biopsychosocial risk factors for the development of MDD. Our analyses suggest that future efforts should be directed towards understanding gender-specific mechanisms underlying recovery and recurrence, including epigenetic and genetic risk, prior and recent socio-environmental adversities and protective factors, comorbid mental and physical health conditions, and personality characteristics.

A second demographic correlate associated with two fold increased odds of MDD was being outside the workforce (but not retired or working as a homemaker). This finding has been reported in population-based studies (e.g., Gallo *et al.* 2006), primary care research (e.g., Rizvi *et al.* 2015), and pre-post studies of plant closings (e.g., Kasl *et al.* 1975). Prospective studies are needed to identify culturally specific protective factors that dampen the association of unemployment on subsequent MDD. Given the growth in unemployment and under-employment in countries around the world, preventing depression, and other adverse health and mental health consequences of unemployment, is a global challenge.

The third demographic variable of special interest was the different relationship of age with MDD in high- and low-income countries, as previously noted in our paper summarizing the epidemiology of major depressive episodes in the WMH (Bromet *et al.* 2011). Prior to the WMH, the majority of epidemiologic studies were conducted in high-income settings, where the rate of depression declines with age. It was widely thus assumed that the negative correlation was universal. The WMH surveys have clarified that this age pattern is specific to higher-income countries. In poor countries, where many older people barely have enough money to subsist on and have chronic medical conditions, coupled with limited or no access to adequate medical care, it appears that depression increases with age. Public-health programmes typically focus on preventing depression in youth. Our findings suggest that in poor countries in particular, comprehensive interventions are needed for older adults.

Despite differences in the prevalence of MDD among the 29 countries, the consistency of the degree and associations of impairment with help-seeking is quite striking. The fact that more than half of WMH respondents were severely impaired by their depressive episode confirms the public-health importance of major depression as a commonly occurring and seriously impairing condition throughout the world. Indeed, the impairment associated with MDD was evident in all domains. It is instructive to juxtapose these findings against the fact that a relatively small proportion of respondents with MDD received any form treatment, especially in low-income countries. The proportion receiving some form of treatment was highest for respondents with the greatest impairment, but even respondents with severe impairment often failed to receive treatment. When mental health-related services were obtained, they were most often from the general medical sector, where providers are rarely trained to recognize and treatment common mental disorders and minimum standards of adequate mental health care are typically lacking (Wang *et al.* 2007). In countries with integrated mental and physical health services, referrals to mental health specialists can more readily take place. In most countries, however, people with MDD are highly stigmatized. Moreover, in many countries, medical school curricula do not include courses on the diagnosis and treatment of common mental conditions, such as MDD, and mental health specialists are not seen as part of mainstream health care. The WMH data regarding treatment in low compared to middle- and high-income countries reflect this underlying stigma towards mental health in most countries in the world.

In conclusion, given the recent GBD report that depression is the second leading cause of YLDs (GBD Collaborators, Vos *et al.* 2015), and in the context of other studies showing links of depression with work impairment, physical health, cognitive impairment, Alzheimer's disease and mortality, the WMH findings on MDD shed light on correlates that may help inform the development and expansion of programmes aimed at early detection and adequate intervention across the life course.

References

Andrade, L., Caraveo-Anduaga, J. J., Berglund P., *et al.* (2003). The epidemiology of major depressive episodes: results from the International Consortium of Psychiatric Epidemiology (ICPE) Surveys. *International Journal of Methods in Psychiatric Research*, 12, 3–21.

Bromet, E., Andrade, L. H., Hwang, I., *et al.* (2011). Cross-national epidemiology of DSM-IV major depressive episode. *BMC Medicine*, 9, 90.

Gallo, W. T., Bradley, E. H., Dubin, J. A., *et al.* (2006). The persistence of depressive symptoms in older workers who experience involuntary job loss: results from the Health and Retirement Survey. *The Journals of Gerontology Series B: Psychological Sciences and Social Sciences*, 61, S221–8.

GBD Collaborators, Vos, T., Barber, R.M., Bell, B. *et al.* (2015). Global, regional, and national incidence, prevalence, and years lived with disability for 301 acute and chronic diseases and injuries in 188 countries, 1990–2013: a systematic analysis for the Global Burden of Disease Study 2013. *Lancet*, 386, 743–800.

Haro, J. M., Arbabzadeh-Bouchez, S., Brugha, T. S., *et al.* (2006). Concordance of the Composite International Diagnostic Interview Version 3.0 (CIDI 3.0) with standardized clinical assessments in the WHO World Mental Health surveys. *International Journal of Methods in Psychiatric Research*, 15, 167–80.

Kasl, S. V., Gore, S., & Cobb, W. (1975). The experience of losing a job: reported changes in health, symptoms and illness behavior. *Psychosomatic Medicine*, 37, 106–22.

Kessler, R. C., Birnbaum, H., Bromet, E., *et al.* (2010). Age differences in major depression: results from the National Comorbidity Survey Replication (NCS-R). *Psychological Medicine*, 40, 225–37.

Kessler, R. C. & Bromet, E. J. (2013). The epidemiology of depression across cultures. *Annual Review of Public Health*, 34, 119–38.

Kessler, R. C., McGonagle, K. A., Zhao, S., *et al.* (1994). Lifetime and 12-month prevalence of DSM-III-R psychiatric disorders in the United States. Results from the National Comorbidity Survey. *Archives of General Psychiatry*, 51, 8–19.

Kessler, R. C. & Üstün, T. B. (2004). The World Mental Health (WMH) Survey Initiative Version of the World Health Organization (WHO) Composite International Diagnostic Interview (CIDI). *International Journal of Methods in Psychiatric Research*, 13, 93–121.

Kessler, R. C., Wittchen, H.-U., Abelson, J. M., *et al.* (1998). Methodological studies of the Composite International Diagnostic Interview (CIDI) in the US National Comorbidity Survey. *International Journal of Methods in Psychiatric Research*, 7, 33–55.

Leon, A. C., Olfson, M., Portera, L., *et al.* (1997). Assessing psychiatric impairment in primary care with the Sheehan Disability Scale. *International Journal of Methods in Psychiatric Research*, 27, 93–105.

Patten, S. B. (2009). Accumulation of major depressive episodes over time in a prospective study indicates that retrospectively assessed lifetime prevalence estimates are too low. *BMC Psychiatry*, 9, 19.

Regier, D. A., Narrow, W. E., Rae, D. S., *et al.* (1993). The de facto US mental and addictive disorders service system. Epidemiologic catchment area prospective 1-year prevalence rates of disorders and services. *Archives of General Psychiatry*, 50, 85–94.

Richards, D. (2011). Prevalence and clinical course of depression: a review. *Clinical Psychology Review*, 31, 1117–25.

Riley, J. C. (2005). Estimates of regional and global life expectancy, 1800-2001. *Population and Development Review*, 31, 537–43.

Rizvi, S. J., Cyriac, A., Grima, E., *et al.* (2015). Depression and employment status in primary and tertiary care settings. *Canadian Journal of Psychiatry*, 60, 14–22.

Robins, L. N., Helzer, J. E., Croughan, J. L., & Ratcliff, K. S. (1981). National Institute of Mental Health Diagnostic Interview Schedule: its history, characteristics and validity. *Archives of General Psychiatry*, 38, 381–9.

Simon, G. E., Goldberg, D. P., Von Korff, M., & Üstün, T. B. (2002). Understanding cross-national differences in depression prevalence. *Psychological Medicine*, 32, 585–94.

Üstün, T. B., Ayuso-Mateos, J. L., Chatterji, S., *et al.* (2004). Global burden of depressive disorders in the year 2000. *British Journal of Psychiatry*, 184, 386–92.

Wang, P. S., Aguilar-Gaxiola, S., Alonso, J., *et al.* (2007). Use of mental health services for anxiety, mood and substance disorders in 17 countries in the WHO World Mental Health surveys. *Lancet*, 370, 841–50.

Weissman, M. M., Bland, R. C., Canino, G. J., *et al.* (1996). Cross-national epidemiology of major depression and bipolar disorder. *Journal of the American Medical Association*, 276, 293–9.

Wells, J. E. & Horwood, L. J. (2004). How accurate is recall of key symptoms of depression? A comparison of recall and longitudinal reports. *Psychological Medicine*, 34, 1001–11.

Chapter 5

Bipolar Spectrum Disorder

Ronald C. Kessler, Elie G. Karam, Sing Lee, Brendan Bunting, Andrew A. Nierenberg

Introduction

This chapter reviews the World Mental Health (WMH) data on bipolar spectrum disorder. We define bipolar spectrum disorder as either bipolar I (BP-I) disorder, bipolar II disorder (BP-II), or subthreshold bipolar disorder (BPD). WMH respondents were classified as having a history of BP-I disorder if they met lifetime DSM-IV/CIDI criteria for a manic episode (at least seven days of either elevated mood in addition to three or more other symptoms of mania or of irritable mood in addition to four or more other symptoms of mania, the symptoms resulting in either marked impairment or need for hospitalization). Respondents were classified as having a history of BP-II if they met lifetime DSM-IV/CIDI criteria for both a major depressive episode and a hypomanic episode (at least four days with the same symptoms as those for BP-I, the symptoms being present to a significant degree but not resulting in marked impairment and never had a lifetime manic episode). The DSM-IV requirement that symptoms do not meet criteria for a mixed episode (DSM-IV Criterion C for mania/hypomania and Criterion B for major depressive episode) was not operationalized in making these diagnoses. Diagnoses of both BP-I and BP-II excluded cases with plausible organic causes.

We included subthreshold BPD in the definition of bipolar spectrum disorder based on evidence that the number of people with a subthreshold manifestation of BPD might be equal to or greater than the number with BP-I and BP-II combined (Akiskal *et al.* 2000) and that these subthreshold cases have levels of impairment comparable to those of other commonly occurring threshold mental disorders (Judd & Akiskal 2003). Perhaps even more importantly, respondents with a history of major depressive episodes and manic-like episodes that did not meet full criteria for either mania or hypomania may run a different course and respond to treatment differently from those with unipolar major depressive disorder. There is no official DSM-IV definition of subthreshold BPD, but DSM-5 has a residual category of *unspecified* bipolar disorder that can be used to characterize patients that do not meet full criteria (American Psychiatric Association 2013). The CIDI allowed us to characterize two subtypes of this sort that have been used to define subthreshold BPD in other empirical studies (Walsh *et al.* 2015; Kim *et al.* 2016). The first included respondents with a history of major depressive episodes and manic-like episodes that did not meet full criteria for either mania or hypomania. The second included respondents who met lifetime DSM-IV/CIDI criteria for a hypomanic episode but never had a lifetime major depressive episode.

Clinical reappraisal interviews for BPD using the lifetime non-patient version of the Structured Clinical Interview for DSM-IV (SCID; First *et al.* 2002) were carried out in a probability subsample of respondents in the American WMH survey. As detailed elsewhere (Kessler *et al.* 2006b), CIDI cases were over-sampled, and the data for these cases were weighted to adjust for this over-sampling in evaluating diagnostic accuracy. CIDI–SCID concordance (AUC) was excellent for BP-I (0.99), with positive predictive value (PPV; the proportion of CIDI cases blindly confirmed by the SCID) of 0.79 and negative predictive value (NPV; the proportion of CIDI non-cases blindly confirmed by the SCID as non-cases) of 1.0. Concordance was lower for BP-II (AUC = 0.83, PPV = 0.41, NPV = 0.99) and subthreshold BPD (AUC = 0.73, PPV = 0.58, NPV = 0.99) due to disagreements between CIDI and SCID diagnoses in which of these two categories the respondent should be classified. There was good CIDI–SCID agreement, though, on whether or not the respondent should be classified in at least one of the two categories. As a result, CIDI–SCID concordance was excellent for whether or not the respondent met criteria for having a BP spectrum disorder (i.e., either BP-I, BP-II, or subthreshold BPD; AUC = 0.99, PPV = 0.85, NPV = 0.99). The McNemar test was consistently insignificant across the individual and composite diagnoses ($\chi^2_1 = 0.1–0.3, P = 0.56–0.75$), showing that prevalence estimates based on the CIDI were unbiased compared to those based on the SCID for these lifetime disorders.

We focus here on BP spectrum disorder overall. In other words, we do not distinguish BP-I, BP-II, and subthreshold BPD. Nor do we present tables on recency of manic, hypomanic, or depressive episodes among respondents with a lifetime history of BP spectrum disorder. The focus on overall BP spectrum disorder is designed both to highlight the overall burden of this set of disorders and to recognize the fact that the CIDI does not distinguish with good accuracy between BP-II and subthreshold BPD. That being said, we note that controversy exists about the validity of extending the definition of bipolar disorder beyond BP-I and BP-II (Patten & Paris 2008) based on the fact that known treatments for BP-I and BP-II have not been found to be effective in treating subthreshold BP disorder (Duffy 2014) and the concern that individuals diagnosed as having subthreshold BP disorder might actually be misdiagnosed cases of borderline personality disorder (Paris 2014), although recent research suggests that the latter concern might be more apparent than real (Zimmerman & Morgan 2013; Ghaemi & Dalley 2014).

Method

BPD was assessed in 21 WMH surveys, including six in low/lower-middle-income countries (the national surveys in Iraq and Peru; the survey of all non-rural areas in Colombia; and the regional surveys in Nigeria, Beijing/Shanghai, and Shenzhen), six in upper-middle-income countries (the national surveys in Bulgaria, Lebanon, and Romania; the survey of all non-rural areas in Mexico; and the regional surveys in São Paulo, Brazil, and Medellin, Colombia), and nine in high-income countries (national surveys in Australia, Israel, New Zealand, Northern Ireland, Poland, Portugal, and the United States; and regional surveys in Japan and in Murcia, Spain). A total of 116,799 respondents participated in these surveys with response rates in the range 50.4% (Poland) and 97.2% (Medellin) and averaging 70.4% across all surveys. Although BPD was a Part I diagnosis, which means that it was assessed for all 116,799 respondents, comorbidities and some other correlates were assessed only among the 64,871 respondents in the Part II sample.

Results

Prevalence

Estimated lifetime prevalence of DSM-IV/CIDI BP spectrum disorder averages 1.9% over all WMH surveys and varies substantially across surveys with a range of 0.1–4.4% and an inter-quartile range (IQR) of 0.6–2.5% ($F = 42.5$, $P < 0.001$) (Table 5.1). These estimates are within the range of the estimates reported in previous studies (reviewed by Dell'Aglio *et al.* 2013). Lifetime prevalence is positively related to country income level (2.5% in high, 1.6% in upper-middle, and 1.0% in low/lower-middle-income countries; $F = 88.6$, $P < 0.001$). Consistent with the variation by country income level, lifetime prevalence is substantially higher in the regions of the Americas (2.8%), the Western Pacific (2.3%), and Western Europe (2.3%) than in other WHO regions (0.1–1.0%; $F = 126.3$, $P < 0.001$). Twelve-month prevalence averages 1.2% and 30-day prevalence 0.4% across surveys and has similar variations across surveys as found for lifetime prevalence (0.1–2.8% range; 0.4–1.5% IQR for 12-month prevalence; 0.0–1.2% range; 0.1–0.6% IQR for 30-day prevalence). The latter prevalence estimates are consistent with those reported in a recent review of the world literature as part of the Global Burden of Disease Study (Ferrari *et al.* 2016). An average of 60.3% of lifetime cases had an episode of major depression, mania, hypomania, or subthreshold hypomania within 12 months of the interview, and 36.4% of 12-month cases had an episode within 30 days of the interview. These indirect measures of persistence are remarkably similar across countries, especially in light of the high cross-national variation in lifetime prevalence. This consistency is indicated by the fact that neither 12-month prevalence among lifetime cases (59.2–62.7%) nor 30-day prevalence among 12-month cases (35.9–41.6%) varies significantly across surveys by country income level ($F = 0.8–1.4$, $P = 0.45–0.25$) even though there is significant variation across WHO regions.

Age-of-Onset

As shown in previous WMH reports (e.g., Kessler *et al.* 2007b) and consistent with other research (Leboyer *et al.* 2005; Kessler *et al.* 2007a), BP spectrum disorder has a median age-of-onset (AOO) in the mid-twenties (Table 5.2). This average is quite consistent across countries, with a median of 24 years of age in both low/lower-middle income and high-income countries and a

Table 5.1 Prevalence of DSM-IV bipolar spectrum disorder in the World Mental Health surveys

Country	Lifetime prevalence		12-month prevalence		30-day prevalence		12-month prevalence among lifetime cases		30-day prevalence among 12-month cases		Sample size used
	%	SE	%	SE	%	SE	%	SE	%	SE	
Low/lower-middle-income countries	**1.0**	**0.1**	**0.6**	**0.1**	**0.2**	**0.0**	**62.3**	**3.1**	**32.2**	**4.6**	**31,773**
Colombia	2.6	0.3	1.5	0.2	0.5	0.2	60.0	5.4	30.6	7.9	4,426
Iraq	0.2	0.1	0.2	0.1	0.1	0.0	77.0	14.2	31.6	22.6	4,332
Nigeria	0.1	0.1	0.1	0.1	–	–	42.6	25.2	–	–	6,752
Peru	1.9	0.3	0.8	0.2	0.3	0.1	45.2	5.9	34.1	10.7	3,930
PRC (Beijing/Shanghai)	0.1	0.0	0.1	0.0	<0.1	0.0	85.2	14.6	9.8	10.5	5,201
PRC (Shenzhen)	1.5	0.2	1.1	0.2	0.4	0.1	75.9	5.2	35.4	7.5	7,132
Upper-middle-income countries	**1.6**	**0.1**	**1.0**	**0.1**	**0.4**	**0.0**	**62.7**	**3.1**	**41.6**	**3.8**	**24,612**
Brazil	2.1	0.2	1.5	0.2	0.7	0.1	69.1	6.2	48.3	7.5	5,037
Bulgaria	0.3	0.1	0.1	0.1	–	–	37.0	20.3	–	–	5,318
Colombia (Medellin)	1.8	0.3	0.8	0.2	0.2	0.1	47.4	8.8	24.8	8.8	3,261
Lebanon	2.4	0.4	1.9	0.4	1.0	0.3	78.9	5.2	53.5	8.7	2,857
Mexico	1.9	0.2	1.1	0.2	0.5	0.1	60.0	5.3	43.2	6.9	5,782
Romania	1.8	0.3	1.0	0.2	0.2	0.1	56.7	9.5	17.9	8.9	2,357
High-income countries	**2.5**	**0.1**	**1.5**	**0.1**	**0.5**	**0.0**	**59.2**	**1.4**	**35.9**	**2.0**	**60,414**
Australia	2.8	0.3	1.8	0.2	0.6	0.1	64.2	4.0	35.4	5.5	8,463
Israel	0.7	0.1	0.5	0.1	0.1	0.1	70.6	8.5	25.2	9.7	4,859
Japan	0.6	0.1	0.2	0.1	0.1	0.0	41.6	11.4	27.7	14.5	4,129
New Zealand	3.9	0.2	2.2	0.2	0.7	0.1	56.6	2.4	30.0	3.3	12,790
Northern Ireland	2.5	0.3	1.6	0.2	0.8	0.1	65.4	4.7	50.0	5.0	4,340
Poland	0.6	0.1	0.4	0.1	0.1	0.0	64.1	5.8	27.8	5.4	10,081
Portugal	2.6	0.3	1.1	0.2	0.2	0.1	42.6	5.2	20.8	6.0	3,849
Spain (Murcia)	1.8	0.5	0.7	0.2	0.3	0.1	37.6	8.1	50.1	14.2	2,621
United States	4.4	0.3	2.8	0.2	1.2	0.1	63.8	2.5	42.6	4.2	9,282
All countries combined	**1.9**	**0.1**	**1.2**	**0.0**	**0.4**	**0.0**	**60.3**	**1.2**	**36.4**	**1.6**	**116,799**

(cont.)

Table 5.1 *(cont.)*

Country	Lifetime prevalence		12-month prevalence		30-day prevalence		12-month prevalence among lifetime cases		30-day prevalence among 12-month cases		Sample size used
	%	SE	%	SE	%	SE	%	SE	%	SE	
WHO regions[a]											
Region of the Americas	2.8	0.1	1.7	0.1	0.7	0.1	60.8	1.9	40.5	2.8	31,718
African region	0.1	0.1	0.1	0.1	–	–	42.6	25.2	–	–	6,752
Western Pacific region	2.3	0.1	1.4	0.1	0.4	0.0	60.8	1.9	32.2	2.7	37,715
Eastern Mediterranean region	1.0	0.1	0.7	0.1	0.3	0.1	76.1	4.4	43.3	6.9	12,048
Western European region	2.3	0.2	1.2	0.1	0.5	0.1	51.2	3.2	40.4	3.9	10,810
Eastern European region	0.6	0.1	0.4	0.0	0.1	0.0	57.9	5.3	22.0	4.6	17,756
Comparison between countries[b]	$F_{20,v} = 42.5^*$, $P < 0.001$		$F_{20,v} = 28.4^*$, $P < 0.001$		$F_{20,v} = 22.1^*$, $P < 0.001$		$F_{20,v} = 2.9^*$, $P < 0.001$		$F_{20,v} = 2.2^*$, $P = 0.002$		
Comparison between low-, middle-, and high-income country groups[b]	$F_{2,v} = 88.6^*$, $P < 0.001$		$F_{2,v} = 51.4^*$, $P < 0.001$		$F_{2,v} = 25.8^*$, $P < 0.001$		$F_{2,v} = 0.8$, $P = 0.446$		$F_{2,v} = 1.4$, $P = 0.246$		
Comparison between WHO regions[b]	$F_{5,v} = 126.3^*$, $P < 0.001$		$F_{5,v} = 80.4^*$, $P < 0.001$		$F_{5,v} = 76.6^*$, $P < 0.001$		$F_{5,v} = 3.5^*$, $P = 0.004$		$F_{5,v} = 3.2^*$, $P = 0.007$		

*Significant at the 0.05 level, two-sided test.

[a]**Region of the Americas** (Colombia, Mexico, Brazil, Peru, United States, Colombia (Medellin)); **African region** (Nigeria); **Western Pacific region** (PRC (Shenzhen), PRC (Beijing and Shanghai), Japan, Australia, New Zealand); **Eastern Mediterranean region** (Israel, Iraq, Lebanon); **Western European region** (Northern Ireland, Portugal, Spain (Murcia)); **Eastern European region** (Romania, Poland, Bulgaria).

[b]Wald design-corrected F-tests were used to determine if there is variation in prevalence estimates across countries. The denominator degree of freedom, v, is 5134.

PRC: People's Republic of China.

Table 5.2 Age at selected percentiles on the standardized age-of-onset distributions of DSM-IV bipolar spectrum disorder with projected lifetime risk at age 75

Country	Ages at selected percentiles								Lifetime prevalence		Projected risk at age 75	
	5	10	25	50	75	90	95	99	%	SE	%	SE
Low/lower-middle-income countries	**12**	**14**	**18**	**24**	**34**	**42**	**46**	**58**	**1.0**	**0.1**	**1.4**	**0.1**
Colombia[a]	11	14	19	28	37	46	58	58	2.6	0.3	3.7	0.5
Iraq	21	22	23	26	36	52	52	52	0.2	0.1	0.4	0.2
Nigeria	15	15	21	21	30	36	39	39	0.1	0.1	0.2	0.1
Peru[a]	15	17	19	25	37	41	46	51	1.9	0.3	2.6	0.3
PRC (Beijing/Shanghai)	14	18	18	25	28	33	33	33	0.1	0.0	0.1	0.1
PRC (Shenzhen)	10	13	17	19	24	29	36	39	1.5	0.2	1.8	0.2
Upper-middle-income countries	**13**	**15**	**18**	**25**	**36**	**46**	**59**	**63**	**1.6**	**0.1**	**2.2**	**0.1**
Brazil	13	15	19	31	40	62	62	68	2.1	0.2	3.3	0.4
Bulgaria	13	13	18	29	34	46	46	49	0.3	0.1	0.3	0.1
Colombia (Medellin)[a]	15	17	20	35	63	63	63	63	1.8	0.3	2.9	0.9
Lebanon	14	14	16	20	27	39	44	46	2.4	0.4	2.9	0.4
Mexico[a]	13	15	19	24	29	44	48	51	1.9	0.2	2.5	0.3
Romania	10	18	21	26	41	47	53	59	1.8	0.3	2.4	0.4
High-income countries	**12**	**14**	**18**	**24**	**39**	**50**	**55**	**63**	**2.5**	**0.1**	**3.4**	**0.1**
Australia	13	15	18	23	34	50	54	57	2.8	0.3	3.7	0.3
Israel	6	13	21	31	48	66	66	66	0.7	0.1	1.2	0.3
Japan	14	19	20	24	31	64	64	64	0.6	0.1	0.8	0.2
New Zealand	12	14	17	23	36	47	53	63	3.9	0.2	5.1	0.3
Northern Ireland	13	14	18	31	41	50	51	58	2.5	0.3	3.5	0.4
Poland[b]	13	14	17	31	43	51	55	55	0.6	0.1	0.8	0.1
Portugal	14	14	18	25	37	47	50	61	2.6	0.3	3.3	0.4
Spain (Murcia)	13	14	23	28	35	44	53	53	1.8	0.5	2.4	0.7
United States	11	13	17	24	41	51	57	65	4.4	0.3	6.1	0.4

(cont.)

Table 5.2 (*cont.*)

Country	Ages at selected percentiles								Lifetime prevalence		Projected risk at age 75	
	5	10	25	50	75	90	95	99	%	SE	%	SE
All countries combined	**13**	**14**	**18**	**25**	**38**	**50**	**56**	**63**	**1.9**	**0.1**	**2.7**	**0.1**
WHO regions												
Region of the Americas	12	14	19	27	41	54	62	65	2.8	0.1	4.0	0.2
African region	15	15	21	21	30	36	39	39	0.1	0.1	0.2	0.1
Western Pacific region	12	14	18	23	36	49	53	63	2.3	0.1	3.1	0.2
Eastern Mediterranean region	11	14	18	23	38	59	66	66	1.0	0.1	1.4	0.2
Western European region	13	14	19	28	39	48	51	61	2.3	0.2	3.2	0.3
Eastern European region	13	14	18	27	41	51	53	59	0.6	0.1	0.9	0.1

[a]The projected risk for these countries is at age 65 because the age range of these surveys is between 18 and 65.
[b]The projected risk for this country is at age 64 because the age range of this survey is between 18 and 64.
PRC: People's Republic of China.

median of 25 years in upper-middle-income countries. The earliest quarter of lifetime cases have onsets by age 18 (equivalent across all country income groups) and the third quarter have onsets by age 38 (in the age range 34–9 across country income groups). Because of this relatively narrow age range of onsets in the third and fourth decades of life, in conjunction with a projected 90% of lifetime cases having onsets by age 50 (in the age range 42–50 across country income groups), projected lifetime morbid risk, which averages 2.7% across countries, is not dramatically higher than the observed 1.9% lifetime prevalence as of the time of interview.

Socio-demographic Correlates

Estimated 30-day prevalence of BP spectrum disorder is very strongly and inversely correlated with respondent age-at-interview (AAI), with odds-ratios (ORs) of 9.0, 6.3, and 3.6, respectively, for respondents in the age ranges 18–29, 30–44, and 45–59, compared to those ages 60+ ($\chi^2_3 = 93.2$, $P < 0.001$) (Table 5.3). This pattern is due to an even more dramatic age gradient in estimates of lifetime prevalence (ORs of 58.2, 18.4, and 6.5, respectively, in the 18–29, 30–44, and 45–59 age ranges compared to 60+; $\chi^2_3 = 838.9$, $P < 0.001$) in conjunction with more complex associations of AAI with our indirect measures of persistence. The latter associations involve a disaggregation of AAI into the two components of AOO and time-since-onset (TSO), where AAI = AOO + TSO. These two components have opposite-sign significant associations with 12-month prevalence among lifetime cases. Specifically, AOO is inversely associated with this measure of persistence, as early onset (first quartile of AOO) has a significantly elevated OR of 2.2, early-average (the second quartile of AOO) a significantly elevated OR of 1.4, and late-average (the third quartile) a non-significantly elevated OR of 1.3 compared to late onset cases ($\chi^2_3 = 30.0$, $P < 0.001$). This opposite-sign pattern would suppress an aggregate association of AAI with 12-month prevalence among lifetime cases. The associations of the two components with 30-day prevalence among 12-month cases are different yet, with AOO not significant and TSO positively and significantly associated with 30-day prevalence among 12-month cases (OR = 1.02). It is difficult to know how to interpret these complex associations, as a number of different substantive and methodological factors could be involved in bringing them about. The dramatic inverse association between AAI and lifetime prevalence is almost certainly an artefact due to a combination of recall error, early mortality, and differential willingness to disclose these disorders to interviewers all positively associated with AAI. Previous methodological studies have found similar age-related biases in lifetime prevalence estimates of mental disorders (Moffitt *et al.* 2010). At the same time, recall bias could not account for the significant inverse association of age with 30-day prevalence, an association that has been documented in a number of other studies (reviewed by Dell'Aglio *et al.* 2013) and that is most plausibly due to early mortality of people with BPD and the resulting right censoring of the age distribution of current cases.

Estimated 30-day prevalence of BP spectrum disorder is marginally higher among women than men, with an OR of 1.4 (Table 5.3). This is true despite a slightly lower lifetime prevalence among women than men (OR 0.9) because the lower lifetime prevalence is more than counter-balanced by a significantly elevated 12-month prevalence among lifetime cases (OR 1.7) and a significantly elevated 30-day prevalence among 12-month cases (OR 1.6) for women compared to men. The somewhat higher 30-day prevalence of BP spectrum disorder among women than men is consistent with considerable evidence showing that while there is no gender difference in prevalence of BP-I, women are considerably more likely than men to have BP-II (reviewed by Vega *et al.* 2011). The even higher indirect estimates of persistence (i.e., 12-month prevalence among lifetime cases and 30-day prevalence among 12-month cases) among women than men are consistent with evidence that women with BPD are more likely than men to be rapid-cyclers (reviewed by Diflorio & Jones 2010). However, a previous WMH report failed to find evidence of a gender difference in rapid cycling the WMH data (Lee *et al.* 2010). Another possibility is related to the fact that a higher proportion of the BPD episodes of women than men are depressive or mixed rather than manic or hypomanic (reviewed by Lopez-Zurbano *et al.* 2015) in conjunction with a difference in the persistence of these different kinds of episodes (Miller *et al.* 2015), but these differences have not been investigated in the WMH data.

Another noteworthy pattern is that BP spectrum disorder is associated with being unmarried – both due to never marrying and to marital disruption – a well-known pattern in the literature (Weissman *et al.* 1988).

Table 5.3 Bivariate associations between socio-demographic correlates and DSM-IV bipolar spectrum disorder, all countries combined

Correlates	30-day bipolar spectrum disorder[a]		Lifetime bipolar spectrum disorder[b]		12-month bipolar spectrum disorder among lifetime cases[c]		30-day bipolar spectrum disorder among 12-month cases[c]	
	OR	(95% CI)	OR	(95% CI)	OR	(95% CI)	OR	(95% CI)
Age-cohort								
18–29	**9.0***	(5.5–15.0)	**58.2***	(43.3–78.3)				
30–44	**6.3***	(3.8–10.5)	**18.4***	(14.1–24.0)				
45–59	**3.6***	(2.1–6.0)	**6.5***	(5.1–8.3)				
60+	**1.0**		**1.0**					
Age-cohort difference[d]	$\chi^2_3 = 93.2^*$, $P < 0.001$		$\chi^2_3 = 838.9^*$, $P < 0.001$					
Age-of-onset								
Early					**2.2***	(1.7–3.0)	**0.9**	(0.6–1.4)
Early-average					**1.4***	(1.0–1.8)	**1.0**	(0.6–1.4)
Late-average					**1.3**	(0.9–1.8)	**1.2**	(0.8–1.7)
Late					**1.0**		**1.0**	
Age-of-onset difference[d]					$\chi^2_3 = 30.0^*$, $P < 0.001$		$\chi^2_3 = 1.4$, $P = 0.716$	
Time since onset (continuous)					**0.98***	(0.97–0.98)	**1.02***	(1.00–1.03)
Gender								
Female	**1.4***	(1.1–1.8)	**0.9***	(0.8–1.0)	**1.7***	(1.4–2.1)	**1.6***	(1.2–2.1)
Male	**1.0**		**1.0**		**1.0**		**1.0**	
Gender difference[d]	$\chi^2_1 = 9.3^*$, $P = 0.002$		$\chi^2_1 = 5.9^*$, $P = 0.015$		$\chi^2_1 = 24.3^*$, $P < 0.001$		$\chi^2_1 = 10.3^*$, $P = 0.001$	
Employment status								
Student	**0.8**	(0.5–1.4)	**1.1**	(0.8–1.4)	**1.2**	(0.7–2.0)	**0.8**	(0.4–1.5)
Homemaker	**1.4***	(1.0–1.9)	**0.9**	(0.8–1.1)	**1.4**	(0.9–2.0)	**1.5**	(1.0–2.4)
Retired	**1.2**	(0.7–2.1)	**0.8**	(0.6–1.2)	**1.2**	(0.7–2.1)	**1.8**	(0.8–4.0)
Other	**2.8***	(2.1–3.6)	**2.0***	(1.7–2.3)	**1.6***	(1.2–2.2)	**1.6***	(1.1–2.3)
Employed	**1.0**		**1.0**		**1.0**		**1.0**	

Table 5.3 (*cont.*)

Correlates	30-day bipolar spectrum disorder[a]		Lifetime bipolar spectrum disorder[b]		12-month bipolar spectrum disorder among lifetime cases[c]		30-day bipolar spectrum disorder among 12-month cases[c]	
	OR	(95% CI)	OR	(95% CI)	OR	(95% CI)	OR	(95% CI)
Employment status difference[d]	$\chi^2_4 = 56.4^*$, $P < 0.001$		$\chi^2_4 = 90.4^*$, $P < 0.001$		$\chi^2_4 = 10.0^*$, $P = 0.040$		$\chi^2_4 = 10.9^*$, $P = 0.028$	
Marital status								
Never married	**1.5***	(1.1–1.9)	**1.6***	(1.4–1.9)	**1.3***	(1.0–1.7)	**1.1**	(0.8–1.5)
Divorced/separated/widowed	**3.1***	(2.3–4.0)	**2.1***	(1.8–2.4)	**1.7***	(1.3–2.2)	**1.2**	(0.8–1.8)
Currently married	**1.0**		**1.0**		**1.0**		**1.0**	
Marital status difference[d]	$\chi^2_2 = 68.9^*$, $P < 0.001$		$\chi^2_2 = 149.8^*$, $P < 0.001$		$\chi^2_2 = 18.0^*$, $P < 0.001$		$\chi^2_2 = 0.8$, $P = 0.662$	
Education level								
No education	**3.8***	(1.3–10.8)	**1.3**	(0.7–2.5)	**2.5**	(0.6–9.7)	**5.6**	(0.9–34.5)
Some primary	**3.1***	(1.7–5.8)	**1.8***	(1.3–2.4)	**1.4**	(0.7–2.6)	**3.3***	(1.6–6.8)
Finished primary	**2.7***	(1.5–4.7)	**2.1***	(1.6–2.6)	**1.2**	(0.7–1.9)	**1.8**	(0.8–3.7)
Some secondary	**2.6***	(1.7–3.9)	**1.8***	(1.5–2.2)	**1.3**	(0.9–1.8)	**1.9***	(1.2–3.1)
Finished secondary	**2.4***	(1.7–3.6)	**1.8***	(1.5–2.2)	**1.6***	(1.1–2.2)	**1.6***	(1.0–2.6)
Some college	**1.8***	(1.2–2.7)	**1.5***	(1.2–1.8)	**1.4**	(1.0–2.0)	**1.3**	(0.8–2.3)
Finished college	**1.0**		**1.0**		**1.0**		**1.0**	
Education level difference[d]	$\chi^2_6 = 28.4^*$, $P < 0.001$		$\chi^2_6 = 52.5^*$, $P < 0.001$		$\chi^2_6 = 8.9$, $P = 0.181$		$\chi^2_6 = 15.0^*$, $P = 0.021$	
Household income								
Low	**1.4***	(1.0–1.9)	**1.4***	(1.2–1.6)	**1.4***	(1.1–1.9)	**1.0**	(0.7–1.4)
Low-average	**1.1**	(0.8–1.5)	**1.2***	(1.0–1.4)	**0.9**	(0.7–1.3)	**0.9**	(0.6–1.4)
High-average	**0.9**	(0.6–1.2)	**1.1**	(0.9–1.3)	**1.3**	(1.0–1.8)	**0.6***	(0.4–0.9)
High	**1.0**		**1.0**		**1.0**		**1.0**	
Household income difference[d]	$\chi^2_3 = 10.1^*$, $P = 0.018$		$\chi^2_3 = 19.0^*$, $P < 0.001$		$\chi^2_3 = 12.5^*$, $P = 0.006$		$\chi^2_3 = 6.4$, $P = 0.092$	
N[e]	**116,799**		**5,012,383**		**2,292**		**1,369**	

*Significant at the 0.05 level, two-sided test.
[a]These estimates are based on logistic regression models adjusted for age, gender, and country.
[b]These estimates are based on survival models adjusted for age-cohorts, gender, person-years, and country.
[c]These estimates are based on logistic regression models adjusted for time since bipolar spectrum disorder onset, age of bipolar spectrum disorder onset, gender, and country.
[d]Chi-square test of significant differences between blocks of socio-demographic variables.
[e]Denominator N: 116,799 = total sample; 5,012,383 = number of person-years in the survival models; 2,292 = number of lifetime bipolar spectrum disorder cases; 1,369 = number of 12-month bipolar spectrum disorder cases.

These associations were examined in more detail in an earlier WMH report (Breslau *et al.* 2011) and have also been documented in previous studies (Forthofer *et al.* 1996; Kessler *et al.* 1998). This finding is consistent with evidence of broader problems in interpersonal functioning described below. A final consistent pattern in Table 5.3 is that BP spectrum disorder is positively associated with disadvantaged socio-economic status as indicated by 'other' (mostly unemployed and disabled) employment status, low educational attainment, and low household income. These associations are for the most part significant both with lifetime prevalence and persistence, resulting in the highest ORs being with 30-day prevalence and with any of the components of 30-day prevalence. It is important to recognize that these indicators of disadvantaged socio-economic status were assessed as of the time of interview, which means that they could have occurred subsequent to the onset of the BP spectrum disorder and could be causes, consequences, or non-causal covariates (Koenders *et al.* 2014). It might be that this point-in-time approach to assessment is responsible for the fact that these associations are stronger and more consistent in the WMH data than in most other studies (reviewed in Eid *et al.* 2013).

Rapid Cycling

The natural history of BPD consists of distinct manic, hypomanic, depressive, and mixed-mood episodes that can switch quickly from one pole to another or are separated by periods of subsyndromal symptoms and euthymia (Judd *et al.* 2008; Alvarez Ariza *et al.* 2009). Polarity, frequency, duration, and intensity of episodes (along with psychosis) are highly variable, both within and between individuals. Rapid cycling has been studied in patients accrued through diverse clinical samples and has been associated with an earlier AOO and greater illness burden (Bauer *et al.* 1994). Clinical samples could be expected, however, to have a greater proportion of patients with rapid cycling than those in the general population, as rapid cycling would be expected to have a higher burden of disease and greater distress and, as a result, a higher probability of seeking help than those without rapid cycling, leading to bias in estimates of prevalence and correlates (Oepen *et al.* 2004).

The prevalence and correlates of rapid cycling in the community are unknown. Assessing rapid cycling in large community samples presents a challenge because it can be difficult to gather the data needed to obtain a precise and valid count of onset and offset of episodes, as well as clearly delineated two-month periods of partial or full remission or a switch to another episode of opposite polarity in community samples. Nevertheless, WMH data provide some relevant information. Although rapid cycling was not operationalized precisely, we were able to define cases with frequent mood episodes (FME) as a proxy measure for rapid cycling. In a pair of prior WMH reports we defined FME simply as self-report of four or more separate major depressive episodes or mania/hypomania episodes within a year (Lee *et al.* 2010; Nierenberg *et al.* 2010). We found that roughly 40% of cases with 12-month BPD and 30% of those with lifetime BPD had FME. Among respondents with a lifetime history of BPD, those with FME had an earlier AOO, higher persistence, more severe depressive symptoms, greater impairment associated with depressive symptoms, more days-out-of-role associated with mania/hypomania, more anxiety disorders, and increased likelihood of using health services.

Comparative Frequency-Intensity of Manic, Hypomanic, and Depressive Episodes

Clinical studies have been quite interested in comparative frequency and severity of manic, hypomanic, depressive, and mixed episodes among patients with BPD (reviewed by Saunders & Goodwin 2010). These studies show that depressive episodes typically have first onsets earlier than manic-hypomanic episodes in BPD; that depressive episodes are more frequent in BPD than mania-hypomania or mixed episodes; that mixed episodes typically have the longest episode duration, depressive episodes intermediate duration, and manic-hypomanic episodes the shortest duration; and that patients report more impairment associated with their depressive than their manic-hypomanic episodes. Little research on these differences has been carried out in the WMH surveys, as the cross-sectional WMH survey design does not lend itself to studying course of illness.

However, a few relevant findings have emerged from WMH studies. First, an analysis of 12-month prevalence among employed respondents with lifetime BPD in the US WMH survey found that number of days depressed in the past year far exceeded number of days with mania or hypomania, that depressive episodes were associated with more severe work role impairment than manic-hypomanic episodes, and, interestingly, that the major depressive episodes of workers with BPD were more persistent and severely impairing than the major depressive episodes of workers with major depressive disorder (Kessler *et al.* 2006a). Another WMH paper found results consistent with prospective clinical studies that depressive episodes in BPD typically have first onsets prior to manic-hypomanic episodes, that the proportion of days depressed in the preceding year is significantly associated with shorter time to depressive recurrence, and that role impairments are more pronounced in depressive than manic-hypomanic episodes. Regarding the latter, the proportion of respondents with 12-month BPD reporting severe role impairment associated with major depressive episode was 74.0% compared to 50.9% associated with mania-hypomania.

Comorbidity

An earlier WMH report documented that the vast majority of WMH respondents with a history of BP spectrum disorder also meet lifetime criteria for at least one of the other DSM-IV/CIDI disorders assessed in the survey (Merikangas *et al.* 2011). As shown in Table 5.4, this high lifetime comorbidity is even a bit higher for people with 12-month BP spectrum disorder (79.5% of whom have at least one lifetime comorbid disorder compared to 77.3% among all respondents with lifetime BP spectrum disorder), suggesting indirectly that lifetime comorbidity is to some extent associated with increased persistence of BP spectrum disorder. We also see in Table 5.4 that BP spectrum disorder typically has a later AOO than comorbid disorders, with only 10.9% of lifetime cases with the relevant comorbidity having onsets prior to first comorbid anxiety disorders, 14.9% before first comorbid disruptive behaviour/impulse-control disorders, and 38.1% before first comorbid substance-use disorders. This consistent temporal priority suggests indirectly that earlier disorders are significant predictors of the subsequent first onset of BP spectrum disorder, but this cannot be evaluated in the table due to the absence of comparison data on prevalence of comorbid disorders among respondents who do not meet criteria for BP spectrum disorder. The same limitation makes it impossible for us to judge the comparative strength of associations of BP spectrum disorder with each of the other kinds of disorder shown in Table 5.4, even though lifetime comorbid anxiety disorders are much more common than lifetime comorbid disruptive behaviour/impulse-control or substance-use disorders (60.4%, 25.8%, and 39.0%, respectively) because anxiety disorders are much more common than these other disorders in the total population (see Chapter 20 for the *associations* between lifetime mental disorders). In a similar way, the results reported in Table 5.4 on 12-month comorbidity among 12-month cases, while useful from the perspective of simple description in telling us that 65.6% of people with 12-month BP spectrum disorder also have at least one other comorbid disorder over the same time period, cannot be used to draw inferences about synchrony of course of illness of BP spectrum disorder and comorbid disorders.

Other WMH analyses reported elsewhere used retrospective AOO reports about each lifetime hierarchy-free disorder assessed in the surveys to investigate predictive associations of temporally prior lifetime disorders with the subsequent first lifetime onset of each other disorder (Kessler *et al.* 2011). The 18 disorders considered in the analysis generated 306 (18×17) time-lagged bivariate associations (survival coefficients) between prior onset of one disorder in the set and subsequent first onset of one of the other disorders. Significant positive time-lagged associations were pervasive, even after adjusting for age, gender, person-year, and survey, with 98.0% of coefficients positive and 95.1% significant at the 0.05 level. This pattern remained in attenuated form in multivariate models where we posited the existence of latent internalizing and externalizing liabilities that were affected by each of the temporally primary disorders. BPD (subthreshold BPD was not assessed in the analysis) was a significant predictor of later disorders with a strength of association in predicting the latent liability (0.18) larger than those of panic disorder and generalized anxiety disorder (nonsignificant), comparable to those of PTSD and major depressive episode (0.21–0.29), but smaller than those of other internalizing disorders: agoraphobia, separation anxiety disorder, social phobia, specific phobia, with coefficients in the range 0.44–1.0. The reciprocal association of the latent liability predicting subsequent first onset of BP disorder was quite comparable in magnitude to the associations of the latent liability with other internalizing disorder outcomes. These results suggest that the major reason for the high comorbidity of BP disorder with many other DSM-IV/CIDI disorders is that prior onset of other disorders predicts subsequent onset of BPD.

Role Impairment

We know from many previous studies that the lives of people with BP disorder are fraught with difficulties. Patients with BP disorder have substantially elevated

Table 5.4 Comorbidity of bipolar spectrum disorder with other DSM-IV disorders, all countries combined

	Bipolar spectrum disorder cases with comorbid disorders							
	Anxiety disorder[a]		Disruptive behaviour/ impulse-control disorder[b]		Substance-use disorder[c]		Any mental disorder[d]	
	%	SE	%	SE	%	SE	%	SE
Lifetime comorbidity[e]								
Lifetime	**60.4**	1.3	**25.8**	1.3	**39.0**	1.4	**77.3**	1.2
12-month	**63.8**	1.8	**27.8**	1.6	**40.2**	1.8	**79.7**	1.5
12-month comorbidity[f]								
12-month	**53.7**	1.8	**19.8**	1.4	**18.9**	1.5	**65.6**	1.8
Temporal priority of bipolar spectrum disorder[g]								
Lifetime	**10.9**	1.1	**14.9**	1.9	**38.1**	2.5	**11.5**	1.1
12-month	**11.0**	1.4	**15.1**	2.2	**41.8**	3.3	**12.0**	1.3

[a]Respondents with panic disorder, generalized anxiety disorder, social phobia, specific phobia, agoraphobia, post-traumatic stress disorder, or separation anxiety disorder.
[b]Respondents with intermittent explosive disorder, conduct disorder, attention-deficit disorder, oppositional-defiant disorder, binge-eating disorder, or bulimia nervosa.
[c]Respondents with alcohol abuse with or without dependence or drug abuse with or without dependence.
[d]Respondents with any disorder listed above.
[e]Percentage of respondents with either lifetime or 12-month bipolar spectrum disorder who also meet lifetime criteria for at least one of the other DSM-IV disorders.
[f]Percentage of respondents with 12-month bipolar spectrum disorder who also meet 12-month criteria for at least one of the other disorders.
[g]Percentage of respondents with either lifetime or 12-month bipolar spectrum disorder and at least one of the other disorders, whose AOO of bipolar spectrum disorder is reported to be younger than the AOO of all comorbid disorders under consideration.

rates of cardiovascular disease and associated mortality (Goldstein *et al.* 2009), high rates of suicide attempts (Tondo *et al.* 2016) and deaths (Pompili *et al.* 2013), and high rates of functional impairment (Miklowitz 2011). Earlier WMH reports, most of them pulled together in an earlier WMH volume on *The Burdens of Mental Disorders* (Alonso *et al.* 2013), documented many of these associations in the WMH data. One great appeal of having epidemiological data on a wide range of mental disorders across a number of countries is that information on these kinds of associations can be compared and contrasted to create a portrait of relative burden across disorders and to investigate the stability of this portrait across countries.

One of the most striking measures of impairment in the WMH surveys are responses to a series of visual analogue ratings based on the Sheehan Disability Scale (SDS; Leon *et al.* 1997). These ratings were administered to each WMH respondent with 12-month prevalence of any DSM-IV/CIDI disorder on a disorder-specific basis and focused on the month in the past 12 months when the disorder was most severe. Separate disorder-specific ratings were obtained on a 0 (*no interference*) to 10 (*very severe interference*) scale for how much the disorder interfered with the respondent's functioning at home, work, in interpersonal relationships, and in social life. The same questions were administered to respondents with any 12-month chronic physical disorder assessed in the surveys about one such random chronic physical disorder. As detailed in an earlier WMH report (Ormel *et al.* 2008), mental disorders were associated with significantly higher impairment scores than physical disorders, and BP disorder (subthreshold BPD was not assessed in that study) was associated with higher scores than any of the other mental disorders assessed in the surveys. And these patterns held both in high-income and in low/middle-income countries. Concretely, more than two-thirds of respondents with 12-month BP disorder in high-income countries reported severe role impairment in at last one of the four domains we considered due to their bipolar disorder compared to only a minority of those with most other DSM-IV/CIDI disorders and no more than about 40% of those with the chronic physical conditions assessed in the surveys (e.g., arthritis, cancer, heart disease).

The stability of these results for BP spectrum disorder across the expanded set of WMH countries considered here (only the first 16 WMH surveys were included in the Ormel *et al.* 2008 report) can be seen in Table 5.5. The proportion of respondents with 12-month BP reporting severe impairment in at least one role decreased from 68.3% in the Ormel *et al.* report to 54.1% in our larger series of surveys with the addition of subthreshold BPD to the definition. The proportion reporting severe impairment ranges between a low of 30.6% in functioning at home to 35.0% for functioning in social life. The proportions with overall severe impairment are highest in high-income countries (59.2%), lower in upper-middle-income countries (50.8%), and considerably lower in low/lower-middle-income countries (35.4%). In terms of WHO regions, the proportions with overall severe impairment are highest in the Eastern Mediterranean (72.4%) and Eastern Europe (66.9%), lower in Western Europe (61.0%), and lowest in the Americas (51.5%) and the Western Pacific (50.0%), with too few cases to calculate a regional average in Africa.

Treatment

Twelve-month treatment of WMH respondents with BP spectrum disorder was 43.0% across all WMH countries and positively associated with country income level (52.5% in high-income countries, 24.0% in upper-middle-income countries, 23.9% in low/lower-middle-income countries; $F = 33.6$, $P < 0.001$) (Table 5.6). The same general pattern between country income level and probability of 12-month treatment held across all treatment sectors ($F = 6.5$–54.4, $P < 0.001$). Treatment was highest overall in the general medical (27.8%) and specialty mental health (26.2%) treatment sectors, but the proportion in treatment was higher in the former than latter sector in high-income countries (37.3% vs. 31.7%) but the reverse in upper-middle and low/lower-middle-income countries (8.0–9.6% vs. 14.7–15.8%). The proportion in treatment was higher overall among cases with severe impairment (50.5%) than those with either moderate (30.8%) or mild (31.5%) impairment. Although not shown in the table, an earlier WMH report showed that treatment rates are considerably higher for people with BP-I and BP-II disorders than those with subthreshold BPD (Merikangas *et al.* 2011).

Although we focused here on 12-month treatment, it is noteworthy that other WMH country-specific reports have shown that the vast majority of people with BPD eventually seek treatment but that delays of a decade or more are not uncommon between AOO of the disorder and age of first seeking treatment (e.g., Wang *et al.* 2007a; Bunting *et al.* 2012; ten Have *et al.*

Table 5.5 Severity of role impairment (Sheehan Disability Scale) associated with 12-month bipolar spectrum disorder, by country

Country	Proportion with severe role impairment (SDS score: 7–10)										Number of 12-month cases
	Home		Work		Relationship		Social		Any[a]		
	%	SE	%	SE	%	SE	%	SE	%	SE	
Low/lower-middle-income countries	**24.1**	**4.7**	**22.1**	**4.7**	**15.9**	**3.3**	**27.8**	**5.2**	**35.4**	**5.2**	**168**
Colombia	38.6	10.0	29.3	10.4	18.8	5.5	33.4	9.9	45.7	9.9	65
Iraq	–	–	–	–	–	–	–	–	–	–	6
Nigeria	–	–	–	–	–	–	–	–	–	–	2
Peru	37.3	10.7	34.8	9.5	34.3	10.5	27.2	7.8	46.0	12.4	30
PRC (Beijing/Shanghai)	–	–	–	–	–	–	–	–	–	–	4
PRC (Shenzhen)	4.8	3.3	6.9	4.1	7.7	4.2	16.2	6.6	19.0	6.7	61
Upper-middle-income countries	**28.4**	**4.6**	**26.8**	**3.8**	**32.0**	**4.5**	**30.2**	**4.2**	**50.8**	**4.5**	**230**
Brazil	27.2	10.9	40.6	8.2	41.2	9.2	40.2	7.7	55.0	8.6	73
Bulgaria	–	–	–	–	–	–	–	–	–	–	3
Colombia (Medellin)	51.6	13.2	23.1	10.6	30.6	11.3	14.4	7.6	61.4	12.8	25
Lebanon	30.0	9.6	26.8	7.9	30.6	9.2	31.3	9.9	58.1	9.1	44
Mexico	18.0	4.7	13.6	4.7	15.5	5.8	12.3	4.1	30.3	6.2	64
Romania	38.2	13.3	34.4	11.3	46.3	13.4	59.4	13.2	58.9	14.2	21
High-income countries	**32.7**	**2.0**	**34.4**	**2.2**	**36.9**	**2.1**	**38.1**	**2.0**	**59.2**	**2.1**	**971**
Australia	23.3	4.4	30.3	6.4	35.6	5.3	30.4	4.9	53.7	5.8	142
Israel	81.1	8.8	86.1	7.6	84.6	8.6	74.2	10.4	100.0	0.0	22
Japan	12.0	11.4	47.1	26.1	12.0	11.4	37.2	18.2	51.6	19.7	9
New Zealand	27.9	3.8	37.1	4.0	32.0	3.6	34.1	3.8	58.0	4.2	351
Northern Ireland	43.2	7.0	39.3	7.5	42.2	7.1	53.0	7.9	65.3	6.9	86
Poland	61.0	9.6	36.8	9.7	56.2	9.7	49.0	10.8	72.9	9.0	35
Portugal	28.1	8.6	30.6	10.2	20.8	7.3	24.9	6.9	55.0	8.6	45
Spain (Murcia)	38.4	11.7	59.9	9.8	41.5	9.8	59.9	9.8	59.9	9.8	19
United States	32.1	3.2	24.5	3.2	36.5	3.8	38.2	3.0	56.6	3.4	262
All countries combined	**30.6**	**1.7**	**31.1**	**1.8**	**32.9**	**1.7**	**35.0**	**1.7**	**54.1**	**1.8**	**1,369**

Table 5.5 (*cont.*)

Country	Proportion with severe role impairment (SDS score: 7–10)										Number of 12-month cases
	Home		Work		Relationship		Social		Any[a]		
	%	SE	%	SE	%	SE	%	SE	%	SE	
WHO regions											
Region of the Americas	31.9	2.8	26.4	2.6	32.1	2.8	32.7	2.5	51.5	2.8	519
African region	–	–	–	–	–	–	–	–	–	–	2
Western Pacific region	22.2	2.5	30.1	2.9	28.2	2.6	29.8	2.7	50.0	3.1	567
Eastern Mediterranean region	54.0	8.2	51.9	7.5	48.1	7.3	48.3	8.1	72.4	6.7	72
Western European region	37.4	5.0	40.3	5.4	35.1	4.7	45.1	5.3	61.0	4.7	150
Eastern European region	47.0	8.4	31.9	7.0	53.1	7.8	53.3	8.4	66.9	7.6	59
Comparison between countries[b]	**$F_{20,v} = 3.2^*$, $P < 0.001$**		**$F_{20,v} = 2.8^*$, $P < 0.001$**		**$F_{20,v} = 2.9^*$, $P < 0.001$**		**$F_{20,v} = 2.6^*$, $P < 0.001$**		**$F_{20,v} = 2.9^*$, $P < 0.001$**		
Comparison between low-, middle-, and high-income countries[b]	**$F_{2,v} = 1.6$, $P = 0.208$**		**$F_{2,v} = 3.6^*$, $P = 0.028$**		**$F_{2,v} = 11.1^*$, $P < 0.001$**		**$F_{2,v} = 2.7$, $P = 0.064$**		**$F_{2,v} = 8.8^*$, $P < 0.001$**		
Comparison between WHO regions[b]	**$F_{5,v} = 4.9^*$, $P < 0.001$**		**$F_{5,v} = 2.6^*$, $P = 0.024$**		**$F_{5,v} = 2.5^*$, $P = 0.029$**		**$F_{5,v} = 3.0^*$, $P = 0.001$**		**$F_{5,v} = 3.0^*$, $P = 0.010$**		

*Significant at the 0.05 level, two-sided test.
A dash indicates low cell counts (<5 cases).
[a]Highest severity category across four SDS role domains.
[b]Wald design-corrected F-tests were used to determine if there is variation in impairment severity across countries. The denominator degree of freedom, v, is 5134.
PRC: People's Republic of China.

Table 5.6 Among those with 12-month bipolar spectrum disorder, percent reporting treatment in the past 12 months by Sheehan impairment severity

Sector of treatment	Sheehan Disability Scale category[a]											
	Mild impairment (score: 1–3)			Moderate impairment (score: 4–6)			Severe impairment (score: 7–10)			Any impairment		
	%	SE	Comparison between country income groups[b]	%	SE	Comparison between country income groups[b]	%	SE	Comparison between country income groups[b]	%	SE	Comparison between country income groups[b]
Specialty mental health[c]												
Low/lower-middle-income countries	–	–	–	–	–	$F_{2,v} = 3.0$, $P = 0.05$	**23.3**	8.8	$F_{2,v} = 3.8^*$, $P = 0.02$	**15.8**	4.2	$F_{2,v} = 16.2^*$, $P < 0.001$
Upper-middle-income countries	–	–		**8.6**	4.3		**19.7**	5.3		**14.7**	2.7	
High-income countries	**22.7**	7.5		**22.6**	3.8		**35.3**	2.8		**31.7**	1.8	
All countries combined	**20.9**	5.7		**18.2**	2.9		**31.4**	2.4		**26.2**	1.4	
General medical[d]												
Low/lower-middle-income countries	–	–	–	–	–	–	**5.5**	2.6	$F_{2,v} = 23.4^*$, $P < 0.001$	**9.6**	3.1	$F_{2,v} = 54.4^*$, $P < 0.001$
Upper-middle-income countries	–	–		–	–		**8.3**	3.8		**8.0**	1.9	
High-income countries	**25.7**	6.6		**25.2**	3.6		**41.5**	2.8		**37.3**	1.8	
All countries combined	**20.6**	5.1		**18.2**	2.6		**32.0**	2.4		**27.8**	1.4	
Any health care[e]												
Low/lower-middle-income countries	–	–	–	–	–	$F_{2,v} = 6.5^*$, $P = 0.002$	**27.3**	8.8	$F_{2,v} = 14.5^*$, $P < 0.001$	**20.8**	4.1	$F_{2,v} = 41.5^*$, $P < 0.001$
Upper-middle-income countries	–	–		**12.5**	5.3		**22.3**	5.3		**19.5**	2.8	
High-income countries	**31.7**	7.7		**35.7**	4.3		**54.9**	2.9		**49.1**	1.9	
All countries combined	**28.6**	5.9		**27.8**	3.2		**46.3**	2.6		**39.4**	1.6	
Human services[f]												
Low/lower-middle-income countries	–	–	–	–	–	–	–	–	–	**3.4**	1.9	$F_{2,v} = 6.5^*$, $P = 0.002$
Upper-middle-income countries	–	–		–	–		–	–		**3.5**	1.2	
High-income countries	–	–		**2.9**	1.0		**11.1**	1.7		**8.7**	1.0	
All countries combined	**9.5**	3.7		**2.1**	0.7		**9.5**	1.4		**7.0**	0.8	
CAM[g]												
Low/lower-middle-income countries	–	–	–	–	–	–	–	–	$F_{2,v} = 5.9^*$, $P = 0.003$	–	–	$F_{2,v} = 21.3^*$, $P < 0.001$
Upper-middle-income countries	–	–		–	–		**4.2**	2.6		**2.7**	1.2	
High-income countries	–	–		**8.8**	2.7		**10.2**	1.7		**10.3**	1.3	
All countries combined	–	–		**5.8**	1.8		**8.3**	1.3		**7.4**	0.9	

Table 5.6 *(cont.)*

Sector of treatment	Sheehan Disability Scale category[a]											
	Mild impairment (score: 1–3)			Moderate impairment (score: 4–6)			Severe impairment (score: 7–10)			Any impairment		
	%	SE	Comparison between country income groups[b]	%	SE	Comparison between country income groups[b]	%	SE	Comparison between country income groups[b]	%	SE	Comparison between country income groups[b]
Any non-health care[h]												
Low/lower-middle-income countries	–	–	–	–	–	–	**9.3**	6.4	$F_{2,v}=3.6^*$, $P=0.03$	**3.7**	2.0	$F_{2,v}=14.5^*$, $P<0.001$
Upper-middle-income countries	–	–		–	–		**8.0**	3.4		**5.9**	1.7	
High-income countries	**13.2**	5.7		**11.1**	2.8		**18.7**	2.4		**16.6**	1.5	
All countries combined	**10.9**	3.8		**7.5**	1.9		**15.9**	1.9		**12.7**	1.1	
Any treatment[i]												
Low/lower-middle-income countries	**32.1**	13.6	$F_{2,v}=0.0$, $P=0.95$	**13.9**	7.0	$F_{2,v}=8.0^*$, $P<0.001$	**34.3**	9.4	$F_{2,v}=8.8^*$ $P<0.001$	**23.9**	4.4	$F_{2,v}=33.6^*$, $P<0.001$
Upper-middle-income countries	**27.6**	12.8		**13.3**	5.3		**28.8**	7.1		**24.0**	3.5	
High-income countries	**32.4**	7.7		**40.0**	4.4		**58.1**	2.9		**52.5**	1.9	
All countries combined	**31.5**	6.1		**30.8**	3.3		**50.5**	2.7		**43.0**	1.6	

*Significant at the 0.05 level, two-sided test.
A dash indicates low cell counts (<5 cases).
[a]Highest severity category across four SDS role domains.
[b]Wald design-corrected F-tests were used to determine if there is variation in treatment estimates across country income groups. The denominator degree of freedom, v, is 5134. Wald tests only generated where there is more than one stable cell (≥5 cases) for each combination of treatment sector and Sheehan impairment.
[c]The mental health specialist sector, which includes psychiatrist and non-psychiatrist mental health specialists (psychiatrist, psychologist or other non-psychiatrist mental health professional; social worker or counsellor in a mental health specialty setting; use of a mental health helpline; or overnight admissions for a mental health or drug or alcohol problems, with a presumption of daily contact with a psychiatrist).
[d]The general medical sector (general practitioner, other medical doctor, nurse, occupational therapist or any healthcare professional).
[e]The mental health specialist sector or the general medical sector.
[f]The human services sector (religious or spiritual advisor or social worker or counsellor in any setting other than a specialty mental health setting).
[g]The CAM (complementary and alternative medicine) sector (any other type of healer, such as herbalist or homeopath, participation in an internet support group, or participation in a self-help group).
[h]The human services sector or CAM.
[i]Any treatment listed above.

2013). There is very little other research on this issue to which the WMH results can be compared, but the small amount of such research, which typically reconstructs 'pathways to care' in interviews with patients seeking treatment, is consistent with the WMH data in suggesting that long delays often exist between onset of BPD and first seeking treatment (Baldessarini *et al.* 1999; Oyffe *et al.* 2015).

Discussion

As noted several times throughout this chapter, the WMH surveys are limited in a number of ways that need to be kept in mind in interpreting results: that response rates varied considerably across surveys; lifetime disorders were assessed retrospectively using fully structured rather than semi-structured interviews, probably leading to under estimation of lifetime prevalence and over-estimation of AOO and of the effects of AAI and comorbidity; and that mixed episodes were not assessed. Nonetheless, the data reported here provide the most complete population-based data on the epidemiology of BP spectrum disorder assembled to date.

Although a previous WMH report suggested that the prevalence estimates of BP spectrum disorder from the first WMH surveys were somewhat lower than those in earlier studies (Merikangas *et al.* 2011), we noted above that the more complete set of WMH estimates reported here are within the range of the estimates reported in previous studies of lifetime (Dell'Aglio *et al.* 2013) and recent (Ferrari *et al.* 2016) prevalence. Our use of a consistent diagnostic assessment tool overcomes the problem of cross-study variation in prevalence estimates due to some of the methodological factors that have been noted by the authors of previous reviews (Waraich *et al.* 2004; Pini *et al.* 2005; Dell'Aglio *et al.* 2013). Our finding that 25% of people in the population with BP spectrum disorder date their onset to the first 18 years of life and that fully half date their onset to the first 25 years of life is consistent with previous research on AOO of BPD (Kessler *et al.* 2007; McGorry *et al.* 2011; de Girolamo *et al.* 2012). Although caution is needed in interpreting retrospective AOO reports (Jones 2013), the consistent evidence across WMH countries that many cases begin in childhood, adolescence, or early adulthood raises the possibility that early interventions might be effective in influencing the course of BPD (McGorry 2015; Srihari *et al.* 2016). This is all the more important given the fact, noted in the treatment section, that long delays are quite common in initial help-seeking for treatment of BPD after first onset.

Unlike earlier WMH reports on BP spectrum disorder, which were designed to evaluate the validity of the spectrum concept (Merikangas *et al.* 2007, 2011), we assumed the validity of this concept in this chapter and consequently reported only aggregated results that combined BP-I, BP-II, and subthreshold BPD into a single category. It is noteworthy, though, that earlier WMH reports that investigated the validity of this concept documented significant gradients from BP-I through BP-II to subthreshold BPD in numerous indicators of clinical severity, including symptom severity, role impairment, comorbidity, and suicidality. For example, Merikangas *et al.* (2011) showed that the proportion of mood episodes rated as clinically severe was 74.5% for BP-I, 68.8% for BP-II, and 42.5% for subthreshold BPD, while the proportion of cases reporting suicidal ideation was 52.2% for BP-I, 50.6% for BP-II, and 36.3% for subthreshold BPD. These disaggregated analyses of the three types of BPD demonstrated patterns of association that lend epidemiological-level support to the concept of bipolar spectrum disorder vis-à-vis unipolar depressive disorder.

Additionally, our finding that the majority of people with lifetime BPD report that their depression started earlier than their mania-hypomania reinforces the concerns expressed by many others about inaccurate diagnosis and treatment of BP depressive episodes as if they were part of a unipolar major depressive disorder; an intervention that can lead to rapid switching that, in turn, can result in increased risk of suicide (Hirschfeld 2007; Nasrallah 2015). In the absence of a history of mania or hypomania, clinicians lack biomarkers that distinguish BP from unipolar depressive episodes. While researchers continue to search for such biomarkers (e.g., genetics and neuroimaging) to avoid a mismatch in treatment, the identification of such biomarkers continues to be elusive.

Caution is needed in interpreting the WMH results regarding rapid cycling due to the limitations of recall in cross-sectional surveys, the inability of a fully-structured lay interview to assess partial remission and switching, and the fact that the CIDI did not assess mixed episodes. Despite these limitations, though, the WMH results confirmed a number of well-documented clinical findings. We found a similar, although somewhat higher, proportion of BP cases with rapid cycling than in clinical studies (e.g., Coryell *et al.* 2003; Cruz *et al.* 2008). We also found a good deal of evidence consistent with the finding in clinical studies (e.g., Schneck *et al.* 2004; Bauer *et al.* 2008) that BPD with rapid cycling is a more severe form of BPD.

Our finding of pervasive comorbidity in BP spectrum disorder is consistent with much previous research on comorbid conditions in BPD (e.g., Grant *et al.* 2005; Keller 2006), but extends this evidence to include subthreshold BPD. As shown in a previous WMH report (Merikangas *et al.* 2011), even though this comorbidity is higher in BP-I and BP-II than in subthreshold BPD, more than two-thirds of the latter have a history of at least one lifetime comorbid DSM-IV/CIDI disorder and nearly one-third have a history of three or more such comorbid disorders. The findings that bipolar disorders typically are temporally secondary and that comorbid anxiety disorders are usually the initial disorders are consistent with more general evidence about the typically early AOOs of anxiety disorders (Kessler *et al.* 2007a,b).

Our finding of high role impairments in BP spectrum disorder is consistent with a great deal of other evidence documenting the fact that BPD is a serious disorder associated not only with impairment in functioning but also with increased risk of early mortality. The WMH data add to earlier evidence along these lines, though, in showing that a similar pattern occurs for subthreshold BPD and in the general population. This evidence of severity makes the WMH data on low treatment of BPD all the more important even though we found that treatment of BPD is much more common than treatment of most other mental disorders (Wang *et al.* 2007b; Thornicroft *et al.* 2016). We also found that substantial delays occur between onset of BPD and first contact with the treatment system. This is an important problem given consistent evidence that BPD treatment is more effective early than late in the course of the disorder (Oyffe *et al.* 2015; Joyce *et al.* 2016). In addition, other WMH analyses not reviewed in this paper revealed another problem of considerable importance regarding treatment: that only a minority of the people treated for mental disorders in the WMH surveys described a type of treatment that met even the most minimal standards of adequacy (Wang *et al.* 2007b). It is unclear how to resolve this problem, but it is clear that earlier recognition, more timely treatment, and treatment of higher quality are needed to address the enormous individual and societal burden of BP spectrum disorder.

While leaving many issues unexamined, the results reviewed in this chapter show that the epidemiological data in the WMH surveys support the validity of the bipolar spectrum disorder concept. Based on this fact, the new version of CIDI being developed to operationalize DSM-5 criteria is including more explicit questions than in the DSM-IV version to assess mixed episodes, to improve the detection of BP-II and distinguish it from subthreshold BPD, and to allow a more nuanced investigation of the bipolar spectrum than in the WMH analyses carried out up to now. We anticipate that the data from future WMH surveys using this revised instrument will shed new light on BP spectrum disorders beyond the results reported here.

References

Akiskal, H. S., Bourgeois, M. L., Angst, J., *et al.* (2000). Re-evaluating the prevalence of and diagnostic composition within the broad clinical spectrum of bipolar disorders. *Journal of Affective Disorders* 59, S5–S30.

Alonso, J., Chatterji, S., & He, Y., eds. (2013). *The Burdens of Mental Disorders: Global Perspectives from the WHO World Mental Health Surveys.* New York Cambridge University Press.

Alvarez Ariza, M., Mateos Alvarez, R., & Berrios, G. E. (2009). A review of the natural course of bipolar disorders (manic-depressive psychosis) in the pre-drug era: review of studies prior to 1950. *Journal of Affective Disorders* 115, 293–301.

American Psychiatric Association (2013). *Diagnostic and Statistical Manual of Mental Disorders, 5th edition, Text Revision.* Washington, DC: American Psychiatric Association.

Baldessarini, R. J., Tondo, L., Hennen, J., & Floris, G. (1999). Latency and episodes before treatment: response to lithium maintenance in bipolar I and II disorders. *Bipolar Disorders* 1, 91–7.

Bauer, M. S., Beaulieu, S., Dunner, D. L., *et al.* (2008). Rapid cycling bipolar disorder–diagnostic concepts. *Bipolar Disorders* 10, 153–62.

Bauer, M. S., Calabrese, J., Dunner, D. L., *et al.* (1994). Multisite data reanalysis of the validity of rapid cycling as a course modifier for bipolar disorder in DSM-IV. *The American Journal of Psychiatry* 151, 506–15.

Breslau, J., Miller, E., Jin, R., *et al.* (2011). A multinational study of mental disorders, marriage, and divorce. *Acta Psychiatrica Scandinavica* 124, 474–86.

Bunting, B. P., Murphy, S. D., O'Neill, S. M., & Ferry, F. R. (2012). Lifetime prevalence of mental health disorders and delay in treatment following initial onset: evidence from the Northern Ireland Study of Health and Stress. *Psychological Medicine* 42, 1727–39.

Coryell, W., Solomon, D., Turvey, C., *et al.* (2003). The long-term course of rapid-cycling bipolar disorder. *Archives of General Psychiatry* 60, 914–20.

Cruz, N., Vieta, E., Comes, M., *et al.* (2008). Rapid-cycling bipolar I disorder: course and treatment outcome of a large sample across Europe. *Journal of Psychiatric Research* 42, 1068–75.

de Girolamo, G., Dagani, J., Purcell, R., Cocchi, A., & McGorry, P. D. (2012). Age of onset of mental disorders and use of mental health services: needs, opportunities and obstacles. *Epidemiology and Psychiatric Sciences* 21, 47–57.

Dell'Aglio, J. C., Jr., Basso, L. A., Argimon, II, & Arteche, A. (2013). Systematic review of the prevalence of bipolar disorder and bipolar spectrum disorders in population-based studies. *Trends in Psychiatry and Psychotherapy* 35, 99–105.

Diflorio, A., & Jones, I. (2010). Is sex important? Gender differences in bipolar disorder. *International Review of Psychiatry* 22, 437–52.

Duffy, A. (2014). Toward a comprehensive clinical staging model for bipolar disorder: integrating the evidence. *Canadian Journal of Psychiatry* 59, 659–66.

Eid, L., Heim, K., Doucette, S., *et al.* (2013). Bipolar disorder and socioeconomic status: what is the nature of this relationship? *International Journal of Bipolar Disorders* 1, 9.

Ferrari, A. J., Stockings, E., Khoo, J. P., *et al.* (2016). The prevalence and burden of bipolar disorder: findings from the Global Burden of Disease Study 2013. *Bipolar Disorders* 18, 440–50.

First, M. B., Spitzer, R. L., Gibbon, M., & Williams, J. B. W. (2002). *Structured Clinical Interview for DSM-IV Axis I Disorders, Research Version, Non-patient Edition (SCID-I/NP).* New York Biometrics Research, New York State Psychiatric Institute.

Forthofer, M. S., Kessler, R. C., Story, A. L., & Gotlib, I. H. (1996). The effects of psychiatric disorders on the probability and timing of first marriage. *Journal of Health and Social Behavior* 37, 121–32.

Frank, E., Nimgaonkar, V. L., Phillips, M. L., & Kupfer, D. J. (2015). All the world's a (clinical) stage: rethinking bipolar disorder from a longitudinal perspective. *Molecular Psychiatry* 20, 23–31.

Ghaemi, S. N., & Dalley, S. (2014). The bipolar spectrum: conceptions and misconceptions. *The Australian and New Zealand Journal of Psychiatry* 48, 314–24.

Goldstein, B. I., Fagiolini, A., Houck, P., & Kupfer, D. J. (2009). Cardiovascular disease and hypertension among adults with bipolar I disorder in the United States. *Bipolar Disorders* 11, 657–62.

Grant, B. F., Stinson, F. S., Hasin, D. S., *et al.* (2005). Prevalence, correlates, and comorbidity of bipolar I disorder and axis I and II disorders: results from the National Epidemiologic Survey on Alcohol and Related Conditions. *The Journal of Clinical Psychiatry* 66, 1205–15.

Hirschfeld, R.M. (2007). Screening for bipolar disorder. *The American Journal of Managed Care* 13 (Suppl 7), S164–9.

Jones, P. B. (2013). Adult mental health disorders and their age at onset. *The British Journal of Psychiatry. Supplement* 54, s5–10.

Joyce, K., Thompson, A., & Marwaha, S. (2016). Is treatment for bipolar disorder more effective earlier in illness course? A comprehensive literature review. *International Journal of Bipolar Disorders* 4, 19.

Judd, L. L., & Akiskal, H. S. (2003). The prevalence and disability of bipolar spectrum disorders in the US population: re-analysis of the ECA database taking into account subthreshold cases. *Journal of Affective Disorders* 73, 123–31.

Judd, L. L., Schettler, P. J., Akiskal, H. S., *et al.* (2008). Residual symptom recovery from major affective episodes in bipolar disorders and rapid episode relapse/recurrence. *Archives of General Psychiatry* 65, 386–94.

Karam, E. G., Sampson, N., Itani, L., *et al.* (2014). Under-reporting bipolar disorder in large-scale epidemiologic studies. *Journal of Affective Disorders* 159, 147–54.

Keller, M. B. (2006). Prevalence and impact of comorbid anxiety and bipolar disorder. *The Journal of Clinical Psychiatry* 67 (Suppl 1), 5–7.

Kessler, R. C., Akiskal, H. S., Ames, M., *et al.* (2006a). Prevalence and effects of mood disorders on work performance in a nationally representative sample of U.S. workers. *The American Journal of Psychiatry* 163, 1561–8.

Kessler, R. C., Akiskal, H. S., Angst, J., *et al.* (2006b). Validity of the assessment of bipolar spectrum disorders in the WHO CIDI 3.0. *Journal of Affective Disorders* 96, 259–69.

Kessler, R. C., Amminger, G. P., Aguilar-Gaxiola, S., *et al.* (2007a). Age of onset of mental disorders: a review of recent literature. *Current Opinion in Psychiatry* 20, 359–64.

Kessler, R. C., Angermeyer, M., Anthony, J. C., *et al.* (2007b). Lifetime prevalence and age-of-onset distributions of mental disorders in the World Health Organization's World Mental Health Survey Initiative. *World Psychiatry* 6, 168–76.

Kessler, R. C., Ormel, J., Petukhova, M., *et al.* (2011). Development of lifetime comorbidity in the World Health Organization World Mental Health Surveys. *Archives of General Psychiatry* 68, 90–100.

Kessler, R. C., Walters, E. E., & Forthofer, M. S. (1998). The social consequences of psychiatric disorders, III: probability of marital stability. *The American Journal of Psychiatry* 155, 1092–6.

Kim, J. H., Chang, S. M., Hong, J. P., *et al.* (2016). Lifetime prevalence, sociodemographic correlates, and diagnostic overlaps of bipolar spectrum disorder in the general population of South Korea. *Journal of Affective Disorders* 203, 248–55.

Koenders, M. A., Giltay, E. J., Spijker, A. T., *et al.* (2014). Stressful life events in bipolar I and II disorder: cause or consequence of mood symptoms? *Journal of Affective Disorders* 161, 55–64.

Leboyer, M., Henry, C., Paillere-Martinot, M. L., & Bellivier, F. (2005). Age at onset in bipolar affective disorders: a review. *Bipolar Disorders* 7, 111–8.

Lee, S., Tsang, A., Kessler, R. C., *et al.* (2010). Rapid-cycling bipolar disorder: cross-national community study. *The British Journal of Psychiatry* 196, 217–25.

Leon, A. C., Olfson, M., Portera, L., Farber, L., & Sheehan, D. V. (1997). Assessing psychiatric impairment in primary care with the Sheehan Disability Scale. *International Journal of Psychiatry in Medicine* 27, 93–105.

Lopez-Zurbano, S., Gonzalez-Pinto, A., & Lopez, P. (2015). Gender differences in bipolar disorder. In M. Sáenz-Herrero, ed., *Psychopathology in Women: Incorporating Gender Perspective into Descriptive Psychopathology*. New York, NY: Springer, pp. 641–59.

McGorry, P. D. (2015). Early intervention in psychosis: obvious, effective, overdue. *The Journal of Nervous and Mental Disease* 203, 310–8.

McGorry, P. D., Purcell, R., Goldstone, S., & Amminger, G. P. (2011). Age of onset and timing of treatment for mental and substance use disorders: implications for preventive intervention strategies and models of care. *Current Opinion in Psychiatry* 24, 301–6.

Merikangas, K., & Pato, M. (2009). Recent developments in the epidemiology of bipolar disorder in adults and children: magnitude, correlates, and future directions. *Clinical Psychology: Science and Practice* 16, 121–33.

Merikangas, K. R., Akiskal, H. S., Angst, J., *et al.* (2007). Lifetime and 12-month prevalence of bipolar spectrum disorder in the National Comorbidity Survey Replication. *Archives of General Psychiatry* 64, 543–52.

Merikangas, K. R., Herrell, R., Swendsen, J., *et al.* (2008). Specificity of bipolar spectrum conditions in the comorbidity of mood and substance use disorders: results from the Zurich Cohort Study. *Archives of General Psychiatry* 65, 47–52.

Merikangas, K. R., Jin, R., He, J. P., *et al.* (2011). Prevalence and correlates of bipolar spectrum disorder in the World Mental Health Survey Initiative. *Archives of General Psychiatry* 68, 241–51.

Miklowitz, D. J. (2011). Functional impairment, stress, and psychosocial intervention in bipolar disorder. *Current Psychiatry Reports* 13, 504–12.

Miller, L. J., Ghadiali, N. Y., Larusso, E. M., *et al.* (2015). Bipolar disorder in women. *Health Care for Women International* 36, 475–98.

Moffitt, T. E., Caspi, A., Taylor, A., *et al.* (2010). How common are common mental disorders? Evidence that lifetime prevalence rates are doubled by prospective versus retrospective ascertainment. *Psychological Medicine* 40, 899–909.

Morgan, V. A., Mitchell, P. B., & Jablensky, A. V. (2005). The epidemiology of bipolar disorder: sociodemographic, disability and service utilization data from the Australian National Study of Low Prevalence (Psychotic) Disorders. *Bipolar Disorders* 7, 326–37.

Nasrallah, H. A. (2015). Consequences of misdiagnosis: inaccurate treatment and poor patient outcomes in bipolar disorder. *The Journal of Clinical Psychiatry* 76, e1328.

Nierenberg, A. A., Akiskal, H. S., Angst, J., *et al.* (2010). Bipolar disorder with frequent mood episodes in the National Comorbidity Survey Replication (NCS-R). *Molecular Psychiatry* 15, 1075–87.

Oepen, G., Baldessarini, R. J., Salvatore, P., & Slater, E. (2004). On the periodicity of manic-depressive insanity, by Eliot Slater (1938): translated excerpts and commentary. *Journal of Affective Disorders* 78, 1–9.

Ormel, J., Petukhova, M., Chatterji, S., *et al.* (2008). Disability and treatment of specific mental and physical disorders across the world. *The British Journal of Psychiatry* 192, 368–75.

Oyffe, I., Shwizer, R., & Stolovy, T. (2015). The association between diagnosis, treatment delay and outcome among patients with bipolar disorders. *The Psychiatric Quarterly* 86, 95–105.

Paris, J. (2014). Problems in the boundaries of bipolar disorders. *Current Psychiatry Reports* 16, 461.

Patten, S. B., & Paris, J. (2008). The bipolar spectrum – a bridge too far? *Canadian Journal of Psychiatry* 53, 762–8.

Pini, S., de Queiroz, V., Pagnin, D., *et al.* (2005). Prevalence and burden of bipolar disorders in European countries. *European Neuropsychopharmacology* 15, 425–34.

Pompili, M., Gonda, X., Serafini, G., *et al.* (2013). Epidemiology of suicide in bipolar disorders: a systematic review of the literature. *Bipolar Disorders* 15, 457–90.

Saunders, K. E. A., & Goodwin, G. M. (2010). The course of bipolar disorder. *Advances in Psychiatric Treatment* 16, 318–28.

Schneck, C. D., Miklowitz, D. J., Calabrese, J. R., *et al.* (2004) Phenomenology of rapid-cycling bipolar disorder: data from the first 500 participants in the Systematic Treatment Enhancement Program. *The American Journal of Psychiatry* 161, 1902–8.

Srihari, V. H., Jani, A., & Gray, M. (2016). Early intervention for psychotic disorders: building population health systems. *JAMA Psychiatry* 73, 101–2.

ten Have, M., de Graaf, R., van Dorsselaer, S., & Beekman, A. (2013). Lifetime treatment contact and delay in treatment seeking after first onset of a mental disorder. *Psychiatric Services* 64, 981–9.

Thornicroft, G., Chatterj, S., Evans-Lacho, S., *et al.* (2016). Undertreatment of people with major depressive disorder in 21 countries. *The British Journal of Psychiatry*, 210, 119–24.

Tondo, L., Pompili, M., Forte, A., & Baldessarini, R. J. (2016). Suicide attempts in bipolar disorders: comprehensive review of 101 reports. *Acta Psychiatrica Scandinavica* 133, 174–86.

Vega, P., Barbeito, S., Ruiz de Azua, S., *et al.* (2011). Bipolar disorder differences between genders: special considerations for women. *Women's Health* 7, 663–74.

Walsh, M. A., DeGeorge, D. P., Barrantes-Vidal, N., & Kwapil, T. R. (2015). A 3-year longitudinal study of risk for bipolar spectrum psychopathology. *Journal of Abnormal Psychology* 124, 486–97.

Wang, P. S., Angermeyer, M., Borges, G., *et al.* (2007a). Delay and failure in treatment seeking after first onset of mental disorders in the World Health Organization's World Mental Health Survey Initiative. *World Psychiatry* 6, 177–85.

Wang, P. S., Aguilar-Gaxiola, S., Alonso, J., *et al.* (2007b). Use of mental health services for anxiety, mood, and substance disorders in 17 countries in the WHO World Mental Health Surveys. *Lancet* 370, 841–50.

Waraich, P., Goldner, E. M., Somers, J. M., & Hsu, L. (2004). Prevalence and incidence studies of mood disorders: a systematic review of the literature. *Canadian Journal of Psychiatry* 49, 124–38.

Weissman, M. M., Leaf, P. J., Tischler, G. L., *et al.* (1988). Affective disorders in five United States communities. *Psychological Medicine* 18, 141–53.

World Health Organization (2002). *The World Health Report 2002: Reducing Risks, Promoting Healthy Life.* Geneva, Switzerland: World Health Organization.

Zimmerman, M., & Morgan, T. A. (2013). Problematic boundaries in the diagnosis of bipolar disorder: the interface with borderline personality disorder. *Current Psychiatry Reports* 15, 422.

Chapter 6

Generalized Anxiety Disorder

Ayelet Meron Ruscio, Lauren S. Hallion, Koen Demyttenaere, Sing Lee, Carmen C. W. Lim

Introduction

Generalized, chronic, 'free-floating' anxiety has been recognized as an important clinical condition for more than a century (Rickels & Rynn 2001). However, while there is strong agreement about the existence of generalized anxiety that is severe enough to warrant diagnosis and treatment, there is far less agreement about the features that define the condition and distinguish it from normal anxiety. This may be because anxiety is experienced occasionally by almost everyone, especially during times of stress. Furthermore, normal expressions of anxiety vary widely, with many people experiencing higher-than-average levels of anxiety without being considered to have a mental disorder.

Due in part to these challenges, the definition of generalized anxiety disorder (GAD) has changed more in the last three decades than perhaps any other mental disorder (Davidson *et al.* 2010). In its original instantiation in DSM-III (APA 1980), GAD was defined as persistent anxiety lasting at least one month and involving associated symptoms from three of four categories. As persistent anxiety is a feature of all anxiety disorders, GAD was treated as a 'wastebasket' or residual diagnostic category. It was assumed to be associated with relatively modest impairment. In DSM-III-R (APA 1987), GAD changed from a residual diagnosis to an independent disorder defined centrally by pathological worry. To facilitate discrimination from normal worry, the worry in GAD was defined as generalized (related to multiple life circumstances), excessive, unrealistic, and accompanied by six of 18 associated symptoms of anxiety. Minimum duration was increased from one to six months to distinguish GAD from transient stress reactions. DSM-IV (APA 1994) established generalized, excessive, uncontrollable worry as the cardinal feature of GAD. To sharpen the separation from other anxiety disorders, associated symptoms were restricted to six symptoms of tension and vigilance that were most frequently observed in GAD patients, with three required for diagnosis. The disturbance was required to last at least six months and to cause clinically significant distress or impairment.

The DSM-IV conceptualization of GAD was widely viewed as an improvement over earlier definitions (Ballenger *et al.* 2001). The emphasis on worry and a streamlined set of associated symptoms aided clinicians in detecting GAD and distinguishing it from closely related disorders (Marten *et al.* 1993; Chelminski & Zimmerman 2003), helping to raise diagnostic reliability up to the level of other anxiety disorders (Brown *et al.* 2001). Despite these improvements, debates have persisted about the validity of GAD (Brown *et al.* 1994; Starcevic *et al.* 2012). A particularly controversial aspect of GAD has been its relationship with mood disorders, especially major depressive disorder (MDD). Although associations are strong between all anxiety and mood disorders, GAD and MDD overlap the most in their comorbidity (Ruscio & Khazanov, 2017), clinical features (Ehring & Watkins 2008; Watson 2009), and genetic risk (Kendler *et al.* 1992), leading some to question the distinctness of these disorders (see Goldberg *et al.*, 2010). DSM-IV dealt with the close relationship between GAD and mood disorders by including a diagnostic hierarchy rule that prohibited a diagnosis of GAD when its symptoms occurred exclusively during episodes of a mood disorder. The rationale was that depressed and manic individuals frequently present with heightened anxiety and agitation and that, when these symptoms wax and wane with other mood symptoms, they should be considered part of the mood disorder rather than an independent disorder (APA 1994). Although the hierarchy rule was intended to avoid extraneous diagnoses of GAD, subsequent clinical research suggested that cases subject to the hierarchy rule resembled patients with comorbid GAD-MDD much more closely than patients with MDD alone (Zimmerman & Chelminski 2003). Largely for this reason (Andrews *et al.* 2010), the hierarchical exclusion with mood disorders was dropped from the definition of GAD in the recently published DSM-5 (APA 2013).

This latest diagnostic revision has reopened questions about the validity of the GAD diagnosis and its separation from other mental disorders. It has also raised new questions about how GAD cases identified by DSM-IV differ from those identified by DSM-5. Comparing individuals diagnosed under the two systems is important not only for establishing the validity of the new GAD criteria, but for determining the likely generalizability of prior research findings and treatment guidelines to DSM-5 GAD, ensuring continuity of research and clinical care (see Abel & Borkovec 1995). To our knowledge, only two studies have compared GAD diagnosed with and without the hierarchy rule, both using outpatient samples in specialty mental health clinics in the United States (Zimmerman & Chelminski 2003; Lawrence *et al.* 2009). Those studies suggested that lifting the hierarchy rule yields a sizable number of new GAD cases and that the new cases are particularly severe, with a high burden of comorbidity and disability.

Although suggestive, these findings are limited in two important respects. First, help-seeking samples are known to differ systematically from the population at large in their severity and comorbidity (Berkson 1946). Representative community samples are not subject to these biases. In addition, because they include individuals who are not in treatment as well as those receiving treatment, community samples are well-suited to describing the proportion of those with a disorder who seek clinical care and the settings in which care is sought. Knowledge of these patterns aids clinicians in assessing and detecting GAD in a variety of service settings and aids policy-makers in estimating unmet need in the community. Second, data from countries other than the United States are needed. Most of what is known about GAD comes from a small number of economically developed countries (cf. Somers *et al.* 2006). Studying GAD in other parts of the globe is necessary, however, for separating universal features of the disorder from those that vary by country or culture (Lewis-Fernández *et al.* 2010). As the DSM system is intended to guide clinical diagnosis, treatment planning, and research and policy efforts around the world, cross-national information about the GAD diagnosis is critical.

In this chapter, we used data from the WMH surveys to describe DSM-IV GAD and compare it to DSM-5 GAD. By lifting the DSM-IV hierarchy rule barring the diagnosis of GAD during a mood disorder, we were able to compare cases identified by the two diagnostic systems within the same sample. We considered the implications of the diagnostic revision for the prevalence of GAD, its comorbidity with other mental disorders, its associations with role impairment and treatment seeking, and its clinical course and socio-demographic correlates. We examined the generalizability of results by performing analyses not only in the large cross-national sample, but within subgroups of countries that differ in economic development.

Methods

Data from all 29 WMH surveys are included in this report. The combined sample included 147,261 respondents from 26 countries. As GAD was assessed in Part I, all analyses used the Part I sample except the comorbidity analyses, which were performed using the Part II sample to allow disorders assessed in Part II to be included.

The Composite International Diagnostic Interview (CIDI) 3.0 generates diagnoses of mental disorders using DSM-IV criteria. In the United States survey, lifetime GAD diagnoses based on the CIDI were shown to have good concordance with clinician-assigned diagnoses based on the Structured Clinical Interview for DSM-IV (SCID; First *et al.* 2002), with an area under the Receiver Operating Characteristic (ROC) curve (AUC) of 0.83 (Ruscio *et al.* 2005). Similar analyses in a subset of four WMH surveys did not evaluate GAD in isolation, but found good concordance between CIDI and SCID diagnoses of any 12-month anxiety disorder including GAD (AUC = 0.88; Haro *et al.* 2006).

CIDI diagnoses of DSM-IV GAD are assigned when excessive, uncontrollable worry is reported about a number of events or activities, accompanied by at least three of six associated symptoms, present more days than not for at least six months, and associated with significant distress or impairment; an additional requirement is that DSM-IV diagnostic hierarchy and organic exclusion rules must be met. DSM-5 GAD diagnoses generated for this chapter were identical to the DSM-IV diagnoses except that they allowed GAD to be diagnosed even when the symptoms occurred exclusively during episodes of a mood disorder.

Results

Prevalence

Prevalence increased substantially from DSM-IV to DSM-5 (Table 6.1). DSM-IV GAD has a lifetime

Table 6.1 Prevalence of DSM-IV and DSM-5 generalized anxiety disorder in the World Mental Health Surveys

Country	Lifetime prevalence					12-month prevalence					30-day prevalence					Sample size used
	DSM-IV		DSM-5		% change	DSM-IV		DSM-5		% change	DSM-IV		DSM-5		% change	
	%	SE	%	SE		%	SE	%	SE		%	SE	%	SE		
Low/lower-middle-income	**1.1**	**(0.1)**	**1.6**	**(0.1)**	**45.5**	**0.6**	**(0.1)**	**0.9**	**(0.1)**	**50.0**	**0.3**	**(0.0)**	**0.5**	**(0.1)**	**66.7**	**36,498**
Colombia	1.3	(0.3)	1.9	(0.3)	46.2	0.6	(0.2)	1.0	(0.2)	66.7	0.3	(0.1)	0.4	(0.1)	33.3	4,426
Iraq	3.7	(0.5)	5.0	(0.6)	35.1	2.3	(0.3)	3.0	(0.4)	30.4	1.4	(0.3)	2.0	(0.3)	42.9	4,332
Nigeria	0.1	(0.0)	0.1	(0.0)	0.0	0.03	(0.0)	0.03	(0.0)	0.0	–	–	–	–	0.0[a]	6,752
Peru	0.7	(0.1)	1.1	(0.1)	57.1	0.2	(0.1)	0.5	(0.1)	150.0	–	–	0.1	(0.0)	–[b]	3,930
PRC (Beijing/Shanghai)	0.8	(0.1)	1.0	(0.1)	25.0	0.5	(0.1)	0.6	(0.1)	20.0	0.3	(0.1)	0.3	(0.1)	0.0	5,201
PRC (Shenzhen)	0.1	(0.0)	0.2	(0.1)	100.0	0.04	(0.0)	0.1	(0.1)	150.0	–	–	–	–	0.0[a]	7,132
Ukraine	2.0	(0.2)	3.3	(0.3)	65.0	1.0	(0.1)	2.1	(0.2)	110.0	0.6	(0.1)	1.3	(0.1)	116.7	4,725
Upper-middle-income	**2.1**	**(0.1)**	**2.8**	**(0.1)**	**33.3**	**1.1**	**(0.1)**	**1.6**	**(0.1)**	**45.5**	**0.4**	**(0.0)**	**0.7**	**(0.1)**	**75.0**	**28,927**
Brazil	3.7	(0.3)	5.1	(0.4)	37.8	2.3	(0.2)	3.3	(0.3)	43.5	1.0	(0.1)	1.8	(0.2)	80.0	5,037
Bulgaria	1.7	(0.2)	2.3	(0.2)	35.3	0.9	(0.1)	1.2	(0.1)	33.3	0.3	(0.1)	0.5	(0.1)	66.7	5,318
Colombia (Medellín)	2.6	(0.4)	3.8	(0.5)	46.2	1.2	(0.3)	2.1	(0.3)	75.0	0.4	(0.1)	0.9	(0.2)	125.0	3,261
Lebanon	2.0	(0.3)	2.3	(0.3)	15.0	1.2	(0.3)	1.5	(0.3)	25.0	0.5	(0.2)	0.6	(0.2)	20.0	2,857
Mexico	0.9	(0.1)	1.1	(0.2)	22.2	0.4	(0.1)	0.6	(0.1)	50.0	0.2	(0.1)	0.3	(0.1)	50.0	5,782
Romania	0.8	(0.2)	1.0	(0.3)	25.0	0.2	(0.1)	0.2	(0.1)	0.0	0.1	(0.1)	0.2	(0.1)	100.0	2,357
South Africa	2.5	(0.3)	3.6	(0.4)	44.0	1.4	(0.2)	1.9	(0.3)	35.7	0.4	(0.1)	0.6	(0.1)	50.0	4,315
High-income	**3.7**	**(0.1)**	**5.0**	**(0.1)**	**35.1**	**1.5**	**(0.1)**	**2.3**	**(0.1)**	**53.3**	**0.6**	**(0.0)**	**0.9**	**(0.0)**	**50.0**	**81,836**
Australia	6.0	(0.4)	8.0	(0.5)	33.3	2.2	(0.3)	3.6	(0.3)	63.6	0.8	(0.2)	1.5	(0.2)	87.5	8,460
Belgium	1.9	(0.4)	2.8	(0.5)	47.4	0.6	(0.2)	0.9	(0.3)	50.0	0.2	(0.1)	0.3	(0.1)	50.0	2,419
France	4.9	(0.5)	6.2	(0.5)	26.5	1.5	(0.3)	2.1	(0.3)	40.0	0.5	(0.2)	0.6	(0.2)	20.0	2,894
Germany	1.1	(0.2)	1.5	(0.2)	36.4	0.3	(0.1)	0.5	(0.1)	66.7	0.2	(0.1)	0.2	(0.1)	0.0	3,555
Israel	3.3	(0.3)	4.4	(0.3)	33.3	2.2	(0.2)	3.1	(0.3)	40.9	0.7	(0.1)	1.1	(0.2)	57.1	4,859
Italy	1.4	(0.2)	2.1	(0.3)	50.0	0.4	(0.1)	0.6	(0.1)	50.0	0.1	(0.0)	0.2	(0.1)	100.0	4,712
Japan	1.9	(0.2)	2.6	(0.3)	36.8	0.9	(0.1)	1.2	(0.2)	33.3	0.1	(0.1)	0.2	(0.1)	100.0	4,129
New Zealand	6.2	(0.3)	7.9	(0.3)	27.4	2.1	(0.2)	3.1	(0.2)	47.6	0.8	(0.1)	1.2	(0.1)	50.0	12,790
Northern Ireland	4.1	(0.4)	6.4	(0.4)	56.1	1.9	(0.3)	2.8	(0.3)	47.4	1.0	(0.2)	1.5	(0.2)	50.0	4,340
Poland	0.7	(0.1)	0.9	(0.1)	28.6	0.5	(0.1)	0.5	(0.1)	0.0	0.2	(0.1)	0.3	(0.1)	50.0	10,081
Portugal	4.3	(0.4)	6.1	(0.5)	41.9	2.1	(0.2)	3.3	(0.3)	57.1	0.7	(0.1)	1.1	(0.2)	57.1	3,849
Spain	1.3	(0.2)	1.9	(0.2)	46.2	0.5	(0.1)	0.8	(0.2)	60.0	0.2	(0.1)	0.4	(0.1)	100.0	5,473
Spain (Murcia)	4.7	(0.8)	7.0	(0.9)	48.9	3.0	(0.7)	4.3	(0.7)	43.3	2.1	(0.5)	3.0	(0.6)	42.9	2,621
Netherlands	2.6	(0.4)	3.6	(0.4)	38.5	0.6	(0.2)	1.0	(0.2)	66.7	0.2	(0.1)	0.4	(0.1)	100.0	2,372
United States	5.7	(0.3)	7.8	(0.3)	36.8	2.7	(0.2)	4.0	(0.2)	48.1	1.0	(0.1)	1.6	(0.2)	60.0	9,282
All countries combined	**2.7**	**(0.1)**	**3.7**	**(0.1)**	**37.0**	**1.2**	**(0.0)**	**1.8**	**(0.1)**	**50.0**	**0.5**	**(0.0)**	**0.8**	**(0.0)**	**60.0**	**147,261**
Comparison between countries[c]	**$F_{28,v}=76.8^*$, $P<0.001$**		**$F_{28,v}=85.8^*$, $P<0.001$**			**$F_{28,v}=38.8^*$, $P<0.001$**		**$F_{28,v}=42.7^*$, $P<0.001$**			**$F_{28,v}=20.5^*$, $P<0.001$**		**$F_{28,v}=29.0^*$, $P<0.001$**			
Comparison low-, middle-, and high-income country groups[c]	**$F_{2,v}=253.3^*$, $P<0.001$**		**$F_{2,v}=311.3^*$, $P<0.001$**			**$F_{2,v}=85.0^*$, $P<0.001$**		**$F_{2,v}=106.5^*$, $P<0.001$**			**$F_{2,v}=16.5^*$, $P<0.001$**		**$F_{2,v}=21.7^*$, $P<0.001$**			

Values represent % (SE).
Dashed lines indicate empty cells.
[a]As the numerator and denominator are both zero, a value of 0.0 is shown for per cent change.
[b]The amount of change is greater than zero, but percent change could not be calculated because the denominator is zero.
[c]Wald design-corrected F-tests were used to determine if there is variation in prevalence estimates across countries. The denominator degree of freedom, v, is 5429.
PRC: People's Republic of China.

prevalence of 2.7%, 12-month prevalence of 1.2%, and 30-day prevalence of 0.5% in the total sample. By contrast, DSM-5 GAD has a lifetime prevalence of 3.7%, an increase of 37% over the rate for DSM-IV GAD. The increases are even larger for recent cases: 12-month prevalence rose to 1.8% (an increase of 50%) and 30-day prevalence rose to 0.8% (an increase of 60%) following the diagnostic revision. Both GAD diagnoses are most prevalent in high-income countries, less prevalent in upper-middle-income countries, and least prevalent in low/lower-middle-income countries. Nevertheless, DSM-5 GAD is more prevalent than DSM-IV GAD in all three country income groups. In fact, with the exception of Nigeria, for which no change was observed, the lifetime prevalence of GAD increased from DSM-IV to DSM-5 in every country examined here.

Comorbidity

Comorbidity also increased from DSM-IV to DSM-5 (Table 6.2). In DSM-IV, more than three-quarters (75.6%) of respondents with lifetime GAD, and more than half (57.1%) of those with 12-month GAD, qualify for at least one other mental disorder assessed by the CIDI. Comorbidity is equally common with mood and anxiety disorders, whether assessed over the respondent's lifetime (50.4% mood vs. 49.2% anxiety) or in the 12 months before interview (33.3% mood vs. 34.5% anxiety); comorbidity is less common with substance-use disorders and least common with disruptive behaviour/impulse-control disorders. Even with the DSM-IV hierarchy rule in effect, MDD is by far the single most common comorbid condition (reported by 42.2% of lifetime DSM-IV GAD cases), followed by social anxiety disorder (25.3%) and specific phobia (24.9%). Interestingly, DSM-IV GAD typically develops later than comorbid disorders: GAD precedes other anxiety disorders in only 12.7% of cases, disruptive behaviour/impulse-control disorders in 33.5% of cases, and mood and substance-use disorders in about 40% of cases.

In DSM-5, rates of comorbidity rose to 81.9% among lifetime cases and to 70.8% among 12-month cases of GAD. As expected, the largest change from DSM-IV is in comorbidity with mood disorders, which are present in the majority of individuals with lifetime (63.0%) and 12-month (51.3%) GAD. Although the number of GAD cases with comorbid MDD far exceeds the number with bipolar spectrum disorder, the percent change in comorbidity is strikingly similar for unipolar and bipolar mood disorders: both increase by nearly 25% among lifetime GAD cases and by more than 50% among 12-month GAD cases when the hierarchy rule is eliminated. As a result, the proportion of GAD cases with comorbid mood disorders outnumbers the proportion with comorbid anxiety disorders in DSM-5. Nevertheless, rates of comorbid anxiety, substance-use, and disruptive behaviour/impulse-control disorders are all higher for DSM-5 than DSM-IV GAD, suggesting that new cases captured by the revised diagnostic criteria have higher overall levels of comorbidity than previously identified cases. The new cases also disproportionately experience GAD as a temporally secondary disorder. For example, under DSM-5, 75% of respondents with a lifetime history of both GAD and a mood disorder report that GAD began after the mood disorder.

Role Impairment

DSM-5 GAD is associated with greater role impairment than DSM-IV GAD. Respondents with DSM-IV GAD report a mean of 33.9 days (SE = 2.6) out of role due to GAD in the past 12 months, compared to a mean of 41.2 days (SE = 2.4) for those with DSM-5 GAD (data not shown). On the Sheehan Disability Scales, severe functional impairment in one or more life domains is reported by 45.7% of those with DSM-IV GAD versus 50.6% of those with DSM-5 GAD (Table 6.3). Severe impairment is most common in the social domain and least common in the home domain, regardless of GAD definition. In addition, GAD is more disabling in high-income countries than in the upper-middle- or low/lower-middle-income countries under both definitions. Interestingly, although the number of GAD cases with severe impairment increased in all three country income groups in DSM-5, the proportion of severely disabled cases increased more in high- and upper-middle-income countries (11–12% higher than in DSM-IV) than in low/lower-middle-income countries (4% higher than in DSM-IV).

Treatment

DSM-5 GAD is associated with a small but consistent increase in treatment seeking over DSM-IV GAD (Table 6.4). A total of 44.1% of respondents with DSM-IV GAD sought treatment for some type of mental health or substance-use problem during the year before interview, compared to 49.2% of those with DSM-5 GAD. Individuals with GAD, regardless of diagnostic definition, sought treatment most often

Table 6.2 Comorbidity of DSM-IV and DSM-5 generalized anxiety disorder with DSM-IV mental disorders, all countries combined

DSM-IV disorder	DSM-IV			DSM-5		
	Lifetime comorbidity[a]	12-month comorbidity[b]	Temporal priority of GAD[c]	Lifetime comorbidity[a]	12-month comorbidity[b]	Temporal priority of GAD[c]
I. Mood disorder						
Major depressive disorder	42.2 (1.1)	26.8 (1.4)		52.6 (0.9)	40.9 (1.3)	
Bipolar spectrum disorder[d]	9.2 (0.6)	7.0 (0.8)		11.4 (0.6)	10.8 (0.8)	
Any mood disorder[e]	50.4 (1.1)	33.3 (1.5)	40.5 (1.6)	63.0 (0.9)	51.3 (1.3)	24.6 (1.1)
II. Anxiety disorder						
Panic disorder	11.3 (0.8)	8.3 (0.9)		12.3 (0.7)	11.8 (0.9)	
Social anxiety disorder	25.3 (1.0)	18.5 (1.3)		26.1 (0.9)	22.6 (1.2)	
Specific phobia	24.9 (1.0)	22.4 (1.4)		25.6 (0.8)	25.2 (1.2)	
Agoraphobia	8.2 (0.6)	6.5 (0.8)		9.4 (0.5)	9.0 (0.7)	
Posttraumatic stress disorder	18.7 (0.8)	3.7 (0.5)		21.0 (0.7)	14.4 (0.8)	
Childhood-onset separation anxiety disorder[f]	8.9 (0.9)	–		8.6 (0.7)	–	
Adult-onset separation anxiety disorder	13.6 (1.0)	5.7 (0.9)		15.8 (0.8)	6.9 (0.8)	
Any anxiety disorder	49.2 (1.1)	34.5 (1.5)	12.7 (1.0)	51.7 (0.9)	44.0 (1.2)	11.6 (0.8)
III. Disruptive behaviour/Impulse-control disorder						
Intermittent explosive disorder	14.4 (1.3)	11.0 (1.7)		15.0 (1.1)	12.1 (1.4)	
Binge-eating disorder	5.8 (0.7)	3.6 (0.9)		6.1 (0.6)	4.3 (0.8)	
Bulimia nervosa	3.8 (0.5)	1.7 (0.5)		3.8 (0.4)	2.4 (0.5)	
Conduct disorder	8.4 (1.0)	0.3 (0.2)		7.8 (0.8)	1.0 (0.3)	
Attention-deficit/hyperactivity disorder	7.0 (0.8)	4.3 (0.9)		7.5 (0.8)	5.8 (0.9)	
Oppositional defiant disorder	10.7 (1.1)	1.8 (0.6)		10.7 (0.9)	3.5 (0.7)	
Any disruptive behaviour/impulse-control disorder	9.9 (0.7)	7.5 (0.9)	33.5 (2.9)	10.1 (0.6)	8.1 (0.8)	29.8 (2.4)
IV. Substance-use disorder						
Alcohol abuse	19.4 (0.9)	4.6 (0.6)		19.6 (0.8)	5.8 (0.6)	
Alcohol dependence	8.2 (0.6)	3.0 (0.5)		8.9 (0.5)	4.4 (0.6)	
Drug abuse	9.6 (0.7)	2.8 (0.6)		10.5 (0.6)	3.6 (0.6)	
Drug dependence	4.4 (0.4)	1.5 (0.3)		5.3 (0.4)	2.5 (0.5)	
Any substance-use disorder	22.6 (1.0)	7.7 (0.9)	40.3 (2.3)	22.5 (0.8)	9.1 (0.8)	37.2 (1.9)
V. Any mental disorder	**75.6 (0.9)**	**57.1 (1.6)**	**16.0 (1.0)**	**81.9 (0.7)**	**70.8 (1.2)**	**11.0 (0.7)**

Values represent % (SE).
[a]Proportion of respondents with lifetime DSM-IV or DSM-5 GAD who also qualified for the lifetime DSM-IV disorder in each row.
[b]Proportion of respondents with 12-month DSM-IV or DSM-5 GAD who also qualified for the 12-month DSM-IV disorder in each row.
[c]Proportion of respondents with lifetime DSM-IV or DSM-5 GAD and at least one disorder in the designated disorder class, whose age of onset of GAD is reported to be younger than the age-of-onset of all comorbid disorders in that class.
[d]Includes bipolar I disorder, bipolar II disorder, or subthreshold bipolar disorder.
[e]Includes major depressive episode and bipolar spectrum disorder.
[f]The surveys did not include a 12-month assessment of childhood-onset separation anxiety disorder.

Table 6.3 Severity of role impairment (Sheehan Disability Scale) associated with 12-month DSM-IV and DSM-5 generalized anxiety disorder, by country income group

Proportion with severe role impairment (SDS score: 7-10)	DSM-IV		DSM-5	
	%	SE	%	SE
Home				
Low/lower-middle-income countries	18.9	3.0	23.2	2.8
Upper-middle-income countries	22.2	3.1	25.8	2.2
High-income countries	26.1	1.6	29.4	1.3
All countries combined	24.7	1.3	28.0	1.1
Comparison between low-, middle-, and high-income countries[a]	$F_{2,v} = 2.4$, $P = 0.092$		$F_{2,v} = 2.5$, $P = 0.081$	
Work				
Low/lower-middle-income countries	22.0	3.7	23.7	3.3
Upper-middle-income countries	21.2	3.0	28.7	3.0
High-income countries	29.7	1.7	34.4	1.4
All countries combined	27.4	1.4	32.1	1.2
Comparison between low-, middle-, and high-income countries[a]	$F_{2,v} = 4.0^*$, $P = 0.018$		$F_{2,v} = 5.4^*$, $P = 0.005$	
Relationship				
Low/lower-middle-income countries	24.7	4.5	26.1	3.4
Upper-middle-income countries	23.6	2.8	26.8	2.2
High-income countries	27.6	1.6	33.0	1.3
All countries combined	26.6	1.4	31.1	1.1
Comparison between low-, middle-, and high-income countries[a]	$F_{2,v} = 0.9$, $P = 0.427$		$F_{2,v} = 4.1^*$, $P = 0.016$	
Social				
Low/lower-middle-income countries	27.3	4.7	24.6	3.7
Upper-middle-income countries	24.2	2.9	28.4	2.8
High-income countries	32.8	1.8	38.1	1.4
All countries combined	30.7	1.5	34.9	1.2
Comparison between low-, middle-, and high-income countries[a]	$F_{2,v} = 3.2^*$, $P = 0.039$		$F_{2,v} = 9.6^*$, $P < 0.001$	
Any[b]				
Low/lower-middle-income countries	37.5	4.7	39.0	3.6
Upper-middle-income countries	38.1	3.4	42.6	3.0
High-income countries	49.0	1.8	54.5	1.4
All countries combined	45.7	1.5	50.6	1.2
Comparison between low-, middle-, and high-income countries[a]	$F_{2,v} = 5.8^*$, $P = 0.003$		$F_{2,v} = 13.0^*$, $P < 0.001$	

*Significant at the 0.05 level, two-sided test.
[a]Wald design-corrected F-tests were used to determine if there is variation in impairment severity across country income groups. The denominator degree of freedom, v, is 5429.
[b]Highest severity category across the four SDS role domains.

in general medical settings, less often in specialty mental health settings, and very rarely in human services or complementary-alternative settings. Help-seeking patterns differ greatly by country income, with very few GAD cases by either definition receiving specialty mental health treatment in low /lower-middle-income countries, and with a far higher rate of treatment overall in high-income than upper-middle- or low/lower-middle-income countries. Despite these broader patterns, treatment seeking is higher for DSM-5 than DSM-IV GAD in all three country income groups.

Course and Correlates

DSM-IV and DSM-5 GAD have a similar course of illness. Median age-of-onset (AOO) (ages 38 and 39 for DSM-IV and DSM-5 GAD, respectively) and cumulative AOO distributions are nearly identical for the two diagnoses (Table 6.5). GAD typically begins after puberty: only 5% of cases develop by age 13. New cases emerge gradually through adolescence and adulthood, with one-quarter of GAD cases beginning by ages 24–25, half

Table 6.4 Among those with 12-month DSM-IV and DSM-5 generalized anxiety disorder, percent reporting treatment in the past 12 months

Sector of treatment	DSM-IV		DSM-5	
	%	SE	%	SE
Specialty mental health[b]				
Low/lower-middle-income countries	1.3	0.6	3.7	1.4
Upper-middle-income countries	12.0	2.1	16.5	2.3
High-income countries	27.4	1.7	32.3	1.3
All countries combined	21.6	1.3	26.0	1.1
Comparison between low-, middle-, and high-income countries[a]	$F_{2,v} = 55.2^*$, $P < 0.001$		$F_{2,v} = 72.1^*$, $P < 0.001$	
General medical[c]				
Low/lower-middle-income countries	11.5	2.9	11.4	2.2
Upper-middle-income countries	13.6	2.1	14.7	2.0
High-income countries	37.2	1.7	41.0	1.4
All countries combined	29.9	1.3	32.8	1.1
Comparison between low-, middle-, and high-income countries[a]	$F_{2,v} = 42.5^*$, $P < 0.001$		$F_{2,v} = 76.8^*$, $P < 0.001$	
Human services[d]				
Low/lower-middle-income countries	5.1	2.8	6.4	2.2
Upper-middle-income countries	3.0	1.1	3.8	1.0
High-income countries	6.4	1.0	7.6	0.8
All countries combined	5.6	0.8	6.8	0.6
Comparison between low-, middle-, and high-income countries[a]	$F_{2,v} = 2.6$, $P = 0.08$		$F_{2,v} = 4.7^*$, $P = 0.01$	
Complementary-alternative medicine[e]				
Low/lower-middle-income countries	3.1	1.4	2.4	0.9
Upper-middle-income countries	2.5	1.0	4.0	1.5
High-income countries	7.2	0.8	8.2	0.8
All countries combined	5.9	0.6	6.8	0.1
Comparison between low-, middle-, and high-income countries[a]	$F_{2,v} = 7.4^*$, $P < 0.001$		$F_{2,v} = 12.0^*$, $P < 0.001$	
Any treatment[f]				
Low/lower-middle-income countries	19.6	4.1	21.7	3.3
Upper-middle-income countries	24.5	2.9	29.1	2.8
High-income countries	53.3	1.6	59.0	1.3
All countries combined	44.1	1.4	49.2	1.2
Comparison between low-, middle-, and high-income countries[a]	$F_{2,v} = 45.3^*$, $P < 0.001$		$F_{2,v} = 73.6^*$, $P < 0.001$	

*Significant at the 0.05 level, two-sided test.
[a]Wald design-corrected F-tests were used to determine if there is variation in treatment estimates across country income groups. The denominator degree of freedom, v, is 5429.
[b]The mental health specialist sector, which includes psychiatrist and non-psychiatrist mental health specialists (psychiatrist, psychologist or other non-psychiatrist mental health professional; social worker or counsellor in a mental health specialty setting; use of a mental health helpline; or overnight admissions for a mental health or drug or alcohol problems, with a presumption of daily contact with a psychiatrist).
[c]The general medical sector (general practitioner, other medical doctor, nurse, occupational therapist or any healthcare professional).
[d]The human services sector (religious or spiritual advisor or social worker or counsellor in any setting other than a specialty mental health setting).
[e]The CAM (complementary and alternative medicine) sector (any other type of healer, such as herbalist or homeopath, participation in an internet support group, or participation in a self-help group).
[f]Any treatment listed above.

beginning by ages 38–39, and three-quarters beginning by age 53. Only 10% of first onsets occur in adults aged 65 or older. Once GAD begins, it often persists: 44.8% of individuals with DSM-IV GAD and 48.8% of individuals with DSM-5 GAD in their lifetime still had the disorder in the year before interview. Onsets are somewhat earlier and course is less persistent in high-income countries than in upper-middle- or low/lower-middle-income countries for both GAD diagnoses (data not shown).

Table 6.5 Cumulative age-of-onset distributions for DSM-IV and DSM-5 generalized anxiety disorder (GAD), by country income group

DSM edition	Ages at selected percentiles								Projected risk at age 75
	5	10	25	50	75	90	95	99	% (SE)
DSM-IV									
Low/lower-middle-income countries	14	18	28	44	56	70	70	74	2.6 (0.4)
Upper-middle-income countries	14	18	29	44	64	72	73	73	5.1 (0.6)
High-income countries	12	14	22	35	50	60	67	73	6.0 (0.2)
All countries combined	13	15	24	38	53	65	71	73	5.1 (0.2)
DSM-5									
Low/lower-middle-income countries	15	18	28	43	56	66	70	74	3.7 (0.4)
Upper-middle-income countries	14	18	29	43	62	72	72	73	6.7 (0.6)
High-income countries	13	14	23	36	50	61	68	74	8.7 (0.4)
All countries combined	13	16	25	39	53	65	70	74	7.3 (0.3)

Values represent ages at selected percentiles on the standardized age-of-onset (AOO) distributions for DSM-IV and DSM-5 GAD. These values, and the projected lifetime risk of GAD at age 75, are based on survival models.

DSM-IV and DSM-5 GAD also have very similar socio-demographic correlates (Table 6.6). Both lifetime diagnoses are more prevalent among young (under age 60), female, and previously married individuals. Both are also more prevalent among individuals with less education, a lower household income, and 'other' employment status (mostly unemployed or disabled), although these three variables are consistently associated with GAD only in high-income countries. Socio-demographic correlates of 30-day GAD are also very similar regardless of how the disorder was defined. Where correlates for 30-day GAD deviate from the profile for lifetime cases (e.g., weaker associations with age; elevated odds among homemakers as well as those of 'other' employment status), the deviations are evident for both DSM-IV and DSM-5 GAD. In spite of these similarities, the associations with socio-demographic variables generally are a bit larger, show a clearer dose-response gradient, and are more consistent across lifetime and 30-day analyses for DSM-5 than DSM-IV GAD. Likewise, socio-demographic predictors of course (disorder persistence) are similar for the two diagnoses, but slightly more robust for DSM-5 GAD. Neither female gender nor previously married status is associated with a more persistent course of illness. Instead, GAD is more persistent among individuals with an earlier onset of GAD, lower education and family income, and – for DSM-5 GAD – lack of employment outside the home ('other' status or homemaker).

Discussion

The challenge of separating clinically significant anxiety from normal anxiety and from other forms of emotional disturbance has spurred repeated revisions of the definition of GAD. The decision in DSM-5 to remove GAD's hierarchical relationship with the mood disorders raises new opportunities for understanding GAD and describing its connections to other disorders. In this chapter we examined the implications of this decision for the epidemiology of GAD in a large, multinational sample. Eliminating the hierarchy rule led to an influx of new GAD cases: prevalence estimates increased by 37% for lifetime GAD, by 50% for 12-month GAD, and by 60% for 30-day GAD compared to DSM-IV estimates in the same surveys. Notably, the prevalence estimates reported here for the broadened DSM-5 diagnosis are still lower than those published for DSM-IV GAD in reviews of previous epidemiological surveys (Somers *et al.* 2006). This appears to be due mainly to the lower prevalence of GAD in low/lower-middle-income countries, which were excluded from earlier reviews. Our results highlight the importance of studying GAD in developing as well as developed countries, given reliable differences not only in prevalence but also in degree of role impairment, patterns of treatment seeking, and course of illness across country groups (see also Ruscio *et al.* 2017). At the same time, the results show consistently that DSM-5 GAD is more prevalent and severe than DSM-IV GAD across countries, irrespective of

Table 6.6 Bivariate associations of socio-demographic correlates with DSM-IV and DSM-5 generalized anxiety disorder (GAD), all countries combined

Variable	DSM-IV						DSM-5					
	Lifetime GAD[a]		30-day GAD[b]		12-month GAD, lifetime cases[c]		Lifetime GAD[a]		30-day GAD[b]		12-month GAD/ lifetime cases[c]	
	OR	(95% CI)	OR	(95% CI)	OR	(95% CI)	OR	(95% CI)	OR	(95% CI)	OR	(95% CI)
Age-cohort											–	
18–29	**4.8***	(4.0–5.7)	**0.9**	(0.7–1.2)	–		**6.0***	(5.1–7.0)	**0.9**	(0.7–1.2)	–	
30–44	**4.0***	(3.5–4.5)	**1.2**	(1.0–1.6)	–		**4.8***	(4.3–5.4)	**1.4***	(1.1–1.6)	–	
45–59	**2.6***	(2.3–2.9)	**1.3**	(1.0–1.6)	–		**3.0***	(2.7–3.3)	**1.4***	(1.2–1.8)	–	
60+	**1.0**		**1.0**		–		**1.0**		**1.0**		–	
χ^2 (P Value)[d]	445.2	(<0.001)	10.9	(0.012)	–		743.8	(<0.001)	32.1	(<0.001)	–	
Age-of-onset												
Early	–		–		**1.7***	(1.3–2.3)	–		–		**1.8***	(1.5–2.3)
Early-average	–		–		**1.4***	(1.1–1.7)	–		–		**1.2***	(1.0–1.5)
Late-average	–		–		**1.1**	(0.8–1.3)	–		–		**1.0**	(0.8–1.2)
Late	–		–		**1.0**		–		–		**1.0**	
χ^2 (P Value)[d]	–		–		20.8	(<0.001)	–		–		45.9	(<0.001)
Gender												
Female	**1.7***	(1.6–1.9)	**1.8***	(1.5–2.2)	**1.1**	(0.9–1.3)	**1.8***	(1.7–2.0)	**1.9***	(1.6–2.3)	**1.1**	(0.9–1.3)
Male	**1.0**		**1.0**		**1.0**		**1.0**		**1.0**		**1.0**	
χ^2 (P Value)[d]	196.9	(<0.001)	32.8	(<0.001)	1.1	(0.306)	313.2	(<0.001)	53.5	(<0.001)	1.3	(0.249)
Marital status												
Never married	**1.1**	(1.0–1.2)	**0.8**	(0.6–1.0)	**0.9**	(0.8–1.2)	**1.2***	(1.1–1.3)	**0.9**	(0.7–1.0)	**1.1**	(0.9–1.3)
Divorced/separated/widowed	**1.5***	(1.3–1.6)	**1.5***	(1.2–1.8)	**1.0**	(0.8–1.2)	**1.6***	(1.5–1.8)	**1.7***	(1.4–2.0)	**1.1**	(0.9–1.3)
Currently married	**1.0**		**1.0**		**1.0**		**1.0**		**1.0**		**1.0**	
χ^2 (P Value)[d]	59.4	(<0.001)	12.3	(0.002)	0.3	(0.871)	131.4	(<0.001)	33.4	(<0.001)	1.0	(0.604)
Education level												
No education	**1.7***	(1.3–2.3)	**3.0***	(1.8–5.2)	**1.5**	(0.8–2.7)	**1.8***	(1.4–2.3)	**3.1***	(2.0–4.8)	**1.4**	(0.8–2.3)
Some primary	**1.4***	(1.2–1.7)	**2.1***	(1.4–3.0)	**1.7***	(1.2–2.4)	**1.4***	(1.2–1.6)	**2.1***	(1.6–2.9)	**1.9***	(1.4–2.5)
Finished primary	**1.5***	(1.3–1.8)	**2.2***	(1.5–3.3)	**1.8***	(1.2–2.7)	**1.6***	(1.3–1.8)	**2.4***	(1.7–3.3)	**1.7***	(1.2–2.3)
Some secondary	**1.3***	(1.2–1.5)	**1.8***	(1.3–2.4)	**1.4***	(1.1–1.8)	**1.4***	(1.3–1.6)	**2.1***	(1.6–2.6)	**1.5***	(1.2–1.8)
Finished secondary	**1.2***	(1.1–1.4)	**1.3**	(0.9–1.8)	**1.4***	(1.1–1.8)	**1.2***	(1.1–1.4)	**1.5***	(1.1–1.9)	**1.3***	(1.0–1.6)
Some college	**1.2***	(1.0–1.3)	**1.2**	(0.9–1.6)	**1.1**	(0.9–1.4)	**1.3***	(1.1–1.4)	**1.4***	(1.1–1.8)	**1.1**	(0.9–1.4)
Finished college	**1.0**		**1.0**		**1.0**		**1.0**		**1.0**		**1.0**	
χ^2 (P Value)[d]	35.6	(<0.001)	36.4	(<0.001)	16.5	(0.011)	54.1	(<0.001)	58.6	(<0.001)	24.2	(0.001)

(cont.)

Table 6.6 ***(cont.)***

Variable	DSM-IV						DSM-5					
	Lifetime GAD[a]		30-day GAD[b]		12-month GAD, lifetime cases[c]		Lifetime GAD[a]		30-day GAD[b]		12-month GAD/ lifetime cases[c]	
	OR	(95% CI)	OR	(95% CI)	OR	(95% CI)	OR	(95% CI)	OR	(95% CI)	OR	(95% CI)
Household income												
Low	**1.2***	(1.1–1.3)	**1.4***	(1.1–1.8)	**1.4***	(1.1–1.8)	**1.3***	(1.1–1.4)	**1.7***	(1.4–2.1)	**1.6***	(1.3–2.0)
Low-average	**1.1**	(1.0–1.3)	**1.2**	(1.0–1.6)	**1.3***	(1.0–1.6)	**1.2***	(1.0–1.3)	**1.3***	(1.0–1.6)	**1.4***	(1.1–1.7)
High-average	**1.1***	(1.0–1.3)	**1.2**	(0.9–1.6)	**1.4***	(1.1–1.7)	**1.1***	(1.0–1.3)	**1.2**	(1.0–1.5)	**1.3***	(1.1–1.6)
High	**1.0**		**1.0**		**1.0**		**1.0**		**1.0**		**1.0**	
χ^2 (P Value)[d]	8.1	(0.045)	6.5	(0.089)	9.0	(0.029)	20.8	(<0.001)	24.8	(<0.001)	22.1	(<0.001)
Employment status												
Student	**1.0**	(0.8–1.3)	**0.9**	(0.6–1.5)	**1.3**	(0.8–2.1)	**1.2**	(0.9–1.5)	**1.1**	(0.7–1.7)	**1.5**	(1.0–2.4)
Homemaker	**1.1**	(0.9–1.2)	**1.5***	(1.1–2.0)	**1.1**	(0.9–1.4)	**1.1**	(1.0–1.2)	**1.5***	(1.2–1.9)	**1.2***	(1.0–1.5)
Retired	**0.9***	(0.7–1.0)	**0.9**	(0.6–1.2)	**1.2**	(0.9–1.6)	**0.9**	(0.8–1.0)	**0.8**	(0.7–1.1)	**1.2**	(1.0–1.5)
Other	**1.6***	(1.4–1.8)	**2.2***	(1.8–2.8)	**1.3**	(1.0–1.6)	**1.7***	(1.5–1.9)	**2.4***	(2.0–2.9)	**1.6***	(1.3–2.0)
Employed	**1.0**		**1.0**		**1.0**		**1.0**		**1.0**		**1.0**	
χ^2 (P Value)[d]	64.6	(<0.001)	51.3	(<0.001)	5.2	(0.272)	113.3	(<0.001)	81.1	(<0.001)	22.7	(<0.001)

*Significant at the 0.05 level, two-sided test.
Dashed lines indicate empty cells.
[a]Based on survival models adjusted for age-cohorts, gender, person-years, and country. The denominator used for these estimates is the number of person-years in the survival models (N = 6,383,860 for DSM-IV models; N = 6,360,664 for DSM-5 models).
[b]Based on logistic regression models adjusted for age, gender, and country. The denominator used for these estimates is the number of respondents in the total sample (N = 147,261).
[c]Based on logistic regression models predicting 12-month GAD among lifetime cases, adjusted for time since GAD onset, age of GAD onset, sex, and country. The denominator used for these estimates is the number of lifetime GAD cases (N = 4,262 for DSM-IV models; *N* = 5,888 for DSM-5 models).
[d]Chi-square test of significant differences between blocks of socio-demographic variables.

economic development. This provides some assurance that the consequences of the latest GAD revision generalize to many parts of the world in which the DSM is used to inform research, policy, and clinical care.

The diagnostic revision led to several alterations in the epidemiology of GAD, suggesting that new cases captured by the revised criteria differ in meaningful ways from cases identified using DSM-IV criteria. Not surprisingly, some of the most notable differences concerned rates and patterns of comorbidity with other disorders. Approximately 82% of individuals with lifetime DSM-5 GAD qualified for another lifetime disorder, a small increase from the 76% comorbidity estimate for DSM-IV GAD. The increase in comorbidity was more striking among 12-month GAD cases, with more than 70% qualifying for another 12-month disorder under DSM-5 compared to 57% under DSM-IV. Although an increase in comorbidity was expected, the relatively larger increase in comorbidity among 12-month cases than lifetime cases warrants some consideration. A possible methodological explanation is that better memory for recent than distant disorders contributed to increased reporting of comorbid disorders, including hierarchy-triggering mood disorders, in the past year (i.e., a recall effect); another possibility is that lifetime comorbidity rates were already so high for DSM-IV GAD that there was relatively little room for comorbidity to increase under DSM-5 (i.e., a ceiling effect). An alternative, more substantive explanation is that individuals with chronic GAD may be more highly concentrated among 12-month cases than among lifetime cases, who include previously remitted cases as well as those whose GAD persisted without remission. There is some evidence that having a comorbid disorder predicts an unremitting course of GAD (Bruce *et al.* 2001). Additionally, unremitting GAD may be a marker of greater clinical severity or of exposure to risk factors that are particularly severe (e.g., strong genetic diathesis) or enduring (e.g., chronic stress), which may themselves increase the likelihood of comorbidity.

Predictably, the most significant change in comorbidity occurred with mood disorders. Even with the DSM-IV hierarchy rule in effect, comorbid MDD was present in more than 40% of lifetime GAD cases. When the hierarchy rule was lifted, comorbidity increased to more than 50%. The increase was even more dramatic among respondents who experienced GAD in the past year, of whom just over one-quarter were in a major depressive episode in the past year under DSM-IV compared to more than 40% under DSM-5. Based on trends observed in previous research (Ruscio & Khazanov 2017), comorbidity rates are likely to be even higher in clinical samples. Nevertheless, the finding that about half of people with lifetime DSM-5 GAD have never had MDD appears to support the continued separation of these disorders (Goldberg *et al.* 2010).

Although our analyses did not directly address the question of whether GAD should be considered an anxiety disorder or depressive disorder, the results do offer some relevant insights. Whereas DSM-IV GAD had roughly equal rates of lifetime comorbidity with mood disorders and other anxiety disorders (50% versus 49%), DSM-5 GAD had higher comorbidity with mood than anxiety disorders (63% versus 52%). Notably, this deviates from the pattern of substantially higher comorbidity with anxiety than mood disorders that was observed for every other anxiety disorder in the WMH surveys except posttraumatic stress disorder, which in DSM-5 is no longer classified as an anxiety disorder (see Chapters 7–12 in this volume). DSM-5 GAD also resembles MDD more closely than other anxiety disorders in these surveys in having a fairly late AOO, slow accumulation of new cases across the lifespan, and relatively less persistent course of illness. These epidemiological results are consistent with results from large factor analytic studies (Krueger 1999; Watson 2005) suggesting a closer relationship of GAD with depressive disorders than with other anxiety disorders. Although the collective findings appear to support a departure of GAD from the family of anxiety disorders, other considerations may support its continued classification with these disorders. For example, in prospective research, psychosocial risk factors for GAD have been shown to align more closely with those for anxiety disorders than depressive disorders (Beesdo *et al.* 2010). From a more pragmatic standpoint, focusing on GAD's prominent anxiety symptoms may help promote clinical detection and accurate diagnosis of the disorder – an important consideration given that GAD remains poorly recognized, especially in general medical settings (Wittchen *et al.* 2002).

Of note, the new cases identified by DSM-5 disproportionately reported that their GAD began after the onset of another mental disorder. This diverges from conventional clinical wisdom which dictates that anxiety typically precedes depression, as well as from prior research which documented a nearly equal number of comorbid cases beginning with GAD versus MDD (Moffitt *et al.* 2007). Our research suggests that once the hierarchy rule is lifted, an imbalance emerges, with mood disorders (typically MDD) tending to onset before GAD. One explanation for this may be methodological; by definition, GAD cases that emerged first would not meet the hierarchy rule and would be diagnosed by the DSM-IV criteria. Nevertheless, substantive interpretations are also possible. For example, GAD may be a complication of, or a reaction to, a major depressive episode, such as when role impairments associated with depression create secondary problems (e.g., job loss, poor grades, relationship strain) that elicit anxiety. A different possibility, consistent with the idea that anxiety precedes depression, is that the propensity to worry emerges early in life but may not be recognized as a problem until a major stressor – or perhaps another disorder – undermines the ability to manage worry successfully. Research collecting more detailed information about the onset of worry as well as GAD, and about the environmental contexts in which GAD and other disorders first emerge, would aid in understanding the causes of GAD and the functional relationships between disorders that could be targeted in treatment.

Several aspects of the GAD diagnosis, including socio-demographic correlates and AOO, remained stable irrespective of the criterion set applied. Consistent with previous epidemiological research (Grant *et al.* 2005; Lieb *et al.* 2005), individuals with GAD were more likely to be young (below age 60), female, and previously married (divorced, separated, or widowed). In high-income countries, GAD was also associated with lower education, lower income, and a lack of full-time employment. These similarities suggest that GAD is fundamentally the same disorder, concentrated in the same segments of the population, under the two diagnostic definitions. At the same time, DSM-5 cases tended to report more significant role impairment due to GAD, especially in upper-middle- and high-income countries, and were correspondingly more likely to seek treatment. Taken together, these results suggest that the revised criteria were successful in capturing clinically significant cases of GAD that were missed by the DSM-IV diagnosis. The greater severity of these cases is consistent with prior studies, which found greater psychopathology (Zimmerman & Chelminski 2003; Lawrence *et al.* 2009) and a more adverse risk profile (Moffitt *et al.* 2007) among comorbid relative to 'pure' GAD and MDD. Importantly, the available findings do not resolve whether the new cases actually involve multiple, distinct disorders (e.g., comorbid GAD and MDD) or a severe form of mood disorder (e.g., an anxious subtype of MDD); these and another possibilities await evaluation using methods appropriate for explicating comorbidity (Klein & Riso 1993; Neale & Kendler 1995; J. Ruscio & Ruscio 2004). Nevertheless, the observed severity underscores the importance of recognizing the significant consequences of co-occurring anxiety in these former hierarchy cases, especially as the presence of comorbid GAD may have implications for treatment (Zimmerman & Chelminski 2003; Coplan *et al.* 2015).

A notable strength of the current study is the large, multinational sample that was representative of the household populations in the countries and regions included here. The large sample size allowed for the detection of subtle changes from DSM-IV to DSM-5 GAD and increased confidence in the reliability of the findings. The use of representative community samples ensured that results were not biased by self-selection into treatment or by features of specific clinical sites. The inclusion of 29 surveys from 26 diverse countries ensured that results were not limited to particular regions, cultures, or strata of economic development. Nevertheless, the study also had several limitations. Perhaps most important, GAD diagnoses were assigned based on fully structured interviews administered by lay interviewers. Although the CIDI shows good concordance with the SCID, it is possible that results would have differed if diagnoses had been assigned by expert clinicians. This is a particular concern given the challenges of differentiating GAD from MDD symptoms and establishing the dates of episode onset and remission, even for experienced clinicians. Another limitation is that symptom onset was assessed retrospectively; consequently, some caution is warranted when interpreting the AOO and temporal priority data. The timing of GAD and mood disorders was determined from these AOO reports along with reports of symptom offset and episode duration, which were rounded to the nearest year and dated separately for each disorder. Consequently, in the common situation of two disorders beginning in the same year (Kessler *et al.* 2008), we were unable to distinguish simultaneous onsets from onsets that were separated within the year. Finally, although considerable effort was made to standardize data collection across surveys, cultural variation in the interpretation of concepts such as 'excessive worry' and 'feeling sad, empty, or depressed' may have contributed to cross-national differences.

This chapter presents the first comparison of DSM-IV and DSM-5 GAD in the general population. In a large, multinational sample, lifting the DSM-IV hierarchy with mood disorders increased the prevalence of GAD substantially. The newly identified GAD cases appeared to be more severe than previously identified cases on several dimensions. DSM-5 GAD was associated with somewhat higher rates of role impairment and treatment seeking than DSM-IV GAD. In addition, DSM-5 GAD was associated more strongly with psychiatric comorbidity in general and MDD comorbidity in particular, with most GAD onsets occurring after the onset of another mental disorder. These patterns of comorbidity are consistent with findings from empirically derived taxonomies, which tend to group GAD with depressive disorders rather than anxiety disorders. Other important correlates of GAD such as female gender, previously married status, lower education and income, and a lack of full-time employment remained unchanged. Whether DSM-IV or DSM-5 criteria are applied, these findings converge on a conceptualization of GAD as a common disorder that is associated with considerable morbidity and disability.

Acknowledgements

This work was supported in part by National Institute of Mental Health Grant R01 MH094425 awarded to Ayelet Meron Ruscio. We are grateful to Courtney Forbes for her assistance in preparing this chapter.

References

Abel, J. L. & Borkovec, T. D. (1995). Generalizability of DSM-III-R generalized anxiety disorders to proposed DSM-IV criteria and cross-validation of proposed changes. *Journal of Anxiety Disorders*, 4, 303–15.

American Psychiatric Association. (1980). *Diagnostic and Statistical Manual of Mental Disorders*. 3rd ed. Washington, DC: Author.

(1987). *Diagnostic and Statistical Manual of Mental Disorders*. 3rd ed., revised. Washington, DC: Author.

(1994). *Diagnostic and Statistical Manual of Mental Disorders*. 4th ed. Washington, DC: Author.

(2013). *Diagnostic and Statistical Manual of Mental Disorders*. 5th ed. Washington, DC: Author.

Andrews, G., Hobbs, M. J., Borkovec, T. D., *et al.* (2010). Generalized worry disorder: a review of DSM-IV generalized anxiety disorder and options for DSM-V. *Depression and Anxiety*, 27, 134–47.

Ballenger, J. C., Davidson, J., Lecrubier, Y., & Wittchen, H. U. (2001). Consensus statement on generalized anxiety disorder from the International Consensus Group on Depression and Anxiety. *The Journal of Clinical Psychiatry*, 62, 53–8.

Beesdo, K., Pine, D. S., Lieb, R., & Wittchen, H. U. (2010). Incidence and risk patterns of anxiety and depressive disorders and categorization of generalized anxiety disorder. *Archives of General Psychiatry*, 67, 47–57.

Berkson, J. (1946). Limitations of the application of the four-fold table analysis to hospital data. *Biometrics Bulletin*, 2, 47–53.

Brown, T. A., Barlow, D. H., & Liebowitz, M. R. (1994). The empirical basis of generalized anxiety disorder. *American Journal of Psychiatry*, 151, 1272–80.

Brown, T. A., DiNardo, P. A., Lehman, C. L., & Campbell, L. A. (2001). Reliability of DSM-IV anxiety and mood disorders: implications for the classification of emotional disorders. *Journal of Abnormal Psychology*, 110, 49–58.

Bruce, S. E., Machan, J. T., Dyck, I., & Keller, M. B. (2001). Infrequency of "pure" GAD: impact of psychiatric comorbidity on clinical course. *Depression and Anxiety*, 14, 219–25.

Chelminski, I. & Zimmerman, M. (2003). Pathological worry in depressed and anxious patients. *Journal of Anxiety Disorders*, 17, 553–46.

Coplan, J. D., Aaronson, C. J., Panthangi, V., & Kim, Y. (2015). Treating comorbid anxiety and depression: psychosocial and pharmacological approaches. *World Journal of Psychiatry*, 5, 366–78.

Davidson, J. R., Zhang, W., Connor, K. M., *et al.* (2010). A psychopharmacological treatment algorithm for generalised anxiety disorder (GAD). *Journal of Psychopharmacology*, 24, 3–26.

Ehring, T. & Watkins, E. R. (2008). Repetitive negative thinking as a transdiagnostic process. *International Journal of Cognitive Therapy*, 1, 192–205.

First, M. B., Spitzer, R. L., Gibbon, M., & Williams, J. B. W. (2002). *Structured Clinical Interview for DSM-IV-TR Axis I Disorders: Research Version, Non-patient Ed.* New York, NY: Biometrics Research, New York State Psychiatric Institute.

Goldberg, D., Kendler, K. S., Sirovatka, P. J., & Regier, D. A., eds. (2010). *Diagnostic Issues in Depression and Generalized Anxiety Disorder: Refining the Research Agenda for DSM-V*. Washington, DC: American Psychiatric Association.

Grant, B. F., Hasin, D. S., Stinson, F. S., *et al.* (2005). Prevalence, correlates, co-morbidity, and comparative disability of DSM-IV generalized anxiety disorder in the USA: results from the National Epidemiologic Survey on Alcohol and Related Conditions. *Psychological Medicine*, 35, 1747–59.

Haro, J. M., Arbabzadeh-Bouchez, S., Brugha, T. S., *et al.* (2006). Concordance of the Composite International Diagnostic Interview Version 3.0 (CIDI 3.0) with standardized clinical assessments in the WHO World Mental Health Surveys. *International Journal of Methods in Psychiatric Research*, 15, 167–80.

Kendler, K. S., Neale, M. C., Kessler, R. C., Heath, A. C., & Eaves, L. J. (1992). Major depression and generalized anxiety disorder: same genes, (partly) different environments? *Archives of General Psychiatry*, 49, 716–22.

Kessler, R. C., Gruber, M., Hettema, J. M., Hwang, I., Sampson, N., & Yonkers, K. A. (2008). Comorbid major depression and generalized anxiety disorders in the National Comorbidity Survey follow-up. *Psychological Medicine*, 38, 365–74.

Klein, D. N., & Riso, L. P. (1993). Psychiatric disorders: Problems of boundaries and comorbidity. In C. G. Costello (Ed.), *Basic Issues in Psychopathology* (pp. 19–66). New York, NY: Guilford Press.

Krueger, R. F. (1999). The structure of common mental disorders. *Archives of General Psychiatry*, 56, 921–6.

Lawrence, A. E., Liverant, G. I., Rosellini, A. J., & Brown, T. A. (2009). Generalized anxiety disorder within the course of major depressive disorder: examining the utility of the DSM-IV hierarchy rule. *Depression and Anxiety*, 26, 909–16.

Lewis-Fernández, R., Hinton, D. E., Laria, A. J., *et al.* (2010). Culture and the anxiety disorders: recommendations for DSM-V. *Depression and Anxiety*, 27, 212–29.

Lieb, R., Becker, E., & Altamura, C. (2005). The epidemiology of generalized anxiety disorder in Europe. *European Neuropsychopharmacology*, 15, 445–52.

Marten, P. A., Brown, T. A., Barlow, D. H., Borkovec, T. D., Shear, M. K., & Lydiard, R. B. (1993). Evaluation of the ratings comprising the associated symptom criterion of DSM-III-R generalized anxiety disorder. *Journal of Nervous and Mental Disease*, 181, 676–82.

Merikangas, K. R., Akiskal, H. S., Angst, J., *et al.* (2007). Lifetime and 12-month prevalence of bipolar spectrum disorder in the National Comorbidity Survey Replication. *Archives of General Psychiatry*, 64, 543–52.

Moffitt, T. E., Caspi, A., Harrington, H., *et al.* (2007). Generalized anxiety disorder and depression: childhood risk factors in a birth cohort followed to age 32. *Psychological Medicine*, 37, 441–52.

Moffitt, T. E., Harrington, H., Caspi, A., *et al.* (2007). Depression and generalized anxiety disorder: cumulative and sequential comorbidity in a birth cohort followed prospectively to age 32 years. *Archives of General Psychiatry*, 64, 651–60.

Neale, M. C., & Kendler, K. S. (1995). Models of comorbidity for multifactorial disorders. *American Journal of Human Genetics*, 57, 935–53.

Rickels, K. & Rynn, M. (2001). Overview and clinical presentation of generalized anxiety disorder. *Psychiatric Clinics of North America*, 24, 1–17.

Ruscio, A. M., Hallion, L. S., Lim, C. C. W., *et al.* (2017). Cross-sectional comparison of the epidemiology of DSM-5 generalized anxiety disorder across the globe. *JAMA Psychiatry*, 74, 465–75.

Ruscio, A. M. & Khazanov, G. K. (2017). Anxiety and depression. In R. J. DeRubeis and D. R. Strunk (eds.), *Oxford Handbook of Mood Disorders* (pp. 313–24). New York, NY: Oxford University Press.

Ruscio, A. M., Lane, M., Roy-Byrne, P., *et al.* (2005). Should excessive worry be required for a diagnosis of generalized anxiety disorder? Results from the US National Comorbidity Survey Replication. *Psychological Medicine*, 35, 1761–772.

Ruscio, J., & Ruscio, A. M. (2004). Clarifying boundary issues in psychopathology: the role of taxometrics in a comprehensive program of structural research. *Journal of Abnormal Psychology*, 113, 24–38.

Somers, J. M., Goldner, E. M., Waraich, P., & Hsu, L. (2006). Prevalence and incidence studies of anxiety disorders: a systematic review of the literature. *The Canadian Journal of Psychiatry*, 51, 100–13.

Starcevic, V., Portman, M. E., & Beck, A. T. (2012). Generalized anxiety disorder: between neglect and an epidemic. *Journal of Nervous and Mental Disease*, 200, 664–7.

The World Bank. (2009). *Data & Statistics, Country Groups by Income.* Retrieved from https://datahelpdesk.worldbank.org/knowledgebase/articles/906519.

Watson, D. (2005). Rethinking the mood and anxiety disorders: A quantitative hierarchal model for DSM-V. *Journal of Abnormal Psychology*, 114, 522–36.

(2009). Differentiating the mood and anxiety disorders: A quadripartite model. *Annual Review of Clinical Psychology*, 5, 221–47.

Wittchen, H. U., Kessler, R. C., Beesdo, K., Krause, P., Höfler, M., & Hoyer, J. (2002). Generalized anxiety and depression in primary care: Prevalence, recognition, and management. *The Journal of Clinical Psychiatry*, 63, 24–34.

Zimmerman, M. & Chelminski, I. (2003). Generalized anxiety disorder in patients with major depression: is DSM-IV's hierarchy correct? *American Journal of Psychiatry*, 160, 504–12.

Chapter 7

Panic Disorder and Panic Attacks

Peter de Jonge, Annelieke M. Roest, Carmen C. W. Lim, Daphna Levinson, Kate M. Scott

Introduction

Panic attacks (PAs) are an important set of anxiety symptoms and are defined in different editions of the *Diagnostic and Statistical Manual*: DSM (APA 1987, 1994). PAs are a common phenomenon that many people will experience at some point during their lives. A distinction is made between PAs and Panic Disorder (PD); the latter being characterized by recurrent PAs (Horwath, Gould & Weissman 2011). Despite some minor changes, the definition of PAs is largely comparable across the recent editions of the DSM (DSM-III, DSM-IV, DSM-5) (APA 1987, 1994, 2013). These are defined as periods of intense fear or discomfort in which at least 4 of the following 13 symptoms develop quickly, reaching a peak within 10 minutes:

(1) palpitations, pounding heart, or accelerated heart rate,
(2) sweating,
(3) trembling or shaking,
(4) sensations of shortness of breath or smothering,
(5) feeling of choking,
(6) chest pain or discomfort,
(7) nausea or abdominal distress,
(8) feeling dizzy, unsteady, lightheaded, or faint,
(9) derealization or depersonalization,
(10) fear of losing control or going crazy,
(11) fear of dying,
(12) numbness or tingling sensations,
(13) chills or hot flushes.

To diagnose PD, PAs should not be attributable to a general medical condition (such as hyperthyroidism or myocardial ischemia) or to substances (such as caffeine or amphetamine; Roberson-Nay & Kendler 2011). It should be noted that in DSM-IV, PAs were only coded in the context of a specific diagnosis, such as PD or agoraphobia. However, in DSM-5 PAs are conceptualized as a generic specifier and prognostic factor for severity of diagnosis, course, and comorbidity across different disorders. Thus, for example, an individual may have a major depressive disorder with PAs. Therefore, although the epidemiological data we present in this chapter are for DSM-IV PD, we also present the epidemiological data on PAs separately from PD (see also de Jonge *et al.* 2016).

In DSM-IV, the essential feature of PD is the presence of recurrent, unexpected PAs. In addition, at least one of the attacks must be followed by one month or more of at least one of the following:

(1) Persistent concern about having additional attacks.
(2) Worry about the implications of the attack or its consequences (such as losing control, having a heart attack, going crazy).
(3) A significant change in behaviour related to the attack.

In DSM-III and DSM-IV, PD was closely linked to the presence of agoraphobia such that explicit distinctions were made between PD with and without agoraphobia, and agoraphobia without PD. Agoraphobia was described as a condition accompanying PD, while agoraphobia without a history of PD described individuals where avoidance was a key symptom. The link between the disorders was based on research in clinical samples (Klein 1993) where agoraphobia mostly occurred after PD or PAs. However, it has become increasingly apparent that PAs may be a marker of psychopathology in general rather than being specific to PD or agoraphobia (Goodwin & Hamilton 2001; Batelaan *et al.* 2007, 2012) and that PD and agoraphobia are not expressions of a single disorder (Wittchen *et al.* 2010). In DSM-5, diagnostic criteria for PD and agoraphobia have therefore been unlinked, to emphasize that they are two independent diagnoses.

Anxiety disorders are among the major contributors to the worldwide burden of disease (Murray *et al.* 2010; Whiteford *et al.* 2013). The epidemiology of PD is well described. Several studies have reported the prevalence rates of PD, including the National Comorbidity Study (NCS), the National Comorbidity Study Replication (NCS-R), the Epidemiological Area Catchment Study (ECA), and the National Epidemiological Survey on Alcohol and Related Conditions (NESARC) (Regier, Narrow & Rae 1990; Kessler & Walters 2002; Kessler & Merikangas 2004; Grant & Dawson 2006). Lifetime rates are generally found in the order of 1–4%, with some exceptions at the higher end in specific studies or countries (e.g. NCS-R: 4.7%) and the lower end (e.g. in Taiwan: <0.5%). As recently summarized, risk factors for PD are fairly consistent and include female gender, smoking and alcohol problems, mental comorbidity, and low socio-economic status (Moreno-Peral *et al.* 2004). Age-of-onset (AOO) of PD is mostly in early to middle adulthood, regardless of presence or absence of agoraphobia (Weissman *et al.* 1997; Kessler *et al.* 2006). In comparison to other mental disorders, PD is characterized by relatively high levels of help-seeking (Iza *et al.* 2013) (see also Chapter 21), predominantly due to the extreme discomfort associated with PAs and the concern among sufferers that the symptoms may indicate a heart attack or some other medical problem.

Several authors have reported high levels of psychiatric comorbidity (Chen & Dilsaver 1995; Roy-Byrne *et al.* 2000; Kessler *et al.* 2006), especially with other anxiety disorders, but also with mood disorders (Grant *et al.* 2005). In the NCS, half of the respondents with lifetime PAs (50.9%) or with lifetime PD (55.6%) also met lifetime criteria for depression (Kessler *et al.* 1998). In addition, personality disorders have been associated with the presence of PD (Grant *et al.* 2005). In the NESARC study, avoidant and dependent personality disorders were strongly associated with PD, but paranoid, schizoid, histrionic, and antisocial personality disorders also had some association with PD.

Prior research based on the WMH survey in the United States (the NCS-R) found that PD is associated with substantial levels of impairment (Kessler *et al.* 2006). As many as 84.7% of individuals with PD and agoraphobia reported severe impairment on at least one of the four Sheehan domains (work, home, social, and personal relationship), while this percentage was 56.2% for people with PD without agoraphobia. Substantially less severe impairment (11.1%) was reported by individuals with PAs without PD and agoraphobia. In the same report, it was found that treatment rates varied in a similar way, in that high lifetime treatment rates were reported for individuals with lifetime PD (84.8% lifetime treatment for PD only and 96.1% for PD with agoraphobia) and somewhat lower rates for people with lifetime PAs (61.1%). Based on several reports it was concluded that most individuals with PD eventually receive treatment. Also, of those with a past 12-month diagnosis of PD, most receive treatment, although it was noted that most treatment fails to meet basic treatment guidelines (Wang *et al.* 2005).

Most of the available epidemiological data on PD and PAs comes from the United States. However, it has been suggested that considerable cross-cultural variation exists in the prevalence and presentation of the anxiety disorders (Marques *et al.* 2011). The first study on the cross-national epidemiology of PD was reported by Weissman *et al.* (1997). It was concluded that the rates and patterns of PD were fairly consistent across countries. However, while the lifetime prevalence rates varied between 1.4% (Alberta) and 3.5% (United States), in Taiwan this was considerably lower (0.4%). Mean AOO of PD was between 23 and 25 years of age and fairly consistent across the samples. Comorbidity with agoraphobia was consistently high, with a 10–20-fold increased risk across the samples. However, comorbidity with depression varied substantially, with ORs of 1.3 and 2.5 for Taiwan and Korea, and 16.0 and 17.3 for the United States and France. Overall, the study revealed a fairly consistent pattern of epidemiological data across countries but several notable differences were also observed. As the authors emphasized, several of the subsamples were fairly small and the methods differed somewhat across sites. Moreover, although this study had coverage of 11 sites including Puerto Rico, Lebanon, Korea, and Taiwan, many of these were Western or high-income countries (e.g. the United States, Canada, Germany, France, Italy, New Zealand). The WMH Surveys Initiative draws from a wider range of countries and employs much greater standardization of methods, thus providing a unique opportunity to study the cross-national epidemiology of both PAs and PD.

Method

The assessment of PD and PAs was included in 28 of the surveys included in this volume, originating from 25 countries and comprising 147,264 participants (Table 7.1). With respect to PD, a blinded clinical reappraisal study using the Structured Clinical Interview for DSM-IV (SCID) (First *et al.* 2002) found good diagnostic concordance between CIDI and SCID diagnoses, indicated by an area under the curve of 0.72 (Haro *et al.* 2006). In addition, while most of the available literature is on PD (and often in conjunction with or without agoraphobia), the WMH surveys have extensive data on PAs as well. Within those reporting PAs, we further distinguish between single and recurrent PAs, in order to evaluate the DSM-5 decision to use PAs as a generic specifier. For analyses examining whether PAs predict onset and course of psychiatric disorders, we used PAs *in the absence of PD*, as otherwise these would count as being part of a comorbid psychiatric disorder (i.e. PD).

Results

Prevalence

Significant differences in prevalence rates of PAs and PD can be observed between country groups based on income level (Table 7.1). Specifically, higher prevalence rates are found in the high-income countries. Overall lifetime prevalence of PAs for all countries combined is 13.2% (Table 7.1), but this figure varies from 2.1% to 18.5% for low/lower-middle-income countries, 6.0% to 20.1% for upper-middle-income countries, and 6.6% to 27.4% for high-income countries. Of the people with lifetime PA, only a minority of 12.8% have a lifetime PD diagnosis. Lifetime prevalence of PD is thus much lower: 1.7%. This percentage varies between 0.8% for the low/lower-middle-income countries to 1.1% for the upper-middle-income countries and 2.2% for the high-income countries. Of people with lifetime PA without PD, about two-thirds (66.5%) have recurrent PAs. This figure is fairly consistent for the three income groups of countries. Overall, differences between countries are driven more by income level than by geographical region.

Twelve-month prevalence rates for PAs and PD (Appendix Table 7A.1) are 4.9% and 1.0%, respectively. Slightly more than a third (34.5%) of people with lifetime PAs, but without lifetime PD, have PAs in the last 12 months. For PD, this figure is 57.1%, indicating a moderate level of disorder persistence. Prevalence rates for 30-day PAs and PD are 1.6% and 0.4% respectively (Appendix Table 7A.2). Of people with 12-month PAs without PD, 29.2% have 30-day PAs. For PD, this figure is 40.6%, which suggests that episode persistence is lower than disorder persistence. Median AOO of PD is 32 years (interquartile range (IQR) 20–47) (Appendix Table 7A.3). The AOO distribution results in a projected lifetime risk of PD at age 75 of 2.7%. Median AOO of PAs is 34 years (IQR 20–51), and for PAs without PD it is 35 years (IQR 20–52), resulting in a projected lifetime risk at age 75 of 23.0% for PAs and 20.6% for PAs without PD.

Role Impairment and Treatment

Severe role impairment in the past 12 months is reported by 45.7% of people with 12-month PD (Table 7.2). Impairment is more or less equally reported for the home (26.9%), work (30.8%), relationship (26.9%), and social domains (30.5%) (Table 7.2). It is notable that relatively fewer respondents from low/lower-middle-income countries and from the African region report impairment.

Of people with 12-month PD with any impairment, 59.8% report seeking treatment, most often consisting of general medical care (44.1%) and specialty mental health care (30.3%) (data not shown). The proportion of treated cases increases as a function of level of impairment, with 74.6% of those reporting severe impairment indicating receipt of any treatment. In low/lower-middle-income countries, only about one-third of people with 12-month PD report seeking treatment, and this proportion is irrespective of the level of associated impairment. Higher treatment proportions are found in the higher-income countries, particularly at higher levels of associated impairment. As another indicator of functional impairment, people with 12-month PD report on average 43.8 days-out-of-role in the past year (data not shown). For those reporting severe impairment on any of the four domains, this figure is 72.9 days.

Comorbidity and Correlates

Lifetime comorbidity with other mental disorders in people with lifetime PD is 80.4%. Comorbidity levels are particularly high for other anxiety disorders (63.1%) and mood disorders (53.7%), but considerably lower for substance-abuse disorders (26.2%) and disruptive behaviour/impulse-control disorders (10.4%). In people with lifetime comorbidity, onset of PD precedes the onset of the other disorders in a minority of cases (15.4%) (data not shown).

Being under the age of 60, having early AOO, being female, being unemployed or disabled ('other' employment status), being divorced/separated/widowed,

Table 7.1 Lifetime prevalence of panic attack (PA) and DSM-IV panic disorder (PD) in the World Mental Health Surveys

Country	Among total population						Among lifetime PA without lifetime PD cases				Part 1 sample sizes	Sample size used[b]
	Lifetime PA		Lifetime PA without lifetime PD cases		Lifetime PD		Proportion with single attack		Proportion with recurrent attacks[a]			
	%	SE	%	SE	%	SE	%	SE	%	SE		
Low/lower-middle-income countries	**6.9**	**0.2**	**6.1**	**0.2**	**0.8**	**0.1**	**29.8**	**1.4**	**61.5**	**1.4**	**36,498**	**36,395**
Colombia	18.5	0.7	17.2	0.8	1.3	0.2	43.4	2.6	52.8	2.5	4,426	4,422
Iraq	7.5	0.6	6.2	0.6	1.4	0.3	27.6	4.8	47.4	5.5	4,332	4,295
Nigeria	2.6	0.3	2.4	0.3	0.2	0.1	25.0	4.9	67.3	5.3	6,752	6,713
Peru	7.1	0.4	6.7	0.4	0.5	0.1	31.2	2.9	62.7	2.6	3,930	3,929
PRC (Beijing/Shanghai)	2.1	0.3	1.7	0.2	0.4	0.1	17.2	4.5	79.5	4.9	5,201	5,197
PRC (Shenzhen)	2.5	0.3	2.2	0.3	0.3	0.1	20.9	5.0	79.1	5.0	7,132	7,129
Ukraine	13.4	0.6	11.2	0.6	2.2	0.3	16.8	1.7	70.4	2.0	4,725	4,710
Upper-middle-income countries	**11.1**	**0.3**	**10.0**	**0.3**	**1.1**	**0.1**	**28.7**	**1.1**	**57.1**	**1.2**	**24,612**	**24,565**
Brazil	11.7	0.6	10.0	0.6	1.7	0.2	26.1	1.7	56.8	2.2	5,037	5,023
Bulgaria	6.0	0.3	5.0	0.3	1.1	0.1	14.7	2.4	53.5	3.9	5,318	5,301
Colombia (Medellin)	20.1	1.3	18.8	1.2	1.3	0.3	39.5	2.4	48.7	2.5	3,261	3,260
Lebanon	13.9	0.9	13.4	0.9	0.5	0.1	32.2	2.9	55.9	2.6	2,857	2,851
Mexico	7.8	0.5	6.8	0.5	1.0	0.2	28.8	3.0	69.5	2.9	5,782	5,781
Romania	13.9	0.8	13.3	0.8	0.7	0.2	19.2	2.9	63.1	3.2	2,357	2,349
High-income countries	**16.6**	**0.2**	**14.4**	**0.2**	**2.2**	**0.1**	**22.5**	**0.5**	**69.4**	**0.5**	**81,839**	**81,754**
Australia	21.5	0.6	17.9	0.6	3.7	0.3	25.6	1.5	71.9	1.7	8,463	8,461
Belgium	10.1	1.0	8.5	0.8	1.6	0.3	27.6	3.2	58.2	3.2	2,419	2,417
France	11.1	0.9	9.0	0.8	2.1	0.3	37.5	3.5	58.9	3.6	2,894	2,894
Germany	10.1	0.6	8.5	0.6	1.6	0.2	29.5	3.9	66.5	3.9	3,555	3,555
Israel	10.0	0.5	9.1	0.5	0.9	0.1	24.3	2.2	55.6	2.5	4,859	4,853
Italy	8.0	0.5	6.4	0.4	1.6	0.2	14.9	2.2	70.0	2.7	4,712	4,708
Japan	6.6	0.4	5.9	0.4	0.8	0.1	28.2	3.2	65.8	3.7	4,129	4,126

Table 7.1 *(cont.)*

Country	Among total population						Among lifetime PA without lifetime PD cases				Part 1 sample sizes	Sample size used[b]
	Lifetime PA		Lifetime PA without lifetime PD cases		Lifetime PD		Proportion with single attack		Proportion with recurrent attacks[a]			
	%	SE	%	SE	%	SE	%	SE	%	SE		
New Zealand	27.4	0.6	24.7	0.5	2.8	0.2	22.8	1.0	74.3	1.0	12,790	12,781
Northern Ireland	24.4	0.8	21.1	0.7	3.3	0.3	23.1	1.8	70.6	2.0	4,340	4,335
Poland	5.9	0.2	5.6	0.2	0.3	0.1	11.3	1.1	47.1	2.1	10,081	10,049
Portugal	19.6	0.7	17.9	0.6	1.7	0.3	21.9	1.9	64.4	2.1	3,849	3,841
Spain	9.6	0.5	8.4	0.5	1.2	0.2	33.5	3.0	54.1	3.2	5,473	5,472
Spain (Murcia)	16.3	1.0	14.7	1.0	1.6	0.4	27.1	2.3	54.5	4.1	2,621	2,617
Netherlands	14.0	0.8	11.0	0.7	3.0	0.4	24.3	3.7	72.3	3.7	2,372	2,370
United States	27.3	0.7	22.6	0.7	4.7	0.2	16.0	0.8	79.2	0.8	9,282	9,275
All countries combined	**13.2**	**0.1**	**11.5**	**0.1**	**1.7**	**0.0**	**24.4**	**0.4**	**66.5**	**0.5**	**147,264**	**142,714**
WHO regions[c]												
Region of the Americas	16.8	0.4	14.6	0.4	2.2	0.1	26.7	0.9	66.6	0.9	31,718	31,690
African region	2.6	0.3	2.4	0.3	0.2	0.1	25.0	4.9	67.3	5.3	11,067	6,713
Western Pacific region	15.6	0.3	13.7	0.2	2.0	0.1	23.7	0.8	73.4	0.8	37,715	37,694
Eastern Mediterranean region	10.0	0.4	9.1	0.4	1.0	0.1	27.9	1.8	53.7	1.9	12,048	11,999
Western European region	13.6	0.2	11.7	0.2	1.9	0.1	25.7	0.9	64.1	1.0	32,235	32,209
Eastern European region	8.4	0.2	7.4	0.2	0.9	0.1	15.0	0.9	58.4	1.3	22,481	22,409
Comparison between countries[d]	**$F_{27,v} = 164.6^*$, $P < 0.001$**		**$F_{27,v} = 143.0^*$, $P < 0.001$**		**$F_{27,v} = 32.4^*$, $P < 0.001$**		**$F_{27,v} = 12.7^*$, $P < 0.001$**		**$F_{27,v} = 16.9^*$, $P < 0.001$**			
Comparison between low-, middle-, and high-income country groups[d]	**$F_{2,v} = 638.7^*$, $P < 0.001$**		**$F_{2,v} = 529.7^*$, $P < 0.001$**		**$F_{2,v} = 130.8^*$, $P < 0.001$**		**$F_{2,v} = 22.5^*$, $P < 0.001$**		**$F_{5,v} = 50.5^*$, $P < 0.001$**			
Comparison between WHO regions[d]	**$F_{5,v} = 320.6^*$, $P < 0.001$**		**$F_{5,v} = 275.2^*$, $P < 0.001$**		**$F_{5,v} = 85.8^*$, $P < 0.001$**		**$F_{5,v} = 20.3^*$, $P < 0.001$**		**$F_{5,v} = 30.8^*$, $P < 0.001$**			

[a] Recurrent panic attacks = at least two panic attacks.
[b] Sample size used after excluding lifetime panic attack cases with missing age-of-onset.
[c] **Region of the Americas** (Colombia, Mexico, Brazil, United States, Colombia (Medellin)); **African region** (Nigeria); **Western Pacific region** (PRC (Shenzhen), PRC Beijing and Shanghai, Japan, Australia, New Zealand); **Eastern Mediterranean region** (Israel, Iraq, Lebanon); **Western European region** (Belgium, France, Germany, Italy, Netherlands, Spain, Northern Ireland, Portugal, Spain (Murcia); **Eastern European region** (Romania, Bulgaria, Poland, Ukraine).
[d] Wald design-corrected F-tests were used to determine if there is variation in prevalence estimates across countries. The denominator degree of freedom, v, is 5367.
PRC: People's Republic of China.

Table 7.2 Severity of role impairment (Sheehan Disability Scale) associated with 12-month panic disorder, by country income groups and WHO region

Country	Proportion with severe role impairment (SDS score: 7–10)										Number of 12-month panic disorder cases
	Home		Work		Relationship		Social		Any[a]		
	%	SE	%	SE	%	SE	%	SE	%	SE	
Country Income groups											
Low/lower-middle-income countries	21.7	3.8	19.0	3.8	17.1	4.0	17.2	3.9	29.9	4.3	204
Upper-middle-income countries	32.5	4.2	30.3	4.5	30.0	3.8	31.1	4.1	42.1	4.5	184
High-income countries	26.9	1.7	32.9	1.9	28.0	1.9	32.4	1.9	49.1	2.0	1,077
WHO regions											
Region of the Americas	27.9	2.6	28.4	2.6	26.9	2.7	31.7	2.9	46.5	3.0	446
African region	8.7	7.0	3.7	4.0	3.7	4.0	3.7	4.0	8.7	7.0	9
Western Pacific region	18.2	2.3	30.7	3.2	24.8	2.8	29.7	2.9	44.3	3.4	454
Eastern Mediterranean region	40.5	7.6	39.5	8.2	28.3	8.4	23.7	7.0	52.1	8.1	78
Western European region	33.7	3.3	35.6	3.4	29.8	3.2	33.7	3.2	48.6	3.4	339
Eastern European region	30.0	4.7	24.9	4.8	27.1	5.0	25.6	5.2	39.3	5.3	139
All countries combined	26.9	1.4	30.8	1.6	26.9	1.6	30.5	1.6	45.7	1.7	1,465
Comparison between low-, middle-, and high-income countries[b]	**$F_{2,v} = 1.9$, $P = 0.154$**		**$F_{2,v} = 5.1^*$, $P = 0.006$**		**$F_{2,v} = 3.4^*$, $P = 0.035$**		**$F_{2,v} = 5.4^*$, $P = 0.004$**		**$F_{2,v} = 7.5^*$, $P < 0.001$**		
Comparison between WHO regions[b]	**$F_{5,v} = 4.6^*$, $P < 0.001$**		**$F_{5,v} = 1.7$, $P = 0.130$**		**$F_{5,v} = 0.9$, $P = 0.483$**		**$F_{5,v} = 1.2$, $P = 0.287$**		**$F_{5,v} = 1.2$, $P = 0.329$**		

[a]Highest severity category across four SDS role domains.
[b]Wald design-corrected F-tests were used to determine if there is variation in impairment severity across countries. The denominator degree of freedom, v, is 5367.

and having lower education or household income are all associated with both PAs without PD and with PD (data not shown). These correlates are largely comparable for the different country income groups, and largely in line with a recent systematic review (Moreno-Peral *et al.* 2014). Few differences are found when comparing risk factors for 30-day, lifetime, 12-month/lifetime, and 30-day/12-month cases, suggesting that similar risk factors may operate for onset and course of PAs and PD. However, as an exception, female gender is associated with increased odds of onset of PAs and PD (lifetime prevalence), but not with episode persistence (30-day/12-month).

Number and Type of PAs

As noted earlier, there are two significant changes in DSM-5 regarding PD and PAs, namely that PD became unlinked from agoraphobia, and that the presence of PAs is a generic specifier that can apply to any mental disorders. This section explores the support for these changes.

In Table 7.3, we distinguish between single and recurrent PAs. Based on the AOO data we were able to determine the presence of a wide range of mental disorders that occurred after the first PA. To be on the safe side, we excluded the onset of a disorder that occurred in the same year as the PA. The findings are quite consistent in that single PAs are generally not associated with subsequent mental disorders. There are only a few exceptions to this general rule, namely that single PAs are associated with an increased risk of disruptive behaviour/impulse-control disorders and alcohol abuse and a decreased risk of specific phobia and any anxiety disorder. In contrast, recurrent PAs are associated with increased odds of all mental disorders. We also examined whether the course of a disorder varied as a function of the presence of single or recurrent PAs. Here we found that single PAs are generally slightly protective against the persistence of disorders while recurrent PAs are associated with a worse course. Specifically, the risk of any 12-month mental disorder given a lifetime disorder is significantly lower (OR 0.7) in the presence of a single PA and significantly higher (OR 1.3) in the presence of recurrent PAs.

In Table 7.4, we distinguish between several subgroups of individuals with combinations of anxiety disorders to evaluate the similarities and dissimilarities in terms of kinds and numbers of PAs. In respondents with a lifetime diagnosis of agoraphobia without PD, 52.4% experienced a PA. For social anxiety disorder and specific phobia without PD, rates of 42.2% and 32.5% are found. Thus even in the absence of PD, many people with anxiety disorders experience PAs. About half of the individuals who experience PAs report unexpected attacks. Remarkably, this ratio between expected and unexpected PAs is relatively stable across individual anxiety disorders, the exception being PD. The number of expected attacks among people experiencing expected attacks is higher than the number of unexpected attacks among those who experience unexpected attacks. This is the case for all groups, although the difference is smallest for individuals with PD. Median AOO of PAs is generally around 20 years, with the exception of people with a single PA in the absence of PD where the median AOO is later (29.5 years, IQR 20–41.6).

Discussion

These analyses of the WMH surveys data on PD and PAs confirm the picture that PAs are a relatively common phenomenon (Von Korff *et al.* 1985; Eaton *et al.* 1994, 1998). In contrast, lifetime prevalence for PD is much lower. For PD, we found a lifetime prevalence of 1.7% and a projected lifetime risk at age 75 of 2.7%. These findings are largely in line with previous cross-national DSM-IV estimates of 1.4–2.9% (Weissman *et al.* 1997) but notably lower than prior estimates exclusively from high-income countries like the United States. Also comparable to previous reports, most PAs actually occur in the absence of PD. While 13.2% of respondents ever experienced one or more PAs, only 1.7% of respondents met criteria for lifetime PD. Similarly, while 23.0% of people are projected to ever experience one or more PAs, 89.6% of these individuals do not fulfil criteria for lifetime PD. Of interest, although there were substantial differences in the prevalence of PAs across countries, this ratio was very stable in that most people experiencing PAs did not develop PD.

Based on the association of PD with impairment, we conclude that this condition is a serious mental disorder with substantial consequences. Almost half of individuals with 12-month PD reported severe limitations in their functioning. It should be noted that this figure was even higher in a previous report on the NCS, namely 56% for PD without agoraphobia and 84.7% for PD with agoraphobia. We also calculated how many days in the past year that respondents with

Table 7.3 Comorbidity of single and recurrent panic attacks (with and without panic disorder) with DSM-IV disorders, all countries combined

Type of comorbid disorder	Panic attack without panic disorder as a predictor of comorbid disorder onset								Panic attack with panic disorder as a predictor of comorbid disorder course							
	Single attack				Recurrent attacks				Single attack				Recurrent attacks			
	% with lifetime single PA onset prior to onset of lifetime disorder		Lifetime single PA predicting lifetime disorder[a]		% with lifetime recurrent PA onset prior to onset of lifetime disorder		Lifetime recurrent PA predicting lifetime disorder[a]		% with lifetime single PA prior to 12-month disorder episode among lifetime disorder cases[b]		Lifetime single PA predicting 12-month disorder episode among lifetime disorder cases[c]		% with lifetime recurrent PA prior to 12-month disorder episode among lifetime disorder cases[b]		Lifetime recurrent PA predicting 12-month disorder episode among lifetime disorder cases[c]	
	%	(SE)	OR	(95% CI)	%	(SE)	OR	(95% CI)	%	(SE)	OR	(95% CI)	%	(SE)	OR	(95% CI)
I. Mood disorder																
Major depressive episode/dysthymia	**17.8**	(1.5)	**1.1**	(0.9–1.3)	**39.2**	(1.0)	**2.0***	(1.9–2.2)	**3.0**	(0.2)	**0.5***	(0.4–0.6)	**22.5**	(0.6)	**1.2***	(1.1–1.3)
Bipolar spectrum disorder	**21.0**	(4.1)	**0.9**	(0.6–1.3)	**54.7**	(2.4)	**2.9***	(2.5–3.4)	**2.2**	(0.4)	**0.4***	(0.2–0.7)	**29.0**	(1.4)	**1.1**	(0.8–1.3)
Any mood disorder	**18.0**	(1.4)	**1.1**	(0.9–1.3)	**39.1**	(1.0)	**2.1***	(2.0–2.2)	**2.9**	(0.2)	**0.5***	(0.4–0.6)	**22.8**	(0.6)	**1.2***	(1.1–1.3)
II. Anxiety disorder																
Generalized anxiety disorder	**17.3**	(2.4)	**0.9**	(0.6–1.2)	**42.7**	(1.6)	**2.3***	(2.0–2.6)	**3.3**	(0.4)	**0.6***	(0.5–0.9)	**25.8**	(1.1)	**0.9**	(0.8–1.1)
Social anxiety disorder	**5.9**	(1.6)	**0.6**	(0.4–1.1)	**19.5**	(1.3)	**2.1***	(1.8–2.4)	**3.4**	(0.4)	**0.9**	(0.6–1.2)	**27.9**	(1.0)	**1.0**	(0.8–1.1)
Specific phobia	**1.9**	(0.7)	**0.5***	(0.2–1.0)	**7.5**	(0.7)	**1.3***	(1.1–1.6)	**3.5**	(0.3)	**0.9**	(0.7–1.2)	**21.5**	(0.6)	**1.0**	(0.8–1.1)
Agoraphobia without panic	**9.9**	(5.6)	**0.8**	(0.3–2.7)	**25.3**	(2.3)	**2.9***	(2.3–3.7)	**4.2**	(1.0)	**1.0**	(0.4–2.4)	**37.1**	(2.3)	**1.2**	(0.8–1.6)
Post-traumatic stress disorder	**12.0**	(2.3)	**0.7**	(0.5–1.0)	**41.0**	(1.8)	**2.4***	(2.1–2.7)	**4.0**	(0.6)	**0.6***	(0.4–1.0)	**31.0**	(1.4)	**1.2**	(0.9–1.4)
Any anxiety disorder	**6.1**	(1.0)	**0.7***	(0.5–1.0)	**18.1**	(0.8)	**1.9***	(1.7–2.1)	**3.5**	(0.2)	**0.7***	(0.5–0.9)	**24.2**	(0.6)	**1.0**	(0.9–1.2)

Table 7.3 *(cont.)*

Type of comorbid disorder	Panic attack without panic disorder as a predictor of comorbid disorder onset								Panic attack with panic disorder as a predictor of comorbid disorder course							
	Single attack				Recurrent attacks				Single attack				Recurrent attacks			
	% with lifetime single PA onset prior to onset of lifetime disorder		Lifetime single PA predicting lifetime disorder[a]		% with lifetime recurrent PA onset prior to onset of lifetime disorder		Lifetime recurrent PA predicting lifetime disorder[a]		% with lifetime single PA prior to 12-month disorder episode among lifetime disorder cases[b]		Lifetime single PA predicting 12-month disorder episode among lifetime disorder cases[c]		% with lifetime recurrent PA prior to 12-month disorder episode among lifetime disorder cases[b]		Lifetime recurrent PA predicting 12-month disorder episode among lifetime disorder cases[c]	
	%	(SE)	OR	(95% CI)	%	(SE)	OR	(95% CI)	%	(SE)	OR	(95% CI)	%	(SE)	OR	(95% CI)
III. Disruptive behaviour/impulse-control disorder																
Intermittent explosive disorder	**15.6**	(3.0)	**1.3**	(0.9–1.9)	**36.9**	(2.1)	**2.7***	(2.3–3.2)	**2.7**	(0.5)	**0.8**	(0.5–1.4)	**20.9**	(1.2)	**1.1**	(0.8–1.4)
Binge-eating disorder	**35.1**	(9.4)	**1.5**	(0.7–3.1)	**62.8**	(4.2)	**2.8***	(2.1–3.6)	**3.8**	(1.1)	**1.2**	(0.4–3.4)	**24.1**	(2.7)	**0.9**	(0.6–1.4)
Bulimia nervosa	**28.7**	(10.6)	**1.5**	(0.6–3.6)	**50.0**	(5.0)	**2.4***	(1.7–3.5)	**6.0**	(2.2)	**2.3**	(0.9–6.1)	**24.8**	(4.4)	**1.0**	(0.6–1.8)
Any disruptive behaviour/impulse-control disorder	**23.1**	(3.9)	**1.5***	(1.0–2.2)	**41.5**	(2.1)	**2.5***	(2.1–2.9)	**3.2**	(0.5)	**1.0**	(0.6–1.6)	**22.2**	(1.2)	**1.0**	(0.8–1.3)
IV. Substance-use disorder																
Alcohol abuse	**25.1**	(2.8)	**1.3***	(1.0–1.8)	**55.6**	(1.6)	**2.3***	(2.1–2.6)	**3.2**	(0.6)	**1.0**	(0.7–1.5)	**16.6**	(1.1)	**1.1**	(0.9–1.3)
Alcohol dependence	**20.0**	(4.3)	**0.9**	(0.6–1.4)	**56.9**	(2.4)	**2.7***	(2.3–3.2)	**3.0**	(1.0)	**0.7**	(0.3–1.7)	**21.0**	(2.0)	**1.0**	(0.8–1.3)
Drug abuse	**22.9**	(4.0)	**1.3**	(0.9–1.9)	**53.1**	(2.4)	**2.6***	(2.2–3.0)	**3.3**	(1.0)	**0.6**	(0.3–1.1)	**25.6**	(2.5)	**1.2**	(0.9–1.7)
Drug dependence	**23.8**	(6.3)	**1.1**	(0.6–2.1)	**57.0**	(3.3)	**3.0***	(2.4–3.8)	**3.3**	(1.3)	**0.5**	(0.2–1.3)	**35.8**	(4.3)	**1.8***	(1.1–2.8)
Any substance-use disorder	**20.8**	(2.4)	**1.2**	(0.9–1.6)	**51.1**	(1.5)	**2.3***	(2.0–2.5)	**3.4**	(0.6)	**1.0**	(0.6–1.6)	**18.3**	(1.0)	**1.2**	(1.0–1.4)
V. Any mental disorder	**10.9**	**(0.9)**	**1.1**	**(0.9–1.3)**	**23.3**	**(0.7)**	**2.0***	**(1.8–2.2)**	**3.4**	**(0.2)**	**0.7***	**(0.6–0.8)**	**21.2**	**(0.4)**	**1.3***	**(1.2–1.4)**

*Significant at the 0.05 level, two-sided test.
[a]Each model was estimated using lifetime panic attack as predictor of lifetime comorbid disorder onset in a separate discrete-time survival model controlling for country, person-years, gender, and age-cohort. Person-years were restricted up to and including the first onset of lifetime comorbid disorder.
[b]Respondents with lifetime PA onset that occurred within 12 months of the age of interview were not included in the numerator.
[c]Each model was estimated using lifetime panic attack as predictor of 12-month comorbid episode among lifetime comorbid disorder cases in a separate logistic regression model controlling for country, gender, age-cohort, time since comorbid disorder onset, and age of comorbid disorder onset. Respondents with lifetime PA onset that occurred within 12 months of the age of interview were not counted among the predictor set.

Table 7.4 Prevalence and age-of-onset of different types of panic attacks, all countries combined

	Any panic attacks		Age-of-onset of attacks	Expected attacks only						Unexpected attacks[b]		Number of expected attacks[c]	Number of unexpected attacks[d]
				Any[a]		Real danger		Strong fear					
	%	(SE)	Median (IQR)	%	(SE)	%	(SE)	%	(SE)	%	(SE)	Median (IQR)	Median (IQR)
Total sample	**13.2**	(0.1)	**21.5** (13.7–34.4)	**6.5**	(0.1)	**3.6**	(0.1)	**3.9**	(0.1)	**6.6**	(0.1)	**2.8** (1.0–8.3)	**1.9** (1.0–4.9)
Panic attack	–	–	**21.5** (13.7–34.4)	**49.5**	(0.5)	**27.2**	(0.4)	**29.4**	(0.4)	**49.6**	(0.5)	**2.8** (1.0–8.3)	**1.9** (1.0–4.9)
Panic attack without panic disorder	**100.0**	(0.0)	**21.5** (13.8–34.6)	**56.6**	(0.5)	**31.1**	(0.5)	**33.6**	(0.5)	**42.3**	(0.5)	**2.4** (1.0–5.9)	**1.2** (1.0–2.5)
Panic attack without panic disorder (single attack)	**100.0**	(0.0)	**29.5** (20.0–41.6)	**49.8**	(1.0)	**32.7**	(0.9)	**17.2**	(0.8)	**48.4**	(1.0)	–	–
Panic attack without panic disorder (recurrent attack)	**100.0**	(0.0)	**19.6** (12.8–31.5)	**49.0**	(0.6)	**24.8**	(0.5)	**32.4**	(0.5)	**50.6**	(0.6)	**3.8** (1.9–9.7)	**2.9** (1.5–7.9)
Panic disorder	**100.0**	(0.0)	**21.2** (13.0–32.3)	–	–	–	–	–	–	**100.0**	(0.0)	**9.6** (4.1–49.2)	**9.2** (4.7–19.8)
Agoraphobia with or without panic disorder	**64.6**	(1.5)	**19.3** (13.0–31.5)	**19.8**	(1.1)	**9.3**	(0.9)	**15.8**	(1.0)	**44.7**	(1.5)	**9.1** (3.0–42.1)	**4.9** (1.6–19.3)
Agoraphobia without panic disorder	**52.4**	(1.8)	**19.0** (12.8–31.5)	**25.9**	(1.4)	**12.0**	(1.1)	**20.5**	(1.3)	**26.4**	(1.6)	**5.4** (2.3–19.9)	**1.4** (1.0–2.6)
Social anxiety disorder	**48.5**	(0.8)	**18.1** (12.4–28.5)	**21.3**	(0.7)	**10.3**	(0.5)	**16.5**	(0.6)	**27.0**	(0.7)	**4.8** (2.1–18.14)	**3.1** (1.2–9.6)
Social anxiety disorder without panic disorder	**42.2**	(0.9)	**18.1** (12.2–28.5)	**23.9**	(0.7)	**11.5**	(0.5)	**18.6**	(0.7)	**17.9**	(0.7)	**4.1** (1.8–10.2)	**1.7** (1.0–2.8)
Specific phobia	**37.5**	(0.7)	**18.9** (12.4–30.4)	**17.1**	(0.5)	**8.5**	(0.4)	**12.3**	(0.4)	**20.2**	(0.5)	**4.1** (1.7–14.4)	**2.7** (1.0–7.3)
Specific phobia without panic disorder	**32.5**	(0.7)	**18.9** (12.5–31.0)	**18.4**	(0.5)	**9.1**	(0.4)	**13.3**	(0.5)	**13.7**	(0.5)	**3.3** (1.4–9.6)	**1.5** (1.0–2.6)

"–" not applicable.
[a]Attacks that occurred in a situation of unreasonably strong fear or in a situation of real danger only.
[b]With or without expected attacks.
[c]Among cases with expected attacks.
[d]Among cases with unexpected attacks.

PD reporting severe impairment were unable to carry out their normal daily roles. We found this to amount to some two to three months in the year on average, suggesting quite substantial role limitations for some individuals with PD.

Comorbidity of PD with other mental disorders was found to be high (80.4% over the lifetime) and particularly so with regard to mood and anxiety disorders. Substantial differences were observed regarding treatment status, which is linearly related to the level of severity and country income level, ranging from 42.2% for individuals reporting no impairments to 74.6% for those reporting severe impairment, and from 35.6% for individuals in low/lower-middle-income countries to 66.9% for those in high-income countries.

Among respondents who ever had at least one PA, the majority had more than one PA. The ratio of recurrent attacks versus single attack was about 2:1 in all countries, apart from Nigeria, Poland, and Colombia (Medellin) where the majority of people experiencing PAs had more than one. Recurrent PAs were associated with a substantially lower AOO than single PAs (19.6 years versus 29.5 years). Remarkably, recurrent PAs were predictive of a broad range of subsequent mental disorders whereas single PAs were not. Significantly increased odds were found for all 14 included disorders, typically around 2. Highest odds were found for subsequent onset of drug dependence, bipolar disorder, agoraphobia (without panic) and binge-eating disorder, which were all about 3. Lowest odds (1.3) were found for specific phobia, which may be due to the low AOO of that disorder. Of interest, recurrent PAs were even associated with an increased odds (1.3) of reporting 12-month disorders among people with a lifetime mental disorder. This suggests that the presence of recurrent PAs may predict a poorer course of mental disorders. This finding therefore supports the DSM-5 decision to frame PAs as a generic severity marker, based on several indications from the literature (Klerman *et al.* 1991; Goodwin *et al.* 2001; Craske *et al.* 2010). Note however, that we found no increased odds of mental disorders for people with a single PA, nor any indication that the presence of single PAs are associated with a poor course of mental disorder among those with a lifetime mental disorder. The message should thus be that only recurrent PAs are a generic specifier for mental disorder severity.

In contrast, we found no support for a distinction between expected and unexpected PAs in the context of being generic specifiers for mental disorder severity. This finding is in line with several others (Craske *et al.* 1995; Bruce *et al.* 2005; Kessler *et al.* 2006). In the total sample, we found that about half of the respondents with lifetime PAs had unexpected PAs. This ratio between expected and unexpected PAs was relatively stable across specific groups of anxiety disorders, the exception, by definition, being individuals diagnosed with PD. Also in individuals with agoraphobia, 44.7% experienced unexpected attacks, and even in people with agoraphobia that did not qualify for PD, 26.4% experienced unexpected attacks. These findings challenge the notion that unexpected PAs are specific to PD, and suggest they are a common phenomenon across a range of mental disorders. We also observed that the numbers of expected and unexpected attacks differed in that expected PAs occurred about three to four times as often as unexpected PAs. This ratio was also relatively stable, although somewhat higher across subgroups of people with agoraphobia, specific phobia, and social anxiety disorder, and somewhat lower for panic disorder.

Returning to the start of this chapter and the definition of PAs and PD, it is clear that WMH data provide a valuable, new perspective. While many of the observations in the literature have been confirmed, there have also been several extensions. Notably, the distinction between expected and unexpected PAs may not be as informative as the distinction between single and recurrent PAs. The presence of recurrent PAs may well serve as a generic marker for psychopathology, associated not only with the presence of a range of other mental disorders but also with their course, an issue deserving more research in the future.

Acknowledgements

Portions of this chapter appeared previously in: de Jonge, P., Roest, A. M., Lim, C. C.W., Florescu, S. E., Bromet, E. J., Stein, D. J., Harris, M., Nakov, V., Caldas-de-Almeida, J. M., Levinson, D., Al-Hamzawi, A. O., Haro, J. M., Viana, M. C., Borges, G., O'Neill, S., de Girolamo, G., Demyttenaere, K., Gureje, O., Iwata, N., Lee, S., Hu, C., Karam, A., Moskalewicz, J., Kovess-Masfety, V., Navarro-Mateu, F., Browne, M. O., Piazza, M., Posada-Villa, J., Torres, Y., ten Have, M. L., Kessler, R. C., & Scott, K. M. (2016). Cross-national epidemiology of panic disorder and panic attacks in the world mental health surveys. *Depression and Anxiety*; 33: 1155–77; used with permission from John Wiley & Sons.

References

American Psychiatric Association (1987). *Diagnostic and Statistical Manual of Mental Disorders Third Edition (DSM-III)*. Washington, DC: American Psychiatric Publishing.

(1994). *Diagnostic and Statistical Manual of Mental Disorders Fourth Edition (DSM-IV)*. Washington, DC: American Psychiatric Publishing.

(2013). *Diagnostic and Statistical Manual of Mental Disorders Fifth Edition (DSM-5)*. Washington, DC: American Psychiatric Publishing.

Batelaan, N., De Graaf, R., Van Balkom, A., Vollebergh, W., & Beekman, A. (2007). Thresholds for health and thresholds for illness: panic disorder versus subthreshold panic disorder. *Psychological Medicine*, 37, 247–56.

Batelaan, N. M., Rhebergen, D., de Graaf, R., *et al.* (2012). Panic attacks as a dimension of psychopathology: evidence for associations with onset and course of mental disorders and level of functioning. *Journal of Clinical Psychiatry*, 73(9), 1195–202.

Bruce, S. E., Yonkers, K. A., Otto, M. W., *et al.* (2005). Influence of psychiatric comorbidity on recovery and recurrence in generalized anxiety disorder, social phobia, and panic disorder: a 12-year prospective study. *American Journal of Psychiatry*, 162, 1179–87.

Chen, Y. W., & Dilsaver, S. C. (1995). Comorbidity of panic disorder in bipolar illness – evidence from The Epidemiologic Catchment-Area Survey. *American Journal of Psychiatry*, 152 (2), 280–2.

Craske, M. G., Glover, D., & DeCola, J. (1995). Predicted versus unpredicted panic attacks: acute versus general distress. *Journal of Abnormal Psychology*, 104(1), 214–23.

Craske, M. G., Kircanski, K., Epstein, A., *et al.* (2010). Panic disorder: a review of DSM-IV panic disorder and proposals for DSM-V. *Depression and Anxiety*, 27(2), 93–112.

de Jonge, P., Roest, A. M., Lim, C. C., *et al.* (2016). Cross-national epidemiology of panic disorder and panic attacks in the world mental health surveys. *Depression and Anxiety*, 33(12), 1155–77.

Eaton, W. W., Anthony, J. C., Romanoski, A., *et al.* (1988). Onset and recovery from panic disorder in the Baltimore Epidemiologic Catchment Area follow-up. *British Journal of Psychiatry*, 173, 501–7.

Eaton, W. W., Kessler, R. C., Wittchen, H. U., *et al.* (1994). Panic and panic disorder in the United States. *American Journal of Psychiatry*, 151(3), 413–20.

First, M. B., Spitzer, R. L., Gibbon, M., & Williams, J. B. W. (2002). *Structured Clinical Interview for DSM-IV Axis I Disorders, Research Version, Non-patient Edition (SCID-I/NP)*. New York, NY: Biometrics Research, New York State Psychiatric Institute.

Goodwin, R. D., Faravelli, C., Rosi, S., *et al.* (2005). The epidemiology of panic disorder and agoraphobia in Europe. *European Neuropsychopharmacology*, 15(4), 435–43.

Goodwin, R. D., & Hamilton, S. P. (2001). Panic attack as a marker of core psychopathological processes. *Psychopathology*, 34(6), 278–88.

Grant, B. F., Hasin, D. S., Stinson, F. S., *et al.* (2005). Co-occurrence of 12-month mood and anxiety disorders and personality disorders in the US: results from the NESARC. *Journal of Psychiatric Research*, 39, 1–9.

(2006). The epidemiology of DSM-IV panic disorder and agoraphobia in the United States: results from the National Epidemiologic Survey on Alcohol and Related Conditions. *Journal of Clinical Psychiatry*, 67, 363–74.

Haro, J. M., Arbabzadeh-Bouchez, S., Brugha, T. S., *et al.* (2006). Concordance of the Composite International Diagnostic Interview Version 3.0 (CIDI 3.0) with standardized clinical assessments in the WHO World Mental Health surveys. *International Journal of Methods in Psychiatric Research*, 15(4), 167–80.

Horwath, E., Gould, F., & Weissman, M. M. (2011). Epidemiology of anxiety disorders. In: *Textbook of Psychiatric Epidemiology*, Third edition. Tsuang, M. T., Tohen, M., Jones, P.B. (eds). New York, NY: John Wiley & Sons.

Huang, B., Dawson, D. A., Stinson, F. S., *et al.* (2006). Prevalence, correlates, and comorbidity of nonmedical prescription drug use and drug use disorders in the United States: results of the National Epidemiologic Survey on Alcohol and Related Conditions. *Journal of Clinical Psychiatry*, 67(7), 1062–73.

Iza, M., Olfson, M., Vermes, D., *et al.* (2013). Probability and predictors of first treatment contact for anxiety disorders in the United States. *Journal of Clinical Psychiatry*, 74(11), 1093–100.

Kessler, R. C., Chiu, W. T., Jin, R., *et al.* (2006). The epidemiology of panic attacks, panic disorder, and agoraphobia in the National Comorbidity Survey Replication. *Archives of General Psychiatry*, 63, 415–24.

Kessler, R. C., & Merikangas, K. R. (2004). The National Comorbidity Survey Replication (NCS-R): background and aims. *International Journal of Methods in Psychiatric Research*, 13(2), 60–8.

Kessler, R. C., Stang, P. E., Wittchen, H. U., *et al.* (1998). Lifetime panic-depression comorbidity in the National Comorbidity Survey. *Archives of General Psychiatry*, 55, 801–8.

Kessler, R. C., & Walters, E. E. (2002). The national comorbidity survey. In: *Textbook in Psychiatric Epidemiology*, 2nd edition. Tsuang, M. T., Tohen, M., Zahner, G.E.P. (eds). New York, NY: John Wiley & Sons.

Klein, D. F. (1993). Panic disorder with agoraphobia. *British Journal of Psychiatry*, 163, 835–7.

Klerman, G. L., Weissman, M. M., Ouellette, R., *et al.* (1991). Panic attacks in the community: social morbidity and health care utilization. *Journal of the American Medical Association*, 265, 742–6.

Marques, L., Robinaugh, D. J., LeBlanc, N. J., & Hinton, D. (2011). Cross-cultural variations in the prevalence and presentation of anxiety disorders. *Expert Review of Neurotherapeutics*, 11(2), 313–22.

Moreno-Peral, P., Conejo-Cerón, S., Motrico, E., *et al.* (2004). Risk factors for the onset of panic and generalised anxiety disorders in the general adult population: a systematic review of cohort studies. *Journal of Affective Disorders*, 168, 337–48.

Murray, C. J., Vos, T., Lozano, R., *et al.* (2010). Disability-adjusted life years (DALYs) for 291 diseases and injuries in 21 regions, 1990–2010: a systematic analysis for the Global Burden of Disease Study. *Lancet*, 380 (9859), 2197–223.

Regier, D. A., Narrow, W. E., & Rae, D. S. (1990). The epidemiology of anxiety disorders: the Epidemiologic Catchment Area (ECA) experience. *Journal of Psychiatric Research*, 24, 3–14.

Roberson-Nay, R., & Kendler, K. S. (2011). Panic disorder and its subtypes: a comprehensive analysis of panic symptom heterogeneity using epidemiological and treatment seeking samples. *Psychological Medicine*, 41, 2411–21.

Roy-Byrne, P. P., Stang, P., Wittchen, H. U., *et al.* (2000). Lifetime panic-depression comorbidity in the National Comorbidity Survey. *British Journal of Psychiatry*, 176, 229–35.

The World Bank. Data and Statistics. Accessed 12 May 2009 at: http://go.worldbank.org/D7SN0B8YU0

Von Korff, M. R., Eaton, W. W., & Keyl, P.M. (1985). The epidemiology of panic attacks and panic disorder: results of three community samples. *American Journal of Epidemiology*, 122 (6), 970–80.

Wang, P. S., Lane, M., Olfson, M., *et al.* (2005). Twelve-month use of mental health services in the United States: results from the National Comorbidity Survey Replication. *Archives of General Psychiatry*, 62(6), 629–40.

Weissman, M. M., Bland, R. C., Canino, G. J., *et al.* (1997). The cross-national epidemiology of panic disorder. *Archives of General Psychiatry*, 54, 305–9.

Whiteford, H. A., Degenhardt, L., Rehm, J., *et al.* (2013). Global burden of disease attributable to mental and substance abuse disorders: findings from the Global Burden of Disease Study 2010. *Lancet*, 382 (9904), 1575–86.

Wittchen, H. U., Gloster, A. T., Beesdo-Baum, K., *et al.* (2010). Agoraphobia: a review of the diagnostic classificatory position and criteria. *Depression and Anxiety*, 27(2), 113–33.

Chapter 8

Agoraphobia

Annelieke M. Roest, Peter de Jonge, Carmen C. W. Lim, Dan J. Stein, Maria Elena Medina-Mora, Kate M. Scott

Introduction

Agoraphobia (AG) is characterized by the avoidance of situations. According to DSM-IV, AG is defined as anxiety about being in places or situations from which escape might be difficult (or embarrassing) or in which help may not be available in the event of having an unexpected or situationally predisposed panic attack or panic-like symptoms. Agoraphobic fears typically involve characteristic clusters of situations that include being outside the home alone; being in a crowd or standing in a line; being on a bridge; and travelling in a bus, train, or automobile. The situations are avoided (e.g., travelling is restricted) or the situations are endured with marked distress or with anxiety about having a panic attack or panic-like symptoms, or the situations require the presence of a companion. AG can be diagnosed as part of panic disorder (PD) (i.e., PD with AG). If individuals have never met criteria for PD, AG is coded as an individual disorder (i.e., AG without a history of PD) (American Psychiatric Association 2000).

While the epidemiology of panic disorder (Chapter 7) has received a great deal of attention, less is known about the epidemiology of AG. A systematic review of 13 studies performed in Europe found a median 12-month prevalence of 1.3% for AG, but there was high variability in the findings. Prevalence rates ranged from 0.4% to 3.1%, probably as a result of some studies presenting rates for total AG while others presented data for AG without a history of PD (Goodwin *et al.* 2005). A report from the National Epidemiologic Survey on Alcohol and Related Conditions, a nationally representative study in the United States, found an extremely low prevalence of AG without a history of PD, a 12-month prevalence of 0.05% and a lifetime prevalence of 0.17% (Grant *et al.* 2006). In contrast, in the Australian National Survey of Mental Health and Well-being (NSMHWB), the 12-month prevalence of AG without a history of PD was 1.6% (Andrews & Slade 2002). The age-of-onset of AG is generally in adolescence or early adulthood and females are twice as likely to develop AG compared to males (Goodwin *et al.* 2005). Although high comorbidity rates between AG and other anxiety and mood disorders have been reported, this has not been studied in detail (Goodwin *et al.* 2005). AG without PD is not typically seen in clinical settings, but has been shown to be as disabling as PD (Andrews & Slade 2002). The low prevalence of AG without PD in the clinic suggests that these patients are not recognized or that individuals suffering from AG only are less likely to seek help (Wittchen *et al.* 1998; Andrews & Slade 2002), potentially as a result of avoidance behaviour (Andrews & Slade 2002). Indeed, in the NSMHWB study, respondents with AG without a history of PD had lower consultation rates for mental health problems than respondents with PD or PD with AG (Andrews & Slade 2002).

Most studies of the epidemiology of AG have only examined individuals with AG who did not have a lifetime history of PD (Goodwin *et al.* 2005) and most have been undertaken in high-income countries. In order to provide a comprehensive account of the epidemiology of AG, this chapter focuses on AG irrespective of the presence of PD and compares AG including and excluding lifetime comorbid PD in samples from high-, upper-middle-, and low/lower-middle-income countries. We present cross-national prevalence rates for total AG (with or without PD) and AG without PD, impairment due to AG and data on the age-of-onset of AG, as well as socio-demographic correlates and comorbidity patterns with other mental disorders.

Method

AG was assessed through a specific section in the Composite International Diagnostic Interview (CIDI). Thus, AG can be separated from PD in order to study total AG (AG with or without PD) and AG without a lifetime diagnosis of PD. For CIDI diagnosed AG (with or without PD), there was good concordance with a diagnosis based on blinded clinical interview, as indicated by an area under the curve of 0.81 (Haro *et al.* 2006).

In the analyses reported in this chapter we include data from 26 of the total of 29 surveys, conducted in low/lower-middle-income countries (Colombia, Iraq, Nigeria, Peru, PRC Shenzhen, Ukraine), upper-middle-income countries (Brazil, Colombia [Medellin], Lebanon, Mexico, Romania), and high-income countries (Australia, Belgium, France, Germany, Israel, Italy, Japan, New Zealand, Northern Ireland, Poland, Portugal, Spain, Spain [Murcia], the Netherlands, the United States). The total sample size is 132,430 respondents (Part I sample).

Results

Prevalence

The prevalence rates of AG (with or without PD) in all surveys are shown in Table 8.1. Prevalence rates differ significantly between the surveys, between the country income groups and between regions. The lifetime prevalence of AG in all surveys combined is 1.2% with a relatively low prevalence rate found in the low/lower-middle-income countries (0.7%), and higher prevalence rates in upper-middle- (1.5%) and high-income countries (1.4%). Across all surveys, the 12-month prevalence of AG is 0.8% and the 30-day prevalence of AG averages 0.4%. We find the same pattern across country income groups for the 12-month and 30-day prevalence rates as for the lifetime prevalence of AG.

The lifetime, 12-month, and 30-day prevalence of AG without PD in all surveys combined is 0.9%, 0.6%, and 0.3%, respectively, indicating that most individuals suffering from AG do not have lifetime comorbid PD (Appendix Table 8A.1).

Persistence

When looking at all surveys combined, lifetime AG (with or without PD) appears to be a moderately persistent disorder. Among lifetime cases of AG, 62.9% also meet criteria for AG in the past 12 months, indicating persistence of the disorder, while among 12-month cases, 56.3% also meet diagnostic criteria in the past 30 days, indicating persistence of the episode. Again there are significant differences across surveys. Disorder persistence is lowest in high-income countries, and higher in low/lower-middle- and upper-middle-income countries. Episode persistence is lowest in low/lower-middle-income countries and highest in upper-middle-income countries (Table 8.1).

Respondents with lifetime AG without PD also suffer from disorder or episode persistence, with 61.9% of lifetime cases having AG in the prior 12 months and 53.5% of 12-month cases having AG in the past 30 days (Appendix Table 8A.1).

Age-of-Onset

The interquartile ranges (IQR), i.e., the number of years between the 25th and 75th percentiles of the age-of-onset distributions, are relatively broad for most surveys and there are substantial differences between surveys in the median age of AG onset (Table 8.2). However, the IQRs for country income groups are fairly similar. Median age-of-onset of AG (with or without PD) is 16 (IQR 11–38) in the low/lower-middle-income countries, 19 (IQR 13–36) in the upper-middle-income countries and 22 (IQR 14–38) in the high-income countries. Combining all surveys, the median age-of-onset is 21 years (IQR 13–38). The projected lifetime risk at age 75 of AG is 1.7%, indicating that 1.7% of the population across these countries will at some point in their life meet criteria for a diagnosis of AG.

For AG without PD the median age-of-onset is somewhat lower, namely 19 years (IQR 13–36) and the projected lifetime risk at age 75 is 1.2% (Appendix Table 8A.2).

Role Impairment

Table 8.3 shows the severity of role impairment in respondents who meet criteria for AG (with or without PD) in the past 12 months. When looking at all surveys combined, 41.9% of respondents report severe impairment in any domain, such as in home management, ability to work, ability to form and maintain close relationships, or social life. This prevalence differs significantly across surveys, with a higher rate for high-income countries (48.5%) compared with upper-middle-income (33.3%), and low/lower-middle-income countries (25.9%). The number of days-out-of-role (days when respondents report that they were unable to function in their usual role due to their anxiety problems) in the past year is 55.3 days for respondents who meet criteria for 12-month AG (data not shown). For those respondents who report severe impairment in any domain, the number of days-out-of-role is higher, namely 83.7.

There is no significant difference in the percent reporting severe impairment by type of domain among

Table 8.1 Prevalence of agoraphobia in the World Mental Health surveys

Country	Lifetime prevalence		12-month prevalence		30-day prevalence		12-month prevalence of agoraphobia among lifetime cases		30-day prevalence of agoraphobia among 12-month cases		Part I sample sizes
	%	SE	%	SE	%	SE	%	SE	%	SE	
Low/lower-middle-income countries	**0.7**	**0.1**	**0.5**	**0.1**	**0.2**	**0.0**	**65.1**	**5.1**	**44.8**	**5.3**	**31,297**
Colombia	2.5	0.3	1.7	0.3	0.7	0.1	67.3	8.0	42.3	6.8	4,426
Iraq	0.9	0.2	0.6	0.2	0.4	0.2	68.3	12.1	61.5	16.9	4,332
Nigeria	0.4	0.1	0.1	0.1	0.1	0.0	38.1	15.5	35.3	18.9	6,752
Peru	0.7	0.1	0.5	0.1	0.2	0.1	69.3	10.7	31.6	12.1	3,930
PRC (Shenzhen)	0.2	0.1	0.1	0.1	<0.1	0.0	64.0	15.2	6.9	5.8	7,132
Ukraine	0.4	0.1	0.3	0.1	0.2	0.1	74.9	11.3	72.3	11.8	4,725
Upper-middle-income countries	**1.5**	**0.1**	**1.1**	**0.1**	**0.7**	**0.1**	**71.1**	**2.9**	**62.9**	**3.5**	**19,294**
Brazil	2.9	0.4	1.9	0.3	1.2	0.2	65.9	4.7	64.6	5.3	5,037
Colombia (Medellin)	1.6	0.3	1.3	0.2	0.7	0.2	79.5	6.0	55.8	9.0	3,261
Lebanon	0.5	0.1	0.3	0.1	0.3	0.1	72.7	13.0	90.3	9.5	2,857
Mexico	1.2	0.2	0.9	0.1	0.5	0.1	75.3	5.2	57.1	6.5	5,782
Romania	0.7	0.3	0.5	0.2	0.4	0.2	71.6	14.5	78.1	12.2	2,357
High-income countries	**1.4**	**0.1**	**0.8**	**0.0**	**0.5**	**0.0**	**60.3**	**1.6**	**56.7**	**2.4**	**81,839**
Australia	2.4	0.3	1.2	0.2	0.5	0.1	52.2	4.4	38.8	7.2	8,463
Belgium	1.1	0.2	0.6	0.2	0.4	0.2	58.1	13.7	66.5	20.1	2,419
France	1.6	0.3	1.0	0.2	0.7	0.2	64.1	6.8	71.3	9.6	2,894
Germany	0.7	0.2	0.5	0.1	0.4	0.1	75.0	7.0	71.6	13.0	3,555
Israel	0.7	0.1	0.4	0.1	0.2	0.1	61.9	9.3	41.0	11.7	4,859
Italy	1.1	0.2	0.6	0.1	0.4	0.1	57.8	6.8	62.5	9.2	4,712
Japan	0.3	0.1	0.2	0.1	0.1	0.1	59.7	10.1	79.7	24.6	4,129
New Zealand	1.7	0.1	1.0	0.1	0.6	0.1	55.5	3.9	58.4	4.9	12,790
Northern Ireland	2.5	0.3	2.0	0.3	1.3	0.2	76.7	4.8	68.0	5.5	4,340
Poland	0.3	0.1	0.1	0.0	0.1	0.0	50.5	9.3	77.1	11.9	10,081
Portugal	1.4	0.2	0.9	0.2	0.7	0.1	66.4	5.2	73.9	6.9	3,849
Spain	0.8	0.2	0.5	0.1	0.3	0.1	68.4	7.3	47.7	11.9	5,473
Spain (Murcia)	0.6	0.1	0.3	0.1	0.2	0.1	45.0	15.3	63.0	8.2	2,621
Netherlands	1.2	0.3	0.7	0.3	0.4	0.2	61.6	10.9	48.8	13.9	2,372
United States	2.4	0.2	1.5	0.1	0.8	0.1	61.3	2.8	51.7	5.0	9,282

Table 8.1 *(cont.)*

Country	Lifetime prevalence		12-month prevalence		30-day prevalence		12-month prevalence of agoraphobia among lifetime cases		30-day prevalence of agoraphobia among 12-month cases		Part I sample sizes
	%	SE	%	SE	%	SE	%	SE	%	SE	
All countries combined	**1.2**	**0.0**	**0.8**	**0.0**	**0.4**	**0.0**	**62.9**	**1.4**	**56.3**	**1.9**	**132,430**
WHO regions[a]											
Region of the Americas	2.0	0.1	1.3	0.1	0.7	0.1	66.8	2.2	53.1	2.7	31,718
African region	0.4	0.1	0.1	0.1	0.1	0.0	38.1	15.5	35.3	18.9	6,752
Western Pacific region	1.4	0.1	0.7	0.1	0.4	0.0	54.3	2.8	48.9	4.5	32,514
Eastern Mediterranean region	0.7	0.1	0.5	0.1	0.3	0.1	66.5	7.0	59.1	9.6	12,048
Western European region	1.2	0.1	0.8	0.1	0.5	0.0	66.9	2.6	65.2	3.4	32,235
Eastern European region	0.3	0.1	0.2	0.0	0.2	0.0	63.7	7.0	75.8	6.9	17,163
Comparison between countries[b]	**$F_{25,v} = 22.0^*$, $P < 0.001$**		**$F_{25,v} = 15.5^*$, $P < 0.001$**		**$F_{25,v} = 18.3^*$, $P < 0.001$**		**$F_{25,v} = 1.6^*$, $P = 0.027$**		**$F_{25,v} = 1.8^*$, $P = 0.010$**		
Comparison between low-, middle-, and high-income country groups[b]	**$F_{2,v} = 32.3^*$, $P < 0.001$**		**$F_{2,v} = 18.3^*$, $P < 0.001$**		**$F_{2,v} = 28.8^*$, $P < 0.001$**		**$F_{2,v} = 5.0^*$, $P = 0.007$**		**$F_{2,v} = 3.8^*$, $P = 0.022$**		
Comparison between WHO regions[b]	**$F_{5,v} = 58.7^*$, $P < 0.001$**		**$F_{5,v} = 43.0^*$, $P < 0.001$**		**$F_{5,v} = 38.2^*$, $P < 0.001$**		**$F_{5,v} = 3.3^*$, $P = 0.005$**		**$F_{5,v} = 3.5^*$, $P = 0.004$**		

*Significant at the 0.05 level, two-sided test.
[a]**Region of the Americas** (Colombia, Mexico, Brazil, Peru, United States, Colombia (Medellin)); **African region** (Nigeria); **Western Pacific region** (PRC (Shenzhen), Japan, Australia, New Zealand); **Eastern Mediterranean region** (Israel, Iraq, Lebanon); **Western European region** (Belgium, France, Germany, Italy, Netherlands, Spain, Northern Ireland, Portugal, Spain (Murcia)); **Eastern European region** (Romania, Poland, Ukraine).
[b]Wald design-corrected F-tests were used to determine if there is variation in prevalence estimates across countries. The denominator degree of freedom, v, is 5287.
PRC: People's Republic of China.

Table 8.2 Age at selected percentiles on the standardized age-of-onset distributions of agoraphobia with projected lifetime risk at age 75

Country	Ages at selected percentiles								Lifetime prevalence of agoraphobia		Projected risk at age 75	
	5	10	25	50	75	90	95	99	%	SE	%	SE
Low/lower-middle-income countries	**5**	**6**	**11**	**16**	**38**	**59**	**59**	**63**	**0.7**	**0.1**	**1.0**	**0.1**
Colombia[a]	5	6	12	19	41	59	63	63	2.5	0.3	3.4	0.5
Iraq	5	8	11	13	14	19	21	31	0.9	0.2	0.9	0.2
Nigeria	5	5	8	9	13	33	33	33	0.4	0.1	0.4	0.1
Peru[a]	7	10	14	26	59	59	59	59	0.7	0.1	1.2	0.5
PRC (Shenzhen)	5	8	13	29	47	47	47	47	0.2	0.1	0.3	0.1
Ukraine	5	5	7	13	18	62	62	62	0.4	0.1	0.5	0.1
Upper-middle-income countries	**5**	**8**	**13**	**19**	**36**	**52**	**61**	**67**	**1.5**	**0.1**	**2.0**	**0.2**
Brazil	5	9	13	19	41	54	67	67	2.9	0.4	3.7	0.4
Colombia (Medellin)[a]	5	5	8	13	19	37	48	49	1.6	0.3	1.8	0.3
Lebanon	13	13	14	18	31	31	41	41	0.5	0.1	0.5	0.2
Mexico[a]	8	9	15	23	41	61	61	61	1.2	0.2	1.8	0.3
Romania	5	5	18	21	35	41	41	41	0.7	0.3	0.9	0.3
High-income countries	**5**	**8**	**14**	**22**	**38**	**51**	**60**	**71**	**1.4**	**0.1**	**1.8**	**0.1**
Australia	7	11	14	23	39	54	66	71	2.4	0.3	3.2	0.3
Belgium	5	5	13	29	46	66	66	66	1.1	0.2	1.7	0.6
France	11	12	15	25	36	45	53	58	1.6	0.3	2.1	0.3
Germany	5	5	19	25	37	51	51	51	0.7	0.2	0.8	0.2
Israel	11	12	14	36	48	65	65	65	0.7	0.1	1.0	0.2
Italy	6	8	16	32	40	58	66	66	1.1	0.2	1.4	0.2
Japan	5	7	21	23	41	42	47	47	0.3	0.1	0.3	0.1
New Zealand	5	7	13	19	30	41	53	59	1.7	0.1	2.1	0.2
Northern Ireland	6	8	14	23	41	50	51	54	2.5	0.3	3.5	0.4
Poland[b]	5	5	7	14	31	49	49	49	0.3	0.1	0.3	0.1
Portugal	5	5	11	21	40	55	62	66	1.4	0.2	1.8	0.3
Spain	11	12	20	42	47	64	73	73	0.8	0.2	1.3	0.3
Spain (Murcia)	10	10	14	26	34	40	40	41	0.6	0.1	0.8	0.2
Netherlands	11	14	26	29	41	47	48	48	1.2	0.3	1.7	0.4
United States	5	7	12	19	31	44	51	54	2.4	0.2	2.9	0.2
All countries combined	**5**	**8**	**13**	**21**	**38**	**51**	**60**	**67**	**1.2**	**0.0**	**1.7**	**0.1**
WHO regions												
Region of the Americas	5	7	13	19	36	51	59	67	2.0	0.1	2.5	0.1
African region	5	5	8	9	13	33	33	33	0.4	0.1	0.4	0.1
Western Pacific region	6	9	14	21	36	50	59	71	1.4	0.1	1.8	0.1
Eastern Mediterranean region	8	11	13	17	36	51	65	65	0.7	0.1	0.9	0.2
Western European region	6	10	14	26	41	53	64	66	1.2	0.1	1.7	0.1
Eastern European region	5	5	7	17	35	49	62	62	0.3	0.1	0.4	0.1

[a]The projected risk for these countries is at age 65 because the age range of these surveys is between 18 and 65.
[b]The projected risk for this country is at age 64 because the age range of this survey is between 18 and 64.

Table 8.3 Severity of role impairment (Sheehan Disability Scale) associated with 12-month agoraphobia, by country

Country	Proportion with severe role impairment (SDS score: 7–10)										Number of 12-month cases
	Home		Work		Relationship		Social		Any[a]		
	%	SE	%	SE	%	SE	%	SE	%	SE	
Low/lower-middle-income countries	**15.5**	**4.0**	**12.7**	**3.2**	**12.3**	**3.2**	**14.1**	**3.5**	**25.9**	**4.9**	**149**
Colombia	15.3	4.9	13.4	4.6	13.6	5.1	18.3	5.7	25.0	6.7	73
Iraq	22.1	13.8	6.7	3.4	11.9	5.8	9.4	4.9	33.4	14.3	25
Nigeria	–	–	–	–	–	–	–	–	–	–	9
Peru	10.7	10.1	20.7	13.2	10.7	10.1	19.8	11.4	29.8	13.0	18
PRC (Shenzhen)	5.3	4.6	1.6	1.8	1.6	1.8	–	–	5.3	4.6	11
Ukraine	24.2	13.8	27.1	14.8	22.0	11.2	10.4	9.7	40.6	16.1	13
Upper-middle-income countries	**17.4**	**3.3**	**21.6**	**3.6**	**27.5**	**4.1**	**25.1**	**3.9**	**33.3**	**4.4**	**233**
Brazil	19.6	5.3	22.3	5.6	28.1	6.2	24.7	5.6	31.8	6.5	107
Colombia (Medellin)	14.9	8.3	35.9	10.5	33.9	10.2	27.3	10.2	48.1	11.2	42
Lebanon	6.9	6.9	–	–	23.2	17.5	23.2	17.5	23.2	17.5	9
Mexico	14.4	4.9	16.5	5.5	19.9	6.3	20.5	6.3	24.7	6.5	67
Romania	26.4	15.7	20.1	14.1	43.6	21.7	43.6	21.7	53.3	21.8	8
High-income countries	**20.9**	**1.8**	**27.2**	**2.1**	**31.8**	**2.1**	**37.5**	**2.2**	**48.5**	**2.4**	**730**
Australia	40.4	7.2	54.8	7.8	44.8	6.6	50.1	7.6	68.1	6.4	117
Belgium	5.7	5.5	32.9	21.4	41.6	21.0	20.1	11.3	47.3	20.6	12
France	8.4	6.9	10.5	5.3	27.1	9.8	21.8	10.1	43.5	11.4	30
Germany	3.4	3.1	9.4	8.5	3.4	3.1	38.7	16.4	42.1	17.3	17
Israel	23.3	10.4	34.4	11.5	36.6	11.5	44.8	11.9	49.0	11.9	19
Italy	36.9	12.1	13.3	5.4	35.7	10.8	36.0	10.1	51.6	11.6	25
Japan	16.1	14.1	16.1	14.1	46.4	24.7	16.1	14.1	46.4	24.7	6
New Zealand	15.1	3.8	19.2	4.5	28.2	4.9	34.5	5.3	44.8	5.2	155
Northern Ireland	23.0	3.7	30.2	4.2	35.6	5.6	57.0	6.4	62.2	5.8	99
Poland	44.7	16.0	76.5	14.3	44.0	16.0	55.2	16.1	67.3	15.1	12
Portugal	11.9	4.7	15.0	4.9	16.6	6.4	18.1	6.6	22.5	7.0	44
Spain	8.7	4.3	13.8	6.2	16.7	6.2	18.1	6.5	23.6	7.6	30
Spain (Murcia)	16.1	11.8	46.7	26.6	95.5	3.4	100.0	0.0	100.0	0.0	8
Netherlands	34.5	12.3	57.9	17.7	26.9	14.9	17.1	7.1	57.9	17.7	14
United States	21.1	3.7	27.4	4.8	33.1	3.9	36.4	4.5	43.5	5.2	142

(cont.)

Table 8.3 (*cont.*)

Country	Proportion with severe role impairment (SDS score: 7–10)										Number of 12-month cases
	Home		Work		Relationship		Social		Any[a]		
	%	SE	%	SE	%	SE	%	SE	%	SE	
All countries combined	**19.3**	**1.5**	**23.8**	**1.7**	**28.0**	**1.7**	**31.4**	**1.8**	**41.9**	**2.0**	**1112**
WHO regions											
Region of the Americas	18.0	2.2	22.5	2.6	25.9	2.6	27.0	2.6	34.7	3.0	449
African region	–	–	–	–	–	–	–	–	–	–	9
Western Pacific region	22.6	3.5	28.9	3.9	33.0	3.9	37.5	4.1	50.8	4.1	289
Eastern Mediterranean region	20.0	7.7	15.3	5.3	22.5	6.4	24.2	6.8	37.1	8.8	53
Western European region	18.0	2.5	23.0	3.1	28.6	3.4	36.0	3.3	47.5	3.8	279
Eastern European region	30.6	9.1	37.0	10.1	35.7	10.0	34.4	10.0	52.4	10.8	33
Comparison between countries[b]	$F_{25,v} = 1.7^*$, $P = 0.014$		$F_{25,v} = 2.2^*$, $P < 0.001$		$F_{25,v} = 2.2^*$, $P < 0.001$		$F_{25,v} = 2.7^*$, $P < 0.001$		$F_{25,v} = 2.5^*$, $P < 0.001$		
Comparison between low-, middle-, and high-income countries[b]	$F_{2,v} = 1.0$, $P = 0.368$		$F_{2,v} = 5.8^*$, $P = 0.003$		$F_{2,v} = 9.0^*$, $P < 0.001$		$F_{2,v} = 12.9^*$, $P < 0.001$		$F_{2,v} = 9.4^*$, $P < 0.001$		
Comparison between WHO regions[b]	$F_{5,v} = 1.5$, $P = 0.203$		$F_{5,v} = 2.0$, $P = 0.078$		$F_{5,v} = 1.6$, $P = 0.162$		$F_{5,v} = 2.4^*$ $P = 0.032$		$F_{5,v} = 3.4^*$, $P = 0.004$		

"–": All 12-month cases associated with role impairment were non-severe.
*Significant at the 0.05 level, two-sided test.
[a]Highest severity category across four SDS role domains.
[b]Wald design-corrected F-tests were used to determine if there is variation in impairment severity across countries. The denominator degrees of freedom, v, is 5287.
PRC: People's Republic of China.

the low/lower-middle-income countries, but in the upper-middle- and high-income countries there is a fairly consistent pattern of impairment being significantly higher in the social and relationship domains than in the home domain.

The severity of role impairment is a little lower in respondents who meet criteria for AG in the past 12 months but without lifetime comorbid PD. Combining all surveys, 35.0% of this group report severe role impairment in at least one of the domains (Appendix Table 8A.3). Similarly, the number of days-out-of-role in the past year is a little lower for this group; 45.3 days for the group as a whole and 75.7 days for those who report severe impairment in at least one domain (data not shown).

Treatment

Almost half of all respondents who meet criteria for AG (with or without PD) in the past 12 months, and are at least mildly impaired, report that they have sought treatment from within the health care or non-health care sectors, namely 49.4% (SE = 1.9) (data not shown). Treatment most often consists of general medical care (33.2% [SE = 1.8]) or specialty mental health care (27.0% [SE = 1.6]). Treatment rates are higher for respondents with more severe AG, i.e., those reporting higher impairment due to AG. Of the respondents who report severe impairment, 65.2% (SE = 2.7) have sought treatment. These rates of treatment seeking are higher than for many of the other disorders included in this volume (see Chapter 21).

Treatment rates are a little lower for respondents who meet criteria for AG in the past 12 months but who do not have comorbid lifetime PD. Of those who are at least mildly impaired, 43.6% (SE = 2.2) report that they have sought treatment. Again, treatment rates are higher for respondents who report higher levels of impairment; of the respondents in this group who report severe impairment, 60.0% (SE = 3.4) have sought treatment.

Socio-demographic Correlates

For these analyses data from all surveys are again combined. Respondents younger than 60 years (ORs ranging from 1.7–3.8) and females (ORs 2.1–2.2) have a higher lifetime and 30-day prevalence of AG (with or without PD) compared to respondents older than 60 years and males (Table 8.4). Employment status, marital status, education level, and household income are also significantly associated with lifetime and 30-day AG. Respondents without paid jobs (categories 'other' and 'homemaker') are more likely to meet criteria for AG compared with employed respondents (ORs 1.7–3.4). Respondents who are divorced, separated, or widowed are at increased odds of both lifetime (OR 1.5) and 30-day AG (OR 1.7), compared to those currently married. However, never being married is only predictive of lifetime AG (OR 1.4). For education and household income, higher levels show a protective association with lifetime and 30-day AG (low education and low household income are associated with the highest odds of AG).

Results are comparable for AG without PD, although marital status is not a statistically significant predictor of 30-day AG without PD.

Compared to the presence of lifetime and 30-day AG, fewer socio-demographic factors are predictive of disorder persistence (12-month/lifetime) and episode persistence (30-day/12month) (Table 8.4). These results suggest that socio-demographic factors predict the first onset of AG, but are not strongly associated with the disorder course. Results are similar for AG without PD.

Comorbidity

Respondents with lifetime AG (with or without PD) are highly likely to have a lifetime diagnosis of another mental disorder as well (88.8%) (Table 8.5). Most often this comorbid disorder is another phobic anxiety disorder, namely social anxiety disorder (50.2%) or specific phobia (41.2%), while the lifetime comorbidity with generalized anxiety disorder (29.4%), posttraumatic stress disorder (21.0%), and also PD (25.5%) is lower. Comorbidity levels are also high for mood disorders (including depression), namely 55.1%, but lower for substance-use disorders (26.3%), and disruptive behaviour/impulse-control disorders (20.6%). We find similar patterns of comorbidity for 12-month AG with lifetime comorbid disorders and 12-month AG with 12-month comorbid disorders (Table 8.5).

Comorbidity levels for AG without PD are generally comparable although slightly lower. Lifetime comorbidity rates with any mental disorder, other anxiety disorders, mood disorders, substance-use disorders, and disruptive behaviour/impulse-control disorders are: 84.5%, 73.8%, 50.5%, 23.3%, 13.9%, respectively.

In respondents who have a comorbid disorder, the onset of AG (with or without PD) is earlier than the

Table 8.4 Bivariate associations between socio-demographic correlates and agoraphobia, all countries combined

Correlates	30-day agoraphobia[a]		Lifetime agoraphobia[b]		12-month agoraphobia among lifetime cases[c]		30-day agoraphobia among 12-month cases[c]	
	OR	(95% CI)	OR	(95% CI)	OR	(95% CI)	OR	(95% CI)
Age-cohort								
18–29	**1.7***	(1.2–2.3)	**3.8***	(3.0–4.8)				
30–44	**1.7***	(1.3–2.4)	**2.9***	(2.4–3.6)				
45–59	**1.8***	(1.3–2.4)	**2.4***	(2.0–3.0)				
60+	**1.0**		**1.0**					
Age-cohort difference[d]	$\chi^2_3 = 15.2^*, P = 0.002$		$\chi^2_3 = 134.1^*, P < 0.001$					
Age-of-onset								
Early					**1.3**	(0.8–2.0)	**1.1**	(0.6–1.8)
Early-average					**0.9**	(0.6–1.3)	**0.7**	(0.5–1.2)
Late-average					**0.9**	(0.6–1.3)	**1.0**	(0.6–1.5)
Late					**1.0**		**1.0**	
Age-of-onset difference[d]					$\chi^2_3 = 3.9, P = 0.279$		$\chi^2_3 = 3.9, P = 0.268$	
Time since onset (continuous)					**0.99**	(0.98–1.00)	**1.00**	(0.99–1.01)
Gender								
Female	**2.1***	(1.7–2.7)	**2.2***	(1.9–2.5)	**0.8**	(0.6–1.1)	**1.1**	(0.8–1.5)
Male	**1.0**		**1.0**		**1.0**		**1.0**	
Gender difference[d]	$\chi^2_1 = 43.0^*, P < 0.001$		$\chi^2_1 = 119.1^*, P < 0.001$		$\chi^2_1 = 2.0, P = 0.153$		$\chi^2_1 = 0.2, P = 0.652$	
Employment status								
Student	**1.2**	(0.7–2.2)	**1.4**	(0.9–1.9)	**1.7**	(0.9–3.5)	**0.8**	(0.3–1.9)
Homemaker	**2.4***	(1.8–3.2)	**1.7***	(1.4–2.0)	**1.7***	(1.2–2.4)	**1.5**	(1.0–2.3)
Retired	**1.1**	(0.7–1.7)	**1.3**	(1.0–1.8)	**1.2**	(0.7–2.1)	**1.6**	(0.8–3.0)
Other	**3.4***	(2.6–4.6)	**2.4***	(2.0–2.9)	**1.9***	(1.3–2.9)	**1.6***	(1.0–2.6)
Employed	**1.0**		**1.0**		**1.0**		**1.0**	
Employment status difference[d]	$\chi^2_4 = 84.6^*, P < 0.001$		$\chi^2_4 = 108.9^*, P < 0.001$		$\chi^2_4 = 16.6^*, P = 0.002$		$\chi^2_4 = 7.5, P = 0.114$	
Marital status								
Never married	**1.2**	(0.9–1.5)	**1.4***	(1.2–1.7)	**0.9**	(0.7–1.3)	**1.3**	(0.9–2.0)
Divorced/separated/widowed	**1.7***	(1.3–2.1)	**1.5***	(1.3–1.8)	**1.2**	(0.8–1.6)	**1.2**	(0.8–1.8)
Currently married	**1.0**		**1.0**		**1.0**		**1.0**	
Marital status difference[d]	$\chi^2_2 = 17.5^*, P < 0.001$		$\chi^2_2 = 41.7^*, P < 0.001$		$\chi^2_2 = 1.2, P = 0.557$		$\chi^2_2 = 2.5, P = 0.289$	

Table 8.4 *(cont.)*

Correlates	30-day agoraphobia[a]		Lifetime agoraphobia[b]		12-month agoraphobia among lifetime cases[c]		30-day agoraphobia among 12-month cases[c]	
	OR	(95% CI)	OR	(95% CI)	OR	(95% CI)	OR	(95% CI)
Education level								
No education	**3.5***	(1.6–7.6)	**2.9***	(1.8–4.7)	**1.5**	(0.6–3.7)	**1.6**	(0.5–4.7)
Some primary	**3.5***	(2.3–5.4)	**2.4***	(1.8–3.2)	**2.7***	(1.5–4.9)	**1.3**	(0.6–2.7)
Finished primary	**3.1***	(2.0–4.9)	**2.8***	(2.1–3.7)	**1.1**	(0.6–2.0)	**1.4**	(0.7–2.9)
Some secondary	**3.1***	(2.1–4.5)	**2.1***	(1.7–2.7)	**1.5**	(1.0–2.3)	**1.7**	(1.0–2.9)
Finished secondary	**1.8***	(1.2–2.6)	**1.5***	(1.2–1.9)	**1.1**	(0.7–1.7)	**1.4**	(0.8–2.5)
Some college	**1.5**	(1.0–2.2)	**1.4***	(1.1–1.7)	**1.1**	(0.7–1.8)	**1.1**	(0.6–2.0)
Finished college	**1.0**		**1.0**		**1.0**		**1.0**	
Education level difference[d]	$\chi^2_6 = 58.2^*$, P < 0.001		$\chi^2_6 = 76.8^*$, P < 0.001		$\chi^2_6 = 14.1^*$, P = 0.028		$\chi^2_6 = 5.1$, P = 0.535	
Household income								
Low	**2.5***	(1.8–3.6)	**1.8***	(1.5–2.1)	**2.3***	(1.6–3.3)	**1.6**	(1.0–2.6)
Low-average	**2.2***	(1.5–3.1)	**1.8***	(1.5–2.2)	**1.6***	(1.1–2.4)	**1.2**	(0.7–2.0)
High-average	**1.5***	(1.0–2.1)	**1.2**	(1.0–1.4)	**1.6***	(1.0–2.3)	**1.3**	(0.8–2.1)
High	**1.0**		**1.0**		**1.0**		**1.0**	
Household income difference[d]	$\chi^2_3 = 35.7^*$, P < 0.001		$\chi^2_3 = 60.9^*$, P < 0.001		$\chi^2_3 = 18.7^*$, P < 0.001		$\chi^2_3 = 4.2$, P = 0.243	
N[e]	**132,430**		**5,759,589**		**1,734**		**1,112**	

*Significant at the 0.05 level, two-sided test.
[a]These estimates are based on logistic regression models adjusted for age, gender, and country.
[b]These estimates are based on survival models adjusted for age-cohorts, gender, person-years, and country.
[c]These estimates are based on logistic regression models adjusted for time since agoraphobia onset, age of agoraphobia onset, gender, and country.
[d]Chi-square test of significant differences between blocks of socio-demographic variables.
[e]Denominator N: 132,430 = total sample; 5,759,589 = number of person-years in the survival models; 1,734 = number of lifetime agoraphobia cases; 1,112 = number of 12-month agoraphobia cases.

Table 8.5 Comorbidity of agoraphobia with other DSM-IV disorders, all countries combined

	Agoraphobia cases with comorbid disorders									
	Mood disorder[a]		Anxiety disorder[b]		Disruptive behaviour/ impulse-control disorder[c]		Substance-use disorder[d]		Any mental disorder[e]	
	%	SE	%	SE	%	SE	%	SE	%	SE
Lifetime comorbidity[f]										
Lifetime	**55.1**	1.8	**81.6**	1.5	**20.6**	1.5	**26.3**	1.5	**88.8**	1.4
12-month	**56.8**	2.4	**85.8**	1.8	**22.4**	1.9	**27.5**	1.9	**91.9**	1.6
12-month comorbidity[g]										
12-month	**44.0**	2.3	**76.7**	2.0	**12.6**	1.5	**8.8**	1.1	**83.5**	1.9
Temporal priority of agoraphobia[h]										
Lifetime	**51.4**	2.0	**14.9**	1.5	**43.7**	3.6	**58.5**	3.0	**17.1**	1.4
12-month	**50.3**	2.4	**13.6**	1.7	**40.7**	3.7	**59.4**	3.5	**15.1**	1.8

[a]Respondents with major depressive episode or bipolar spectrum disorder.
[b]Respondents with panic disorder, generalized anxiety disorder, social phobia, specific phobia, posttraumatic stress disorder, or separation anxiety disorder.
[c]Respondents with intermittent explosive disorder, attention deficit disorder, conduct disorder, oppositional defiant disorder, binge-eating disorder, or bulimia nervosa.
[d]Respondents with alcohol abuse with or without dependence or drug abuse with or without dependence.
[e]Respondents with any disorder listed above.
[f]Percentage of respondents with either lifetime or 12-month agoraphobia who also meet lifetime criteria for at least one of the other DSM-IV disorders.
[g]Percentage of respondents with 12-month agoraphobia who also meet 12-month criteria for at least one of the other disorders.
[h]Percentage of respondents with either lifetime or 12-month agoraphobia and at least one of the other disorders, whose age-of-onset of agoraphobia is reported to be younger than the age-of-onset of all comorbid disorders under consideration.

onset of other disorders ('any mental disorder') in only a minority of cases (17.1%). However, this is probably due to other phobic disorders, such as social anxiety disorder and specific phobia, preceding the development of AG. The prevalence of cases in which AG preceded the comorbid disorder is indeed substantially higher for PD (42.6%), mood disorders (51.4%), substance-use disorders (58.5%), and disruptive behaviour/impulse-control disorders (43.7%). This pattern is again similar for respondents with 12-month AG (Table 8.5).

In respondents who have AG without PD, the onset of AG preceded the onset of other disorders somewhat more often. For any lifetime mental disorder this percentage is 19.0%, and for other anxiety disorders, mood disorders, substance-use disorders, and disruptive behaviour/impulse-control disorders the percentages are 15.6%, 55.4%, 62.2%, and 62.7%, respectively.

Discussion

As noted elsewhere in this volume, the WMH surveys data have the important limitation of being cross-sectional. Therefore, information on the prevalence of mental disorders and on the temporal order of these disorders is based on retrospective information regarding self-reported age-of-onset, which could be biased (for example as a result of forgetting). In addition, the cross-sectional nature of the WMH surveys means that the indicators of disorder and episode persistence of AG are proxy indicators and may also be biased (see Chapters 3 and 22 for discussion of the implications of these biases). However, the WMH surveys also have several strengths. The surveys used a common methodology and diagnostic instrument to assess AG; this instrument allowed assessment of AG separately from PD; and the surveys allow us to provide estimates on AG for a wide variety of countries with different income ranges and from different continents. In addition, the number of respondents was large enough to examine not only lifetime and 12-month prevalence of AG, but also the point prevalence of AG (i.e., 30-day AG).

These data from 26 WMH surveys show that total AG (with or without PD) is not a rare disorder, with a cross-national lifetime prevalence of 1.2%, and 12-month and 30-day prevalence rates of 0.8% and 0.4%, respectively. AG has a rather early median age-of-onset of 21 years, and the results regarding the course of AG suggest that most individuals with AG suffer from recurrent or persistent episodes. Not surprisingly, AG was shown to be associated with severe role impairment in a substantial number of individuals, most of whom sought some form of treatment. Comorbidity rates with other mental disorders were very high, especially for other phobic anxiety disorders. Although other anxiety disorders often precede AG, it is of interest to note that this is not necessarily the case for PD, since AG preceded PD in 42.6% of cases.

When comparing total AG to AG without PD we found some differences. Respondents with AG without PD had a slightly lower age-of-onset of AG (i.e., 19 years). Also, fewer respondents with this condition reported severe impairment and treatment rates and comorbidity rates were a little lower. Nevertheless, 35.0% of respondents with AG in the past 12 months but without lifetime PD reported severe impairment and 84.5% of respondents with lifetime AG but without lifetime PD had another lifetime comorbid mental disorder.

The 12-month prevalence rate of total AG reported here (0.8%) is comparable, although somewhat lower, than the 12-month prevalence rate of 1.3% for AG without a history of PD found in European countries (Goodwin *et al.* 2005). It is interesting to note that although our 12-month prevalence rate of AG increased somewhat by including AG with PD, most respondents (75%) with AG actually did not meet criteria for lifetime PD. This percentage is comparable to that found for 12-month AG in an Australian survey, in which 64% did not have a history of PD (Andrews & Slade 2002). Also, the socio-demographic predictors of AG found in the WMH surveys are comparable to those found in previous work in Australia, where female gender, younger age, being widowed, separated or divorced, not well educated, and unemployed predicted the presence of AG, PD, or comorbid PD and AG (Andrews & Slade 2002). Respondents meeting criteria for PD, AG, or PD and AG have also previously been found likely to have a comorbid affective, anxiety, or substance-use disorder, as found in the WMH surveys (Andrews & Slade 2002).

DSM-IV AG can be diagnosed as part of PD or in the absence of PD. In DSM-5, there is an emphasis on AG as an independent disorder that may or may not occur together with PD (American Psychiatric Association 2013). One of the reasons for the decision to classify AG as a disorder that exists separately from PD was based on studies indicating that in many cases PD or panic attacks do not precede AG. One study in adolescents and young adults showed that a substantial percentage of individuals with clinically confirmed AG did not have a history of panic attacks, or did not even experience symptoms of panic (Wittchen *et al.* 1998). After 10-year follow-up, panic attack and PD seemed to only moderately increase the risk of AG (Wittchen *et al.* 2008). In these studies the focus was only on the avoidance of feared situations, and not on a fear of the development of panic-like symptoms, a criterion included in DSM-IV criteria for AG. Still, these studies suggest that, although panic attacks precipitate AG in some individuals, this is not always the case (Wittchen *et al.* 2008; 2010). Consistent with this, the median age-of-onset of AG (without PD) appears to be lower than the age-of-onset of PD (Wittchen *et al.* 1998; Kessler *et al.* 2005). In this way AG is more comparable to other phobic disorders, such as social anxiety disorder, which also have early onsets (Kessler *et al.* 2005). In our results AG preceded PD in 42.6% of the cases, consistent with prior evidence (Wittchen *et al.* 2008; 2010). Similarly, our finding that the majority of respondents with AG did not have lifetime PD supports the decision in DSM-5 to separate AG from PD.

The question of whether AG can be regarded as an independent disorder has been the subject of debate in recent decades (e.g., Wittchen *et al.*, 1998, 2008; Grant *et al.* 2006; Stein 2012). Since AG without a history of PD is not typically seen in clinical settings, it has been argued that most individuals diagnosed with AG in epidemiological studies actually suffer from specific phobia (Horwath *et al.* 1993). However, the low percentage of patients with AG seen in clinical care may also be the result of individuals suffering from AG being less likely to seek treatment (Wittchen *et al.* 1998; Andrews & Slade 2002), which would make sense since their disorder is characterized by avoidance behaviour. One study validated the existence of AG in the absence of panic attacks in a community survey using re-interviews performed by clinical psychiatrists (Faravelli *et al.* 2008). In addition, recent epidemiological surveys used better measurements of AG than older surveys, which likely improved the validity of the AG diagnosis in this work (Andrews & Slade 2002; Wittchen *et al.* 2010). This point also applies to the methods used in the WMH surveys, for example, in order to meet criteria for AG, agoraphobic anxiety had to apply to at least two different situations.

In the WMH surveys, participants had to report experiencing strong fear of having a panic attack in a situation in which it might be difficult or embarrassing to escape, in concordance with DSM-IV criteria (American Psychiatric Association 2000). However, DSM-5 criteria are reworded, broadening this criterion to a fear or avoidance of situations because of thoughts that escape might be difficult or help might not be available in the event of developing panic-like symptoms or other incapacitating or embarrassing symptoms (e.g., fear of falling in the elderly; fear of incontinence) (American Psychiatric Association 2013). This is in line with the proposed *International Classification of Diseases* (ICD) diagnostic guidelines in which AG is conceptualized as the consequence, not only of fear of panic attacks/panic-like symptoms, but of a broader range of fears (Wittchen *et al.* 2010; Stein 2012). It is plausible that the prevalence of AG will be higher with the criterion of fear of panic attacks/panic-like symptoms being expanded in this way. However, it is important to keep in mind that fear of becoming physically ill, or having a heart attack may be realistic and not a sign of a psychiatric disorder, especially in older individuals.

The prevalence of AG and the associated impairment differed across countries and was lower for the low/lower-middle-income countries than for the other countries. The finding of lower impairment in low/lower-middle-income countries may be unexpected, but this finding is consistent with other reports based on WMH data for depression (Bromet *et al.* 2011) and PD (de Jonge *et al.* 2016). Differences in impairment rates due to AG across countries may be the result of social structures and legislation. For example, in lower-income countries in which women are more likely to be at home, the percentage of women reporting work impairment may be lower. In addition, the ability to take sick leave in higher-income countries may lead to higher impairment rates on the work domain. Bromet *et al.* (2011) showed that functional impairment in individuals *without* lifetime depression was also higher in respondents from high-income countries compared with respondents from low- and middle-income countries, suggesting that higher impairment rates in high-income countries may represent a general finding that is not only related to the presence of mental disorders (see also Chapter 22).

To conclude, this chapter has provided comprehensive cross-national epidemiological data for AG. AG is an impairing disorder with an early age-of-onset, is often comorbid with other mental disorders, especially phobic and mood disorders, and does not occur just as a result of PD.

References

American Psychiatric Association (2000). *Diagnostic and Statistical Manual of Mental Disorders. 4th ed., text revision*. Washington, DC: American Psychiatric Press.

(2013). *Diagnostic and Statistical Manual of Mental Disorders. 5th ed.* Washington, DC: American Psychiatric Press.

Andrews, G. & Slade, T. (2002). Agoraphobia without a history of panic disorder may be part of the panic disorder syndrome. *The Journal of Nervous and Mental Disease* 190, 624–30.

Bromet, E., Andrade, L. H., Hwang, I., *et al.* (2011). Cross-national epidemiology of DSM-IV major depressive episode. *BMC Medicine* 9, 90.

de Jonge, P., Roest, A. M., Lim, C. W., *et al.* (2016). Cross-national epidemiology of DSM-5 panic disorder and panic attacks in the World Mental Health Surveys. *Depression and Anxiety* 33, 1155–77.

Faravelli, C., Cosci, F., Rotella, F., Faravelli, L., & Catena Dell'osso, M. (2008). Agoraphobia between panic and phobias: clinical epidemiology from the Sesto Fiorentino Study. *Comprehensive Psychiatry* 49, 283–7.

Goodwin, R. D., Faravelli, C., Rosi, S., *et al.* (2005). The epidemiology of panic disorder and agoraphobia in Europe. *European Neuropsychopharmacology* 15, 435–43.

Grant, B. F., Hasin, D. S., Stinson, F. S., *et al.* (2006). The epidemiology of DSM-IV panic disorder and agoraphobia in the United States: results from the National Epidemiologic Survey on Alcohol and Related Conditions. *The Journal of Clinical Psychiatry* 67, 363–74.

Haro, J. M., Arbabzadeh-Bouchez, S., Brugha, T. S., *et al.* (2006). Concordance of the Composite International Diagnostic Interview Version 3.0 (CIDI 3.0) with standardized clinical assessments in the WHO World Mental Health surveys. *International Journal of Methods in Psychiatric Research* 15, 167–80.

Horwath, E., Lish, J. D., Johnson, J., Hornig, C. D., & Weissman, M. M. (1993). Agoraphobia without panic: clinical reappraisal of an epidemiologic finding. *The American Journal of Psychiatry* 150, 1496–501.

Kessler, R. C., Berglund, P., Demler, O., *et al.* (2005). Lifetime prevalence and age-of-onset distributions of DSM-IV disorders in the National Comorbidity Survey Replication. *Archives of General Psychiatry* 62, 593–602.

Stein, D. J. (2012). Agoraphobia and panic disorder: options for ICD-11. *World Psychiatry 2012* 11 (suppl 1), 88–92.

Wittchen, H. U., Gloster, A. T., Beesdo-Baum, K., Fava, G. A., & Craske, M. G. (2010). Agoraphobia: a review of the diagnostic classificatory position and criteria. *Depression and Anxiety* 27, 113–33.

Wittchen, H. U., Nocon, A., Beesdo, K., *et al.* (2008). Agoraphobia and panic. Prospective-longitudinal relations suggest a rethinking of diagnostic concepts. *Psychotherapy and Psychosomatics* 77, 147–57.

Wittchen, H. U., Reed, V., & Kessler, R. C. (1998). The relationship of agoraphobia and panic in a community sample of adolescents and young adults. *Archives of General Psychiatry* 55, 1017–24.

Chapter 9

Social Anxiety Disorder

Dan J. Stein, Norito Kawakami, Giovanni de Girolamo, Jean-Pierre Lépine

Introduction

Social anxiety disorder (SAD) is a relatively new nosological construct. Anxiety and phobias have been recognized since the time of Hippocrates, but are often conceptualized as part of broader conditions such as depression. Early editions of the *Diagnostic and Statistical Manual of Mental Disorders* (DSM) and the *International Classification of Disease* (ICD) recognized the phobic disorders, but did not subdivide these conditions. In his early paper on the classification of phobic disorders, Marks noted some distinctions between social phobia and other phobias, but emphasized the need for more research (Marks 1970). The third edition of the DSM included diagnostic criteria for social phobia, but shortly thereafter, in their review of the literature, Liebowitz and colleagues emphasized that this was a 'neglected disorder' about which little was known (Liebowitz *et al.* 1985). Not all patients demonstrate the avoidance that the term 'phobia' may imply (Bogels *et al.* 2010), and DSM-IV used the rubric 'social phobia (social anxiety disorder)', with DSM-5 changing the name to 'social anxiety disorder (social phobia)'. As the field has increasingly adopted the term 'social anxiety disorder', we use it in this chapter.

The inclusion of SAD in DSM-III did, however, give important impetus to further study, including epidemiological research. Early work with the Diagnostic Interview Schedule, which generated a DSM-III diagnosis, allowed prevalence estimates to be ascertained both in the United States (Myers *et al.* 1984) and in a small number of other countries (Weissman *et al.* 1996). Subsequent work in the National Comorbidity Survey and the National Epidemiological Study of Alcohol and Related Conditions in the United States used the DSM-IV criteria for SAD, and provided information not only on the prevalence of the condition, but also on its socio-demographic correlates, its extensive comorbidity with other anxiety disorders, mood disorders, and substance-use disorders (Magee *et al.* 1996; Buckner *et al.* 2012), as well as on its associated impairment (Kessler 2003). Subtyping of SAD has also been extensively explored in the United States and elsewhere (Ruscio *et al.* 2008; Stein *et al.* 2010).

By 2005, a systematic review of community studies of social phobia found 21 surveys, with median 12-month and lifetime prevalence rates of 2.0% and 6.7%, respectively, with higher rates in women and in younger individuals (Fehm *et al.* 2005). Social phobia was accompanied by significant comorbidity, as well as associated impairment (Fehm *et al.* 2005). Subsequent reviews of the epidemiology of anxiety disorders (Somers *et al.* 2006; Kessler *et al.* 2010) and of mental disorders across the globe (Steel *et al.* 2014) have emphasized the high prevalence of anxiety disorders, the early age-of-onset of phobias including SAD, and the chronic-recurrent course of this condition. These findings, as well as data on the high economic costs of anxiety disorders (Greenberg *et al.* 1999), suggest that early interventions might not only be useful in preventing and treatment of SAD, but also in addressing comorbid conditions.

Still, much remains to be understood about the community epidemiology of SAD. The majority of community surveys reported are from high-income countries, where only a minority of the world's population lives, and it has been suggested that the prevalence and phenomenology of SAD may differ across cultures (Stein 2009). High-income countries tend to be Westernized, educated, industrialized, rich, and democratic (WEIRD) (Henrich *et al.* 2010), so that the socio-demographic correlates of SAD globally have not been well delineated. In addition, few surveys have included detailed assessment of the impulse-control disorders, so that comorbidity of SAD with these conditions is not well documented. The World Mental Health (WMH) Surveys Initiative provides a unique opportunity to address limitations in the current literature, and to provide rigorous data on the prevalence and correlates of SAD across the world.

Methods

All WMH countries except Israel assessed SAD so this chapter is based on thirteen countries classified by the World Bank as high-income (Australia, Belgium, France, Germany, Italy, Japan, New Zealand, Northern Ireland, Poland, Portugal, Spain, the Netherlands, the United States), seven as upper-middle income (Brazil, Bulgaria, Colombia (Medellin), Lebanon, Mexico, Romania, South Africa) and six as low/lower-middle-income (Colombia, Iraq, Nigeria, Peru, People's Republic of China [PRC], Ukraine).

SAD and other DSM-IV anxiety, mood, disruptive behaviour/impulse-control, and substance-use disorders were assessed using version 3.0 of the WHO Composite International Diagnostic Interview (CIDI 3.0) (Kessler & Üstün 2004). Respondents were administered the full SAD section if they endorsed a diagnostic stem question for one or more performance or interactional fears described as excessive and causing substantial distress or avoidance. The SAD section assessed lifetime experiences of shyness, fear, and discomfort associated with each of 14 social situations.

Respondents endorsing one or more such questions were asked about all DSM-IV criteria. These criteria include: (1) a marked and persistent fear of one or more social or performance situations with exposure to unfamiliar people or to potential scrutiny, and fear of humiliation/embarrassment; (2) exposure to these situations almost invariably results in anxiety; (3) the person recognizes that the fear is excessive or unreasonable, and either avoids these situations or endures them with intense distress; (4) there is significant interference or marked distress; and (5) the symptoms are not due to a substance-use disorder, a general medical condition, or another mental disorder.

As detailed elsewhere, good CIDI-SCID diagnostic concordance was found for SAD and most other DSM-IV/CIDI disorders (Haro *et al.* 2006).

Results

Prevalence

On average, the estimated lifetime, 12-month, and 30-day prevalence of SAD is highest in high-income countries (5.5%, 3.1%, 1.7%), intermediate in upper-middle-income countries (2.9%, 2.1%, 1.3%), and lowest in low/lower-middle-income countries (1.6%, 1.0%, 0.5%) (Table 9.1). Prevalence rates are highest in the Americas and the Western Pacific region, and lowest in Africa and the Eastern Mediterranean region. In all countries combined, the lifetime, 12-month and 30-day rates for SAD (4.0%, 2.4%, 1.3%, respectively) indicate that it is a prevalent disorder. Similar prevalence patterns are seen in males and females across the globe, with higher prevalence in females and lower prevalence in males (data not shown).

The ratio of the 12-month prevalence to lifetime prevalence is an indirect indicator of disorder persistence. This ratio is lowest in high-income countries (57.3%) and the Western Pacific region (54.5%), and highest in upper-middle-income countries (72.4%), Africa (71.1%), and the Eastern Mediterranean region (74.2%). Across all countries, SAD is a persistent disorder (60.2%). The ratio of the 30-day prevalence to 12-month prevalence is an indirect indicator of episode persistence amongst those with recent disorder. This ratio is again lowest in the Western Pacific region (49.4%), and highest in upper-middle-income countries (61.4%), Africa (66.7%), and the Eastern Mediterranean region (66.0%).

Age-of-Onset

Table 9.2 and Figure 9.1 indicate that the median estimated age-of-onset (AOO) is similar for high-income, upper-middle-income, and low/lower-middle-income countries. Across all countries, onset of SAD ranges from the mid-late adolescence to the early 40s. In high-income countries, the earliest median AOO estimates occurred in Poland (50% by age 11), whereas the latest are in the Netherlands (50% by age 17). In upper-middle-income countries, the earliest median AOO estimates are in Colombia (50% by age 13), and the latest in South Africa (50% by age 26). In low/lower-middle-income countries, the earliest median AOO estimates are in Nigeria (50% by age 11), and the latest in Peru (50% by age 16). Projected lifetime risk for SAD by age 75 across the globe is 4.4%.

Role Impairment

SAD is associated with substantial impairment in multiple domains of role functioning in the WMH data, with 37.6% of those with 12-month SAD, in all countries combined, reporting severe impairment on the Sheehan Disability Scale (SDS) in at least one domain (Table 9.3). In the vast majority of countries, the proportion of respondents with 12-month SAD and severe role impairment is, however, higher in the relationship and social domains than in the domains of home and

Table 9.1 Prevalence of DSM-IV social anxiety disorder (SAD) in the World Mental Health surveys

Country	Lifetime prevalence		12-month prevalence		30-day prevalence		12-month prevalence of SAD among lifetime cases		30-day prevalence of SAD among 12-month cases		Sample size used
	%	SE	%	SE	%	SE	%	SE	%	SE	
Low/lower-middle-income countries	**1.6**	**0.1**	**1.0**	**0.1**	**0.5**	**0.0**	**62.6**	**2.5**	**52.0**	**3.4**	**36,498**
Colombia	5.0	0.5	2.9	0.3	1.6	0.3	58.0	4.6	54.9	6.1	4,426
Iraq	0.8	0.2	0.7	0.2	0.5	0.2	86.0	7.5	72.0	6.9	4,332
Nigeria	0.2	0.1	0.2	0.1	0.1	0.1	96.3	3.9	83.3	11.7	6,752
Peru	2.6	0.3	1.4	0.1	0.5	0.1	54.2	3.2	35.5	6.8	3,930
PRC (Beijing/Shanghai)	0.5	0.1	0.4	0.1	0.2	0.1	66.6	11.9	52.8	13.7	5,201
PRC (Shenzhen)	0.9	0.2	0.7	0.1	0.2	0.1	76.5	6.0	29.3	9.9	7,132
Ukraine	2.6	0.2	1.5	0.2	1.0	0.2	59.9	4.9	62.3	7.8	4,725
Upper-middle-income countries	**2.9**	**0.1**	**2.1**	**0.1**	**1.3**	**0.1**	**72.4**	**2.1**	**61.4**	**2.6**	**28,927**
Brazil	5.6	0.4	3.9	0.3	2.7	0.3	70.8	4.5	67.5	5.2	5,037
Bulgaria	0.8	0.2	0.6	0.2	0.4	0.1	74.7	7.0	58.9	9.4	5,318
Colombia (Medellin)	4.6	0.5	3.8	0.5	2.2	0.4	82.7	3.8	58.3	6.5	3,261
Lebanon	1.9	0.4	1.3	0.3	0.8	0.2	67.0	7.0	61.3	9.4	2,857
Mexico	2.9	0.2	2.0	0.2	1.1	0.2	69.4	4.0	53.4	4.9	5,782
Romania	1.3	0.3	1.0	0.2	0.6	0.2	74.7	8.3	60.1	12.2	2,357
South Africa	2.8	0.4	1.9	0.3	1.2	0.2	68.7	5.8	64.4	5.6	4,315
High-income countries	**5.5**	**0.1**	**3.1**	**0.1**	**1.7**	**0.1**	**57.3**	**1.0**	**53.1**	**1.2**	**76,980**
Australia	8.5	0.4	4.2	0.3	1.9	0.2	49.8	2.9	44.7	3.3	8,463
Belgium	2.0	0.4	1.2	0.2	0.7	0.2	59.8	7.2	58.4	13.5	2,419
France	4.3	0.5	2.6	0.4	1.8	0.3	59.3	5.2	71.8	6.7	2,894
Germany	2.5	0.3	1.5	0.2	1.0	0.2	60.4	6.0	63.7	7.7	3,555
Italy	1.9	0.2	1.1	0.2	0.6	0.1	60.0	5.4	52.8	8.6	4,712
Japan	1.4	0.2	0.7	0.2	0.5	0.1	51.9	8.1	68.4	9.3	4,129
New Zealand	9.5	0.3	5.3	0.3	2.8	0.2	56.0	1.8	52.5	2.5	12,790
Northern Ireland	6.0	0.4	4.0	0.3	2.5	0.3	65.8	2.9	63.4	4.6	4,340
Poland	1.4	0.1	0.9	0.1	0.5	0.1	63.4	3.8	55.1	4.5	10,081
Portugal	4.7	0.5	3.1	0.4	1.7	0.2	67.1	3.9	54.2	4.8	3,849
Spain	1.2	0.2	0.7	0.1	0.4	0.1	56.3	6.9	58.6	12.4	5,473
Spain (Murcia)	1.7	0.2	1.2	0.2	0.9	0.2	67.7	11.0	74.4	10.3	2,621
Netherlands	2.6	0.4	1.3	0.3	1.0	0.3	50.8	9.3	73.9	8.1	2,372
United States	12.1	0.4	7.1	0.3	3.5	0.2	58.8	1.7	48.9	1.9	9,282

Table 9.1 (*cont.*)

Country	Lifetime prevalence		12-month prevalence		30-day prevalence		12-month prevalence of SAD among lifetime cases		30-day prevalence of SAD among 12-month cases		Sample size used
	%	SE	%	SE	%	SE	%	SE	%	SE	
All countries combined	**4.0**	**0.1**	**2.4**	**0.1**	**1.3**	**0.0**	**60.2**	**0.8**	**54.5**	**1.0**	**142,405**
WHO regions[a]											
Region of the Americas	6.4	0.2	4.0	0.1	2.1	0.1	62.8	1.3	53.1	1.6	31,718
African region	1.2	0.2	0.9	0.1	0.6	0.1	71.1	5.5	66.7	5.3	11,067
Western Pacific region	5.5	0.2	3.0	0.1	1.5	0.1	54.5	1.5	49.4	1.9	37,715
Eastern Mediterranean region	1.2	0.2	0.9	0.2	0.6	0.1	74.2	5.7	66.0	6.1	7,189
Western European region	3.0	0.1	1.9	0.1	1.2	0.1	62.4	1.8	62.3	2.5	32,235
Eastern European region	1.5	0.1	1.0	0.1	0.6	0.1	64.7	2.7	58.6	3.7	22,481
Comparison between countries[b]	**$F_{27,v} = 78.6^*$, $P < 0.001$**		**$F_{27,v} = 46.3^*$, $P < 0.001$**		**$F_{27,v} = 25.7^*$, $P < 0.001$**		**$F_{27,v} = 3.3^*$, $P < 0.001$**		**$F_{27,v} = 2.4^*$, $P < 0.001$**		
Comparison between low-, middle-, and high-income country groups[b]	**$F_{2,v} = 387.5^*$, $P < 0.001$**		**$F_{2,v} = 224.2^*$, $P < 0.001$**		**$F_{2,v} = 121.7^*$, $P < 0.001$**		**$F_{2,v} = 21.3^*$, $P < 0.001$**		**$F_{2,v} = 4.5^*$, $P = 0.01$**		
Comparison between WHO regions[b]	**$F_{5,v} = 207.5^*$, $P < 0.001$**		**$F_{5,v} = 118.4^*$, $P < 0.001$**		**$F_{5,v} = 53.2^*$, $P < 0.001$**		**$F_{5,v} = 6.1^*$, $P < 0.001$**		**$F_{5,v} = 5.2^*$, $P < 0.001$**		

*Significant at the 0.05 level, two-sided test.

[a]**Region of the Americas** (Colombia, Mexico, Brazil, Peru, United States, Columbia (Medellin)); **African region** (Nigeria, South Africa); **Western Pacific region** (PRC (Shenzhen), PRC (Beijing and Shanghai), Japan, Australia, New Zealand); **Eastern Mediterranean region** (Iraq, Lebanon); **Western European region** (Belgium, France, Germany, Italy, Netherlands, Spain, Northern Ireland, Portugal, Spain (Murcia)); **Eastern European region** (Romania, Bulgaria, Poland, Ukraine).

[b]Wald design-corrected F-tests were used to determine if there is variation in prevalence estimates across countries. The denominator degree of freedom, v, is 1535.

PRC: People's Republic of China.

Table 9.2 Age at selected percentiles on the standardized age-of-onset distributions of DSM-IV social anxiety disorder (SAD) with projected lifetime risk at age 75

Country	Ages at selected percentiles								Lifetime prevalence of SAD		Projected risk at age 75	
	5	10	25	50	75	90	95	99	%	SE	%	SE
Low/lower-middle-income countries	**7**	**8**	**11**	**15**	**19**	**26**	**36**	**57**	**1.6**	**0.1**	**1.7**	**0.1**
Colombia[a]	6	8	11	15	19	26	31	39	5.0	0.5	5.3	0.5
Iraq	7	9	13	14	18	23	36	36	0.8	0.2	0.8	0.2
Nigeria	7	7	7	11	19	23	24	24	0.2	0.1	0.2	0.1
Peru[a]	9	10	13	16	19	27	34	41	2.6	0.3	2.7	0.3
PRC (Beijing/Shanghai)	8	12	14	14	17	19	37	37	0.5	0.1	0.5	0.1
PRC (Shenzhen)	5	7	11	14	18	26	31	41	0.9	0.2	1.0	0.2
Ukraine	7	8	11	14	16	25	37	57	2.6	0.2	2.9	0.3
Upper-middle-income countries	**5**	**7**	**11**	**15**	**20**	**36**	**49**	**67**	**2.9**	**0.1**	**3.4**	**0.2**
Brazil	5	7	11	14	17	29	41	54	5.6	0.4	6.1	0.4
Bulgaria	8	8	11	14	18	24	31	38	0.8	0.2	0.9	0.2
Colombia (Medellin)[a]	5	5	8	13	16	21	31	41	4.6	0.5	4.7	0.5
Lebanon	6	7	11	14	18	20	26	30	1.9	0.4	2.0	0.4
Mexico[a]	6	7	11	15	19	26	40	54	2.9	0.2	3.2	0.3
Romania	10	13	14	21	36	58	58	58	1.3	0.3	1.8	0.4
South Africa	11	13	16	26	49	67	67	67	2.8	0.4	4.7	1.2
High-income countries	**5**	**6**	**9**	**13**	**17**	**29**	**42**	**59**	**4.0**	**0.1**	**6.0**	**0.1**
Australia	5	6	9	14	20	37	46	68	8.5	0.4	9.6	0.5
Belgium	5	5	7	13	17	25	36	36	2.0	0.4	2.2	0.4
France	7	8	11	14	20	31	45	57	4.3	0.5	4.9	0.5
Germany	7	9	11	14	35	50	62	62	2.5	0.3	3.0	0.5
Italy	5	7	13	15	20	28	36	56	1.9	0.2	2.0	0.3
Japan	5	5	9	13	16	29	43	48	1.4	0.2	1.6	0.2
New Zealand	5	6	8	13	17	27	38	57	9.5	0.3	10.4	0.4
Northern Ireland	5	6	10	14	20	40	49	54	6.0	0.4	7.1	0.5
Poland[b]	5	5	8	11	14	17	19	21	1.4	0.1	1.4	0.1
Portugal	5	5	9	14	18	29	43	61	4.7	0.5	5.2	0.5
Spain	5	5	9	13	19	22	48	48	1.2	0.2	1.3	0.2
Spain (Murcia)	5	5	5	13	18	33	37	40	1.7	0.2	1.9	0.3
Netherlands	5	7	11	17	29	41	49	52	2.6	0.4	3.1	0.5
United States	5	6	8	13	15	23	32	51	12.1	0.4	13.0	0.5
All countries combined	**5**	**6**	**9**	**14**	**18**	**31**	**44**	**62**	**4.0**	**0.1**	**4.4**	**0.1**
WHO regions												
Region of the Americas	5	6	9	13	17	26	36	52	6.4	0.2	6.9	0.2
African region	7	13	15	23	47	67	67	67	1.2	0.2	2.0	0.5
Western Pacific region	5	6	9	14	18	33	46	66	5.5	0.2	6.1	0.2
Eastern Mediterranean region	6	8	11	14	18	23	26	36	1.2	0.2	1.3	0.2
Western European region	5	6	10	14	20	36	45	61	3.0	0.1	3.4	0.1
Eastern European region	5	7	9	13	17	24	38	58	1.5	0.1	1.7	0.1

[a]The projected risk for these countries is at age 65 because the age range of these surveys is between 18 and 65.
[b]The projected risk for this country is at age 64 because the age range of this survey is between 18 and 64.
PRC: People's Republic of China.

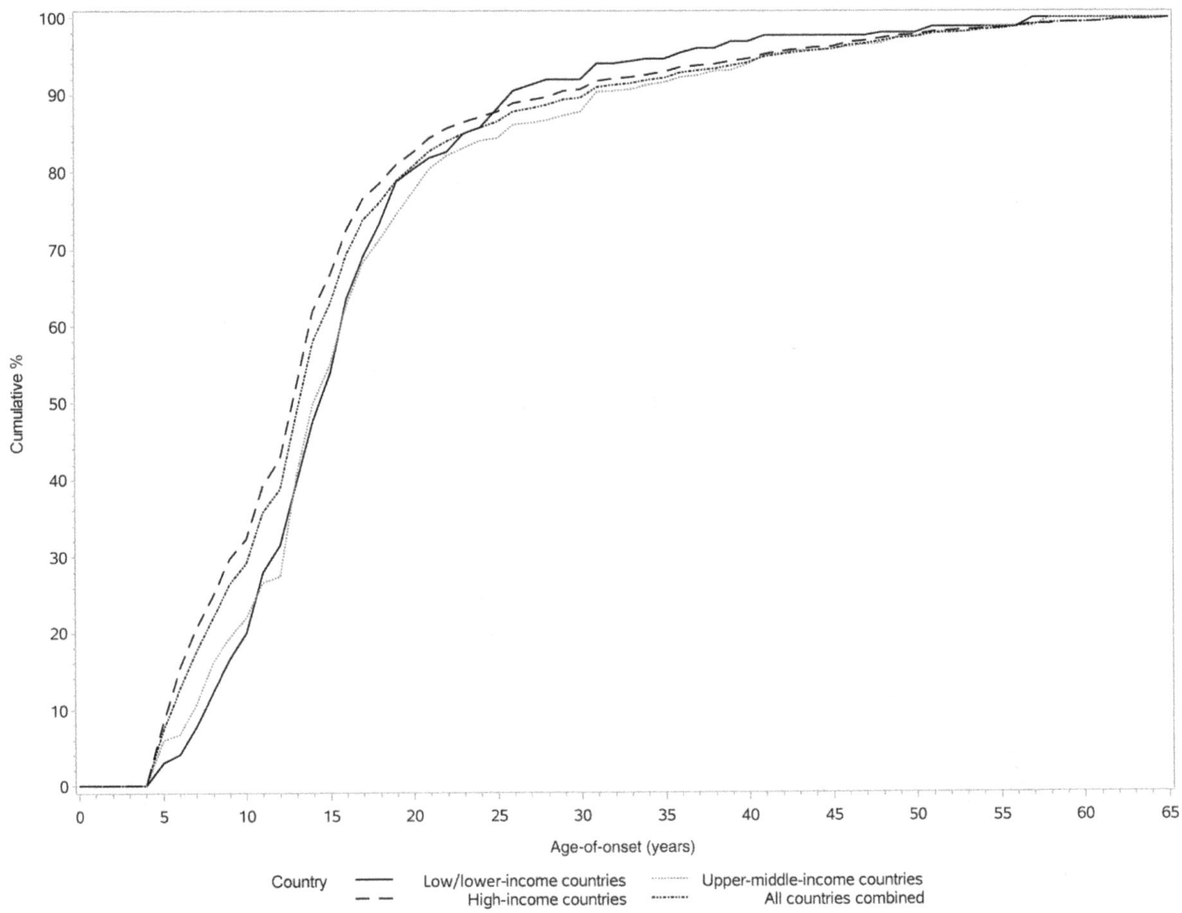

Figure 9.1 Cumulative age-of-onset distribution for social anxiety disorder by country income groups and in all countries combined

work. Furthermore, in the vast majority of countries, between one-third and one-half of respondents with 12-month SAD have severe role impairment in at least one domain. Notably, there are no significant differences between low/lower-middle-, upper-middle-, and high-income country groups, nor between different WHO regions, in the proportion of respondents with severe role impairment in at least one domain. However, there are significant differences among countries in the proportion of 12-month SAD respondents with severe role impairment in any domain, ranging from 9.4% in Shenzhen to 71.6% in Spain, Murcia (Table 9.3). Finally, using a different indicator of impairment (days-out-of-role): people with 12-month SAD report an average of 24.7 days in the year when they are unable to carry out their normal role functions due to their problems with social anxiety (data not shown).

Socio-demographic Correlates

Table 9.4 shows the bivariate associations of the socio-demographic characteristics with SAD in the combined sample. Both 30-day and lifetime SAD are associated with younger AOO, female gender, not being employed, being unmarried (never married or divorced/widowed/separated), lower educational status, and low household income. SAD persistence (12-month SAD/lifetime) is associated with female gender, earlier AOO, and not being married – while episode persistence (30-day SAD/12-month) is associated with

Table 9.3 Severity of role impairment (Sheehan Disability Scale) associated with 12-month social anxiety disorder, by country

Country	Proportion with severe role impairment (SDS score: 7–10)										Number of 12-month cases
	Home		Work		Relationship		Social		Any[a]		
	%	SE	%	SE	%	SE	%	SE	%	SE	
Low/lower-middle-income countries	**9.3**	**1.6**	**14.1**	**2.4**	**18.0**	**2.6**	**21.2**	**2.8**	**34.3**	**3.2**	**349**
Colombia	8.1	2.3	18.1	5.2	22.5	4.9	32.3	5.0	43.2	5.3	133
Iraq	18.0	9.2	9.0	5.4	31.6	12.7	22.7	8.3	48.0	12.6	28
Nigeria	7.8	7.8	28.2	15.7	24.1	13.9	24.1	13.9	36.3	17.4	9
Peru	13.7	4.7	13.4	5.2	11.7	4.0	20.6	7.7	33.0	7.9	51
PRC (Beijing/Shanghai)	4.9	4.8	4.6	4.6	4.6	4.6	17.4	12.1	26.9	13.0	16
PRC (Shenzhen)	2.1	1.9	1.4	1.2	1.2	1.2	6.1	3.5	9.4	4.2	45
Ukraine	11.5	4.1	18.4	5.6	23.1	5.8	12.2	4.7	33.0	6.4	67
Upper-middle-income countries	**12.7**	**1.8**	**17.0**	**2.5**	**28.5**	**2.2**	**28.5**	**2.2**	**39.3**	**2.6**	**601**
Brazil	13.9	4.0	20.5	6.1	25.8	3.5	27.7	3.9	36.7	4.7	186
Bulgaria	5.3	2.9	2.5	1.0	23.2	11.0	10.0	4.7	25.8	10.8	27
Colombia (Medellin)	12.5	4.0	19.8	4.6	33.5	6.1	33.6	6.0	43.2	6.1	110
Lebanon	14.1	6.4	7.9	5.5	43.7	10.0	33.8	9.8	45.8	9.6	35
Mexico	7.3	2.0	11.9	3.2	23.4	3.7	28.1	4.2	35.2	4.4	134
Romania	26.0	10.9	31.5	11.9	40.4	12.9	32.0	11.0	56.2	9.8	22
South Africa	16.6	5.2	17.9	6.0	27.4	6.1	28.1	5.9	43.6	8.1	87
High-income countries	**11.0**	**0.7**	**16.8**	**0.8**	**23.6**	**1.0**	**29.8**	**1.1**	**37.7**	**1.1**	**2,510**
Australia	17.2	2.7	24.3	2.8	37.2	3.9	43.1	4.2	50.1	4.0	381
Belgium	9.6	6.9	28.1	10.7	37.0	13.1	38.4	8.8	54.9	8.3	28
France	9.9	5.1	11.0	4.3	17.5	4.0	24.0	5.3	32.9	5.9	72
Germany	4.0	3.0	14.1	4.9	20.0	5.9	28.0	7.9	42.2	7.9	58
Italy	15.9	6.1	7.9	3.9	23.3	6.0	17.1	6.3	33.1	6.9	53
Japan	6.5	5.9	26.2	8.3	20.4	8.0	25.7	9.4	37.8	8.8	25
New Zealand	6.1	1.1	12.3	1.3	18.8	1.9	26.7	2.1	32.5	2.1	720
Northern Ireland	19.6	2.7	24.7	3.0	31.4	3.4	41.4	4.3	52.3	4.1	183
Poland	14.2	4.6	21.3	4.8	18.6	4.5	21.4	5.2	32.4	5.6	91
Portugal	7.2	2.1	13.4	2.5	15.8	2.7	19.4	3.2	25.1	3.9	124
Spain	8.2	5.4	15.6	7.3	21.2	9.8	17.0	8.2	26.3	10.5	33
Spain (Murcia)	25.8	8.9	41.7	12.7	67.2	11.0	62.4	6.8	71.6	9.4	33
Netherlands	41.9	11.2	56.8	12.7	46.8	13.9	56.1	11.1	63.6	12.0	30
United States	10.9	1.3	15.4	1.4	22.6	1.6	28.8	1.4	36.5	1.7	679

Table 9.3 *(cont.)*

Country	Proportion with severe role impairment (SDS score: 7–10)										Number of 12-month cases
	Home		Work		Relationship		Social		Any[a]		
	%	SE	%	SE	%	SE	%	SE	%	SE	
All countries combined	**11.1**	**0.7**	**16.5**	**0.8**	**23.9**	**0.9**	**28.6**	**0.9**	**37.6**	**1.0**	**3,460**
WHO regions											
Region of the Americas	11.0	1.0	16.5	1.4	23.7	1.3	29.0	1.3	37.5	1.5	1,293
African region	15.6	4.7	19.1	5.6	27.0	5.6	27.6	5.4	42.7	7.4	96
Western Pacific region	8.1	1.0	14.2	1.1	21.4	1.6	28.7	1.8	34.9	1.8	1,187
Eastern Mediterranean region	15.8	5.4	8.4	3.9	38.4	7.9	28.9	7.0	46.8	7.7	63
Western European region	14.4	1.7	20.2	2.0	26.7	2.0	31.4	2.2	41.7	2.4	614
Eastern European region	13.2	2.6	18.3	3.1	23.4	3.6	17.6	3.1	34.2	3.7	207
Comparison between countries[b]	$F_{27,v} = 2.3^*$, $P < 0.001$		$F_{27,v} = 2.9^*$, $P < 0.001$		$F_{27,v} = 3.0^*$, $P < 0.001$		$F_{27,v} = 2.8^*$, $P < 0.001$		$F_{27,v} = 2.6^*$, $P < 0.001$		
Comparison between low-, middle-, and high-income country groups[b]	$F_{2,v} = 1.0$, $P = 0.371$		$F_{2,v} = 0.6$, $P = 0.561$		$F_{2,v} = 4.7^*$, $P = 0.008$		$F_{2,v} = 4.1^*$, $P = 0.016$		$F_{2,v} = 0.8$, $P = 0.463$		
Comparison between WHO regions[b]	$F_{5,v} = 2.9^*$, $P = 0.013$		$F_{5,v} = 2.3^*$, $P = 0.042$		$F_{5,v} = 1.5$, $P = 0.180$		$F_{5,v} = 2.7^*$, $P = 0.020$		$F_{5,v} = 1.5$, $P = 0.175$		

*Significant at the 0.05 level, two-sided test.
[a]Highest severity category across four SDS role domains.
[b]Wald design-corrected F-tests were used to determine if there is variation in impairment severity across countries. The denominator degree of freedom, v, is 1535.
PRC: People's Republic of China.

Table 9.4 Bivariate associations between socio-demographic correlates and DSM-IV social anxiety disorder (SAD), all countries combined

Correlates	30-day SAD[a]		Lifetime SAD[b]		12-month SAD among lifetime cases[c]		30-day SAD among 12-month cases[c]	
	OR	(95% CI)	OR	(95% CI)	OR	(95% CI)	OR	(95% CI)
Age-cohort								
18–29	**3.2***	(2.6–3.9)	**3.6***	(3.2–4.0)				
30–44	**2.8***	(2.3–3.4)	**2.9***	(2.6–3.2)				
45–59	**2.5***	(2.0–3.1)	**2.4***	(2.1–2.6)				
60+	**1.0**		**1.0**					
Age-cohort difference[d]	$\chi^2_3 = 145.4^*$, P < 0.001		$\chi^2_3 = 547.3^*$, P < 0.001					
Age-of-onset								
Early					**1.5***	(1.2–1.8)	**1.0**	(0.7–1.2)
Early-average					**1.4***	(1.1–1.7)	**0.9**	(0.7–1.2)
Late-average					**1.1**	(0.9–1.3)	**0.9**	(0.8–1.2)
Late					**1.0**		**1.0**	
Age-of-onset difference[d]					$\chi^2_3 = 15.4^*$, P = 0.002		$\chi^2_3 = 0.5$, P = 0.926	
Time since onset (continuous)					**0.98***	(0.98–0.99)	**1.01***	(1.00–1.01)
Gender								
Female	**1.7***	(1.5–1.9)	**1.3***	(1.2–1.4)	**1.3***	(1.2–1.5)	**1.2***	(1.0–1.4)
Male	**1.0**		**1.0**		**1.0**		**1.0**	
Gender difference[d]	$\chi^2_1 = 65.3^*$, P < 0.001		$\chi^2_1 = 61.5^*$, P < 0.001		$\chi^2_1 = 15.7^*$, P < 0.001		$\chi^2_1 = 5.9^*$, P = 0.015	
Employment status								
Student	**1.4***	(1.1–1.9)	**1.2**	(1.0–1.4)	**1.1**	(0.8–1.6)	**2.1***	(1.4–3.0)
Homemaker	**1.5***	(1.3–1.7)	**1.2***	(1.1–1.3)	**1.4***	(1.1–1.7)	**1.4***	(1.1–1.8)
Retired	**0.6***	(0.5–0.8)	**0.9**	(0.7–1.0)	**1.0**	(0.7–1.3)	**0.9**	(0.6–1.3)
Other	**1.8***	(1.5–2.1)	**1.5***	(1.3–1.6)	**2.0***	(1.6–2.6)	**1.0**	(0.8–1.3)
Employed	**1.0**		**1.0**		**1.0**		**1.0**	
Employment status difference[d]	$\chi^2_4 = 81.8^*$, P < 0.001		$\chi^2_4 = 63.6^*$, P < 0.001		$\chi^2_4 = 36.9^*$, P < 0.001		$\chi^2_4 = 20.4^*$, P < 0.001	

(cont.)

Table 9.4 (*cont.*)

Correlates	30-day SAD[a]		Lifetime SAD[b]		12-month SAD among lifetime cases[c]		30-day SAD among 12-month cases[c]	
	OR	(95% CI)	OR	(95% CI)	OR	(95% CI)	OR	(95% CI)
Marital status								
Never married	**1.2***	(1.1–1.4)	**1.4***	(1.3–1.5)	**1.3***	(1.1–1.6)	**1.0**	(0.8–1.2)
Divorced/separated/widowed	**1.5***	(1.3–1.7)	**1.3***	(1.2–1.5)	**1.4***	(1.1–1.6)	**1.0**	(0.8–1.3)
Currently married	**1.0**		**1.0**		**1.0**		**1.0**	
Marital status difference[d]	$\chi^2_2 = 26.6^*, P < 0.001$		$\chi^2_2 = 75.7^*, P < 0.001$		$\chi^2_2 = 18.4^*, P < 0.001$		$\chi^2_2 = 0.2, P = 0.887$	
Education level								
No education	**1.3**	(0.8–2.2)	**0.8**	(0.6–1.2)	**5.6***	(2.2–14.4)	**1.2**	(0.6–2.6)
Some primary	**1.8***	(1.3–2.4)	**1.1**	(0.9–1.3)	**3.0***	(2.1–4.3)	**1.7***	(1.1–2.8)
Finished primary	**1.5***	(1.2–2.0)	**1.2**	(1.0–1.4)	**2.0***	(1.4–2.8)	**1.1**	(0.7–1.8)
Some secondary	**1.4***	(1.1–1.7)	**1.2***	(1.1–1.3)	**1.6***	(1.3–2.0)	**1.0**	(0.8–1.4)
Finished secondary	**1.0**	(0.8–1.2)	**1.1**	(1.0–1.2)	**1.3***	(1.1–1.6)	**0.8**	(0.6–1.0)
Some college	**1.0**	(0.8–1.2)	**1.1**	(1.0–1.2)	**1.3***	(1.0–1.6)	**0.8**	(0.6–1.0)
Finished college	**1.0**		**1.0**		**1.0**		**1.0**	
Education level difference[d]	$\chi^2_6 = 33.6^*, P < 0.001$		$\chi^2_6 = 16.2^*, P = 0.013$		$\chi^2_6 = 54.1^*, P < 0.001$		$\chi^2_6 = 14.8^*, P = 0.022$	
Household income								
Low	**1.4***	(1.2–1.7)	**1.1***	(1.0–1.2)	**1.6***	(1.3–1.9)	**1.4***	(1.0–1.8)
Low-average	**1.3***	(1.0–1.5)	**1.0**	(0.9–1.1)	**1.4***	(1.1–1.7)	**1.3**	(1.0–1.7)
High-average	**1.1**	(0.9–1.3)	**1.0**	(0.9–1.1)	**1.1**	(0.9–1.4)	**1.1**	(0.9–1.4)
High	**1.0**		**1.0**		**1.0**		**1.0**	
Household income difference[d]	$\chi^2_3 = 19.4^*, P < 0.001$		$\chi^2_3 = 10.5^*, P = 0.015$		$\chi^2_3 = 23.1^*, P < 0.001$		$\chi^2_3 = 6.9, P = 0.077$	
N[e]	**142,405**		**6,081,561**		**5,758**		**3,460**	

*Significant at the 0.05 level, two-sided test.

[a]These estimates are based on logistic regression models adjusted for age, gender, and country.

[b]These estimates are based on survival models adjusted for age-cohorts, gender, person-years, and country.

[c]These estimates are based on logistic regression models adjusted for time since SAD onset, age of SAD onset, gender, and country.

[d]Chi-square test of significant differences between blocks of socio-demographic variables.

[e]Denominator N: 142,405 = total sample; 6,081,561 = number of person-years in the survival models; 5,758 = number of lifetime SAD cases; 3,460 = number of 12-month SAD cases.

female gender but not with earlier age-of-onset or marital status. SAD persistence is particularly highly associated with lower education (with no education having an OR of 5.6), while episode persistence is particularly associated with being a student (OR of 2.1), and both indicators of persistence are associated with being a homemaker. Similar patterns are seen when the data are separately examined in low/lower-middle-, upper-middle-, and high-income countries, although associations less commonly reach significance in the first group of countries and most commonly reach significance in the last group of countries (where the associations of 30-day and lifetime SAD with younger AOO, female gender, not being employed, being unmarried, lower educational status, and lower household income are particularly apparent) (Appendix Tables 9A.1–9A.3).

Comorbidity

Respondents with either lifetime or 12-month SAD are most likely to meet lifetime criteria for other anxiety disorders (59.8% and 64.9%), less likely to meet lifetime criteria for mood and substance-use disorders, and least likely to meet lifetime criteria for disruptive behaviour/impulse-control disorders (19.3% and 21.9%) (Table 9.5); in both cases around 80% of such respondents meet lifetime criteria for any other mental disorder. Similarly, respondents with 12-month SAD are most likely to meet 12-month criteria for other anxiety disorders (52.7%), less likely to meet 12-month criteria for mood and disruptive behaviour/impulse-control disorders, and least likely to meet 12 month criteria for substance-use disorders (10.2%); with 66.9% of such respondents meeting 12-month criteria for any other disorder. In both lifetime and 12-month SAD, SAD begins earlier in only 31.4% to 35.4% of cases of comorbid anxiety disorder, but SAD begins earlier in 48.8% to 80.9% of cases of comorbid mood disorder, substance-use disorder, or disruptive behaviour/impulse-control disorder.

Treatment

Among those with 12-month SAD, the percentage reporting treatment of any kind (i.e., specialty mental health, general medical care, health care, human services, complementary, and alternative medicine, non-health care) in the past 12 months differs significantly by impairment, with 38% receiving any treatment (Appendix Table 9A.4). Across all countries, any treatment is lowest in those with moderate impairment (27.4%), and highest in those with severe impairment (46.9%). This pattern holds true for specialty mental health, general medical care, and health care, but human services, complementary and alternative medicine, and non-health care are most commonly used by those with mild impairment. Treatment rates for those with any impairment are lowest in low/lower-income countries (18.0%), and highest in high-income countries (44.2%). This pattern holds true for patients with any impairment across all treatment sectors, and for almost all treatment sectors across different levels of impairment.

Discussion

It is important to emphasize a number of limitations related to the data from the WMH surveys, including the data on SAD. Arguably, a particularly important limitation is that probes for SAD were not modified to address possible cross-cultural differences in the expression and experience of social anxiety (Stein & Matsunaga; 2001; Hofmann *et al.* 2010). It is notable that DSM-5 now includes an emphasis on 'negative evaluation', which is a somewhat broader construct than the DSM-IV operationalization, and which may include 'fear of offending' which is thought to be part of the phenomenology of SAD in several parts of the world (Stein 2009; Lewis-Fernandez *et al.* 2010). However, in countries where blinded clinical reappraisal interviews with subsamples of WMH respondents were undertaken, there was no evidence for systematic bias in the diagnostic threshold for SAD (Haro *et al.* 2006). Still, the possibility that a more valid assessment of the construct of SAD would have altered prevalence rates in some regions where the phenomenology of SAD may differ in subtle but important ways from that ordinarily seen in Western contexts cannot be ruled out.

Other pertinent limitations of WMH surveys data include those related to sampling. While response rates do not appear to be related to SAD prevalence, it is possible that in some settings, particularly those where treatment is unavailable, those with the most severe SAD symptoms were unable to participate in the WMH surveys. Some surveys only included metropolitan areas, whereas others involved national samples, and such differences may also have affected estimates of cross-national variation in prevalence. The surveys did not include a number of different segments of society, including institutionalized patients, people in jails and prisons, people in the military, people who were too intoxicated to be interviewed, or people with severe cognitive or physical disabilities. In addition,

Table 9.5 Comorbidity of social anxiety disorder (SAD) with other DSM-IV disorders, all countries combined

	SAD cases with comorbid disorders									
	Mood disorder[a]		Anxiety disorder[b]		Disruptive behaviour/impulse-control disorder[c]		Substance-use disorder[d]		Any mental disorder[e]	
	%	SE	%	SE	%	SE	%	SE	%	SE
Lifetime comorbidity[f]										
Lifetime	**47.0**	1.0	**59.8**	1.0	**19.3**	0.8	**26.7**	0.8	**78.8**	0.8
12-month	**49.8**	1.2	**64.9**	1.2	**21.9**	1.1	**27.0**	1.0	**81.8**	1.0
12-month comorbidity[g]										
12-month	**33.4**	1.1	**52.7**	1.2	**12.7**	0.9	**10.2**	0.7	**66.9**	1.2
Temporal priority of SAD[h]										
Lifetime	**71.8**	1.1	**35.4**	1.2	**49.8**	2.3	**80.9**	1.3	**40.4**	1.1
12-month	**69.1**	1.5	**31.4**	1.4	**48.8**	2.3	**79.7**	1.6	**35.2**	1.2

[a]Respondents with major depressive episode or bipolar spectrum.
[b]Respondents with panic disorder, generalized anxiety disorder, specific phobia, agoraphobia, posttraumatic stress disorder, or separation anxiety disorder.
[c]Respondents with intermittent explosive disorder, conduct disorder, attention-deficit disorder, oppositional defiant disorder, binge-eating disorder, or bulimia nervosa.
[d]Respondents with alcohol abuse with or without dependence or drug abuse with or without dependence.
[e]Respondents with any disorder listed above.
[f]Percentage of respondents with either lifetime or 12-month SAD who also meet lifetime criteria for at least one of the other DSM-IV disorders.
[g]Percentage of respondents with 12-month SAD who also meet 12-month criteria for at least one of the other disorders.
[h]Percentage of respondents with either lifetime or 12-month SAD and at least one of the other disorders, whose age-of-onset of SAD is reported to be younger than the age-of-onset of all comorbid disorders under consideration.

the samples also reflect survivor bias; this may be pertinent to interpreting differences between high-income and low/lower-middle-income countries, as there is gap in life expectancy of 10 to 15 years across these contexts (Bromet *et al.* 2011). Taken together, therefore, the rates reported here arguably provide conservative estimates of SAD prevalence.

That said, the data presented here provide the most comprehensive picture of the epidemiology of SAD to date. Cross-national differences in SAD prevalence have been noted in the literature, and the current data extend this work by rigorously exploring role impairment. Proportions of SAD respondents with any severe role impairment do not significantly differ by country income and geographic groupings, suggesting that differences in prevalence are not simply due to regional differences in diagnostic thresholding. In higher-income countries and in particular regions of the globe such as the Americas, Western Pacific, and Western Europe there is a higher prevalence of SAD, and SAD is associated with more impairment in the social domain than in other domains, suggesting high demands for social performance in such contexts. Persistence of SAD is highest in upper-middle-income countries, the African and Eastern Mediterranean regions (with non-statistically significant elevations of the proportion with severe role impairment in these countries and regions also), perhaps pointing to growing performance demands in these regions, but with fewer treatment resources than in higher-income countries.

WMH data on the epidemiology of SAD demonstrate a number of uniform patterns across the globe. For example, the socio-demographic correlates of SAD are remarkably similar by country income level and geographic region. SAD is associated with specific socio-demographic features (younger age, female gender, unmarried status, lower education, and lower income), with similar patterns of comorbidity (typically beginning later than specific phobia, but earlier than other anxiety disorders, mood, substance-use, or disruptive behaviour/impulse-control disorders), with a persistent course, with impairment in different areas of functioning, and with common patterns of health care utilization. Taken together, these findings are important in emphasizing the public health significance of a condition that continues to be somewhat neglected, three decades after Liebowitz and colleagues advocated for better recognition and intervention (Nagata *et al.* 2015). Causal mechanisms underlying these associations deserve further investigation: they may reflect psychobiological mechanisms underpinning anxiety (e.g., contributing to increased social anxiety after the onset of adolescence), and they may reflect the consequences of anxiety (e.g., social anxiety may lead to reduced academic and occupational performance, particularly in the context of high-income economies).

Perhaps the very universality of social anxiety as an experience that all individuals are familiar with has contributed to some of the controversy about its diagnosis as a mental disorder (Stein and Stein 2008). Data from the WMH surveys have, however, emphasized that social fears fall on a spectrum (from minimal to extreme), and that above a particular threshold, such fears begin to be associated with significant impairment (Stein *et al.* 2010). In deciding whether or not an individual with such fears suffers from a mental disorder, it is clearly relevant to note the growing database of research on the effectiveness and cost-efficiency of pharmacotherapies and psychotherapies for anxiety symptoms, as well as the growing voice of consumer advocates who assert the rights of individuals with anxiety disorder to treatment. The data in this chapter are important in demonstrating the extent to which SAD is associated with disability, but remains underdiagnosed and under-treated, particularly in less well-resourced contexts. Given our growing understanding that SAD often precedes other psychiatric disorders, and given the availability of effective treatments for this condition, there is a clear need to increase awareness of SAD as an important public health concern across the globe.

Acknowledgements

This chapter is based on: Stein D. J., Lim C. C. W., Roest A. M., de Jonge P., Aguilar-Gaxiola S., Al-Hamzawi A., Alonso J., Benjet C., Bromet E. J., Bruffaerts R., de Girolamo G., Florescu S., Gureje O., Maria Haro J., Harris M. G., He Y., Hinkov H., Horiguchi I., Hu C., Karam A., Karam E. G., Lee S., Lepine J.-P., Navarro-Mateu F., Pennell B. E., Piazza M., Posada-Villa J., ten Have M., Torres Y., Viana M. C., Wojtyniak B., Xavier M., Kessler R. C., Scott K. M. (2017). The cross-national epidemiology of social anxiety disorder: data from the World Mental Health Survey Initiative, *BMC Medicine*, 15, 143, used with permission from BioMed Central.

References

Bogels, S. M., Alden, L., Beidel, D. C., *et al.* (2010). Social anxiety disorder: questions and answers for the DSM-V. *Depression and Anxiety*, 27, 168–89.

Bromet, E., Andrade, L. H., Hwang, I., *et al.* (2011). Cross-national epidemiology of DSM-IV major depressive episode. *Biomedical Central Medicine*, 9, 90.

Buckner, J. D., Heimberg, R. G., Schneier, F., *et al.* (2012). The relationship between cannabis use disorders and social anxiety disorder in the National Epidemiological Study of Alcohol and Related Conditions (NESARC). *Drug and Alcohol Dependence*, 124, 128–34.

Fehm, L., Pelissolo, A., Furmark, T. *et al.* (2005). Size and burden of social phobia in Europe. *European Neuropsychopharmacology*, 15, 453–62.

Greenberg, P. E., Sisitsky, T., Kessler, R. C., *et al.* (1999). The economic burden of anxiety disorders in the 1990s. *Journal of Clinical Psychiatry*, 60, 427–35.

Haro, J. M., Arbabzadeh-Bouchez, S., Brugha, T. S., *et al.* (2006). Concordance of the Composite International Diagnostic Interview Version 3.0 (CIDI 3.0) with standardized clinical assessments in the WHO World Mental Health surveys. *International Journal of Methods in Psychiatric Research*, 15, 167–80.

Henrich, J., Heine, S. J. & Norenzayan, A. (2010). Most people are not WEIRD. *Nature*, 466, 29.

Hofmann, S. G., Anu Asnaani, M. A. & Hinton, D. E. (2010). Cultural aspects in social anxiety and social anxiety disorder. *Depression and Anxiety*, 27, 1117–27.

Kessler, R. C. (2003). The impairments caused by social phobia in the general population: implications for intervention. *Acta Psychiatrica Scandinavica Supplementum*, 19–27.

Kessler, R. C., Ruscio, A. M., Shear, K., *et al.* (2010). Epidemiology of anxiety disorders. *Current Topics of Behavioral Neurosciences*, 2, 21–35.

Kessler, R. C. & Üstün, T. B. (2004). The World Mental Health (WMH) Survey Initiative Version of the World Health Organization (WHO) Composite International Diagnostic Interview (CIDI). *International Journal of Methods in Psychiatric Research*, 13, 93–121.

Lewis-Fernandez, R., Hinton, D. E., Laria, A. J., *et al.* (2010). Culture and the anxiety disorders: recommendations for DSM-V. *Depression and Anxiety*, 27, 212–29.

Liebowitz, M. R., Gorman, J. M., Fyer, A. J., *et al.* (1985). Social phobia. Review of a neglected anxiety disorder. *Archives of General Psychiatry*, 42, 729–36.

Magee, W. J., Eaton, W. W., Wittchen, H. U., *et al.* (1996). Agoraphobia, simple phobia, and social phobia in the National Comorbidity Survey. *Archives of General Psychiatry*, 53, 159–68.

Marks, I. M. (1970). The classification of phobic disorders. *British Journal of Psychiatry*, 116, 377–86.

Myers, J. K., Weissman, M. M., Tischler, G. L., *et al.* (1984). Six-month prevalence of psychiatric disorders in three communities 1980 to 1982. *Archives of General Psychiatry*, 41, 959–67.

Nagata, T., Suzuki, F. & Teo, A. R. (2015). Generalized social anxiety disorder: A still-neglected anxiety disorder 3 decades since Liebowitz's review. *Psychiatry and Clinical Neuroscience*, 69, 724–40.

Ruscio, A. M., Brown, T. A., Chiu, W. T., *et al.* (2008). Social fears and social phobia in the USA: results from the National Comorbidity Survey Replication. *Psychological Medicine*, 38, 15–28.

Somers, J. M., Goldner, E. M., Waraich, P. *et al.* (2006). Prevalence and incidence studies of anxiety disorders: a systematic review of the literature. *Canadian Journal of Psychiatry*, 51, 100–13.

Steel, Z., Marnane, C., Iranpour, C., *et al.* (2014). The global prevalence of common mental disorders: a systematic review and meta-analysis 1980–2013. *International Journal of Epidemiology*, 43, 476–93.

Stein, D. J. (2009). Social anxiety disorder in the West and in the East. *Annals of Clinical Psychiatry*, 21, 109–17.

Stein, D. J. & Matsunaga, H. (2001). Cross-cultural aspects of social anxiety disorder. *Psychiatric Clinics of North America*, 24, 773–82.

Stein, D. J., Ruscio, A. M., Lee, S., *et al.* (2010). Subtyping social anxiety disorder in developed and developing countries. *Depression and Anxiety*, 27, 390–403.

Stein, M. B. & Stein, D. J. (2008). Social anxiety disorder. *Lancet*, 371, 1115–25.

Weissman, M. M., Bland, R. C., Canino, G. J., *et al.* (1996). The cross-national epidemiology of social phobia: a preliminary report. *International Clinical Psychopharmacology*, 11 (Suppl 3), 9–14.

Chapter 10

Specific Phobia

Klaas J. Wardenaar, Corina Benjet, Maria Carmen Viana, Peter de Jonge

Introduction

DSM-defined specific phobia is characterized by the presence of a significant level of anxiety provoked by exposure to a specific object or situation, which often leads to avoidance behaviour. In DSM-IV, several diagnostic criteria are used. The first criterion is that an individual has a persistent and marked fear that is provoked by the presence or anticipation of a discernable object or situation. Second, the exposure to the phobic stimulus should almost always lead to an immediate anxiety response in the affected individual. Third, adults older than 18 years should recognize that their fear or anxiety is excessive and/or unreasonable given the actual danger posed by the specific stimulus. Fourth, the exposure to the phobic stimulus is avoided or only endured by the affected individual with intense anxiety or distress. Fifth, the avoidance and fear of the phobic stimulus should lead to marked distress and/or should interfere with an individual's normal routines, occupational functioning, social life and/or relationships. Sixth, the duration of specific phobia should be at least six months in persons under 18. Finally, the avoidance and fear should not be better accounted for by another mental disorder. With the move from the DSM-IV to DSM-5, most diagnostic features have remained the same, but people are no longer required to recognize that their fear is excessive or unreasonable and the duration requirement of six months applies to all ages in DSM-5. Based on the nature of the feared object, DSM-IV/-5 specifies the following subtypes: animal (e.g. snakes, dogs, spiders), natural environment (e.g. weather, heights, water), blood-injection-injury, situational (e.g. enclosed spaces, flying in an airplane), and other (e.g. vomiting, choking).

Prior research has found that the onset of specific phobia is usually in childhood or early adolescence (Kessler *et al.* 2005; Stinson *et al.* 2007), although the age-of-onset (AOO) can vary across subtypes (Becker *et al.* 2007). Epidemiological surveys have shown that specific phobia is common, with reported prevalence rates of 9.4% (lifetime) and 7.1% (12-month) in the National Epidemiologic Survey on Alcohol and Related Conditions (NESARC; Stinson *et al.* 2007), 10.1% (lifetime), and 7.1% (12-month) in the Netherlands Mental Health Survey and Incidence Initiative (NEMESIS; Bijl *et al.* 1998), and 11.3% (lifetime), and 8.8% (12-month) in the National Comorbidity Study (NCS; Kessler *et al.* 1994; Magee *et al.* 1996). In prospective research, specific phobia has been shown to have a high incidence rate, with studies showing a cumulative incidence of 26.9% between ages 20 and 50 (Angst *et al.* 2016), a one-year incidence rate of 0.44 new cases per 100 person years (Grant *et al.* 2009), and an incidence rate of 2.20 new cases per 100 person years (Bijl *et al.* 2002). Almost all studies have found that the prevalence and incidence rates of specific phobia are higher in females than in males (Kessler *et al.* 1994; Bijl *et al.* 1998, 2002; Stinson *et al.*, 2007; Angst *et al.* 2016). In addition, several studies have shown that specific phobia prevalence decreases with increasing age (e.g. Stinson *et al.* 2007; Sigström *et al.* 2016), although research also indicates that when they persist into adulthood, most untreated specific phobias tend to become chronic (e.g. Goisman *et al.* 1998; Sigström *et al.* 2011).

Because of its high prevalence, persistence, and high rates of comorbidity with other disorders, specific phobia is of considerable interest to psychopathology researchers and clinicians. A range of studies have shown specific phobia to be associated with considerable impairment. Magee *et al.* (1996) showed that 34.2% of specific phobia patients reported role impairments in their daily life, which was comparable to the impairment reported in social phobia (33.5%) but higher than for agoraphobia (26.5%). Depla *et al.* (2008) showed that, depending on the specific phobia subtype, a considerable percentage of patients reported serious interference in their daily life (up to 59.2%) and work/social situations (up to 43.8%). In addition, Stinson *et al.* (2007) showed that impairment levels in specific phobia were comparable with those observed in substance-use disorders and other anxiety disorders. It has been suggested that the observed impairment in specific phobia could be partly explained by its frequent co-occurrence with other mental disorders (Comer *et al.* 2011) and there are also studies that found specific phobia to be associated with lower impairment than other disorders (Wells *et al.* 2006; Ormel *et al.* 2008). However, even if comorbid disorders explain part of the reported impairment, the specific symptoms of specific phobia can by themselves also lead to a restricted lifestyle that interferes with patients' professional functioning, social lives, and physical health. For instance, a fear of flying can seriously restrict an individual's mobility and a blood-injection-injury fear could lead patients to avoid necessary medical or dental treatment.

Previous surveys have shown that specific phobia often co-occurs with other mental disorders. Magee *et al.* (1996) showed that 83.4% of lifetime specific phobia cases reported another mental disorder, with the highest comorbidity rates with anxiety disorders (68.7%) and affective disorders (46.8%). In line with this, Stinson *et al.* (2007) showed that 12-month specific phobia was associated with increased odds of the presence of other mental disorders. The strongest association was observed between specific phobia and other anxiety disorders, followed by the presence of mood disorders and substance-use disorders. For lifetime diagnoses, they found similar patterns of comorbidity. An important observation with regard to comorbidity in specific phobia patients is that the specific phobia preceded the other disorder(s) in the majority of cases (e.g. Magee *et al.* 1996; Kessler *et al.* 1997). These cross-sectional findings align with the known early AOO of specific phobia and have led researchers to view specific phobia as a potential early vulnerability marker for later mental problems. Prospective work has been done that provides more insight into the development of comorbid disorders in individuals with specific phobia. Several studies have indeed shown specific phobia to be associated with increased odds of later depressive disorders, anxiety disorders, and eating disorders (Goodwin 2002; Bittner *et al.* 2004; Trumpf *et al.* 2010; Lieb *et al.* 2016). However, one study found specific phobia not to be associated with increased odds of later substance-use disorders (Zimmermann *et al.* 2003). In another prospective study, specific phobia at baseline was shown to be associated with an increased incidence of other anxiety disorders during follow-up, although these associations could also be explained by the presence of other disorders at baseline and/or several socio-demographic factors (Grant *et al.* 2009).

Relatively effective psychological interventions are available for the treatment of specific phobia, such as behaviour therapy and cognitive therapy (Choy *et al.* 2007). However, despite the fact that many specific phobia patients have a clear need for care, only a minority of patients actually seek treatment. The observed treatment rates among specific phobia patients have been varied. One study reported that 8.0% of specific phobia cases received treatment specifically for the disorder (Stinson *et al.* 2007). Another study found that, depending on the phobia subtype, 26.8% to 57.0% of specific phobia patients sought professional help and 13.0% to 36.2% used medication (Depla *et al.* 2008). Finally, Magee *et al.* (1996) found that 30.2% of all specific phobia cases sought help and 8.0% used medication. Other studies have shown that individuals who do seek treatment for specific phobia take a long time to do so compared to other anxiety disorders, such as panic disorder, agoraphobia, and generalized anxiety disorder (Iza *et al.* 2013; ten Have *et al.* 2013).

As described above, there are different specific phobia subtypes. These subtypes have previously been shown to differ in terms of their prevalence, (Fredrikson *et al.* 1996; Becker *et al.* 2007; Depla *et al.* 2008; LeBeau *et al.* 2010), their associated impairment levels, their rates of comorbidity with other mental disorders (Depla *et al.* 2008; LeBeau *et al.* 2010), and their associated treatment use (Depla *et al.* 2008). Most specific phobia patients have more than one subtype (Curtis *et al.* 1998; Stinson *et al.* 2007; Depla *et al.* 2008; Burstein *et al.* 2012). In specific phobia patients, increasing numbers of subtypes have been shown to be associated with higher rates of comorbidity with other disorders, higher levels of impairment, and more treatment seeking (e.g. Curtis *et al.* 1998; Stinson *et al.* 2007; Burstein *et al.* 2012).

The above literature suggests that, although often overlooked, specific phobia deserves the attention of both researchers and clinicians. Compared to other mental disorders, epidemiological research on specific phobia has been rather limited and mostly based on surveys in Western, high-income countries. Therefore, this chapter aims to provide a more comprehensive overview of the cross-national epidemiology of specific phobia based on the World Mental Health (WMH) surveys.

Methods

As described in Chapter 3, specific phobia and other DSM-IV disorders were assessed with the World Health Organization Composite International Diagnostic Interview (CIDI 3.0; Kessler & Üstün 2004); specific phobia was assessed in 25 of the 29 surveys included in this volume (see Table 10.1). The WMH-CIDI has been shown to have adequate concordance with the Structured Clinical Interview for DSM-IV (SCID) for specific phobia (Haro *et al.* 2006).

In the specific phobia section, respondents were shown six groups of fears (animals, still water/weather events, blood/injuries/medical experiences, closed spaces, high places, flying) and asked if they had ever had a strong fear of any of these things. If participants reported one or more fears in this screening part, the interviewer administered the full specific phobia section.

Analyses were conducted to investigate the overall epidemiology of specific phobia. In addition, because previous work has shown the importance of looking at the type and number of reported fears, analyses were conducted to investigate the prevalence and characteristics of (1) lifetime fear subtypes and (2) numbers of lifetime phobia subtypes (one, two, three, four, or more).

Results

Prevalence and Persistence

The lifetime prevalence of specific phobia differs significantly across countries, ranging from 2.6% to 12.5% (Table 10.1), with a cross-national prevalence of 7.4%. The cross-national lifetime prevalence rates for males and females are 4.9% and 9.8%, respectively. The 12-month prevalence of specific phobia ranges from 1.7% to 10.6% across countries, with an overall cross-national prevalence of 5.5%. The 12-month prevalence rates for males and females are 3.3% and 7.7%, respectively. Both the lifetime and 12-month prevalence rates differ significantly across country income groups, with the low/lower-middle-income countries showing lower prevalence rates (lifetime: 5.7%; 12-month: 4.0%) than the upper-middle- (lifetime: 8.0%; 12-month: 6.4%) and high-income countries (lifetime: 8.1%; 12-month: 5.9%). The lifetime and 12-month prevalence rates also differ across regions in the world, with the highest prevalence in the region of the Americas (lifetime: 10.5%; 12-month: 8.0%), followed by the Western European region (lifetime: 7.7%; 12-month: 5.8%) and the Western Pacific region (lifetime: 6.7%; 12-month: 4.5%). The lowest prevalence rates are observed in the Eastern European region (lifetime: 4.2%; 12-month: 3.0%).

The lifetime prevalence rates of different fear subtypes are presented in Table 10.2. Animal fear is the most common subtype with a lifetime cross-national prevalence of 3.8%. Fear of blood, injections, and medical experiences is the next most common subtype with a cross-national prevalence of 3.0% and a median prevalence across countries of 2.4%. Fears of the natural environment show slightly lower lifetime prevalence rates with fear of high places having a cross-national prevalence of 2.8% and fear of still water or weather events having a cross-national prevalence of 2.3%. Fear of closed spaces shows a cross-national prevalence of 2.2% and fear of flying has the lowest cross-national prevalence (1.3%). All fear subtypes have a higher lifetime prevalence among females (1.8–5.4% across subtypes) than males (0.8–2.2% across subtypes). The subtype prevalence rates also differ across country income groups, with the lowest rates in the low/lower-middle-income countries (0.6–3.4% across subtypes) and higher rates in the upper-middle- (1.2–4.4%) and high-income countries (1.7–3.7%). The difference between country income groups is most pronounced for the fear of flying subtype, which shows a prevalence of 0.6% in the low/lower-middle-income countries and a more than two fold higher prevalence in the high-income countries (1.7%). Of the cross-national sample, 3.4% report having a single fear subtype, but the majority report more than one subtype, with 1.8% reporting two subtypes, 1.1% reporting three subtypes and 1.1% reporting four or more subtypes.

Persistence of specific phobia, as represented by the 12-month prevalence among lifetime specific phobia cases (see Table 10.1), is observed in 74.2% of the complete sample. Symptom (episode) persistence, as represented by 30-day prevalence among 12-month cases, is observed in 70.2% of the sample. Both disorder and symptom persistence are more common in females (disorder persistence: 78.2%; symptom persistence: 72.4%) than in males (disorder persistence: 65.8%; symptom persistence: 64.7%) and also differ across country income groups, with disorder persistence and symptom persistence being most common in the upper-middle-income countries (disorder persistence: 80.6%; symptom persistence: 75.1%) and least common in the low/lower-middle-income countries (disorder persistence: 70.6%; symptom persistence: 58.7%). Comparison of regions of the world shows that

Table 10.1 Prevalence of DSM-IV specific phobia (SP) in the World Mental Health surveys

Country	Lifetime prevalence		12-month prevalence		30-day prevalence		12-month prevalence of SP among lifetime cases		30-day prevalence of SP among 12-month cases		Part 1 sample sizes
	%	SE	%	SE	%	SE	%	SE	%	SE	
Low/lower-middle-income countries	**5.7**	**0.2**	**4.0**	**0.2**	**2.4**	**0.1**	**70.6**	**1.6**	**58.7**	**1.8**	**31,773**
Colombia	12.5	0.8	8.9	0.8	5.7	0.5	71.5	2.6	64.2	3.2	4,426
Iraq	4.2	0.4	3.8	0.4	3.2	0.4	90.4	3.5	82.4	4.2	4,332
Nigeria	5.9	0.5	4.4	0.3	2.2	0.2	74.5	3.2	49.6	3.8	6,752
Peru	6.6	0.4	4.6	0.3	2.5	0.2	69.7	4.8	54.4	3.6	3,930
PRC (Beijing/Shanghai)	2.6	0.3	1.7	0.3	1.0	0.2	63.2	3.6	56.9	8.0	5,201
PRC (Shenzhen)	4.0	0.3	2.2	0.3	0.9	0.1	54.9	5.4	42.6	4.1	7,132
Upper-middle-income countries	**8.0**	**0.2**	**6.4**	**0.2**	**4.8**	**0.2**	**80.6**	**1.1**	**75.1**	**1.5**	**24,612**
Brazil	12.5	0.6	10.6	0.5	8.8	0.5	85.2	1.6	82.9	2.6	5,037
Bulgaria	5.8	0.3	3.9	0.3	3.1	0.3	68.1	3.3	78.3	2.9	5,318
Colombia (Medellin)	10.2	0.8	8.3	0.7	6.4	0.6	81.7	3.1	76.9	3.0	3,261
Lebanon	7.1	0.6	6.6	0.5	5.0	0.5	93.0	1.7	75.9	3.8	2,857
Mexico	7.0	0.5	5.2	0.4	2.8	0.2	74.3	2.6	54.3	3.9	5,782
Romania	3.8	0.5	3.3	0.5	2.8	0.5	86.1	4.9	84.3	5.2	2,357
High-income countries	**8.1**	**0.1**	**5.9**	**0.1**	**4.2**	**0.1**	**73.2**	**0.8**	**71.9**	**0.8**	**68,517**
Belgium	6.8	1.0	5.0	0.7	3.6	0.5	73.2	3.5	71.1	5.4	2,419
France	10.7	0.6	7.7	0.7	6.0	0.5	71.7	3.8	78.3	3.3	2,894
Germany	9.9	0.7	6.9	0.6	4.8	0.3	69.5	2.6	70.6	3.5	3,555
Italy	5.4	0.5	3.9	0.4	2.8	0.3	72.6	2.2	72.6	2.8	4,712
Japan	3.4	0.3	2.3	0.2	1.8	0.2	68.0	4.5	77.9	4.7	4,129
New Zealand	10.9	0.4	7.6	0.3	5.2	0.3	70.2	1.4	68.6	2.1	12,790
Northern Ireland	9.7	0.6	7.2	0.5	5.2	0.4	74.6	2.1	71.6	2.7	4,340
Poland	3.4	0.2	2.5	0.2	1.7	0.1	72.8	2.9	67.6	3.0	10,081
Portugal	10.6	0.6	8.6	0.5	7.0	0.5	81.3	1.8	81.1	2.0	3,849
Spain	4.8	0.4	3.8	0.4	2.9	0.3	80.1	3.3	74.6	3.2	5,473
Spain (Murcia)	5.4	0.5	4.7	0.4	3.7	0.3	86.9	2.5	78.4	3.5	2,621
Netherlands	7.6	0.7	5.4	0.6	4.3	0.6	70.5	3.2	79.4	3.9	2,372
United States	12.5	0.4	9.1	0.4	6.3	0.4	73.0	2.2	68.8	1.9	9,282

(cont.)

Table 10.1 *(cont.)*

Country	Lifetime prevalence		12-month prevalence		30-day prevalence		12-month prevalence of SP among lifetime cases		30-day prevalence of SP among 12-month cases		Part 1 sample sizes
	%	SE	%	SE	%	SE	%	SE	%	SE	
All countries combined	**7.4**	**0.1**	**5.5**	**0.1**	**3.9**	**0.1**	**74.2**	**0.6**	**70.2**	**0.7**	**124,902**
WHO regions[a]											
Region of the Americas	10.5	0.2	8.0	0.2	5.5	0.2	75.8	1.1	69.2	1.2	31,718
African region	5.9	0.5	4.4	0.3	2.2	0.2	74.5	3.2	49.6	3.8	6,752
Western Pacific region	6.7	0.2	4.5	0.2	2.9	0.1	67.3	1.4	65.5	1.8	29,252
Eastern Mediterranean region	5.4	0.4	4.9	0.3	3.9	0.3	91.8	1.9	78.9	2.8	7,189
Western European region	7.7	0.2	5.8	0.2	4.4	0.1	75.3	0.9	75.3	1.1	32,235
Eastern European region	4.2	0.2	3.0	0.2	2.2	0.1	72.4	2.0	74.2	2.0	17,756
Gender											
All males	4.9	0.1	3.3	0.1	2.1	0.1	65.8	1.2	64.7	1.4	56,526
All females	9.8	0.1	7.7	0.1	5.5	0.1	78.2	0.6	72.4	0.8	68,376
Comparison between countries[b]	$F_{24,v} = 47.7^*$ $P < 0.001$		$F_{24,v} = 39.4^*$ $P < 0.001$		$F_{24,v} = 39.4^*$ $P < 0.001$		$F_{24,v} = 7.8^*$ $P < 0.001$		$F_{24,v} = 7.2^*$ $P < 0.001$		
Comparison between low-, middle-, and high-income country groups[b]	$F_{2,v} = 51.1^*$ $P < 0.001$		$F_{2,v} = 56.8^*$ $P < 0.001$		$F_{2,v} = 103.8^*$ $P < 0.001$		$F_{2,v} = 19.1^*$ $P < 0.001$		$F_{2,v} = 26.4^*$ $P < 0.001$		
Comparison between WHO regions[a]	$F_{5,v} = 103.3^*$ $P < 0.001$		$F_{5,v} = 77.1^*$ $P < 0.001$		$F_{5,v} = 63.8^*$ $P < 0.001$		$F_{5,v} = 16.8^*$ $P < 0.001$		$F_{5,v} = 12.0^*$ $P < 0.001$		
Gender comparison[b]	$F_{1,v} = 722.1^*$ $P < 0.001$		$F_{1,v} = 855.3^*$ $P < 0.001$		$F_{1,v} = 735.5^*$ $P < 0.001$		$F_{1,v} = 84.2^*$ $P < 0.001$		$F_{1,v} = 23.7^*$ $P < 0.001$		

*Significant at the 0.05 level, two-sided test.

[a]**Region of the Americas** (Colombia, Mexico, Brazil, Peru, United States, Colombia (Medellin)); **African region** (Nigeria); **Western Pacific region** (PRC (Shenzhen), PRC Beijing and Shanghai, Japan, New Zealand); **Eastern Mediterranean region** (Iraq, Lebanon); **Western European region** (Belgium, France, Germany, Italy, Netherlands, Spain, Northern Ireland, Portugal, Spain (Murcia)); **Eastern European region** (Romania, Bulgaria, Poland).

[b]Wald design-corrected F-tests were used to determine if there is variation in prevalence estimates across countries and gender. The denominator degree of freedom, v, is 1377.

PRC: People's Republic of China.

Table 10.2 Lifetime prevalence of DSM-IV specific phobia subtypes and cases with different numbers of co-occurring subtypes in the World Mental Health surveys

Country	Kinds of subtypes												Numbers of subtypes								
	Animal		Still water, weather events		Blood, injuries, medical experiences		Closed spaces		High places		Flying		1 subtype		2 subtypes		3 subtypes		≥4 subtypes		Part 1 sample sizes
	%	SE	%	SE	%	SE	%	SE	%	SE	%	SE	%	SE	%	SE	%	SE	%	SE	
Low/lower-middle-income	**3.4**	**0.1**	**2.1**	**0.1**	**2.2**	**0.1**	**1.6**	**0.1**	**2.0**	**0.1**	**0.6**	**0.1**	**2.7**	**0.1**	**1.3**	**0.1**	**0.8**	**0.1**	**0.9**	**0.1**	**31,773**
Colombia	8.1	0.6	6.2	0.5	6.0	0.5	5.2	0.4	7.1	0.6	2.2	0.3	3.1	0.4	3.0	0.4	2.3	0.3	4.1	0.4	4,426
Iraq	2.3	0.3	1.3	0.3	1.4	0.3	0.7	0.2	0.9	0.2	0.3	0.1	2.8	0.4	0.7	0.1	0.4	0.1	0.3	0.1	4,332
Nigeria	3.7	0.3	2.2	0.3	1.6	0.2	1.4	0.3	1.0	0.1	0.4	0.1	3.4	0.3	1.4	0.2	0.6	0.1	0.5	0.1	6,752
Peru	3.6	0.3	2.0	0.2	2.6	0.2	1.4	0.2	1.7	0.2	0.6	0.2	3.7	0.4	1.4	0.2	0.9	0.1	0.6	0.1	3,930
PRC (Beijing/Shanghai)	1.4	0.2	0.4	0.1	0.9	0.2	0.4	0.1	1.0	0.2	0.2	0.1	1.5	0.3	0.7	0.2	0.3	0.1	0.1	0.1	5,201
PRC (Shenzhen)	2.1	0.2	1.0	0.2	1.8	0.2	1.0	0.2	1.3	0.2	0.4	0.1	2.1	0.2	1.0	0.1	0.4	0.1	0.4	0.1	7,132
Upper-middle-income	**4.4**	**0.2**	**2.8**	**0.1**	**3.0**	**0.2**	**2.3**	**0.1**	**3.0**	**0.1**	**1.2**	**0.1**	**3.6**	**0.2**	**2.0**	**0.1**	**1.0**	**0.1**	**1.3**	**0.1**	**24,612**
Brazil	7.0	0.4	3.7	0.3	4.4	0.5	3.4	0.3	4.8	0.4	1.8	0.2	5.9	0.3	3.1	0.3	1.7	0.2	1.8	0.2	5,037
Bulgaria	3.0	0.3	2.2	0.3	2.4	0.2	1.0	0.1	1.7	0.2	0.4	0.1	2.6	0.3	2.0	0.2	0.6	0.1	0.6	0.1	5,318
Colombia (Medellin)	6.5	0.6	4.4	0.5	4.5	0.5	4.6	0.5	5.7	0.6	2.5	0.3	2.9	0.4	2.1	0.4	1.8	0.3	3.3	0.4	3,261
Lebanon	2.8	0.2	2.9	0.4	2.1	0.4	1.1	0.3	1.0	0.2	0.5	0.1	4.9	0.5	1.5	0.2	0.5	0.2	0.2	0.0	2,857
Mexico	4.0	0.3	2.2	0.3	2.4	0.3	2.1	0.3	2.7	0.3	1.1	0.2	3.4	0.4	1.7	0.2	0.9	0.1	1.1	0.2	5,782
Romania	1.7	0.4	2.0	0.4	2.0	0.4	1.1	0.3	1.8	0.3	0.4	0.2	1.3	0.3	1.2	0.2	0.6	0.2	0.7	0.2	2,357
High-income	**3.7**	**0.1**	**2.2**	**0.1**	**3.4**	**0.1**	**2.4**	**0.1**	**3.1**	**0.1**	**1.7**	**0.1**	**3.7**	**0.1**	**2.0**	**0.1**	**1.3**	**0.1**	**1.1**	**0.1**	**68,517**
Belgium	2.5	0.5	1.7	0.4	2.2	0.4	1.3	0.5	2.3	0.6	0.8	0.2	4.4	0.6	1.3	0.3	0.9	0.3	0.3	0.2	2,419
France	3.8	0.4	2.8	0.3	3.9	0.4	2.7	0.4	3.6	0.4	1.3	0.3	6.2	0.5	2.3	0.4	1.4	0.2	0.8	0.2	2,894
Germany	3.5	0.4	1.7	0.4	3.9	0.4	2.0	0.3	2.5	0.2	1.7	0.2	6.0	0.5	2.7	0.3	0.9	0.2	0.3	0.1	3,555
Italy	2.0	0.2	1.3	0.2	2.2	0.3	1.5	0.2	1.4	0.2	1.0	0.2	3.0	0.3	1.3	0.2	0.7	0.2	0.4	0.1	4,712
Japan	2.0	0.2	1.5	0.2	1.4	0.2	1.1	0.2	1.2	0.2	0.7	0.1	1.3	0.2	0.9	0.1	0.5	0.1	0.7	0.2	4,129
New Zealand	5.0	0.3	2.2	0.2	4.7	0.2	3.4	0.2	4.7	0.2	2.2	0.2	4.7	0.2	3.0	0.2	2.0	0.2	1.2	0.1	12,790
Northern Ireland	4.6	0.4	3.9	0.4	4.8	0.4	3.5	0.4	4.6	0.4	2.3	0.3	3.3	0.4	2.3	0.2	1.7	0.2	2.4	0.3	4,340
Poland	1.5	0.1	0.9	0.1	1.3	0.1	0.8	0.1	1.4	0.1	0.6	0.1	1.7	0.1	0.8	0.1	0.5	0.1	0.4	0.1	10,081
Portugal	6.1	0.5	4.1	0.4	4.6	0.4	3.6	0.3	4.3	0.3	1.9	0.2	3.8	0.4	2.8	0.3	1.9	0.2	2.2	0.3	3,849
Spain	2.1	0.2	1.1	0.2	1.4	0.2	1.3	0.2	1.1	0.2	0.7	0.1	3.0	0.4	1.0	0.2	0.4	0.1	0.3	0.1	5,473
Spain (Murcia)	2.6	0.3	0.9	0.2	0.7	0.2	1.7	0.4	1.5	0.3	0.7	0.2	3.5	0.3	1.1	0.3	0.6	0.2	0.1	0.1	2,621
Netherlands	2.4	0.4	1.5	0.3	2.9	0.5	1.4	0.3	1.7	0.3	1.0	0.3	5.4	0.6	1.4	0.3	0.7	0.2	0.1	0.1	2,372
United States	6.6	0.3	4.3	0.2	6.0	0.3	4.4	0.2	5.9	0.3	3.8	0.2	4.1	0.3	3.1	0.2	2.3	0.2	2.9	0.2	9,282
All countries combined	**3.8**	**0.1**	**2.3**	**0.1**	**3.0**	**0.1**	**2.2**	**0.1**	**2.8**	**0.1**	**1.3**	**0.0**	**3.4**	**0.1**	**1.8**	**0.0**	**1.1**	**0.0**	**1.1**	**0.0**	**124,902**
All males	2.0	0.1	1.3	0.1	2.2	0.1	1.2	0.1	2.0	0.1	0.8	0.0	2.5	0.1	1.2	0.1	0.6	0.0	0.6	0.0	56,526
All females	5.4	0.1	3.3	0.1	3.7	0.1	3.1	0.1	3.6	0.1	1.8	0.1	4.3	0.1	2.4	0.1	1.5	0.1	1.6	0.1	68,376
Comparison between countries[a]	$F_{24,v}=27.4^*$, $P<0.001$		$F_{24,v}=23.7^*$, $P<0.001$		$F_{24,v}=28.1^*$, $P<0.001$		$F_{24,v}=32.7^*$, $P<0.001$		$F_{24,v}=33.6^*$, $P<0.001$		$F_{24,v}=18.2^*$, $P<0.001$		$F_{24,v}=20.8^*$, $P<0.001$		$F_{24,v}=15.5^*$, $P<0.001$		$F_{24,v}=14.5^*$, $P<0.001$		$F_{24,v}=22.4^*$, $P<0.001$		
Comparison between low-, middle-, and high-income country groups[a]	$F_{2,v}=12.2^*$, $P<0.001$		$F_{2,v}=11.4^*$, $P<0.001$		$F_{2,v}=33.0^*$, $P<0.001$		$F_{2,v}=25.2^*$, $P<0.001$		$F_{2,v}=37.6^*$, $P<0.001$		$F_{2,v}=63.6^*$, $P<0.001$		$F_{2,v}=21.0^*$, $P<0.001$		$F_{2,v}=20.3^*$, $P<0.001$		$F_{2,v}=20.9^*$, $P<0.001$		$F_{2,v}=5.4^*$, $P=0.005$		
Gender comparison[a]	$F_{1,v}=658.1^*$, $P<0.001$		$F_{1,v}=420.2^*$, $P<0.001$		$F_{1,v}=153.6^*$, $P<0.001$		$F_{1,v}=333.4^*$, $P<0.001$		$F_{1,v}=187.2^*$, $P<0.001$		$F_{1,v}=190.1^*$, $P<0.001$		$F_{1,v}=188.0^*$, $P<0.001$		$F_{1,v}=203.0^*$, $P<0.001$		$F_{1,v}=167.5^*$, $P<0.001$		$F_{1,v}=191.2^*$, $P<0.001$		

*Significant at the 0.05 level, two-sided test.

[a]Wald design-corrected F-tests were used to determine if there is variation in prevalence estimates across countries and gender. The denominator degree of freedom, v, is 1377.

PRC: People's Republic of China.

disorder persistence is by far the highest in the Eastern Mediterranean region (91.8%), and ranges from 67.3% to 75.8% across the other regions, with the lowest rates in the Western Pacific region. Symptom persistence is most common in the Eastern Mediterranean region (78.9%), followed by the Western European region (75.3%), Eastern European region (74.2%) and region of the Americas (69.2%). Symptom persistence is least common in the African region (49.6%).

Age-of-Onset

Specific phobia has a young AOO (cross-national median AOO = 8 years; interquartile range (IQR) 5-13) with the median AOO showing little variation across countries (IQR 8–9 years) (data not shown). The young AOO distribution is further reflected in the observation that the cross-national projected lifetime risk at age 75 (8.1%) is only slightly higher than the observed cross-national lifetime prevalence (7.4%). Of the four possible AOO categories, early AOO is most common for fear of still water/weather (37.1%), animals (36.6%), and closed spaces (35.2%) (Table 10.4). Fear of flying and fear of high places both show a slightly older AOO distribution. Rates of early onset increase with increasing numbers of fear subtypes, from 23.1% in those with one subtype to 43.1% in cases with four or more fear subtypes. Conversely, percentages of cases with late-average and late onset decrease with increasing numbers of fear subtypes.

Comorbidity

Of all lifetime specific phobia cases, 60.5% meet criteria for another mental disorder (see Appendix Table 10A.1). Most lifetime specific phobia cases have another anxiety disorder (41.2%) or mood disorder (34.3%). Of 12-month specific phobia cases respectively 62.0% and 42.2% meet criteria for other lifetime and 12-month disorders. Most 12-month cases have a comorbid anxiety disorder (lifetime: 42.9%; 12-month: 29.6%) or mood disorder (lifetime: 35.9%; 12-month: 21.0%). Comorbidity with disruptive behaviour/impulse-control disorders (lifetime: 18.1%; 12-month: 10.1%) and substance-use disorders (lifetime: 15.6%; 12-month: 5.3%) is considerably lower. Of lifetime specific phobia cases with a comorbid diagnosis, the AOO of specific phobia precedes the other disorder's AOO in the majority of cases (72.6%). Temporally primary specific phobia is most often observed for comorbidity with substance-use disorders (92.2%) and mood disorders (89.3%), which are known to have a comparatively older AOO, but also often for comorbidity with other anxiety disorders (71.6%) and impulse-control disorders (72.5%), which are known to have a fairly young AOO distribution. Lifetime comorbidity rates with any other disorder show some variation across fear subtypes, ranging from 60.6% for animal fear to 73.0% for fear of flying (Table 10.4). Comorbidity is highest with anxiety (41.9–58.3% across subtypes) and mood disorders (34.7–43.6% across subtypes) and considerable lower with disruptive behaviour/impulse-control disorders (18.3–23.6%) and substance-use disorders (14.9–20.5%). Comorbidity rates with all disorders increase with the number of subtypes from 49.7% with any comorbid disorder in cases with a single subtype to 82.1% with any comorbid disorder in cases with four or more subtypes.

Socio-demographic Correlates of Onset and Prevalence

In the cross-national sample, the presence of current (30-day) specific phobia (Table 10.3) is associated with being younger than 60 years (OR 1.4–1.5), female gender (OR 2.7), being a homemaker (OR 1.3), having employment status 'other' (unemployed and disabled) (OR 1.6), being divorced/separated/widowed (OR 1.2), having less than a college education (OR 1.4–2.2), and having a low (OR 1.4) or low-average (OR 1.2) income. The same socio-demographic factors are associated with the first onset of specific phobia.

These socio-demographic associations with specific phobia show some variation across country income groups (data not shown). The directions of association are generally consistent across country income groups and differences are mostly observed in their magnitude or the involved categories per socio-demographic factor. Marital status only shows an association with 30-day and lifetime specific phobia in the high-income countries (ORs 1.4 and 1.3). Employment status only shows associations with 30-day specific phobia in the low/lower-middle- (OR 1.5–1.6) and high-income (ORs 1.3–2.0) countries and only the 'other' employment category is associated with lifetime specific phobia onset in all country income groups (ORs 1.3–1.5). Household income only shows associations with 30-day specific phobia in the low/lower-middle- countries (low income: OR 1.4) and high-income countries (low: OR 1.5; low-average: OR 1.2) and only with lifetime specific phobia in the high-income countries (OR 1.3). Education level shows different associations with 30-day specific phobia in the low/lower-middle-income countries (some primary: OR 1.7; finished primary: OR 1.8) and upper-middle-income countries (some primary: OR 1.8; finished primary: OR 1.4; some secondary: OR 1.5) compared with the high-income countries (less than finished college: OR 1.4–2.4). Associations between education level and lifetime specific phobia are more similar across country income groups, with most or all education levels lower than college being associated with increased odds of lifetime specific phobia.

The age-group distribution varies across subtypes (Table 10.4), with most young persons being concentrated among those with the animal fear subtype (34.1%) and with fear of blood, injections, and medical experiences (32.4%). Employment status shows limited variation across the different fear subtypes, but does show some variation across individuals with different numbers of fears: the percentage of working persons is markedly lower (53.1%) in those with four or more subtypes compared to those with one to three subtypes (57.7–60.8%). The percentage of cases with completed college shows some variation across subtypes (8.8–12.3%), but a more striking difference can be seen in the percentages of cases with completed college between those with more than four subtypes (7.6%) and those with one to three subtypes (12.1–13.8%). Household income distributions show limited variation across the different fear subtypes, but do show some variation across cases with different numbers of fear subtypes, with percentages of cases in the low- or low-mid-income categories increasing with increasing number of fear subtypes.

Socio-demographic Correlates of Persistence

In the cross-national sample, increased odds of disorder persistence (12-month/lifetime) are associated with early AOO (OR 1.4), being female (OR 1.8), being retired (OR 1.3), having 'other' employment status (OR 1.5), having less than a completed college education (OR 1.3–1.7), and having a low household income (OR 1.4) (Table 10.3). The odds of symptom persistence (30-day/12-month) are negatively associated with having a late-average AOO (OR 0.8) and are positively associated with being female (OR 1.3), being a homemaker (OR 1.3), having 'other' employment status (OR 1.3), having no education (OR 1.7), having only primary education (OR 1.4), having finished secondary education (OR 1.3), and having a low household income (OR 1.3).

The associations of socio-demographic factors with disorder persistence show several differences across country income groups (data not shown). In the high-income countries, disorder persistence is associated with early AOO (OR 1.5), female gender (OR 1.9), employment status (retired: OR 1.3; 'other': OR 1.5), less than a completed college education (ORs 1.4–2.7), and low household income (OR 1.7). In the upper-middle-income countries, disorder persistence is only associated with early AOO (OR 1.7) and female gender (OR 1.8). In the low/lower-middle-income countries, disorder persistence is only associated with female gender (OR 1.5) and 'other' employment status (OR 1.8).

When considering symptom persistence, its associations with socio-demographic factors also show some differences across country income groups (data not shown). In the high-income countries, symptom persistence is associated with female gender (OR 1.2), employment status (homemaker: OR 1.4; 'other': OR 1.5), being divorced/separated/widowed (OR 1.3), lower education (OR 1.4–1.7), and low-average household income (OR 1.4). In the upper-middle-income countries, symptom persistence is associated with female gender (OR 1.9) and negatively associated with employment status 'student' (OR 0.5). In the low/lower-middle-income countries, symptom persistence is only negatively associated with a late-average AOO (OR 0.6).

Role Impairment

On the Sheehan Disability Scales (SDS), 18.7% of the cross-national 12-month specific phobia cases report severe role impairment in any domain (Table 10.5). The highest percentage of severe impairment is reported for the home domain (10.3%), followed by the work domain (9.6%), the social domain (9.0%), and the relationship domain (7.9%). The mean number of days-out-of-role (unable to function in usual role) in the past year due to 12-month specific phobia is 12.2, with a considerably higher number of days-out-of-role in those with severe impairment (29.1 days) (Appendix Table 10A.2) compared with those with mild/moderate impairment (3.8 days). Reports of severe role impairment differ significantly between country income groups, with the lowest percentages of impairment in the low/lower-middle-income countries and the highest percentages in the upper-middle-income countries. In addition, reports of severe role impairment

Table 10.3 Bivariate associations between socio-demographic correlates and DSM-IV specific phobia (SP), all countries combined

Correlates	30-day SP[a]		Lifetime SP[b]		12-month SP among lifetime cases[c]		30-day SP among 12-month cases[c]	
	OR	(95% CI)	OR	(95% CI)	OR	(95% CI)	OR	(95% CI)
Age-cohort								
18–29	**1.5***	(1.3–1.6)	**1.8***	(1.7–2.0)	–	–	–	–
30–44	**1.4***	(1.3–1.6)	**1.6***	(1.4–1.7)	–	–	–	–
45–59	**1.4***	(1.2–1.6)	**1.5***	(1.4–1.6)	–	–	–	–
60+	**1.0**		**1.0**		–	–	–	–
Age-cohort difference[d]	$\chi^2_3 = 54.5^*$, $P < 0.001$		$\chi^2_3 = 208.2^*$, $P < 0.001$					
Age-of-onset								
Early	–	–	–	–	**1.4***	(1.2–1.7)	**0.9**	(0.8–1.1)
Early-average	–	–	–	–	**1.1**	(0.9–1.3)	**0.9**	(0.7–1.0)
Late-average	–	–	–	–	**1.1**	(0.9–1.3)	**0.8***	(0.7–1.0)
Late	–	–	–	–	**1.0**		**1.0**	
Age-of-onset difference[d]					$\chi^2_3 = 20.7^*$, $P < 0.001$		$\chi^2_3 = 7.4$, $P = 0.061$	
Time since onset (continuous)	–	–	–	–	**1.00***	(0.99–1.00)	**1.01***	(1.01–1.01)
Gender								
Female	**2.7***	(2.5–3.0)	**2.0***	(1.9–2.2)	**1.8***	(1.6–2.1)	**1.3***	(1.2–1.5)
Male	**1.0**		**1.0**		**1.0**		**1.0**	
Gender difference[d]	$\chi^2_1 = 617.2^*$, $P < 0.001$		$\chi^2_1 = 635.9^*$, $P < 0.001$		$\chi^2_1 = 88.1^*$, $P < 0.001$		$\chi^2_1 = 15.7^*$, $P < 0.001$	
Employment status								
Student	**1.0**	(0.8–1.2)	**1.1**	(1.0–1.3)	**1.2**	(0.9–1.7)	**0.9**	(0.7–1.2)
Homemaker	**1.3***	(1.2–1.5)	**1.2***	(1.1–1.3)	**1.2**	(1.0–1.5)	**1.3***	(1.1–1.6)
Retired	**1.1**	(0.9–1.2)	**1.1**	(1.0–1.3)	**1.3***	(1.0–1.6)	**0.9**	(0.7–1.2)
Other	**1.6***	(1.5–1.8)	**1.4***	(1.3–1.5)	**1.5***	(1.2–1.8)	**1.3***	(1.1–1.6)
Employed	**1.0**		**1.0**		**1.0**		**1.0**	
Employment status difference[d]	$\chi^2_4 = 90.4^*$, $P < 0.001$		$\chi^2_4 = 69.9^*$, $P < 0.001$		$\chi^2_4 = 21.0^*$, $P < 0.001$		$\chi^2_4 = 15.5^*$, $P = 0.004$	
Marital status								
Never married	**1.0**	(0.9–1.1)	**1.1**	(1.0–1.1)	**1.1**	(0.9–1.2)	**1.0**	(0.9–1.2)
Divorced/separated/widowed	**1.2***	(1.1–1.3)	**1.2***	(1.1–1.3)	**1.1**	(0.9–1.3)	**1.1**	(0.9–1.3)
Currently married	**1.0**		**1.0**		**1.0**		**1.0**	

Table 10.3 (*cont.*)

Correlates	30-day SP[a]		Lifetime SP[b]		12-month SP among lifetime cases[c]		30-day SP among 12-month cases[c]	
	OR	(95% CI)	OR	(95% CI)	OR	(95% CI)	OR	(95% CI)
Marital status difference[d]	$\chi^2_2 = 16.1^*$, $P < 0.001$		$\chi^2_2 = 23.0^*$, $P < 0.001$		$\chi^2_2 = 1.0$, $P < 0.614$		$\chi^2_2 = 1.0$, $P = 0.619$	
Education level								
No education	**1.7***	(1.3–2.2)	**1.4***	(1.1–1.6)	**1.7***	(1.1–2.6)	**1.7***	(1.1–2.6)
Some primary	**2.2***	(1.9–2.5)	**1.7***	(1.6–1.9)	**1.7***	(1.2–2.2)	**1.4***	(1.0–1.8)
Finished primary	**1.9***	(1.6–2.3)	**1.5***	(1.4–1.7)	**1.5***	(1.1–2.0)	**1.4**	(1.0–1.8)
Some secondary	**1.7***	(1.5–1.9)	**1.5***	(1.4–1.6)	**1.3***	(1.1–1.7)	**1.2**	(0.9–1.5)
Finished secondary	**1.5***	(1.3–1.7)	**1.3***	(1.2–1.4)	**1.3***	(1.1–1.6)	**1.3***	(1.0–1.6)
Some college	**1.4***	(1.2–1.6)	**1.3***	(1.2–1.4)	**1.3***	(1.0–1.6)	**1.1**	(0.8–1.4)
Finished college	**1.0**		**1.0**		**1.0**		**1.0**	
Education level difference[d]	$\chi^2_6 = 117.8^*$, $P < 0.001$		$\chi^2_6 = 131.6^*$, $P < 0.001$		$\chi^2_6 = 16.7^*$, $P = 0.010$		$\chi^2_6 = 11.1$, $P = 0.086$	
Household income								
Low	**1.4***	(1.2–1.6)	**1.2***	(1.1–1.3)	**1.4***	(1.1–1.6)	**1.3***	(1.1–1.6)
Low-average	**1.2***	(1.1–1.4)	**1.1***	(1.0–1.2)	**1.2**	(1.0–1.4)	**1.2**	(1.0–1.5)
High-average	**1.1**	(1.0–1.2)	**1.0**	(1.0–1.1)	**1.1**	(0.9–1.2)	**1.1**	(0.9–1.4)
High	**1.0**		**1.0**		**1.0**		**1.0**	
Household income difference[d]	$\chi^2_3 = 38.7^*$, $P < 0.001$		$\chi^2_3 = 28.1^*$, $P < 0.001$		$\chi^2_3 = 14.4^*$, $P = 0.003$		$\chi^2_3 = 7.7$, $P = 0.053$	
N[e]	124,902		5,130,258		9,583		7,140	

*Significant at the 0.05 level, two-sided test.
[a]Based on logistic regression adjusted for age, gender, and country.
[b]Based on survival models adjusted for age-cohorts, gender, person-years, and country.
[c]Based on logistic regression adjusted for time since SP onset, age-of-onset, gender, and country.
[d]Chi-square test of significant differences between blocks of socio-demographic variables.
[e]Denominator N: 124,902 = total sample; 5,130,258 = number of person-years in the survival models; 9,583 = number of lifetime SP cases; 7,140 = number of 12-month SP cases.

Table 10.4 Socio-demographic characteristics, impairment, comorbidity, and service use for each specific phobia subtype and for groups of patients with different numbers of phobias

	Kinds of lifetime phobias												Number of lifetime phobias							
	Animal		Still water, weather		Blood, injection, medical experiences		Closed spaces		High places		Flying		1 phobia		2 phobias		3 phobias		≥4 phobias	
	%	SE	%	SE	%	SE	%	SE	%	SE	%	SE	%	SE	%	SE	%	SE	%	SE
Age																				
18–29	34.1	0.9	27.5	1.1	32.4	1.0	24.1	1.0	23.4	0.9	23.4	1.3	32.6	0.9	28.8	1.3	25.2	1.5	27.9	1.4
30–44	33.1	0.8	30.0	1.0	32.7	0.9	33.6	1.1	34.6	1.0	33.0	1.4	31.3	0.9	33.0	1.2	35.5	1.5	32.1	1.5
45–59	22.0	0.8	27.3	1.0	24.4	0.9	28.3	1.0	29.1	0.9	29.4	1.3	22.5	0.7	23.4	1.1	27.9	1.5	29.1	1.4
60+	10.8	0.5	15.2	0.8	10.5	0.6	14.0	0.7	12.8	0.7	14.3	0.9	13.6	0.6	14.7	0.9	11.5	1.0	11.0	0.9
Gender																				
Male	25.3	0.8	26.5	1.0	35.7	1.0	27.7	1.1	34.8	1.0	29.6	1.3	36.0	0.9	31.0	1.2	28.3	1.5	26.5	1.4
Female	74.7	0.8	73.5	1.0	64.3	1.0	72.3	1.1	65.2	1.0	70.4	1.3	64.0	0.9	69.0	1.2	71.7	1.5	73.5	1.4
Marital status																				
Married	58.6	0.9	61.7	1.1	58.4	1.0	60.3	1.2	61.4	1.0	63.9	1.4	59.6	0.9	59.6	1.3	61.8	1.5	60.4	1.6
Never married	28.1	0.9	22.0	1.1	28.4	0.9	22.9	1.0	23.3	1.0	20.1	1.3	28.1	0.9	26.1	1.2	23.9	1.4	22.9	1.5
Separated/ widowed/divorced	13.2	0.6	16.2	0.8	13.2	0.6	16.7	0.8	15.2	0.6	16.0	0.9	12.3	0.6	14.3	0.8	14.2	1.1	16.7	1.0
Employment status																				
Student	5.3	0.6	3.9	0.6	4.9	0.6	3.7	0.5	3.0	0.4	3.6	0.6	6.5	0.7	5.1	0.7	3.6	0.8	2.4	0.6
Working	57.2	1.1	53.9	1.3	59.6	1.2	55.1	1.3	58.1	1.1	55.4	1.7	57.7	1.4	58.4	1.5	60.8	1.7	53.1	1.8
Retired	8.1	0.6	11.3	0.8	9.1	0.8	10.4	0.9	10.1	0.7	10.3	1.0	10.9	0.8	10.1	0.9	10.5	1.3	7.9	0.9
Homemaker	16.9	0.8	18.1	1.0	13.9	0.8	17.3	1.0	15.4	0.7	17.2	1.3	13.7	0.9	14.2	1.0	13.9	1.2	20.9	1.4
Other	12.5	0.8	12.8	0.9	12.6	0.8	13.6	1.0	13.4	0.8	13.4	1.2	11.1	0.9	12.2	1.0	11.1	0.9	15.7	1.4
Household Income																				
Low	30.1	1.1	31.4	1.2	31.1	1.1	32.5	1.3	30.7	1.1	33.2	1.8	27.0	1.2	29.0	1.5	32.7	1.6	34.6	1.7
Low-mid	25.4	1.0	26.2	1.2	25.1	1.1	24.9	1.1	25.9	1.1	23.7	1.5	23.8	1.1	23.8	1.4	25.3	1.6	27.8	1.6
Mid-high	24.3	1.0	24.5	1.2	23.8	1.0	22.4	1.1	24.6	1.0	22.7	1.5	27.5	1.1	26.3	1.6	22.8	1.5	20.4	1.4
High	20.2	0.9	17.9	1.0	20.0	1.0	20.2	1.1	18.8	0.9	20.4	1.4	21.7	1.2	20.9	1.3	19.2	1.3	17.2	1.4
Education level																				
None	2.6	0.3	3.1	0.3	1.8	0.3	2.0	0.3	1.8	0.2	1.1	0.2	2.6	0.3	2.4	0.3	2.0	0.4	1.8	0.3
Some primary	10.1	0.5	11.7	0.7	9.4	0.6	10.8	0.7	10.6	0.6	9.6	0.9	8.0	0.5	10.0	0.9	9.4	0.9	12.8	1.0
Complete primary	8.2	0.5	10.1	0.7	6.9	0.5	9.1	0.7	8.1	0.5	7.3	0.8	7.0	0.5	7.9	0.7	7.5	0.8	9.9	1.0
Some secondary	21.0	0.7	22.2	1.0	22.1	0.8	23.4	0.9	22.3	0.8	23.3	1.4	19.0	0.8	21.4	1.1	22.5	1.4	24.4	1.4
Complete secondary	27.8	0.8	29.4	1.0	31.5	1.0	27.6	1.0	29.5	0.9	29.1	1.4	31.1	0.9	29.0	1.1	31.9	1.5	26.3	1.4
Some college	16.9	0.7	13.7	0.8	16.2	0.8	15.2	0.8	14.3	0.7	16.1	1.2	16.6	0.7	15.1	1.0	13.6	1.1	16.4	1.2
Complete college	11.8	0.6	8.8	0.6	11.0	0.6	10.8	0.7	12.1	0.7	12.3	0.9	13.8	0.6	13.0	0.8	12.1	1.1	7.6	0.9

Table 10.4 (*cont.*)

	Kinds of lifetime phobias												Number of lifetime phobias							
	Animal		Still water, weather		Blood, injection, medical experiences		Closed spaces		High places		Flying		1 phobia		2 phobias		3 phobias		≥4 phobias	
	%	SE	%	SE	%	SE	%	SE	%	SE	%	SE	%	SE	%	SE	%	SE	%	SE
Age-of-onset																				
Early	36.6	0.9	37.1	1.1	33.4	0.9	35.2	1.0	32.6	1.0	32.9	1.4	23.1	0.8	31.3	1.2	37.7	1.6	43.1	1.6
Early-average	30.4	0.8	28.5	1.0	29.3	1.0	27.9	1.0	27.0	0.9	27.0	1.3	21.8	0.8	27.4	1.1	29.4	1.4	33.6	1.5
Late-average	23.8	0.8	24.4	0.9	23.8	0.9	21.8	1.0	23.1	0.8	21.5	1.2	26.9	0.8	25.6	1.1	23.0	1.3	19.6	1.2
Late	9.2	0.5	10.0	0.6	13.5	0.7	15.1	0.8	17.4	0.7	18.6	1.1	28.1	0.8	15.7	0.9	9.9	0.9	3.7	0.5
Comorbidity (lifetime)																				
Mood disorder	34.7	1.0	39.9	1.3	40.0	1.2	43.6	1.3	41.3	1.1	43.5	1.6	26.5	1.0	34.3	1.4	41.0	1.8	51.0	1.9
Anxiety disorder	41.9	1.1	51.2	1.4	48.1	1.3	55.5	1.4	52.3	1.2	58.3	1.8	28.9	1.0	39.9	1.5	53.7	1.8	67.5	1.7
Impulse-control disorder	18.3	0.9	21.1	1.2	21.7	1.0	22.0	1.2	22.4	1.1	23.6	1.5	13.2	1.0	16.0	1.2	20.4	1.6	30.2	1.7
Substance-use disorder	14.9	0.8	15.6	0.9	19.2	0.9	17.4	1.0	20.5	0.9	17.3	1.3	13.9	0.9	14.9	1.0	18.2	1.6	21.1	1.4
Any mental disorder	60.6	1.1	69.4	1.4	67.2	1.3	71.0	1.4	71.7	1.2	73.0	1.6	49.7	1.3	59.9	1.7	72.5	1.9	82.1	1.4
Any impairment	55.3	0.9	57.3	1.1	52.1	1.0	54.8	1.1	53.6	1.0	56.4	1.4	46.4	1.0	48.8	1.3	56.1	1.6	63.0	1.5
Severe impairment (SDS: 7–10)[a]	16.1	0.6	16.2	0.8	15.2	0.7	15.9	0.8	15.0	0.7	17.0	1.1	11.6	0.6	12.0	0.8	16.3	1.2	20.6	1.3
Moderate impairment (SDS: 4–6)	17.5	0.7	19.3	0.9	16.7	0.8	16.8	0.9	17.8	0.7	17.0	1.1	16.2	0.7	16.2	0.9	17.6	1.2	19.3	1.1
Mild impairment (SDS: 1–3)	21.6	0.8	21.7	0.9	20.2	0.8	22.2	0.9	20.7	0.8	22.4	1.2	18.7	0.8	20.6	1.0	22.2	1.3	23.1	1.3
Use of any services[b]	20.4	0.6	21.7	0.8	24.5	0.8	27.5	1.0	26.0	0.9	28.4	1.2	16.7	0.7	21.2	0.9	27.5	1.3	29.2	1.3

[a]Highest severity category across four Sheehan Disability Scale (SDS) role domains.
[b]Specialty mental health care, general medical care, human services, or complementary/alternative medicine.

Table 10.5 Severity of role impairment (Sheehan Disability Scale) associated with 12-month specific phobia (SP), by country

Country	Proportion with severe role impairment (SDS score: 7–10)										Number of 12-month SP cases
	Home		Work		Relationship		Social		Any[a]		
	%	SE	%	SE	%	SE	%	SE	%	SE	
Low/lower-middle-income	**8.3**	**1.1**	**7.9**	**0.9**	**5.0**	**0.7**	**5.9**	**0.8**	**13.3**	**1.1**	**1,254**
Colombia	10.5	2.2	11.7	1.7	6.5	1.3	7.0	1.4	17.8	2.4	398
Iraq	15.3	4.0	11.2	3.9	10.7	3.2	11.4	3.5	18.3	3.6	163
Nigeria	2.0	1.2	3.7	1.6	1.3	0.6	2.1	1.3	4.5	1.6	266
Peru	10.0	2.3	9.4	2.6	6.6	1.6	6.6	1.6	21.2	3.1	178
PRC (Beijing/Shanghai)	12.5	4.4	8.2	3.1	3.1	1.6	9.6	4.0	16.0	4.5	99
PRC (Shenzhen)	3.2	1.3	1.2	0.6	2.0	0.9	2.1	1.0	4.2	1.5	150
Upper-middle income	**14.4**	**1.2**	**11.3**	**1.1**	**9.9**	**0.8**	**10.6**	**0.9**	**21.9**	**1.3**	**1,630**
Brazil	20.7	2.6	14.7	2.3	13.1	1.4	13.5	1.8	27.7	2.7	572
Bulgaria	10.7	1.9	9.2	1.6	7.7	1.7	10.3	2.3	16.2	2.2	218
Colombia (Medellin)	16.8	2.9	18.9	3.2	11.0	2.9	10.6	2.9	28.2	3.9	271
Lebanon	8.2	2.2	1.0	0.8	3.3	1.7	3.5	1.8	13.9	3.4	185
Mexico	8.7	1.9	6.6	1.7	8.5	1.5	10.3	1.9	15.2	2.3	302
Romania	10.9	4.4	12.6	4.5	11.3	3.9	10.0	3.1	23.0	5.3	82
High-income	**9.3**	**0.5**	**9.5**	**0.6**	**8.0**	**0.5**	**9.4**	**0.6**	**19.2**	**0.7**	**4,256**
Belgium	15.9	2.7	6.4	2.5	15.5	5.5	14.5	5.3	30.7	5.5	117
France	11.4	2.5	15.2	2.7	10.4	2.4	11.0	2.5	21.6	3.2	226
Germany	7.0	1.9	8.4	1.8	7.3	1.9	12.2	2.2	18.1	2.8	248
Italy	13.5	3.0	7.1	2.5	10.6	2.7	9.0	2.3	20.9	3.2	181
Japan[d,e]	11.5	3.5	7.7	2.8	2.7	1.5	2.5	1.9	17.4	4.1	96
New Zealand	6.8	0.9	7.2	1.0	6.1	0.8	7.1	0.9	15.5	1.2	1,098
Northern Ireland	9.4	1.8	12.3	2.7	8.9	1.8	12.8	2.1	22.4	2.8	336
Poland	11.3	2.2	7.6	2.1	6.3	1.7	8.6	2.2	16.9	2.5	250
Portugal	7.6	1.4	9.9	1.6	7.5	1.2	7.8	1.5	19.0	2.4	370
Spain	13.1	2.8	13.8	3.6	9.5	3.0	8.4	2.5	26.0	4.3	206
Spain (Murcia)	10.9	4.9	15.0	4.9	14.4	5.1	15.5	4.3	17.7	4.4	118
Netherlands	13.3	2.4	11.8	2.5	7.0	2.1	5.3	2.3	22.6	3.7	135
United States	8.6	1.2	9.2	1.1	7.8	1.2	10.7	1.4	18.7	1.8	875

Table 10.5 *(cont.)*

Country	Proportion with severe role impairment (SDS score: 7–10)										Number of 12-month SP cases
	Home		Work		Relationship		Social		Any[a]		
	%	SE	%	SE	%	SE	%	SE	%	SE	
All countries combined	**10.3**	**0.5**	**9.6**	**0.4**	**7.9**	**0.4**	**9.0**	**0.4**	**18.7**	**0.6**	**7,140**
WHO regions											
Region of the Americas	12.4	0.9	11.4	0.8	9.1	0.7	10.4	0.8	21.2	1.1	2,596
African region	2.0	1.2	3.7	1.6	1.3	0.6	2.1	1.3	4.5	1.6	266
Western Pacific region	7.1	0.8	6.6	0.8	5.1	0.6	6.3	0.7	14.4	1.0	1,443
Eastern Mediterranean region	11.5	2.3	5.7	1.9	6.7	1.8	7.2	2.0	16.0	2.5	348
Western European region	10.6	0.8	11.1	0.9	9.5	0.9	10.5	0.8	21.7	1.1	1,937
Eastern European region	11.0	1.4	9.1	1.3	7.7	1.2	9.5	1.4	17.5	1.6	550
Comparison between countries[b]	$F_{24,v} = 4.0$* $P < 0.001$		$F_{24,v} = 4.8$* $P < 0.001$		$F_{24,v} = 4.5$* $P < 0.001$		$F_{24,v} = 3.5$* $P < 0.001$		$F_{24,v} = 4.9$* $P < 0.001$		
Comparison between low-, middle- and high-income country groups[b]	$F_{2,v} = 9.2$* $P < 0.001$		$F_{2,v} = 2.8$ $P = 0.059$		$F_{2,v} = 11.2$* $P < 0.001$		$F_{2,v} = 8.6$* $P < 0.001$		$F_{2,v} = 13.5$* $P < 0.001$		
Comparison between WHO regions[b]	$F_{5,v} = 10.5$* $P < 0.001$		$F_{5,v} = 7.5$* $P < 0.001$		$F_{5,v} = 14.4$* $P < 0.001$		$F_{5,v} = 8.5$* $P < 0.001$		$F_{5,v} = 16.2$* $P < 0.001$		

*Significant at the 0.05 level, two-sided test.
[a]Highest severity category across four SDS role domains.
[b]Wald design-corrected F-tests were used to determine if there is variation in impairment severity across countries. The denominator degree of freedom, v, is 1377.
PRC: People's Republic of China.

differ across WHO regions, with the highest percentages in the region of the Americas (9.1–12.4%) and the Western European region (9.5–10.6%) and the lowest percentages in the Western Pacific (5.1–7.1%) and African regions (1.3–3.7%). The percentage of cases reporting any impairment varies somewhat across subtypes (52.1–57.3%; Table 10.4). However, clearer variation in impairment is seen across cases with different numbers of fear subtypes with 11.6% reporting severe impairment in those with one subtype and 20.6% in those with four or more subtypes.

Treatment

Of all 12-month specific phobia cases with any impairment, 23.1% report seeking treatment (Appendix Table 10A.3). Of those with severe impairment, 32.5% report receiving any treatment, which is considerably more than those with moderate (22.8%) and mild impairment (21.1%). This pattern is seen across all different sectors of treatment. Of all 12-month specific phobia cases in the cross-national sample that report any impairment, most receive their treatment in the general medical sector (14.9%) or in the specialty mental health sector (10.4%). CAM and human services are used considerably less often (3.0% and 2.6%, respectively). Treatment rates differ across country income groups. Of all 12-month specific phobia cases with any impairment, 9.6% report treatment in the low/lower-middle-income countries, 16.0% report treatment in the upper-middle-income countries, and 30.1% report treatment in the high-income countries. Overall service use showed some variation across subtypes (Table 10.4), with the highest rates of service use in cases with fear of flying (28.4%), closed spaces (27.5%), and high places (26.0%). In addition, the percentages of service use increase from 16.7% in those with one subtype to 29.2% in those with four or more subtypes.

Discussion

In the WMH surveys we found DSM-IV specific phobia to be very common, with cross-national lifetime and 12-month prevalence rates of 7.4% and 5.5%, respectively. In addition, specific phobia was found to have a high persistence rate and to often be long-lasting. Although these findings with regard to persistence of specific phobia align with previous work (Goisman *et al.* 1998; Sigström *et al.* 2011), the observed prevalence rates in the WMH surveys are lower than the rates found in previous population surveys (Magee *et al.* 1996; Bijl *et al.* 1998; Stinson *et al.* 2007). One explanation could lie in differences between assessment methods (e.g., the lists of assessed subtypes). Another likely explanation could be that previous surveys were limited to Western, high-income countries, whereas the WMH survey results show that specific phobia prevalence varies across countries, country income groups, and regions of the world. Several factors could explain this. First, the degree to which symptoms of specific phobia are recognized or attributed to a mental disorders, as well as tendencies to have catastrophic cognitions about phobic anxious symptoms, could differ across countries (Hinton & Pollack 2009; Marques *et al.* 2011; Hofmann & Hinton 2014). Second, there could be differences between countries and/or regions in how interview questions are interpreted, and in the social norms, attitudes, and stigmas surrounding mental health problems (Angermeyer & Dietrich 2006; Lee *et al.* 2009). Third, prevalence differences could also reflect differences across countries with regard to the kinds and/or frequencies of reported phobic stimuli. For instance, fear of flying is much more likely to manifest itself in higher-income countries where travelling by plane is more common than in lower-income countries. Although the exact reasons for cross-national differences could not be fully investigated in the WMH surveys, the results suggest that the phenomenology and/or underlying processes of specific phobia may vary across countries and/or regions of the world.

In our WMH findings, females have a higher prevalence of specific phobia than males and this was found for all kinds and numbers of fear subtypes. These gender differences fit with previous studies (e.g. Stinson *et al.* 2007; LeBeau *et al.* 2010). We found that younger age was associated with higher odds of specific phobia (lifetime and 30-day), aligning with findings in previous work (Stinson *et al.* 2007; Sigström *et al.* 2016). Lower education than finished college was also associated with higher odds of lifetime and 30-day specific phobia. This association with education level has been observed previously by some (Magee *et al.* 1996) but not by others (Stinson *et al.* 2007). Those with employment status 'other' (e.g., being disabled, looking for a job) showed higher odds of specific phobia than employed individuals. Magee *et al.* (1996) found a similar association, but other surveys did not investigate this. When compared across country income groups, education, employment, gender, and age were the factors that showed similar associations with lifetime and/or 30-day specific phobia across the WMH surveys, whereas other socio-demographic factors only showed associations with specific phobia in one or two country income groups. For instance, marital status was only associated with specific phobia in the high-income countries and household income was unrelated to specific phobia in the upper-middle-income countries. Some of these differences across country income groups may be due to random variation, but there could also be true differences in the socio-demographic profile of specific phobia cases across country income groups, or differences attributable to cultural variation in the reporting of fear/avoidance. Taken together, the results suggest that of all investigated socio-demographic characteristics, female gender and younger age are most consistently associated with specific phobia.

As noted above, the association of age with lifetime specific phobia prevalence has been observed previously in surveys and it has been suggested that this could reflect underreporting of early-life fear or avoidance in older cohorts due to poor recall (Stinson *et al.* 2007). However, such a recall effect cannot explain the association that we found between younger age and 30-day prevalence of specific phobia. Previously, Magee *et al.* (1996) suggested that higher prevalence in younger age groups could be attributed to an age-cohort effect. However, longitudinal data are needed to gain more insight into the association between age or age-cohorts and specific phobia.

Specific phobia is a rather heterogeneous disorder in terms of the involved specific kinds of fears and the number/intensity of the fears. The current results showed that of all assessed fear subtypes, animal phobia has the highest cross-national prevalence (3.8%), with prevalence rates ranging from 1.4% to 8.1% across countries. Previous studies also found this fear subtype to be common and report prevalence rates ranging from 3.3% to 7.0% (Curtis *et al.* 1998; Depla *et al.* 2008; LeBeau *et al.* 2010). In the WMH data, fear of still water or weather events has a cross-national prevalence of 2.3%, with prevalence rates ranging from 0.4% to 6.2% across countries. This overall prevalence in the WMH surveys is in line with previously reported prevalence rates for 'storm' phobia (2.0–2.9%) and 'water' phobia (2.2–3.4%; LeBeau *et al.* 2010). For fear of heights, the cross-national prevalence (2.8%) is somewhat lower than reported previously (3.1–5.3%; LeBeau *et al.* 2010). The observed prevalence rates in the WMH surveys differ considerably across the individual countries, with some countries showing prevalence rates in line with the above-mentioned previous work (3.6–7.1%) and others showing considerably lower prevalence rates (0.9–2.7%). Fear of blood, injections, and medical experiences has a cross-national prevalence of 3.0%. This cross-national prevalence is somewhat lower than previous estimates (3.2–4.5%; LeBeau *et al.* 2010), possibly because of the fact that there is quite some variation across WMH surveys in the prevalence rates of fear of blood, injury, and medical experiences (0.7–6.0%). The cross-national prevalence rates for fear of closed spaces (2.2%) and fear of flying (1.3%) are also both lower than reported previously (closed spaces: 3.2–3.3%; flying: 2.5–2.9%; LeBeau *et al.* 2010). These differences between WMH and previously reported prevalence rates of fear subtypes could partly stem from methodological differences. However, as shown above, the prevalence rates of fear subtypes show quite some variation across the individual surveys, with some surveys showing prevalence rates that are much lower than previously reported and other surveys showing comparable or higher prevalence rates. These differences could be explained by cultural differences and differences in the rates of exposure to the sources of fear, as noted above. Investigation of subtype co-occurrence showed that more than half of all respondents with specific phobia have two or more lifetime fear subtypes (cross-national prevalence: 4.0%). Previous studies also found that the majority of patients had more than one fear subtype (Curtis *et al.* 1998; Stinson *et al.* 2007; Depla *et al.* 2008).

The WMH surveys showed a young AOO distribution for specific phobia, which was relatively stable across countries. This finding is in line with previous work (Becker *et al.* 2007), although the estimated median AOO of 8 years is lower than that found in previous surveys (11.2 years: Stinson *et al.* 2007; 15 years: Magee *et al.* 1996). This could be attributable to differences in sample composition or assessment methods (Stinson *et al.* 2007). Consistent with previous work, the AOO distribution was not the same for all measured fear subtypes (e.g. Burstein *et al.* 2012). For animal fears and fears of natural phenomena an early AOO was more often observed than for fear of closed spaces and fear of flying. In addition, the percentage of cases with an early AOO increased with the number of fear subtypes, which is also in line with observations in previous work (Burstein *et al.* 2012).

Comorbidity is very common in those with specific phobia. In the WMH surveys, the highest comorbidity was observed with other anxiety disorders and with mood disorders, similar to previous studies (e.g. Magee *et al.* 1996; Stinson *et al.* 2007). In line with previous work (Magee *et al.* 1996), the results showed that specific phobia was the temporally primary disorder in most comorbid cases, even when the comorbid disorder(s) are known to have a relatively young AOO (anxiety and disruptive behaviour/impulse-control disorders). The percentages of reported comorbidity varied somewhat across fear subtypes, but showed a more notable variation across cases with increasing numbers of fear subtypes, similar to findings by Curtis *et al.* (1998). Together with the young observed AOO distribution, the observed high comorbidity rates in individuals with specific phobia support the idea that specific phobia may be an early-life vulnerability marker for later psychopathology (Kessler *et al.* 1996, 1997, 2011; Magee *et al.* 1996).

A little under a fifth (18.7%) of 12-month specific phobia cases reported severe role impairment. This finding suggests that specific phobia can have serious impact on people's lives, corroborating previous findings (Bijl & Ravelli 2000; Stinson *et al.* 2007), although relative to other mental disorders specific phobia is among the least impairing (see Chapter 22). However, the WMH survey results also showed that reported impairment differed across countries, which could be related to the previously described between-country differences in how mental health problems are perceived. In addition, the level of impairment depends on the likelihood of and exposure to the feared object, which can differ strongly between countries. Interestingly, analyses of the subtypes showed that the percentages of reported 12-month impairment increased with the number of reported fear subtypes, in line with previous findings (Curtis *et al.* 1998). This indicates that the presence of multiple fear subtypes can be seen as a marker of increased clinical severity.

Only 23.1% of all 12-month specific phobia cases reported any treatment. This percentage of service use is low compared to other anxiety disorders (Magee *et al.* 1996; Iza *et al.* 2013) and compared to other mental disorders in general (Bijl & Ravelli 2000; Stinson *et al.* 2007) (see also Chapters 21 and 22). In high-income countries, treatment use was much higher (30.1%) than in low/lower-middle-income countries (9.6%), which could be ascribed to differences in the availability of care, financial resources (Saxena *et al.* 2007; McBain *et al.* 2012), the perceived need for treatment (Andrade *et al.* 2014), knowledge about mental healthcare (Palazzo *et al.* 2014), and prejudice/stigma (Clement *et al.* 2015; Semrau *et al.* 2015).

There are some methodological factors that could have influenced the prevalence rates for specific phobia. First, not all phobia types were systematically assessed in the WMH-CIDI (e.g., fear of choking, vomiting, contacting an illness), which could have led to some underreporting of specific phobia. Second, DSM-IV diagnoses were used in the current analyses. Although limited changes were made to the criteria in the DSM-5, it is possible that estimated prevalence rates would be somewhat different for DSM-5-based diagnoses. Removal of the criterion that persons should recognize that their fear/avoidance is excessive and/or unreasonable could lead to more individuals meeting criteria for specific phobia, but the added requirement that the fear/avoidance should have a duration of at least six months could lead to a lower prevalence. Based on this, it is likely that DSM-5-based prevalence rates could be somewhat different from the DSM-IV rates provided here, but that very large differences would be unlikely.

In conclusion, although its prevalence, associated impairment, and treatment rates differ across countries, it is clear that specific phobia is a persistent disorder that can be associated with considerable impairment and that it is often is a precursor to other mental problems. Given its high prevalence and its likely role in the development of other psychopathology, it is important to pay attention to specific phobia both in clinical settings and in scientific research.

Acknowledgements

Portions of this chapter appeared previously in: Wardenaar, K. J., Lim, C., Al-Hamzawi, A., Alonso, J., Andrade, L. H., Benjet, C., Bunting, B., de Girolamo, G., Demyttenaere, K., Florescu, S., Gureye, O., Hisateru, T., Hu, C., Huang, Y., Karam, E., Kiejna, A., Lepine, J. P., Navarro-Mateu, F., Oakley Browne, M., Piazza, M., Posada-Villa, J., ten Have, M. L., Torres, Y., Xavier, M., Zarkov, Z., Kessler, R. C., Scott, K. M., de Jonge, P. (2017). The cross-national epidemiology of specific phobia in the World Mental Health Surveys, *Psychological Medicine*, 47, 1744–1760, used with permission from Cambridge University Press.

References

Andrade, L. H., Alonso, J., Mneimneh, Z., *et al.* (2014). Barriers to mental health treatment: results from the WHO World Mental Health surveys. *Psychological Medicine*, 44(6), 1303–17.

Angermeyer, M. C. & Dietrich, S. (2006). Public beliefs about and attitudes towards people with mental illness: a review of population studies. *Acta Psychiatrica Scandinavica*, 113, 163–79.

Angst, J., Paksarian, D., Cui, L., *et al.* (2016). The epidemiology of common mental disorders from age 20 to 50: results from the prospective Zurich cohort Study. *Epidemiology and Psychiatric Science*, 25(1), 24–32.

Becker, E. S., Rinck, M., Türke, V., *et al.* (2007). Epidemiology of specific phobia subtypes: findings from the Dresden Mental Health Study. *European Psychiatry*, 22(2), 69–74.

Bijl, R. V., De Graaf, R., Ravelli, A., Smit, F., Vollebergh, W. A. M., *et al.* (2002). Gender and age-specific first incidence of DSM-III-R psychiatric disorders in the general population. Results from the Netherlands Mental Health Survey and Incidence Study (NEMESIS). *Social Psychiatry and Psychiatric Epidemiology*, 37(8), 372–9.

Bijl, R. V. & Ravelli, A. (2000). Current and residual functional disability associated with psychopathology: findings from the Netherlands Mental Health Survey and Incidence Study (NEMESIS). *Psychological Medicine*, 30(3), 657–68.

Bijl, R. V., Ravelli, A., & van Zessen, G. (1998). Prevalence of psychiatric disorder in the general population: results of the Netherlands Mental Health Survey and Incidence Study (NEMESIS). *Social Psychiatry and Psychiatric Epidemiology*, 33, 587–95.

Bittner, A., Goodwin, R. D., Wittchen, H. U., *et al.* (2004). What characteristics of primary anxiety disorders predict subsequent major depressive disorder? *Journal of Clinical Psychiatry*, 65, 618–26.

Burstein, M., Georgiades, K., He, J. P., *et al.* (2012). Specific phobia among U.S. adolescents: phenomenology and typology. *Depression and Anxiety*, 29, 1072–82.

Choy, Y., Fyer, A. J., & Lipsitz, J. D. (2007). Treatment of specific phobia in adults. *Clinical Psychology Review*, 27(3), 266–86.

Clement, S., Schauman, O., Graham, T., *et al.* (2015). What is the impact of mental health related stigma on help-seeking? A systematic review of quantitative and qualitative studies. *Psychological Medicine*, 45(1), 11–27.

Comer, J. S., Blanco, C., Hasin, D. S., *et al.* (2011). Health-related quality of life across the anxiety disorders: results from the national epidemiologic survey on alcohol and related conditions (NESARC). *Journal of Clinical Psychiatry*, 72(1), 43–50.

Curtis, G. C., Magee, W. J., Eaton, W. W., Wittchen, H. U., & Kessler, R. C. (1998). Specific fears and phobias. Epidemiology and classification. *British Journal of Psychiatry*, 173, 212–17.

Depla, M. F., ten Have, M. L., van Balkom, A. J., *et al.* (2008). Specific fears and phobias in the general population: results from the Netherlands Mental Health Survey and Incidence Study (NEMESIS). *Social Psychiatry and Psychiatric Epidemiology*, 43(3), 200–8.

Fredrikson, M., Annas, P., Fischer, H., Wik, G. (1996). Gender and age differences in the prevalence of specific fears and phobias. *Behaviour Research and Therapy*, 34(1), 33–9.

Goisman, R. M., Allsworth, J., Rogers, M. P., *et al.* (1998). Simple phobia as a comorbid anxiety disorder. *Depression and Anxiety*, 7(3), 105–12.

Goodwin, R. D. (2002). Anxiety disorders and the onset of depression among adults in the community. *Psychological Medicine*, 32, 1121–4.

Grant, B. F., Goldstein, R. B., Chou, S. P., *et al.* (2009) Sociodemographic and psychopathologic predictors of first incidence of DSM-IV substance use, mood and anxiety disorders: results from the Wave 2 National Epidemiologic Survey on Alcohol and Related Conditions. *Molecular Psychiatry*, 14(11), 1051–66.

Haro, J. M., Arbabzadeh-Bouchez, S., Brugha, T. S. *et al.* (2006). Concordance of the Composite International Diagnostic Interview Version 3.0 (CIDI 3.0) with standardized clinical assessments in the WHO World Mental Health surveys. *International Journal of Methods in Psychiatric Research*, 15, 167–80.

Hinton, D. E. & Pollack, M. H. (2009). Introduction to the special issue: anxiety disorders in cross-cultural perspective. *CNS Neuroscience & Therapeutics*, 15(3), 207–9.

Hofmann, S. G. & Hinton, D. E. (2014). Cross-cultural aspects of anxiety disorders. *Current Psychiatry Reports*, 16(6), 450.

Iza, M., Olfson, M., Vermes, D., *et al.* (2013). Probability and predictors of first treatment contact for anxiety disorders in the United States: analysis of data from the National Epidemiologic Survey on Alcohol and Related Conditions (NESARC). *Journal of Clinical Psychiatry*, 74(11), 1093–100.

Kessler, R. C., Berglund, P., Demler, O., Jin, R., Merikangas, K. R., Walters, E. E. (2005). Lifetime prevalence and age-of-onset distributions of DSM-IV disorders in the National Comorbidity Survey Replication. *Archives of General Psychiatry*, 62(6), 593–602.

Kessler, R. C., Crum, R. M., Warner, L. A., *et al.* (1997). Lifetime co-occurrence of DSM-III-R alcohol abuse and dependence with other psychiatric disorders in the National Comorbidity Survey. *Archives of General Psychiatry*, 54(4), 313–21.

Kessler, R. C., McGonagle, K. A., Zhao, S., *et al.* (1994). Lifetime and 12 month prevalence of DSM-III-R psychiatric disorders in the United States: results from the National Comorbidity Survey. *Archives of General Psychiatry*, 51, 8–19.

Kessler, R. C., Nelson, C. B., McGonagle, K. A., *et al.* (1996). Comorbidity of DSM-III-R major depressive disorder in the general population: results from the US National Comorbidity Survey. *British Journal of Psychiatry Supplement*, 30, 17–30.

Kessler, R. C., Ormel, J., Petukhova, M., *et al.* (2011). Development of lifetime comorbidity in the World Health Organization world mental health surveys. *Archives of General Psychiatry*, 68(1), 90–100.

Kessler, R. C. & Üstün, T. B. (2004). The World Mental Health (WMH) Survey Initiative Version of the World Health Organization (WHO) Composite International Diagnostic Interview (CIDI). *International Journal of Methods in Psychiatric Research*, 13, 93–121.

Lee, S., Juon, H. S., Martinez, G., *et al.* (2009). Model minority at risk: expressed needs of mental health by Asian American young adults. *Journal of Community Health*, 34(2), 144–52.

LeBeau, R. T., Glenn, D., Liao, B., *et al.* (2010). Specific phobia: a review of DSM-IV specific phobia and preliminary recommendations for DSM-V. *Depression and Anxiety*, 27, 148–67.

Lieb, R., Miché, M., Gloster, A. T., *et al.* (2016). Impact of specific phobia on the risk of onset of mental disorders: a 10-year prospective longitudinal community study of adolescents and young adults. *Depression and Anxiety*, 33(7), 667–75.

Magee, W. J., Eaton, W. W., Wittchen, H. U., *et al.* (1996). Agoraphobia, simple phobia, and social phobia in the national comorbidity survey. *Archives of General Psychiatry*, 53, 159–68.

Marques, L., Robinaugh, D. J., LeBlanc, N. J., *et al.* (2011). Cross-cultural variations in the prevalence and presentation of anxiety disorders. *Expert Review of Neurotherapeutics*, 11(2), 313–22.

McBain, R., Norton, D. J., Morris, J., *et al.* (2012). The role of health systems factors in facilitating access to psychotropic medicines: a cross-sectional analysis of the WHO-AIMS in 63 low- and middle-income countries. *PLoS Medicine*, 9(1), e1001166.

Mendlowicz, M. V. & Stein, M. B. (2000). Quality of life in individuals with anxiety disorders. *American Journal of Psychiatry*, 157, 669–82.

Ormel, J., Petukhova, M., Chatterji, S., *et al.* (2008). Disability and treatment of specific mental and physical disorders across the world. *British Journal of Psychiatry*, 192(5), 368–75.

Palazzo, M. C., Dell'Osso, B., Altamura, A. C., *et al.* (2014). Health literacy and the pharmacological treatment of anxiety disorders: a systematic review. *Human Psychopharmacology*, 29(3), 211–5.

Saxena, S., Thornicroft, G., Knapp, M., *et al.* (2007) Resources for mental health: scarcity, inequity, and inefficiency. *The Lancet*, 370(9590), 878–89.

Semrau, M., Evans-Lacko, S., Koschorke, M., *et al.* (2015). Stigma and discrimination related to mental illness in low- and middle-income countries. *Epidemiology and Psychiatric Science*, 24(5), 382–94.

Sigström, R., Östling, S., Karlsson, B., *et al.* (2011). A population-based study on phobic fears and DSM-IV specific phobia in 70-year olds. *Journal of Anxiety Disorders*, 25(1), 148–53.

Sigström, R., Skoog, I., Karlsson, B., Nilsson, J., & Östling, S. (2016). Nine-year follow-up of specific phobia in a population sample of older people. *Depression and Anxiety*, 33, 339–46.

Stinson, F. S., Dawson, D. A., Chou, S. P., *et al.* (2007). The epidemiology of DSM-IV specific phobia in the USA: results from the National Epidemiologic Survey on Alcohol and Related Conditions. *Psychological Medicine*, 37(7), 1047–59.

ten Have, M., de Graaf, R., van Dorsselaer, S., & Beekman, A. (2013). Lifetime treatment contact and delay in treatment seeking after first onset of a mental disorder. *Psychiatric Services*, 64(10), 981–9.

Trumpf, J., Margraf, J., Vriends, N., Meyer, A. H., & Becker, E. S. (2010). Specific phobia predicts psychopathology in young women. *Social Psychiatry and Psychiatric Epidemiology*, 45(12), 1161–6.

Wells, J. E., Browne, M. A., Scott, K. M., *et al.* (2006). Prevalence, interference with life and severity of 12 month DSM-IV disorders in Te Rau Hinengaro: the New Zealand Mental Health Survey. *Australian and New Zealand Journal of Psychiatry*, 40(10), 845–54.

Zimmermann, P., Wittchen, H. U., Höfler, M., *et al.* (2003). Primary anxiety disorders and the development of subsequent alcohol use disorders: a 4-year community study of adolescents and young adults. *Psychological Medicine*, 33(7), 1211–22.

Chapter 11

Posttraumatic Stress Disorder

Andrew Ratanatharathorn, Lauren C. Ng, Fernando Navarro-Mateu, Karestan C. Koenen

Introduction

Posttraumatic stress disorder (PTSD) is a trauma- and stressor-related disorder characterized by re-experiencing, avoidance, and hyper-arousal symptoms along with alterations in cognition and mood following a traumatic event (TE). Potential TEs include actual or threatened death, serious injury, or sexual violence, and may be directly experienced, witnessed, experienced by a close friend or family member, or experienced through repeated in-person exposure to aversive details of TEs (American Psychiatric Association 2013). Under the Fourth Edition of the *Diagnostic and Statistical Manual* (DSM-IV) (American Psychiatric Association 2013), to qualify for a diagnosis of PTSD, individuals have to endorse one of five re-experiencing symptoms (e.g., having recurrent and distressing dreams of the event), three of seven avoidance symptoms (e.g., diminished interest in significant activities), and two of five hyper-arousal symptoms (e.g., difficulty falling or staying asleep). In addition, symptoms must be present for at least one month and cause clinically significant distress or impairment in functioning.

National epidemiological studies have found wide variation in lifetime prevalence of trauma exposure from lows of 24% in Germany (Hauffa *et al.* 2011) to highs of 83% in the United States (US) (Alegria *et al.* 2013). However, we can infer little about the cross-national prevalence of trauma as the method of assessing TEs has varied across studies, which could account for the variation in prevalences. PTSD prevalence has similarly been shown to vary widely across countries. Part of the variation in estimated PTSD prevalences stems from the index TE that interviewers have used to assess PTSD when respondents report multiple TEs. Respondents may be asked to identify either the 'worst event' (where among the list of TEs endorsed, the respondent chooses the one they consider to have been the 'worst' or most traumatic) or the interviewer may randomly select one event from among the endorsed TEs and assess PTSD in relation to that TE. TEs identified as 'worst' are not representative of all TEs as these events usually represent atypical circumstances, which confer higher conditional risk of PTSD than random events in the same class.

Results from nationally representative samples of adults that used the Composite International Diagnostic Interview (CIDI) to assess PTSD pegged to the worst event experienced have found lifetime rates of PTSD diagnoses ranging from 1.7% in South Korea (Jeon *et al.* 2007) to 9.2% in Canada (Van Ameringen *et al.* 2008). When using the CIDI with an unspecified or random event, results from nationally representative samples have found lifetime rates of 2.3% in South Africa (Atwoli *et al.* 2013), 2.5% in Iraq (Alhasnawi *et al.* 2009), and 3.4% in Lebanon (Karam *et al.* 2008).

Despite PTSD being prevalent and debilitating, many people with PTSD do not seek treatment, and even then only do so after experiencing symptoms for extended periods of time (Wang *et al.* 2007). In the US where services are more widely available than in most of the world (Roberts *et al.* 2011), only about half of those with PTSD seek treatment. In addition, the National Comorbidity Replication Study estimated that individuals on average delay 12 years to seek treatment (Wang *et al.* 2005). Furthermore, among those seeking treatment, only 58% receive care from a mental health professional (Kessler 2000). Although research on treatment seeking among people with PTSD in the general population is limited outside of the US and Western Europe, we expect that rates would be even lower given limited access to mental health care in most regions of the world (World Health Organization 2014).

In this chapter, we provide a summary of the cross-national epidemiology of PTSD including estimates of age-of-onset (AOO), socio-demographic correlates, comorbidity, and treatment seeking. The results we present below provide the most detailed picture of the global burden of PTSD.

Methods

TEs and PTSD were assessed in 26 of the 29 surveys included in this volume and PTSD was a Part II diagnosis. Because of these restrictions, the number of respondents assessed was only n = 71,083 across the 26 surveys.

The WMH surveys assessed 29 TEs across six categories: seven war-related events (e.g., combatant, civilian in a war zone), five types of physical assault (e.g., beaten by a caregiver as a child, mugged), three types of sexual assault (e.g., stalked, attempted rape, rape), six events involving threats to physical integrity excluding violence (e.g., life-threatening accidents, natural disasters), five events involving threats to loved ones (e.g., life-threatening illness/injury), and the traumatic death of loved one. In addition, respondents were asked an open-ended question about TEs not listed during the interview as well as a question for TEs that respondents did not wish to describe in detail. Respondents were asked about both the number of lifetime occurrences of each TE type and age when each TE type first occurred (Benjet *et al.* 2016). Respondents reporting more than one qualifying TE were assessed for PTSD twice: once for the self-nominated lifetime TE with the largest number of symptoms of PTSD and a second time for one TE randomly selected from all those reported (Breslau & Kessler 2001). This approach was used to create a weighted dataset that was representative of all lifetime TEs that occurred among the respondents (Kessler & Üstün 2004).

PTSD was assessed in the CIDI using DSM-IV criteria (Kessler & Üstün 2004). Respondents who experienced a qualifying TE were asked about re-experiencing, avoidance, and hyper-arousal symptoms regardless of the whether the TE involved intense fear, helplessness, or horror. Respondents meeting these criteria were then assessed for whether the symptoms lasted longer than one month and caused clinically significant distress and impairment. Lifetime prevalence of PTSD was estimated in the whole population and among those exposed to a TE. The prevalences of PTSD in the 12 months and 30 days prior to the survey were estimated in the whole population.

Results

TE Prevalence

The prevalence of trauma exposure is presented in Table 11.1. Trauma exposure varies significantly across countries, country income groups, and regions. An average of 69.7% of respondents report experiencing a TE over their lifetime with the reported exposures ranging from 28.6% in Bulgaria to 84.6% in the Ukraine. 72.4% of the respondents in high-income countries reported being exposed to trauma, followed by respondents in upper-middle-income countries (63.2%) and in low/lower-middle-income countries (69.1%) ($F = 74.5$, $P < 0.001$). More detailed reporting of TEs in the WMH surveys can be found in Benjet *et al.* (2016).

PTSD Prevalence

PTSD prevalence results are presented in Table 11.1. Lifetime prevalence of PTSD captures the proportion of persons who develop PTSD in the population while the lifetime prevalence among the exposed is the prevalence of PTSD among respondents who reported at least one TE. Lifetime prevalence among the exposed will vary both with the overall lifetime prevalence of PTSD and the prevalence of trauma exposure in a country. For example, lifetime prevalence of PTSD is 2.2% in Spain and 2.3% in South Africa, but the lifetime prevalence rate of PTSD among the exposed is 1% higher in Spain (4%) compared to South Africa (3%). This is because the prevalence of trauma is 20% higher in South Africa. Among respondents who experienced a TE, the prevalence of PTSD is 5.6% while the population prevalence is 3.9% with significant variation in PTSD prevalence across countries ($F = 32.7$ and $F = 33.7$, $P < 0.001$). Among those exposed to TEs, lifetime prevalence of PTSD varies significantly across countries, country income groups, and WHO regions (F ranging between 32.7 and 115.3, $P < 0.001$) with lifetime prevalence in high-income countries (6.9%) approximately twice that of low/lower-middle-income countries (3.0%) and upper-middle-income countries (3.9%). Overall PTSD prevalence in high-income countries (5.0%) remains twice that of upper-middle-income (2.3%) and low/low-middle-income countries (2.1%).

Across all countries, the 12-month prevalence of PTSD is 2.0% and ranges from 0.2% in Peru and the People's Republic of China (PRC) to 5.1% in Northern Ireland. High-income countries (2.6%) have a 12-month prevalence of PTSD, more than twice that of upper-middle-(1.0%) and low/lower-middle-income countries (1.0%). The 12-month prevalence of PTSD among lifetime cases, which is an indirect indicator of the proportion of PTSD cases with a persistent course of PTSD, ranges from 23.1% in Peru to 82.1% in the PRC. While both Peru and the PRC have 12-month prevalences of 0.2%, the lifetime prevalences are 0.7% and 0.3%, respectively. Thus, although the PRC has a

Table 11.1 Prevalence of DSM-IV posttraumatic stress disorder (PTSD) in the World Mental Health surveys

Country	Trauma exposure		Lifetime prevalence among exposed		Lifetime prevalence		12-month prevalence		30-day prevalence		12-month prevalence of PTSD among lifetime cases		30-day prevalence of PTSD among 12-month cases		Sample size used
	%	SE	%	SE	%	SE	%	SE	%	SE	%	SE	%	SE	
Low/lower-middle-income countries	**69.1**	**0.7**	**3.0**	**0.2**	**2.1**	**0.2**	**1.0**	**0.1**	**0.4**	**0.1**	**47.8**	**3.9**	**43.2**	**5.4**	**11,862**
Colombia	82.7	1.4	2.2	0.5	1.8	0.4	0.6	0.2	0.2	0.1	34.2	9.6	29.2	13.7	2,381
Iraq	56.0	0.8	4.4	0.4	2.5	0.2	1.1	0.2	0.4	0.1	46.1	6.2	33.7	9.4	4,332
Peru	83.1	0.8	0.8	0.2	0.7	0.1	0.2	0.1	0.1	0.1	23.1	8.9	37.5	26.1	1,801
PRC (Beijing/Shanghai)	52.5	2.6	0.5	0.2	0.3	0.1	0.2	0.1	0.0	0.0	82.1	11.5	17.9	14.0	1,628
Ukraine	84.6	1.7	5.7	0.7	4.8	0.6	2.8	0.5	1.7	0.4	58.9	5.3	59.2	7.5	1,720
Upper-middle-income countries	**63.2**	**0.6**	**3.6**	**0.2**	**2.3**	**0.1**	**1.0**	**0.1**	**0.4**	**0.1**	**43.5**	**2.7**	**44.3**	**4.5**	**16,913**
Brazil	73.8	1.5	4.3	0.3	3.2	0.2	1.6	0.2	0.7	0.2	48.8	4.9	44.8	8.4	2,942
Bulgaria	28.6	1.3	6.5	1.1	1.9	0.3	1.1	0.2	0.8	0.2	61.9	4.9	69.3	10.4	2,233
Colombia (Medellin)	75.1	2.6	4.9	0.8	3.7	0.6	1.0	0.2	0.3	0.1	26.4	5.3	26.9	9.2	1,673
Lebanon	81.1	2.7	4.2	0.7	3.4	0.6	2.0	0.6	1.2	0.6	58.2	11.2	62.3	12.6	1,031
Mexico	68.8	1.8	2.1	0.4	1.5	0.3	0.6	0.1	0.2	0.1	39.2	8.6	40.3	11.9	2,362
Romania	41.5	1.1	2.8	0.7	1.2	0.3	0.7	0.3	0.4	0.2	64.6	8.7	47.7	14.1	2,357
South Africa	73.8	1.2	3.0	0.4	2.3	0.3	0.7	0.2	0.1	0.1	31.7	5.5	20.0	7.4	4,315
High-income countries	**72.4**	**0.4**	**6.9**	**0.2**	**5.0**	**0.1**	**2.6**	**0.1**	**1.3**	**0.1**	**52.1**	**1.2**	**51.3**	**1.8**	**42,308**
Australia	76.2	0.7	9.6	0.5	7.3	0.4	4.4	0.3	2.5	0.2	60.0	2.2	56.6	3.3	8,463
Belgium	65.8	3.1	4.1	0.8	2.7	0.5	0.8	0.1	0.2	0.1	28.0	6.2	29.7	9.5	1,043
France	72.7	2.3	5.4	0.7	3.9	0.6	2.3	0.4	1.0	0.3	59.5	6.8	44.8	8.0	1,436
Germany	67.3	2.2	2.5	0.5	1.7	0.3	0.7	0.2	0.2	0.1	40.9	8.3	36.9	11.5	1,323
Israel	74.8	0.7	2.1	0.3	1.6	0.2	0.6	0.1	0.3	0.1	37.3	5.9	44.1	10.3	4,859
Italy	56.1	2.2	4.3	1.0	2.4	0.6	0.7	0.2	0.4	0.1	30.0	7.6	48.8	13.1	1,779
Japan	60.7	1.7	2.1	0.4	1.3	0.2	0.7	0.2	0.2	0.1	55.4	7.1	35.0	14.0	1,682
New Zealand	79.3	0.8	7.6	0.4	6.1	0.3	3.0	0.2	1.7	0.2	50.0	2.5	54.9	3.8	7,312
Northern Ireland	60.6	1.7	14.5	1.1	8.8	0.7	5.1	0.6	2.4	0.4	57.5	3.8	48.0	6.4	1,986
Portugal	69.0	1.7	7.7	0.7	5.3	0.5	2.3	0.3	1.0	0.2	42.6	4.5	42.3	6.5	2,060
Spain	54.0	1.7	4.0	0.8	2.2	0.4	0.6	0.1	0.2	0.0	26.1	6.7	33.5	9.0	2,121
Spain (Murcia)	62.4	1.9	4.5	0.7	2.8	0.5	0.9	0.3	0.4	0.1	32.1	8.5	47.4	9.5	1,459
Netherlands	65.6	2.8	6.7	1.2	4.4	0.8	2.7	0.7	1.1	0.3	62.0	8.3	39.3	10.8	1,093
United States	82.7	0.9	8.3	0.5	6.9	0.4	3.6	0.3	1.8	0.2	52.4	2.9	49.3	4.1	5,692

(cont.)

Table 11.1 *(cont.)*

Country	Trauma exposure		Lifetime prevalence among exposed		Lifetime prevalence		12-month prevalence		30-day prevalence		12-month prevalence of PTSD among lifetime cases		30-day prevalence of PTSD among 12-month cases		Sample size used
	%	SE	%	SE	%	SE	%	SE	%	SE	%	SE	%	SE	
All countries combined	**69.7**	**0.3**	**5.6**	**0.1**	**3.9**	**0.1**	**2.0**	**0.1**	**1.0**	**0.0**	**50.5**	**1.0**	**49.8**	**1.6**	**71,083**
WHO regions[a]															
Region of the Americas	78.5	0.6	4.8	0.2	3.8	0.2	1.8	0.1	0.8	0.1	46.9	2.2	45.9	3.3	16,851
African region	73.8	1.2	3.0	0.4	2.3	0.3	0.7	0.2	0.1	0.1	31.7	5.5	20.0	7.4	4,315
Western Pacific region	74.0	0.5	7.7	0.3	5.7	0.2	3.2	0.1	1.8	0.1	56.0	1.6	55.3	2.5	19,085
Eastern Mediterranean region	67.5	0.6	3.2	0.2	2.1	0.1	1.0	0.1	0.4	0.1	44.9	4.2	42.6	6.7	10,222
Western European region	63.0	0.7	6.3	0.3	4.0	0.2	1.9	0.1	0.8	0.1	46.7	2.3	44.1	3.3	14,300
Eastern European region	48.7	1.0	4.9	0.5	2.4	0.2	1.5	0.2	0.9	0.1	60.7	3.6	59.8	5.7	6,310
Comparison between countries[b]	$F_{25,v}=81.8^*$, $P<0.001$		$F_{25,v}=32.7^*$, $P<0.001$		$F_{25,v}=33.7^*$, $P<0.001$		$F_{25,v}=24.5^*$, $P<0.001$		$F_{25,v}=13.0^*$, $P<0.001$		$F_{25,v}=4.0^*$, $P<0.001$		$F_{25,v}=1.7^*$, $P=0.021$		
Comparison between low-, middle-, and high-income country groups[b]	$F_{2,v}=74.5^*$, $P<0.001$		$F_{2,v}=115.3^*$, $P<0.001$		$F_{2,v}=135.8^*$, $P<0.001$		$F_{2,v}=104.4^*$, $P<0.001$		$F_{2,v}=58.2^*$, $P<0.001$		$F_{2,v}=4.3^*$, $P=0.013$		$F_{2,v}=1.8$, $P=0.158$		
Comparison between WHO regions[b]	$F_{5,v}=148.2^*$, $P<0.001$		$F_{5,v}=40.7^*$, $P<0.001$		$F_{5,v}=46.3^*$, $P<0.001$		$F_{5,v}=37.9^*$, $P<0.001$		$F_{5,v}=35.2^*$, $P<0.001$		$F_{5,v}=7.1^*$, $P<0.001$		$F_{5,v}=4.1^*$, $P=0.001$		

*Significant at the 0.05 level, two-sided test.

[a]**Region of the Americas** (Colombia, Mexico, Brazil, Peru, United States, Colombia (Medellin)); **African region** (South Africa); **Western Pacific region** (PRC Beijing and Shanghai, Japan, Australia, New Zealand); **Eastern Mediterranean region** (Israel, Iraq, Lebanon); **Western European region** (Belgium, France, Germany, Italy, Netherlands, Spain, Northern Ireland, Portugal, Spain (Murcia)); **Eastern European region** (Romania, Bulgaria, Ukraine).

[b]Wald design-corrected F-tests were used to determine if there is variation in prevalence estimates across countries. The denominator degree of freedom, v, is 5212.

PRC: People's Republic of China.

lower lifetime prevalence of PTSD than Peru, among PTSD cases in the PRC the disorder is more likely to be persistent.

The 30-day prevalence represents the population burden of PTSD at the specific time each country's survey was conducted. The worldwide 30-day prevalence is 1.0%, but varies significantly across country income groups ($F = 13.0$, $P < 0.001$) with the prevalence in high-income countries (1.3%) three times that of upper-middle-income countries (0.4%) and low/lower-middle-income countries (0.4%). Thirty-day prevalence also varies across WHO regions with the Eastern European region reporting the highest 30-day prevalence (0.9%), which is nine times the prevalence in the Africa region (0.1%).

Thirty-day prevalence of PTSD among 12-month cases is an indicator of the persistence of PTSD symptoms. For example, in Iraq the 30-day prevalence is 0.4% and the 12-month prevalence is 1.1%, which yields a 30-day prevalence of PTSD among the 12-month cases of 33.7% (0.4%/1.1%). Since these are proportions, countries can have a similar 30-day prevalence of PTSD among 12-month cases, but with significantly different rates of 12-month prevalence or 30-day prevalence. Similarly to Iraq, Spain has a 30-day prevalence of PTSD among 12-month cases of 33.5% but half the rate of 30-day prevalence (0.2%) and 12-month prevalence (0.6%). Overall, almost half (49.8%) of 12-month cases report PTSD symptoms in the 30 days before their interview with a range of 17.9% in the PRC to 69.3% in Bulgaria. The 30-day prevalence of PTSD among 12-month cases also varies significantly by country ($F = 1.7$, $P < 0.021$) and WHO regions ($F = 4.1$, $P < 0.001$), but does not vary by country income level ($F = 1.8$, $P = 0.158$).

The 12-month prevalence of PTSD among lifetime cases and 30-day prevalence of PTSD among 12-month cases give insight into how the burden of PTSD across countries varies, even those with a similar prevalence of lifetime PTSD. For example, Colombia (Medellin) and Lebanon have a lifetime prevalence of PTSD of 3.7% and 3.4%, respectively. However, Lebanon's 12-month prevalence of PTSD among lifetime cases (58.2%) is more than twice that of Colombia's (26.4%). As a result, the 12-month prevalence of PTSD in Lebanon is twice (2.0%) that of Colombia's (1.0%). Furthermore, the 30-day prevalence of PTSD among 12-month PTSD cases is twice as high in Lebanon (62.3%) as it is in Colombia (26.9%). Since both the 12-month prevalence of PTSD among lifetime cases and the 30-day prevalence of PTSD among 12-month cases are twice as large in Lebanon compared to Colombia, the 30-day prevalence in Lebanon is four times that of Colombia. This indicates that more respondents in Lebanon are suffering from PTSD, and that their PTSD symptoms are more persistent than in Colombia despite both having a similar lifetime prevalence of PTSD. In summary, Lebanon has a higher burden of PTSD than Colombia.

Age-of-Onset

The cumulative distributions for the age of PTSD onset stratified by income group are presented in Figure 11.1. Onset of PTSD is earlier on average in high-income countries than in low/lower-middle- and upper-middle-income countries, with half of respondents in high-income countries reporting PTSD onset before age 30 compared to age 43 for low/lower-middle-income countries. Within income groups, AOO also varies significantly across countries. Across the low/lower-middle-income countries, 50% of respondents in Peru report PTSD onset before the age of 28 compared to 14% in Colombia. Age-of-onset is similarly wide across high-income countries with 50% of US respondents reporting PTSD onset by age 21 compared to less than 10% in Japan. The AOO distributions vary less widely among upper-middle-income countries compared to other income groups with half of respondents in Colombia reporting PTSD onset by 25 years of age compared to 24% in Brazil.

Socio-demographic Correlates

Associations of socio-demographic correlates with PTSD and TEs are presented in Table 11.2. Age-cohort is a significant correlate ($\chi^2 = 1063.8$, $P < 0.001$) of experiencing a TE, with the 18–29-year-old cohort having twice the odds of the 60+ cohort. Females are less likely to experience a TE ($\chi^2 = 146.0$, $P < 0.001$). People who are divorced, separated, or widowed are more likely to report experiencing a TE compared to those who never or are currently married ($\chi^2 = 67.2$, $P < 0.001$). The odds of experiencing a TE vary significantly by employment status, with homemakers less likely to experience a TE compared with students, retirees, or employed respondents. No education, some primary school, or finished primary school are associated with significantly lower odds of experiencing a TE compared with those who had some or finished secondary school ($\chi^2 = 85.7$, $P < 0.001$). In addition, low household income is associated with decreased likelihood of experiencing a TE compared with other income groups ($\chi^2 = 13.3$, $P = 0.004$).

The associations between socio-demographic factors and PTSD onset, persistence, and burden vary.

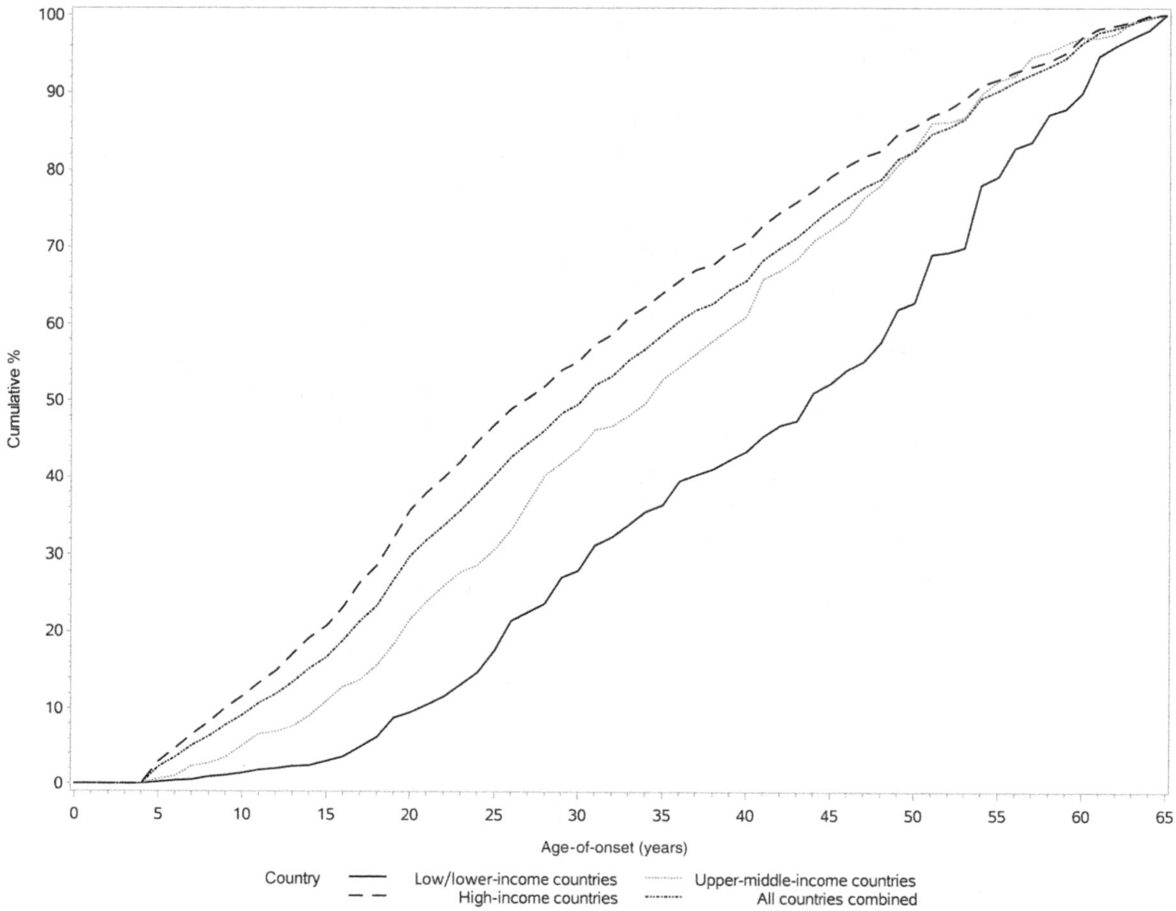

Figure 11.1 Cumulative age-of-onset distributions of DSM-IV posttraumatic stress disorder by country income groups and in all countries combined.

For example, female gender is significantly associated with PTSD onset (lifetime PTSD among exposed and overall) as well as with PTSD burden (30-day PTSD) with females having over twice the odds as males. However, female gender is not associated with disorder persistence (12-month PTSD/lifetime) or symptom persistence (30-day PTSD/12-month). Similarly, marital status is associated with of PTSD onset and burden, but is not significantly associated with disorder persistence ($\chi^2 = 3.8$, $P = 0.152$) or symptom persistence ($\chi^2 = 1.5$, $P = 0.472$). In contrast, lower household income and employment status are significantly associated with the likelihood of PTSD onset, burden, and disorder persistence, but not symptom persistence. Finally, education level is associated only with PTSD onset, but is not associated with burden ($\chi^2 = 3.3$, $P = 0.772$), disorder persistence ($\chi^2 = 5.8$, $P = 0.447$), or symptom persistence ($\chi^2 = 3.3$, $P = 0.764$).

Socio-demographic correlates stratified by country income groups are presented in Appendix Tables 11A.1–11A.3. Gender, marital status, and household income are significant correlates of PTSD onset across all country income groups, while employment status and education are significant in only low/lower-middle-income countries and high-income countries. In high-income countries, no correlates are significantly associated with symptom persistence, while employment status is associated with persistence in both low/lower-middle-income and upper-middle-income countries.

Comorbidity

Comorbidities of PTSD with other DSM-IV disorders are presented in Table 11.3. Among those with a lifetime diagnosis of PTSD, 78.1% meet the criteria for at

Table 11.2 Bivariate associations between socio-demographic correlates and DSM-IV posttraumatic stress disorder (PTSD), all countries combined

Correlates	Exposure to TE[b,f]		Lifetime PTSD among exposed[b,f]		30-day PTSD[a]		Lifetime PTSD[b]		12-month PTSD among lifetime cases[c]		30-day PTSD among 12-month cases[c]	
	OR	(95% CI)	OR	(95% CI)	OR	(95% CI)	OR	(95% CI)	OR	(95% CI)	OR	(95% CI)
Age-cohort												
18–29	**2.0***	(1.9–2.1)	**2.5***	(2.1–3.0)	**1.1**	(0.9–1.5)	**4.3***	(3.6–5.2)				
30–44	**1.6***	(1.5–1.6)	**2.1***	(1.8–2.4)	**1.5***	(1.2–1.9)	**3.5***	(3.0–4.1)				
45–59	**1.3***	(1.2–1.3)	**1.8***	(1.6–2.1)	**1.7***	(1.3–2.2)	**2.5***	(2.1–2.9)				
60+	**1.0**		**1.0**		**1.0**		**1.0**					
Age-cohort difference[d]	$\chi^2_3 = 1{,}063.8^*$, $P < 0.001$		$\chi^2_3 = 122.1^*$, $P < 0.001$		$\chi^2_3 = 24.1^*$, $P < 0.001$		$\chi^2_3 = 278.9^*$, $P < 0.001$					
Age-of-onset												
Early									**1.1**	(0.9–1.5)	**0.7**	(0.5–1.0)
Early-average									**0.8***	(0.6–1.0)	**0.7**	(0.5–1.0)
Late-average									**0.7***	(0.5–0.9)	**0.7***	(0.5–0.9)
Late									**1.0**		**1.0**	
Age-of-onset difference[d]									$\chi^2_3 = 21.7^*$, $P < 0.001$		$\chi^2_3 = 5.9$, $P = 0.115$	
Time since onset (continuous)									**0.97***	(0.97–0.98)	**1.01**	(1.00–1.02)
Gender												
Female	**0.9***	(0.8–0.9)	**2.6***	(2.4–2.9)	**2.4***	(1.9–2.9)	**2.3***	(2.1–2.5)	**1.1**	(0.9–1.3)	**0.9**	(0.7–1.3)
Male	**1.0**		**1.0**		**1.0**		**1.0**		**1.0**		**1.0**	
Gender difference[d]	$\chi^2_1 = 146.0^*$, $P < 0.001$		$\chi^2_1 = 321.8^*$, $P < 0.001$		$\chi^2_1 = 56.4^*$, $P < 0.001$		$\chi^2_1 = 252.0^*$, $P < 0.001$		$\chi^2_1 = 0.5$, $P = 0.477$		$\chi^2_1 = 0.2$, $P = 0.698$	
Employment status												
Student	**1.0**	(0.9–1.1)	**1.0**	(0.7–1.3)	**1.1**	(0.6–2.2)	**1.0**	(0.8–1.4)	**1.7**	(1.0–3.0)	**1.2**	(0.6–2.5)
Homemaker	**0.9***	(0.8–0.9)	**1.2***	(1.0–1.4)	**1.4***	(1.1–1.8)	**1.1**	(0.9–1.2)	**1.2**	(0.9–1.6)	**1.2**	(0.8–1.7)
Retired	**1.0**	(0.9–1.1)	**1.3***	(1.1–1.6)	**1.0**	(0.7–1.4)	**1.1**	(0.9–1.3)	**1.1**	(0.8–1.5)	**1.5**	(1.0–2.4)
Other	**1.1***	(1.0–1.1)	**1.7***	(1.5–2.0)	**2.4***	(1.9–3.0)	**1.7***	(1.5–2.0)	**1.5***	(1.2–1.9)	**1.3**	(0.9–1.9)
Employed	**1.0**		**1.0**		**1.0**		**1.0**		**1.0**		**1.0**	
Employment status difference[d]	$\chi^2_4 = 39.2^*$, $P < 0.001$		$\chi^2_4 = 77.7^*$, $P < 0.001$		$\chi^2_4 = 50.2^*$, $P < 0.001$		$\chi^2_4 = 66.5^*$, $P < 0.001$		$\chi^2_4 = 12.3^*$, $P = 0.015$		$\chi^2_4 = 5.3$, $P = 0.259$	

(cont.)

Table 11.2 *(cont.)*

Correlates	Exposure to TE[b,f]		Lifetime PTSD among exposed[b,f]		30-day PTSD[a]		Lifetime PTSD[b]		12-month PTSD among lifetime cases[c]		30-day PTSD among 12-month cases[c]	
	OR	(95% CI)	OR	(95% CI)	OR	(95% CI)	OR	(95% CI)	OR	(95% CI)	OR	(95% CI)
Marital status												
Never married	**1.0**	(1.0–1.0)	**1.3***	(1.1–1.5)	**1.0**	(0.8–1.2)	**1.3***	(1.1–1.5)	**1.1**	(0.8–1.4)	**0.8**	(0.6–1.1)
Divorced/separated/widowed	**1.2***	(1.1–1.2)	**1.7***	(1.5–1.9)	**2.0***	(1.6–2.6)	**1.8***	(1.6–2.0)	**1.2**	(1.0–1.5)	**0.9**	(0.7–1.2)
Currently married	**1.0**		**1.0**		**1.0**		**1.0**		**1.0**		**1.0**	
Marital status difference[d]	$\chi^2_2 = 67.2$, P < 0.001		$\chi^2_2 = 70.8$*, P < 0.001		$\chi^2_2 = 29.7$*, P < 0.001		$\chi^2_2 = 109.3$*, P < 0.001		$\chi^2_2 = 3.8$, P = 0.152		$\chi^2_2 = 1.5$, P = 0.472	
Education level												
No education	**0.7***	(0.6–0.8)	**1.5**	(0.9–2.7)	**0.8**	(0.4–1.6)	**1.1**	(0.7–1.6)	**0.6**	(0.3–1.2)	**1.2**	(0.4–3.5)
Some primary	**0.9***	(0.8–0.9)	**1.4***	(1.2–1.8)	**1.3**	(0.9–2.0)	**1.2**	(1.0–1.5)	**1.0**	(0.7–1.5)	**1.2**	(0.6–2.3)
Finished primary	**0.9***	(0.8–0.9)	**1.7***	(1.3–2.1)	**1.1**	(0.7–1.7)	**1.4***	(1.1–1.7)	**1.2**	(0.8–1.8)	**0.7**	(0.4–1.3)
Some secondary	**1.0**	(0.9–1.0)	**1.4***	(1.2–1.6)	**1.2**	(0.9–1.6)	**1.3***	(1.1–1.5)	**0.9**	(0.7–1.2)	**1.1**	(0.7–1.6)
Finished secondary	**1.0**	(1.0–1.0)	**1.1**	(0.9–1.3)	**1.1**	(0.8–1.5)	**1.1**	(0.9–1.2)	**1.1**	(0.8–1.5)	**1.1**	(0.7–1.6)
Some college	**1.1***	(1.0–1.1)	**1.1**	(0.9–1.3)	**1.1**	(0.8–1.5)	**1.1**	(0.9–1.3)	**1.1**	(0.8–1.5)	**1.0**	(0.7–1.5)
Finished college	**1.0**		**1.0**		**1.0**		**1.0**		**1.0**		**1.0**	
Education level difference[d]	$\chi^2_6 = 85.7$, P < 0.001		$\chi^2_6 = 36.9$*, P < 0.001		$\chi^2_6 = 3.3$, P = 0.772		$\chi^2_6 = 15.2$, P = 0.019		$\chi^2_6 = 5.8$, P = 0.447		$\chi^2_6 = 3.3$, P = 0.764	
Household income												
Low	**0.9***	(0.9–1.0)	**1.7***	(1.5–1.9)	**2.0***	(1.6–2.6)	**1.6***	(1.4–1.8)	**1.5***	(1.2–1.9)	**1.3**	(0.9–1.8)
Low-average	**1.0**	(0.9–1.0)	**1.5***	(1.3–1.7)	**1.9***	(1.4–2.6)	**1.5***	(1.3–1.7)	**1.3**	(1.0–1.7)	**1.5***	(1.0–2.1)
High-average	**1.0**	(1.0–1.0)	**1.4***	(1.3–1.7)	**1.4***	(1.1–1.9)	**1.4***	(1.3–1.7)	**1.0**	(0.8–1.3)	**1.0**	(0.7–1.5)
High	**1.0**		**1.0**		**1.0**		**1.0**		**1.0**		**1.0**	
Household income difference[d]	$\chi^2_3 = 13.3$*, P = 0.004		$\chi^2_3 = 55.2$*, P < 0.001		$\chi^2_3 = 34.8$*, P < 0.001		$\chi^2_3 = 50.2$*, P < 0.001		$\chi^2_3 = 15.8$*, P = 0.001		$\chi^2_3 = 6.0$, P = 0.113	
N[e]	**1,310,008**		**3,072,041**		**71,083**		**3,067,607**		**4,103**		**2,086**	

*Significant at the 0.05 level, two-sided test.

[a]These estimates are based on logistic regression models adjusted for age, gender, and country.

[b]These estimates are based on survival models adjusted for age-cohorts, gender, person-years, and country.

[c]These estimates are based on logistic regression models adjusted for time since PTSD onset, age of PTSD onset, gender, and country.

[d]Chi-square test of significant differences between blocks of socio-demographic variables.

[e]Denominator N: 71,083 = total sample; 3,072,041 = number of person-years in the survival models; 4,103 = number of lifetime PTSD cases; 2,086 = number of 12-month PTSD cases.

[f]Iraq is not included into the analysis related to exposure to TEs because the age of first exposure to TEs is not available in Iraq. Excluding Iraq, there were 49,339 people exposed to TEs and 3,963 people with PTSD.

Table 11.3 Comorbidity of posttraumatic stress disorder (PTSD) with other DSM-IV disorders, all countries combined

	PTSD cases with comorbid disorders									
	Mood disorder[a]		Anxiety disorder[b]		Disruptive behaviour/impulse-control disorder[c]		Substance-use disorder[d]		Any mental disorder[e]	
	%	SE	%	SE	%	SE	%	SE	%	SE
Lifetime comorbidity[f]										
Lifetime	**55.0**	1.1	**50.6**	1.2	**9.5**	0.5	**26.6**	1.0	**78.1**	1.1
12-month	**59.8**	1.6	**56.3**	1.6	**10.5**	0.8	**29.0**	1.3	**80.7**	1.5
12-month comorbidity[g]										
12-month	**38.3**	1.4	**42.9**	1.5	**6.5**	0.7	**9.0**	1.0	**60.3**	1.6
Temporal priority of PTSD[h]										
Lifetime	**35.6**	1.2	**22.3**	1.1	**41.8**	2.7	**48.2**	2.2	**23.7**	1.0
12-month	**34.0**	1.6	**20.4**	1.5	**40.7**	3.5	**45.6**	2.9	**20.4**	1.3

[a]Respondents with major depressive episode or bipolar spectrum disorder.
[b]Respondents with panic disorder, generalized anxiety disorder, social phobia, specific phobia, or separation anxiety disorder.
[c]Respondents with intermittent explosive disorder, attention deficit disorder, conduct disorder, oppositional defiant disorder, binge-eating disorder, or bulimia nervosa.
[d]Respondents with alcohol abuse with or without dependence or drug abuse with or without dependence.
[e]Respondents with any disorder listed above.
[f]Percentage of respondents with either lifetime or 12-month PTSD who also meet lifetime criteria for at least one of the other DSM-IV disorders.
[g]Percentage of respondents with 12-month PTSD who also meet 12-month criteria for at least one of the other disorders.
[h]Percentage of respondents with either lifetime or 12-month PTSD and at least one of the other disorders, whose AOO of PTSD is reported to be younger than the AOO of all comorbid disorders under consideration.

least one other DSM-IV disorder compared to 80.1% of those who meet the 12-month criteria for PTSD. Only 20.4% of 12-month PTSD respondents and 23.7% of lifetime respondents report PTSD onset before any other mental disorder. The most commonly reported comorbid disorders are mood disorder (55–59.8% lifetime comorbidity, 38.3% 12-month comorbidity) and anxiety disorders (50.6–56.3% lifetime comorbidity and 42.9% 12-month comorbidity). While only 9% of 12-month PTSD respondents meet the criteria for substance-use disorder, 45.6% of respondents report PTSD onset before substance-use disorder. Similarly, 6.5% of 12-month respondents meet the criteria for impulse-control disorder with 40.7% reporting PTSD as the first disorder of onset.

Treatment

The percentages of respondents with a diagnosis of 12-month PTSD reporting treatment across levels of impairment and treatment type are presented in Table 11.4. Overall, fewer than half of respondents report seeking any type of treatment. For any type of treatment, individuals in high-income countries were approximately twice as likely to seek treatment (53.5%) compared to low/lower-middle-income (22.8%) and upper-middle-income countries (28.7%). These disparities are observed across all treatment types with low/lower-middle-income country and upper-middle-income country respondents less likely to report treatment than high-income country respondents. The one exception was human services, which includes religious or spiritual advisors, social workers, and counsellors, where respondents in upper-middle income countries (2.5%) are significantly less likely to report treatment than low/lower-middle-income (7.1%) and high-income country respondents (7.0%) (F = 4.3, P = 0.01). For mental health treatment, where, averaged across countries, a quarter (25.3%) of those with PTSD report receiving mental health treatment in the past 12 months, only 3.2% of respondents in low/lower-middle-income countries report receiving mental health treatment.

Discussion

There are two limitations in the WMH surveys that should be considered when interpreting results about trauma exposure and PTSD. First, TE exposure and PTSD were assessed using retrospective reports, which may lead to underreporting of the lifetime prevalence of TE exposure and PTSD, as well as inaccuracies in AOO of PTSD symptoms. Second, while the WMH surveys used standardized instruments across all countries, cultural differences may have affected respondents' willingness to discuss sensitive issues especially stigmatizing TEs. We attempted to reduce underreporting of TEs by including an open-ended question on 'private' TEs that respondents did not want to describe; this was endorsed by 6.1% of the total sample.

The WMH surveys assessed a large representative sample within each of the countries using the same assessment instruments, which enabled us to estimate the 30-day prevalence in all countries in addition to 12-month and lifetime prevalences. For many countries, these will be the first reported 30-day prevalences of PTSD. Across all countries, we found that on average 4% of respondents have a lifetime diagnosis of PTSD, with prevalences ranging from 0.3% to 8.8%. Half of these respondents had symptoms in the 12 months prior to interview, which indicates a high level of disorder persistence, and among these respondents almost half reported symptoms in the 30 days prior to interview.

The decline in PTSD prevalence from 12-month to 30-day is, however, not likely due to full remittance of PTSD symptoms, but rather to individuals with lifetime PTSD having relapsing and remitting symptoms over the year rather than continuous symptoms, which is a course of PTSD that has been documented in several longitudinal studies (Osenbach *et al.* 2014; Bryant *et al.* 2015). The DSM-IV diagnostic system does not distinguish between those who fully remit and those whose symptoms are only sensitive to flaring up again with reminders. The 30-day prevalence of PTSD then, which represents the burden of PTSD at the specific time the survey was conducted, may underestimate the burden of PTSD.

The WMH surveys included several countries with recent mass violence and armed conflict including Iraq, Lebanon, and Northern Ireland. Counterintuitively, with the exception of Northern Ireland, these countries have lower lifetime prevalences of PTSD and rates of exposure to TEs than many non-conflict-affected countries. This result contradicts previous epidemiological studies of conflict-affected populations in Algeria, Cambodia, Ethiopia, and Gaza that used the CIDI to estimate lifetime PTSD prevalence rates and which found significantly higher rates ranging from 15.8% in Ethiopia to 37.4% in Algeria (de Jong *et al.* 2001). These prevalences, however, were based on population level

Table 11.4 Among those with 12-month posttraumatic stress disorder, percent reporting treatment in the past 12 months

Sector of treatment	Low/lower-middle-income countries		Upper-middle-income countries		High-income countries		All countries combined		Comparison between country income groups[a]
	%	SE	%	SE	%	SE	%	SE	
Specialty mental health[b]	**3.2**	1.9	**11.8**	2.7	**28.7**	1.6	**25.3**	1.3	$F_{2,v} = 27.8^*$, $P < 0.001$
General medical[c]	**14.5**	4.5	**16.8**	3.9	**36.0**	1.7	**32.4**	1.5	$F_{2,v} = 15.6^*$, $P < 0.001$
Health care[d]	**16.8**	4.6	**24.6**	4.3	**49.3**	1.8	**44.4**	1.6	$F_{2,v} = 23.6^*$, $P < 0.001$
Human services[e]	**7.1**	2.2	**2.5**	1.2	**7.0**	0.9	**6.4**	0.8	$F_{2,v} = 4.3^*$, $P = 0.01$
CAM[f]	–	–	**4.2**	2.1	**9.9**	1.0	**8.8**	0.9	$F_{2,v} = 12.3^*$, $P < 0.001$
Non-health care[g]	**7.6**	2.2	**6.6**	2.4	**14.7**	1.2	**13.3**	1.0	$F_{2,v} = 6.4^*$, $P < 0.001$
Any treatment[h]	**22.8**	5.5	**28.7**	4.6	**53.5**	1.8	**48.8**	1.6	$F_{2,v} = 19.9^*$, $P < 0.001$

*Significant at the 0.05 level, two-sided test.
A dash indicates low cell counts (<5 cases).
[a]Wald design-corrected F-tests were used to determine if there is variation in treatment estimates across country income groups. The denominator degree of freedom, v, is 5212.
[b]The mental health specialist sector, which includes psychiatrist and non-psychiatrist mental health specialists (psychiatrist, psychologist, or other non-psychiatrist mental health professional; social worker or counsellor in a mental health specialty setting; use of a mental health helpline; or overnight admissions for a mental health or drug or alcohol problems, with a presumption of daily contact with a psychiatrist).
[c]The general medical sector (general practitioner, other medical doctor, nurse, occupational therapist, or any healthcare professional).
[d]The mental health specialist sector or the general medical sector.
[e]The human services sector (religious or spiritual advisor or social worker or counsellor in any setting other than a specialty mental health setting).
[f]The CAM (complementary and alternative medicine) sector (any other type of healer such as herbalist or homeopath, participation in an internet support group, or participation in a self-help group).
[g]The human services sector or CAM.
[h]Any treatment listed above.

samples that were thought to be directly exposed to conflict, such as people living in refugee camps, resettlement zones, and regions that had been targeted in recent terrorist attacks. In addition, rather than pegging PTSD symptoms to a random or worst TE event, these studies assessed PTSD symptoms in relation to adverse events rather than specifically TEs. The combination of specifically targeting segments of a country's population affected by conflict and using a broad definition of trauma exposure may be driving some of the disparities in the literature on the prevalence of PTSD in conflict-affected countries.

While the PTSD prevalences presented here are based on the DSM-IV, factor analyses conducted in 13 WMH countries have shown that over 75% of those who are diagnosed with DSM-IV PTSD would also meet the DSM-5 criteria with few differences in socio-demographic, trauma-related, or prior lifetime risk factors for PTSD found between the two criteria sets (Stein *et al.* 2014). Similar concordance between DSM-IV and DSM-5 diagnoses has also been found in a study of US soldiers (Hoge *et al.* 2014), and in a study of US civilians that found the lifetime DSM-IV prevalence of PTSD only 1% higher than the DSM-5 prevalence (Kilpatrick *et al.* 2013). Thus while the prevalences of PTSD reported in this chapter may differ slightly from those found using DSM-5 criteria, the demographic correlates, comorbidities, and treatment-seeking behaviours would likely remain the same.

We found wide-variations in AOO across all countries and country income groups with PTSD onset occurring significantly earlier in high-income countries (median age 25–28) compared to low/lower-middle-income- (median age 43) and upper-middle-income countries (median age 30). These results confirm earlier reports that PTSD onset occurs later than in life than other anxiety and mood orders (Kessler *et al.* 2005, 2007). However, we note that the PTSD AOO curves contrast with the findings of an earlier WMH report for AOO of TE exposure, where incident TE exposure was more common among children, adolescents, and young adults (Benjet *et al.* 2016). While the difference in these two risks may imply that conditional risk for developing PTSD is higher in older adults exposed to trauma, results presented in this chapter show that younger respondents are at greater risk for developing PTSD. One possible reason for this discrepancy may be that younger people are more likely to be exposed to the types of TEs that have greater risk for the development of PTSD. Exploring this issue was beyond the scope of this chapter but we plan on addressing it in future analyses of WMH data.

We also examined socio-demographic correlates for associations with PTSD onset, persistence, and burden. We found that female gender and being divorced/separated or widowed were both associated with PTSD onset (lifetime prevalence) and burden (30-day prevalence), but not with course (disorder or symptom persistence). These differences across gender are consistent with a large literature on gender differences in risk for PTSD, which has found women are at increased risk for developing PTSD (Tolin & Foa 2006). We also found that being non-employed and having a lower household income, which are two measures of social disadvantage previously found to be associated with PTSD (Brewin *et al.* 2000), were both associated with PTSD onset, burden, and disorder persistence, but not with symptom persistence. Lower levels of educational attainment, which have also been associated with PTSD in past studies (Brewin *et al.* 2000), were only associated with PTSD onset and not with burden, disorder persistence, or symptom persistence. Our analyses do not allow determination of whether these socio-economic factors are risk factors for or consequences of the disorder. However, we can conclude that among the socially disadvantaged, PTSD is more prevalent and persistent.

We found that globally 78.1% of respondents with PTSD met lifetime criteria for at least one other mental disorder, with the most common comorbidities being mood and anxiety disorders. These findings are similar to an earlier report (Karam *et al.* 2014) that found PTSD be comorbid with mood and anxiety disorders with stronger associations among respondents reporting four or more TEs associated with their PTSD symptoms. In addition, while 23.7% of respondents with PTSD reported onset of PTSD symptoms prior to any other mental disorder, 48.2% reported PTSD onset before development of a substance-use disorder, which confirms PTSD as a significant risk factor for developing a substance-use disorder (Breslau *et al.* 2003; Koenen *et al.* 2006). One complicating factor not explored here is the role of trauma (both type and severity) in relation to both PTSD and comorbid disorder onset. PTSD has been found to predict multiple mental disorders, however, these associations have attenuated in the presence of control for TE type (Perkonigg *et al.* 2000).

Finally, our findings are also among the first reports of treatment seeking for PTSD in countries outside of the US and Western Europe. Across all countries, only half of all respondents reported seeking any type of treatment. We found that respondents in high-income countries were almost twice as likely to seek treatment as those in low/lower-middle- and upper-middle-income countries. These results extend the findings from a previous WMH report of 15 countries, which found significant variation in treatment during the year of disorder onset with 0.8% to 36.4% of respondents reporting treatment for anxiety disorders and a median delay of three to 30 years before treatment contact (Wang *et al.* 2007).

The WMH surveys show that half of PTSD is persistent, and among respondents reporting PTSD symptoms in the last 12 months only half are receiving any type of treatment. This gap in treatment is even larger in low/lower-middle-income countries and upper-middle-income countries where less than a quarter of respondents reported any kind of treatment. Our results indicate two potential targets for intervention. The first would be to reduce the high prevalence of TEs, which would result in a decreased prevalence of PTSD. However, as pointed out by Benjet *et al.*, the high prevalence of TEs show that experiencing trauma is a common and perhaps inescapable part of life (Benjet *et al.* 2016). A second and more reasonable target for intervention would be to reduce the psychological sequelae of trauma by increasing treatment seeking and treatment availability among those with PTSD. The low reported rates of treatment, especially among those in low/lower-income countries presents a clear target for reducing the burden of PTSD. We hope that the information contained in this chapter encourages policy-makers, researchers, and health care professionals to address these issues and decrease the global burden of PTSD.

Acknowledgements

Portions of the results appearing in this chapter appeared previously in: Koenen, K.C., Ratanatharathorn, A., Ng, L., McLaughlin, K., Bromet, E.J., Stein, D.J., Karam, E.G., Ruscio, A.M., Benjet, C., Scott, K.M., Atwoli, L., Petukhova, M., Lim, C.C.W., Aguilar-Gaxiola, S., Al-Hamzawi, A., Alonso, J., Bunting, B., Ciutan, M., de Girolamo, G., Degenhardt, L., Gureje, O., Haro, J.M., Huang, Y., Kawakami, N., Lee, S., Navarro-Mateu, F., Pennell, B. E., Piazza, M., Sampson, N., ten Have, M., Torres, Y., Viana, M.C., Williams, D., Xavier, M., Kessler, R.C., on behalf of the WHO World Mental Health Survey collaborators. (2017). Posttraumatic Stress Disorder in the World Mental Health Surveys. Psychological Medicine, 47, 2260–2274, used with permission from Cambridge University Press, 2016.

References

Alegria, M., Fortuna, L. R., Lin, J. Y., *et al.* (2013). Prevalence, risk, and correlates of posttraumatic stress disorder across ethnic and racial minority groups in the United States. *Medical Care*, 51, 1114–23.

Alhasnawi, S., Sadik, S., Rasheed, M., *et al.* (2009). The prevalence and correlates of DSM-IV disorders in the Iraq Mental Health Survey (IMHS). *World Psychiatry*, 8, 97–109.

American Psychiatric Association (2013). *Diagnostic and Statistical Manual of Mental Disorders, Fifth Edition.* Arlington, VA: American Psychiatric Publishing.

Atwoli, L., Stein, D. J., Williams, D. R., *et al.* (2013). Trauma and posttraumatic stress disorder in South Africa: analysis from the South African Stress and Health Study. *BMC Psychiatry*, 13, 182.

Benjet, C., Bromet, E., Karam, E., *et al.* (2016). The epidemiology of traumatic event exposure worldwide: results from the World Mental Health Survey Consortium. *Psychological Medicine*, 46, 327–43.

Breslau, N., Davis, G. C., & Schultz, L. R. (2003). Posttraumatic stress disorder and the incidence of nicotine, alcohol, and other drug disorders in persons who have experienced trauma. *Archives of General Psychiatry*, 60, 289–94.

Breslau, N., & Kessler, R. C. (2001). The stressor criterion in DSM-IV posttraumatic stress disorder: an empirical investigation. *Biological Psychiatry*, 50, 699–704.

Brewin, C. R., Andrews, B., & Valentine, J. D. (2000). Meta-analysis of risk factors for posttraumatic stress disorder in trauma-exposed adults. *Journal of Consulting and Clinical Psychology*, 68, 748–66.

Bryant, R. A., Nickerson, A., Creamer, M., *et al.*(2015). Trajectory of post-traumatic stress following traumatic injury: 6-year follow-up. *The British Journal of Psychiatry*, 206, 417–23.

de Jong, J. T., Komproe, I. H., Van Ommeren, M., *et al.* (2001). Lifetime events and posttraumatic stress disorder in 4 postconflict settings. *JAMA*, 286, 555–62.

Hauffa, R., Rief, W., Brahler, E., *et al.* (2011). Lifetime traumatic experiences and posttraumatic stress disorder in the German population: results of a representative population survey. *The Journal of Nervous and Mental Disease*, 199, 934–9.

Hoge, C. W., Riviere, L. A., Wilk, J. E., *et al.* (2014). The prevalence of post-traumatic stress disorder (PTSD) in US combat soldiers: a head-to-head comparison of DSM-5 versus DSM-IV-TR symptom criteria with the PTSD checklist. *The Lancet Psychiatry*, 1, 269–77.

Jeon, H. J., Suh, T., Lee, H. J., *et al.* (2007). Partial versus full PTSD in the Korean community: prevalence, duration, correlates, comorbidity, and dysfunctions. *Depression and Anxiety*, 24, 577–85.

Karam, E. G., Friedman, M. J., Hill, E. D., *et al.* (2014). Cumulative traumas and risk thresholds: 12-month PTSD in the World Mental Health (WMH) surveys. *Depression and Anxiety*, 31, 130–42.

Karam, E. G., Mneimneh, Z. N., Dimassi, H., *et al.* (2008). Lifetime prevalence of mental disorders in Lebanon: first onset, treatment, and exposure to war. *PLoS Medicine*, 5, e61.

Kessler, R. C. (2000). Posttraumatic stress disorder: the burden to the individual and to society. *Journal of Clinical Psychiatry*, 61 (Suppl 5), 4–12; discussion 13–14.

Kessler, R. C., Amminger, G. P., Aguilar-Gaxiola, S., *et al.* (2007). Age of onset of mental disorders: a review of recent literature. *Current Opinion in Psychiatry*, 20, 359–64.

Kessler, R. C., Berglund, P., Demler, O., *et al.* (2005). Lifetime prevalence and age-of-onset distributions of DSM-IV disorders in the National Comorbidity Survey Replication. *Archives of General Psychiatry*, 62, 593–602.

Kessler, R. C., & Üstün, T. B. (2004). The world mental health (WMH) survey initiative version of the world health organization (WHO) composite international diagnostic interview (CIDI). *International Journal of Methods in Psychiatric Research*, 13, 93–121.

Kilpatrick, D. G., Resnick, H. S., Milanak, M. E., *et al.* (2013). National estimates of exposure to traumatic events and PTSD prevalence using DSM-IV and DSM-5 criteria. *Journal of Traumatic Stress*, 26, 537–47.

Koenen, K. C., Hitsman, B., Lyons, M. J., *et al.* (2006). Posttraumatic stress disorder and late-onset smoking in the Vietnam era twin registry. *Journal of Consulting and Clinical Psychology*, 74, 186–90.

Osenbach, J. E., Lewis, C., Rosenfeld, B., *et al.* (2014). Exploring the longitudinal trajectories of posttraumatic stress disorder in injured trauma survivors. *Psychiatry*, 77, 386–97.

Perkonigg, A., Kessler, R. C., Storz, S., *et al.* (2000). Traumatic events and post-traumatic stress disorder in the community: prevalence, risk factors and comorbidity. *Acta Psychiatrica Scandinavica*, 101, 46–59.

Roberts, A. L., Gilman, S. E., Breslau, J., *et al.* (2011). Race/ethnic differences in exposure to traumatic events, development of post-traumatic stress disorder, and treatment-seeking for post-traumatic stress disorder in the United States. *Psychological Medicine*, 41, 71–83.

Stein, D. J., McLaughlin, K. A., Koenen, K. C., *et al.* (2014). DSM-5 and ICD-11 definitions of posttraumatic stress disorder: Investigating "narrow" and "broad" approaches. *Depression and Anxiety*, 31, 494–505.

Tolin, D. F., & Foa, E. B. (2006). Sex differences in trauma and posttraumatic stress disorder: a quantitative review of 25 years of research. *Psychological Bulletin*, 132, 959–92.

Van Ameringen, M., Mancini, C., Patterson, B., *et al.* (2008). Post-traumatic stress disorder in Canada. *CNS Neuroscience and Therapeutics*, 14, 171–81.

Wang, P. S., Angermeyer, M., Borges, G., *et al.* (2007). Delay and failure in treatment seeking after first onset of mental disorders in the World Health Organization's World Mental Health Survey Initiative. *World Psychiatry*, 6, 177–85.

Wang, P. S., Berglund, P., Olfson, M., *et al.*(2005). Failure and delay in initial treatment contact after first onset of mental disorders in the National Comorbidity Survey Replication. *Archives of General Psychiatry*, 62, 603–13.

World Health Organization (2014). *Mental Health Atlas*. Geneva: WHO Press.

Chapter 12

Separation Anxiety Disorder

Derrick Silove, Yanling He, Marina Piazza Ferrand, Kate M. Scott

Introduction

Separation anxiety disorder (SEPAD) has been characterized as "a dysfunctional exaggeration, both in duration and intensity, of the otherwise adaptive, physiological and self-limiting separation anxiety (SA) behaviour shared by most mammals" (Battaglia 2015). Although a common diagnosis amongst children attending specialist anxiety clinics in high-income countries (Last *et al.* 1987), SEPAD has not been routinely considered in making a diagnosis of an anxiety disorder in adults. Modifications to the criteria for SEPAD in DSM-5 therefore reflect a milestone by explicitly allowing onset and expression of the disorder to occur at any age in the life course. It is timely therefore, to assess key aspects of the epidemiology of SEPAD as it manifests in adulthood, a task we undertake by analysing pooled data from national population studies conducted across a wide range of countries worldwide.

Like its predecessor classification systems until that time, DSM-IV maintained the convention of restricting the onset of SEPAD to childhood (here used broadly to include children and adolescents up until the age of 18 years). Consistent with this emphasis, SEPAD was categorized as a disorder that usually manifests in childhood and adolescence. In DSM-5, three major changes were made to the criteria of SEPAD, including removal of the age-of-onset restriction, rewording symptoms so that they are applicable to adults and children, and relocating the category from the childhood disorders section to the general section of the anxiety disorders. By defining SEPAD as a disorder that can have its onset or expression at any point in the life course, DSM-5 has aligned the category with other common anxiety disorders such as panic disorder and agoraphobia.

It is important to consider why there has been such a long delay in acknowledging that SEPAD can manifest and indeed have its onset in adulthood. A tenet of attachment theory is that SA is quintessentially a response pattern shown by children, representing an age-dependent survival mechanism that protects the young from harm during the prolonged period of dependency on adult caretakers, usually the parents (Bowlby 1960; Milrod *et al.* 2014; Battaglia 2015). It makes sense that in the early phylogenesis of the species, when our ancestors lived in hunter-gatherer bands, the child's capacity to emit alarm signals (crying, clinging, searching) was essential to ensure that parents and other adult caregivers responded rapidly to the ever-present threats to children arising from predators or attack or abduction by other tribes. In keeping with this conceptualization of SA, descriptions of the pathological form, SEPAD, have emphasized the childhood characteristics of symptoms, core descriptors typically including clinging or shadowing parents; reluctance or refusal to attend school; protests at being left to sleep alone at night; tantrums at times of imminent separation; and non-verbal fears expressed in nightmares, drawings, and fantasy play, of being attacked or abducted by monsters or strangers.

An influential developmental theory of anxiety postulating a biological association between early SEPAD and later panic disorder-agoraphobia in adulthood further strengthened the canon that the former was a disorder restricted to childhood (Klein 1964, 1995; Silove *et al.* 1995a). The hypothesis was supported by early clinic studies reporting that adults with agoraphobia differed from those with other anxiety disorders in recounting high rates of school refusal (a proxy index of SA) in their early years (Klein 1964, 1995; Silove *et al.* 1995a; Kossowsky *et al.* 2013). In addition, laboratory studies have documented a common and distinctive pattern of arousal to carbon dioxide inhalation in individuals with SEPAD and panic disorder-agoraphobia (Battaglia *et al.* 2009; Roberson-Nay *et al.* 2010, 2013) a psychophysiological reaction that may reflect a common genetic diathesis underlying both sets of disorders (Battaglia *et al.* 2009).

Nevertheless, several lines of evidence have converged to challenge two of the conventional canons concerning SEPAD, that is, that the diagnosis should be limited to childhood, and that SEPAD is the early precursor of, and shares a common biological foundation with, later panic disorder-agoraphobia in adulthood. Clinical observations extending over the past two decades have identified SEPAD amongst adults and a substantial portion of these cases reported onset of the disorder after 18 years of age. Studies at clinics at the University of New South Wales in Australia, and later at the University of Pisa in Italy, recorded the phenomenology of SEPAD symptoms in adulthood, the foundation for developing measures to assess the disorder in a systematic and reliable manner (Manicavasagar *et al.* 2003; Pini *et al.* 2010). The core SEPAD concerns in adults were consistent with those of children in that they experienced overwhelming and unrealistic anxieties about the safety, health, and survival of attachment figures, coupled with fears of being personally abandoned, abducted or harmed in the absence of these persons. The surface features of symptoms in adults corresponded with their phase of maturation, anxieties often extending to a wider range of attachment figures (partners, children, friends) and contact being maintained in more subtle ways than in children, for example, by the use of pretexts to make repeated phone calls to close others throughout the day.

Clinic-based studies indicated that adult SEPAD may represent a continuation or recurrence of symptoms commencing in childhood, but in a substantial number of cases new onset of the disorder occurred after 18 years, a pattern not acknowledged in DSM-IV (Manicavasagar *et al.* 2000). Other findings from clinic studies include a greater prevalence of adult SEPAD amongst women, high levels of comorbidity with other anxiety disorders and depression, and a substantial degree of functional impairment associated with the disorder (Pini *et al.* 2010; Silove *et al.* 2010). Clinical impressions suggest that persons with SEPAD may not express their fears directly, are less likely than persons with other anxiety disorders to seek treatment, and are frequently misdiagnosed, commonly with primary panic disorder or agoraphobia (Milrod *et al.* 2014; Manicavasagar *et al.* 2016; Silove *et al.* 2016a). In addition, a recent review of the relevant literature found that although childhood SEPAD is associated with risk of later panic disorder-agoraphobia, the relationship may not be specific; instead, SEPAD in early life may be the harbinger of a range of other anxiety disorders in adulthood (Kossowsky *et al.* 2013). These studies did not take into account, however, the possibility of continuity or recurrence of childhood SEPAD in adulthood.

A limitation of the existing body of research investigating the adult form of SEPAD is that the vast majority of studies have been undertaken amongst clinic populations. The only exception is an epidemiological study undertaken in the United States, which offered important data, albeit limited to a high-income country, that SEPAD can have its onset in adulthood (Shear *et al.* 2006). An important next step, therefore, is to extend inquiry to a wider range of countries covering a diversity of socio-economic and cultural backgrounds. The inclusion of a module for assessing adult and (retrospectively assessed) child SEPAD in the Composite International Diagnostic Instrument (CIDI) used in the World Mental Health (WMH) surveys offers a unique opportunity to examine key aspects of SEPAD as it manifests across countries, both according to pooled data and by country income groups. In this chapter we focus specifically on the epidemiology of SEPAD, particularly the adult form. We assess the lifetime and 12-month prevalence of SEPAD, its age-of-onset across the life course, associations of the disorder with socio-demographic characteristics, comorbidity with other common disorders, and the extent and nature of associated functional impairment. Finally, we assess rates and types of help-seeking amongst those with SEPAD, stratified according to country income groups.

Method

SEPAD was assessed in 20 of the 29 WMH surveys included in this volume, 10 in high-income countries (Belgium, France, Germany, Italy, the Netherlands, Northern Ireland, Portugal, Spain, United States, Spain (Murcia)), 6 in upper-middle-income countries (Brazil, Bulgaria, Lebanon, Mexico, Romania, Colombia (Medellin)), and 4 in low/lower-middle-income countries (Colombia, Nigeria, the People's Republic of China (PRC)-Beijing/Shanghai, and Peru). A total of 44,304 respondents were assessed. As described in Chapter 3, the WMH interview was administered in two parts to reduce respondent burden. SEPAD was typically assessed in Part II but in some countries was assessed in Part I. In half the surveys the assessment of SEPAD was restricted to respondents in the age range 18–39 or 18–44 (Nigeria, PRC-Beijing/Shanghai, Lebanon, Belgium, France, Italy, the Netherlands, Spain, and Germany), while in the other surveys there was no such age restriction.

The CIDI module for SEPAD departed from DSM-IV in assessing lifetime onset of symptoms not only as of age 18 but also separately for onsets that occurred at ages 19 or later, thereby corresponding broadly with DSM-5 criteria. A SEPAD diagnosis required endorsement of at least three of the eight DSM-IV symptoms (listed below), having symptoms for at least one month, and experiencing associated clinically significant distress or role impairment. In DSM-IV, SEPAD is defined as a developmentally inappropriate and excessive anxiety concerning separation from home or from those to whom the individual is attached, the wording of items being modified slightly in DSM-5. For a diagnosis (according to DSM-IV), three (or more) of the following symptoms need to be present:

- recurrent excessive distress when separation from home or major attachment figures occurs or is anticipated;
- persistent and excessive worry about losing, or about possible harm befalling, major attachment figures;
- persistent and excessive worry that an untoward event will lead to separation from a major attachment figure (e.g. getting lost or kidnapped);
- reluctance or refusal to go to school or elsewhere because of fear of separation;
- persistently and excessively fearful or reluctant to be alone or without major attachment figures at home or without significant adults in other settings;
- persistent reluctance or refusal to go to sleep without being near a major attachment figure or to sleep away from home;
- repeated nightmares involving the theme of separation;
- repeated complaints of physical symptoms (such as headaches, stomachaches, nausea, or vomiting) when separation from major attachment figures occurs or is anticipated.

As noted earlier, in this chapter we predominantly focus on adult SEPAD but we also report some data for 'adult and child' (i.e., total) SEPAD. The definition of total SEPAD is broadly consistent with the DSM-5 definition of SEPAD, which has removed the age-of-onset criterion, noting however that it is recommended in DSM-5 that the duration of symptoms for adult diagnosis should be six months.

Results

Prevalence and Persistence

The lifetime prevalence of adult SEPAD is 3.1% for all countries combined, and does not significantly vary across countries grouped by income level. It does vary significantly across individual countries and survey sites, ranging from 0.1% in Nigeria and the Murcia region of Spain up to 7.9% in Colombia (Table 12.1). Twelve-month and 30-day prevalence of adult SEPAD are much lower than lifetime prevalence, being 1.0% and 0.4%, respectively, in all countries combined, and consistent with this the current burden of SEPAD in the population (represented by 30-day prevalence) is not high. The 12-month/lifetime column is a proxy indicator of disorder persistence, and at 30.8% in all countries combined this is not high – for most other mental disorders this figure is around 50–60% (see Chapter 22). The 30-day/12-month column indicates that 42.7% of those with episodes in the past 12 months are still symptomatic at the time of interview, which indicates an intermediate level of episode persistence. When child SEPAD is also included (final column of Table 12.1), the lifetime prevalence of the disorder as a whole increases by approximately 50% to 4.6%, though again with significant variation across countries. This figure is at slight variance with the prevalence reported in prior WMH publications (Silove *et al.* 2015) because of the inclusion of additional countries and other minor differences in the present analysis. The projected lifetime risk of adult SEPAD is slightly higher (5.0%) than the lifetime prevalence (4.6%) (data not shown).

Age-of-Onset

Adult SEPAD typically begins in early adulthood, with median onset at age 27 in all countries combined (interquartile range [IQR] of 19–40 years. The median age-of-onset (AOO) is similar across country income groups although there is substantial variation across individual countries and survey sites (Figure 12.1). A third (33%) of adult cases have their onset in childhood suggesting that a sizeable minority experience an early onset and show persistence of the disorder over an extended period of time into later life. The data also support previous findings that the majority of adult cases have onset after 18 years of age. It is noteworthy that 25% of adult onsets occur amongst those aged 40 years and older indicating that, although not the

Table 12.1 Prevalence of DSM-IV separation anxiety disorder (SEPAD) in the World Mental Health surveys

Country	Adult SEPAD										Adult and child SEPAD		Sample size used for	
	Lifetime prevalence		12-month prevalence		30-day prevalence		12-month prevalence of SEPAD among lifetime cases		30-day prevalence of SEPAD among 12-month cases		Lifetime prevalence		Adult SEPAD	Adult and Child SEPAD
	%	SE	%	SE	%	SE	%	SE	%	SE	%	SE		
Low/lower-middle-income countries	**3.4**	**0.3**	**1.1**	**0.2**	**0.4**	**0.1**	**31.9**	**3.4**	**40.1**	**8.2**	**5.6**	**0.4**	**7,953**	**5,955**
Colombia	7.9	0.8	2.7	0.5	1.3	0.5	33.8	4.5	47.9	9.7	9.8	0.8	2,381	2,381
Nigeria[a,b]	0.1	0.0	<0.1	0.0	–	–	13.4	13.5	–	–	0.2	0.1	2,143	1,203
Peru	4.1	0.5	1.2	0.2	0.2	0.1	28.6	4.6	18.2	9.2	6.1	0.7	1,801	1,801
PRC (Beijing/Shanghai)[b]	0.5	0.2	0.1	0.1	<0.1	0.0	22.0	12.6	26.9	20.5	1.4	0.5	1,628	570
Upper-middle-income countries	**3.2**	**0.2**	**1.1**	**0.1**	**0.6**	**0.1**	**35.0**	**2.7**	**51.3**	**4.2**	**4.7**	**0.2**	**16,281**	**15,845**
Brazil	5.3	0.3	2.0	0.3	1.2	0.2	38.5	4.3	59.4	5.8	7.7	0.4	5,037	5,037
Bulgaria	1.2	0.4	0.4	0.3	0.1	0.1	34.7	15.6	32.5	15.2	1.4	0.4	2,233	2,233
Colombia (Medellin)	3.3	0.4	0.9	0.2	0.3	0.1	26.4	5.0	33.1	10.0	4.7	0.6	3,261	3,261
Lebanon[b]	4.6	0.9	1.6	0.3	0.5	0.2	34.9	6.2	28.9	8.2	7.0	1.3	1,031	595
Mexico	2.7	0.3	0.9	0.2	0.5	0.1	34.2	5.0	54.9	8.2	4.5	0.4	2,362	2,362
Romania	0.7	0.3	0.3	0.1	0.2	0.1	36.3	12.3	75.2	18.0	0.9	0.3	2,357	2,357
High-income countries	**2.9**	**0.2**	**0.8**	**0.1**	**0.3**	**0.0**	**27.1**	**1.8**	**35.3**	**3.5**	**4.3**	**0.2**	**22,504**	**22,504**
Belgium[b]	0.5	0.2	0.2	0.1	0.1	0.1	27.4	18.2	31.7	19.7	1.5	0.3	1,133	1,133
France[b]	2.0	0.4	0.9	0.3	0.1	0.1	48.3	14.2	6.7	6.7	3.6	0.6	1,398	1,398
Germany[b]	1.6	0.4	0.5	0.2	–	–	28.8	11.8	–	–	2.1	0.4	1,653	1,653
Italy[b]	0.5	0.2	<0.1	0.0	–	–	7.4	7.4	–	–	1.5	0.4	2,282	2,282
Northern Ireland	3.5	0.5	0.4	0.1	0.3	0.1	11.7	3.5	66.3	13.9	5.1	0.5	1,986	1,986
Portugal	5.6	0.8	1.2	0.3	0.3	0.1	21.1	5.0	24.4	6.6	6.4	0.8	2,060	2,060
Spain[b]	0.5	0.1	0.3	0.1	0.1	0.1	51.2	14.0	30.2	18.3	1.3	0.3	2,617	2,617
Spain (Murcia)[a]	0.1	0.1	–	–	–	–	–	–	–	–	0.5	0.2	2,621	2,621
Netherlands[b]	1.2	0.5	0.6	0.4	0.4	0.3	50.9	20.9	70.8	22.0	3.1	0.6	1,062	1,062
United States	6.6	0.3	1.9	0.2	0.8	0.1	28.9	1.9	39.6	4.3	9.2	0.4	5,692	5,692

Table 12.1 (*cont.*)

Country	Adult SEPAD										Adult and child SEPAD		Sample size used for	
	Lifetime prevalence		12-month prevalence		30-day prevalence		12-month prevalence of SEPAD among life-time cases		30-day prevalence of SEPAD among 12-month cases		Lifetime prevalence		Adult SEPAD	Adult and Child SEPAD
	%	SE	%	SE	%	SE	%	SE	%	SE	%	SE		
All countries combined	**3.1**	**0.1**	**1.0**	**0.1**	**0.4**	**0.0**	**30.8**	**1.5**	**42.7**	**2.7**	**4.6**	**0.1**	**46,738**	**44,304**
WHO regions[c]														
Region of the Americas	5.2	0.2	1.7	0.1	0.8	0.1	32.2	1.7	46.1	3.1	7.4	0.2	20,534	20,534
African region	0.1	0.0	<0.1	0.0	–	–	13.4	13.5	–	–	0.2	0.1	2,143	1,203
Western Pacific region	0.5	0.2	0.1	0.1	<0.1	0.0	22.0	12.6	26.9	20.5	1.4	0.5	1,628	570
Eastern Mediterranean region	4.6	0.9	1.6	0.3	0.5	0.2	34.9	6.2	28.9	8.2	7.0	1.3	1,031	595
Western European region	1.7	0.1	0.4	0.1	0.1	0.0	24.7	3.4	28.6	6.1	2.7	0.2	16,812	16,812
Eastern European region	0.9	0.2	0.3	0.2	0.2	0.1	35.3	10.7	49.5	17.7	1.1	0.3	4,590	4,590
Comparison between countries[d]	**$F_{19,v} = 41.7$*, $P < 0.001$**		**$F_{19,v} = 17.7$*, $P < 0.001$**		**$F_{19,v} = 8.8$*, $P < 0.001$**		**$F_{19,v} = 1.7$*, $P = 0.033$**		**$F_{19,v} = 2.4$*, $P = 0.001$**		**$F_{19,v} = 42.2$*, $P < 0.001$**			
Comparison between low-, middle-, and high-income country groups[d]	**$F_{2,v} = 2.1$, $P = 0.120$**		**$F_{2,v} = 4.7$*, $P = 0.010$**		**$F_{2,v} = 7.5$*, $P = 0.001$**		**$F_{2,v} = 3.0$, $P = 0.050$**		**$F_{2,v} = 4.2$*, $P = 0.016$**		**$F_{2,v} = 5.3$* $P = 0.005$**			
Comparison between WHO regions[d]	**$F_{5,v} = 138.9$*, $P < 0.001$**		**$F_{5,v} = 52.8$*, $P < 0.001$**		**$F_{5,v} = 22.0$*, $P < 0.001$**		**$F_{5,v} = 1.1$, $P = 0.339$**		**$F_{5,v} = 1.9$, $P = 0.086$**		**$F_{5,v} = 131.1$*, $P < 0.001$**			

*Significant at the 0.05 level, two-sided test.
[a]Further analyses involving adult SEPAD excluded Nigeria and Murcia due to small number of lifetime cases (<5 cases) in both surveys.
[b]Assessment of SEPAD was restricted to respondents in the age range 18–39 or 18–44.
[c]**Region of the Americas** (Colombia, Mexico, Brazil, Peru, United States, Colombia (Medellin)); **Western Pacific region** (PRC: Beijing and Shanghai); **Eastern Mediterranean region** (Lebanon); **African region** (Nigeria); **Western European region** (Belgium, France, Germany, Italy, Netherlands, Northern Ireland, Spain, Spain (Murcia), Portugal); **Eastern European region** (Romania, Bulgaria).
[d]Wald design-corrected F-tests were used to determine if there is variation in prevalence estimates across countries. The denominator degree of freedom, v, is 956.
PRC: People's Republic of China.

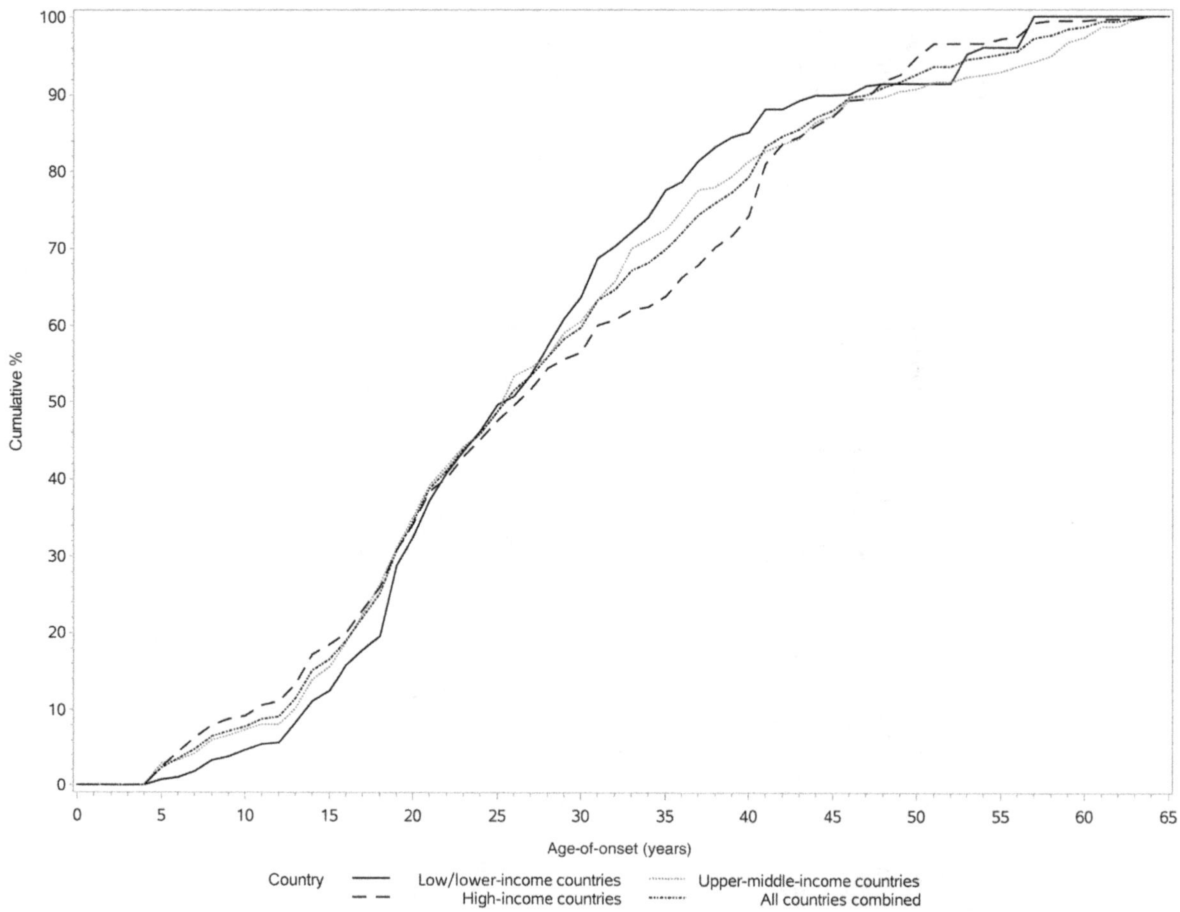

Figure 12.1 Cumulative age-of-onset distributions of adult SEPAD, by country income groups and in all countries combined.

most common age period of onset, the disorder can occur for the first time in middle to later life.

When considering adult and child SEPAD together, the AOO distribution shows somewhat more (although still not pronounced) variation across country income groups (Figure 12.2), with median AOO in the high teenage years in high- and upper-middle-income countries and in the early-20s in low/lower-middle-income countries. As would be expected for a disorder with both child and adult onset, the interquartile range of the AOO distribution for total SEPAD is quite wide (9–33 years in all countries combined). Taken together, these findings further support the removal of the age 18 upper AOO restriction for diagnosis in DSM-5, confirming that SEPAD can occur for the first time across a wide age range extending well into the adult years.

Role Impairment

The small numbers of SEPAD cases makes estimates unstable in several countries so that the averages across all countries, or in country income groups, are a better guide to impairment associated with adult SEPAD. The proportion of those with 12-month adult SEPAD who report severe impairment in at least one domain varies significantly from 19.0% in low/lower-middle-income countries to 39.9% and 46.3% in upper-middle and high-income countries respectively, suggesting that in the latter two country income groups SEPAD is a moderately impairing disorder. Severe impairment is reported significantly more frequently in the social (25.4%) and relationship (24.8%) than in the work (20.0%) and home (18.7%) domains, a differential pattern that is accentuated in high-income countries.

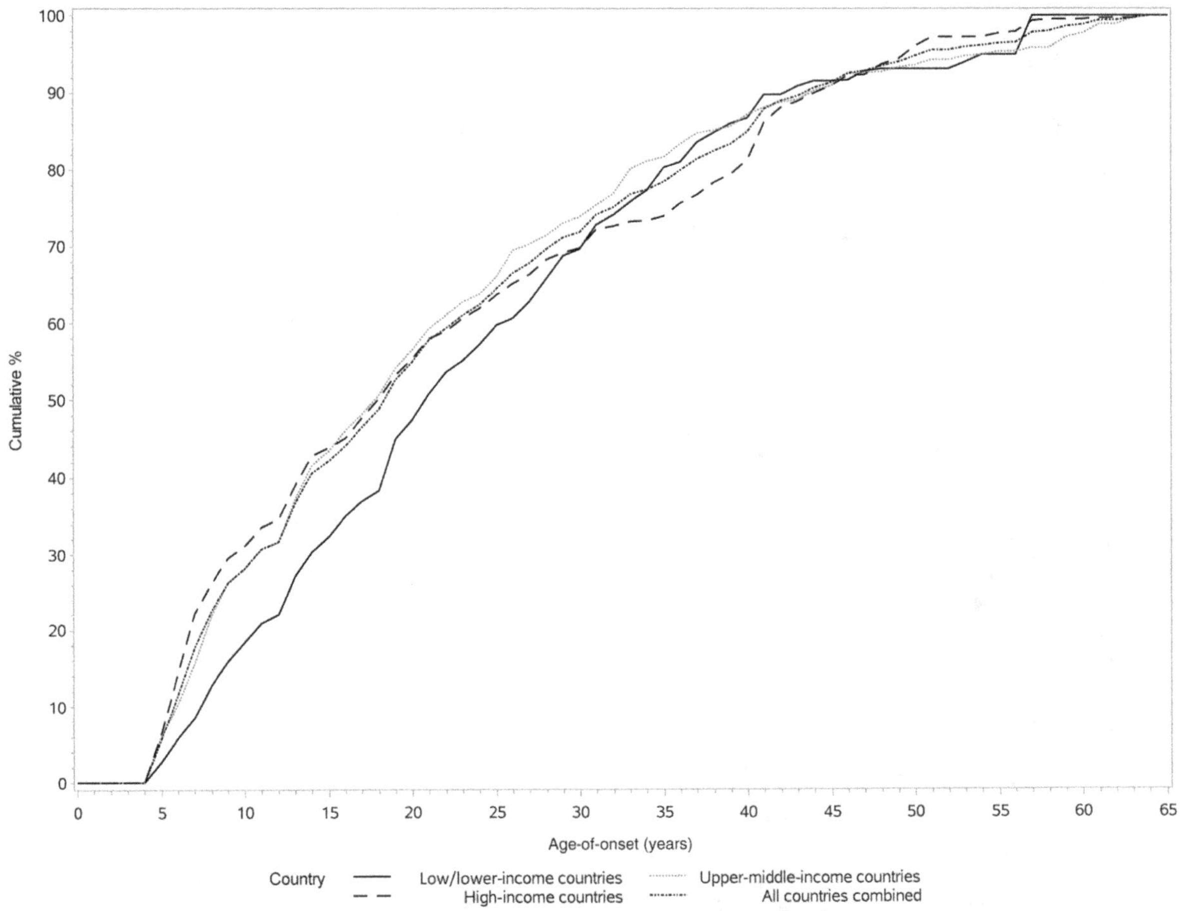

Figure 12.2 Cumulative age-of-onset distributions of total (child + adult) SEPAD, by country income groups and in all countries combined.

Socio-demographic Correlates

In all countries combined, the socio-demographic pattern of total (child and adult combined) SEPAD is similar to that for adult SEPAD. Many of the correlates are only relevant for adults, so we focus here on adult SEPAD. As shown in the third column of Table 12.3, the odds of lifetime adult SEPAD are higher among younger adults, women, the unemployed (though interestingly, not among homemakers), the divorced or separated, those with lower educational attainment (a strong graded pattern for education), and those with lower income. These same patterns are evident for 30-day SEPAD (first column of Table 12.3) so this means that the current burden of SEPAD in the population is more pronounced among those generally considered to be the most vulnerable members of society (young adults, the less well educated, the unemployed, the divorced or separated, and those with least income). However, it is interesting to note that almost none of these socio-demographic correlates are associated with disorder persistence (12-month/lifetime), with the one exception of low household income, nor are any of these socio-demographic factors associated with episode persistence (30-day/12-month). So although general socio-economic vulnerability increases odds of *onset* of SEPAD, it exerts much less influence on the *course* of SEPAD (recurrence and persistence of episodes) once the disorder manifests.

Being female is associated with higher SEPAD onset, a consistent finding across the three country income groups. In contrast, some of the other socio-demographic correlates show greater variation, for

Table 12.2 Severity of role impairment by the Sheehan Disability Scale associated with 12-month adult separation anxiety disorder (SEPAD), by country

Country	Proportion with severe role impairment (SDS score: 7–10)										Number of 12-month adult SEPAD cases
	Home		Work		Relationship		Social		Any[a]		
	%	SE	%	SE	%	SE	%	SE	%	SE	
Low/lower-middle-income countries	**7.3**	**2.7**	**10.2**	**3.4**	**13.5**	**3.7**	**10.9**	**3.2**	**19.0**	**4.5**	**126**
Colombia	8.4	3.6	10.7	4.3	15.3	4.9	11.7	4.1	21.2	6.2	89
Peru	4.3	4.1	9.2	5.5	9.1	5.1	9.1	5.1	14.1	5.3	31
PRC (Beijing/Shanghai)	6.5	7.3	4.9	5.4	4.9	5.4	4.9	5.4	4.9	5.4	6
Upper-middle-income countries	**18.7**	**3.4**	**22.1**	**4.3**	**24.2**	**4.1**	**25.8**	**4.1**	**39.9**	**4.2**	**241**
Brazil	26.8	5.3	26.8	6.7	27.8	5.9	28.0	6.2	42.5	5.8	111
Bulgaria	20.2	15.8	20.2	15.8	38.3	21.8	64.2	18.7	68.1	18.3	8
Colombia(Medellin)	11.4	5.1	10.0	4.8	16.3	8.9	14.0	8.8	26.3	9.8	35
Lebanon	7.5	5.3	45.2	13.6	27.0	9.7	45.4	10.6	66.0	10.1	33
Mexico	3.1	1.8	12.7	5.5	17.4	7.6	13.0	5.2	28.7	7.8	47
Romania	5.7	6.1	5.7	6.1	5.7	6.1	5.7	6.1	5.7	6.1	7
High-income countries	**24.2**	**3.3**	**22.9**	**4.0**	**31.1**	**4.0**	**32.3**	**3.8**	**46.3**	**4.1**	**249**
Belgium	–	–	–	–	–	–	–	–	–	–	3
France	12.3	9.6	3.0	3.1	3.0	3.1	6.3	4.3	15.6	9.8	10
Germany	–	–	18.0	16.8	46.8	24.2	46.8	24.2	46.8	24.2	6
Italy	–	–	–	–	–	–	–	–	–	–	1
Northern Ireland	32.8	12.1	34.1	13.5	45.0	13.2	55.7	12.4	61.9	11.9	16
Portugal	23.2	6.2	15.4	5.4	32.0	11.6	20.7	5.0	40.8	12.2	45
Spain	25.1	20.9	25.1	20.9	31.9	21.1	31.9	21.1	31.9	21.1	7
Netherlands	83.4	16.8	92.7	8.4	70.8	22.0	70.8	22.0	83.4	16.8	5
United States	22.4	3.2	22.6	5.0	29.2	4.5	33.5	4.6	48.1	5.0	156
All countries combined	**18.7**	**2.0**	**20.0**	**2.5**	**24.8**	**2.5**	**25.4**	**2.4**	**38.3**	**2.7**	**616**
WHO regions											
Region of the Americas	17.6	2.2	18.9	2.9	23.1	2.7	23.3	2.7	36.2	3.0	469
Western Pacific region	6.5	7.3	4.9	5.4	4.9	5.4	4.9	5.4	4.9	5.4	6
Eastern Mediterranean region	7.5	5.3	45.2	13.6	27.0	9.7	45.4	10.6	66.0	10.1	33
Western European region	27.2	6.5	23.3	6.6	33.7	7.3	30.5	6.5	43.7	7.3	93
Eastern European region	11.8	8.1	11.8	8.1	19.5	11.8	30.5	14.8	32.1	15.0	15
Comparison between countries[b]	**$F_{17,v}$ = 2.5*, P = 0.001**		**$F_{17,v}$ = 1.2, P = 0.251**		**$F_{17,v}$ = 1.5, P = 0.087**		**$F_{17,v}$ = 2.5*, P = 0.001**		**$F_{17,v}$ = 2.5*, P = 0.001**		
Comparison between low-, middle-, and high-income countries[b]	**$F_{2,v}$ = 5.6*, P = 0.004**		**$F_{2,v}$ = 2.7, P = 0.065**		**$F_{2,v}$ = 3.9*, P = 0.021**		**$F_{2,v}$ = 6.5*, P = 0.002**		**$F_{2,v}$ = 5.9*, P = 0.003**		
Comparison between WHO regions[b]	**$F_{4,v}$ = 1.4, P = 0.240**		**$F_{4,v}$ = 1.2, P = 0.307**		**$F_{4,v}$ = 0.9, P = 0.438**		**$F_{4,v}$ = 1.6, P = 0.165**		**$F_{4,v}$ = 2.0, P = 0.098**		

*Significant at the 0.05 level, two-sided test.
A dash indicates low cell count <5.
[a]Highest severity category across four SDS role domains.
[b]Wald design-corrected F-tests were used to determine if there is variation in impairment severity across countries. The denominator degree of freedom, v, is 887.
PRC: People's Republic of China.

Table 12.3 **Bivariate associations between socio-demographic correlates and DSM-IV separation anxiety disorder (SEPAD), all countries combined**

Correlates	30-day adult SEPAD[a]		Lifetime adult and child SEPAD[b]		Lifetime adult SEPAD[b]		12-month adult SEPAD among lifetime cases[c]		30-day adult SEPAD among 12-month cases[c]	
	OR	(95% CI)	OR	(95% CI)	OR	(95% CI)	OR	(95% CI)	OR	(95% CI)
Age-cohort										
18–29	**6.6***	(3.4–12.8)	**5.1***	(3.8–6.9)	**13.1***	(8.8–19.4)				
30–44	**4.6***	(2.4–9.0)	**4.6***	(3.4–6.1)	**6.8***	(4.7–9.8)				
45–59	**2.5***	(1.2–5.1)	**3.0***	(2.0–4.1)	**3.4***	(2.4–4.8)				
60+	**1.0**		**1.0**		**1.0**					
Age-cohort difference[d]	$\chi^2_3 = 39.9^*, P < 0.001$		$\chi^2_3 = 144.9^*, P < 0.001$		$\chi^2_3 = 227.6^*, P < 0.001$					
Age-of-onset										
Early							**1.1**	(0.8–1.6)	**1.3**	(0.6–2.8)
Early-average							**1.0**	(0.7–1.5)	**1.0**	(0.5–1.9)
Late-average							**0.8**	(0.6–1.2)	**1.1**	(0.5–2.3)
Late							**1.0**		**1.0**	
Age-of-onset difference[d]							$\chi^2_3 = 2.3, P = 0.513$		$\chi^2_3 = 1.0, P = 0.812$	
Time since onset (continuous)							**0.95***	(0.94–0.97)	**0.98**	(0.95–1.00)
Gender										
Female	**1.5***	(1.1–2.2)	**1.4***	(1.2–1.7)	**1.4***	(1.2–1.5)	**1.1**	(0.8–1.4)	**1.2**	(0.8–1.7)
Male	**1.0**		**1.0**		**1.0**		**1.0**		**1.0**	
Gender difference[d]	$\chi^2_1 = 6.1^*, P = 0.014$		$\chi^2_1 = 23.3^*, P < 0.001$		$\chi^2_1 = 28.4^*, P < 0.001$		$\chi^2_1 = 0.1, P = 0.744$		$\chi^2_1 = 0.6, P = 0.444$	
Employment status										
Student	**2.0**	(0.8–5.0)	**1.2**	(0.9–1.6)	**1.4**	(1.0–2.0)	**1.3**	(0.6–2.6)	**2.8**	(1.0–8.2)
Homemaker	**1.2**	(0.7–2.0)	**1.1**	(0.9–1.3)	**1.1**	(0.9–1.3)	**1.2**	(0.8–1.7)	**1.0**	(0.5–2.1)
Retired	**0.5**	(0.2–1.2)	**0.8**	(0.5–1.1)	**0.9**	(0.6–1.3)	**0.7**	(0.3–1.5)	**0.8**	(0.2–3.2)
Other	**1.6***	(1.0–2.6)	**1.6***	(1.4–1.9)	**1.7***	(1.5–2.1)	**1.1**	(0.8–1.5)	**1.2**	(0.7–2.0)
Employed	**1.0**		**1.0**		**1.0**		**1.0**		**1.0**	
Employment status difference[d]	$\chi^2_4 = 8.7, P = 0.069$		$\chi^2_4 = 39.7^*, P < 0.001$		$\chi^2_4 = 41.7^*, P < 0.001$		$\chi^2_4 = 2.6, P = 0.634$		$\chi^2_4 = 3.9, P = 0.423$	
Marital status										
Never married	**0.9**	(0.6–1.4)	**1.0**	(0.9–1.2)	**1.2**	(1.0–1.3)	**1.3**	(0.9–1.8)	**1.0**	(0.6–1.8)
Divorced/separated/widowed	**2.1***	(1.3–3.3)	**1.3***	(1.1–1.5)	**1.6***	(1.4–1.9)	**1.2**	(0.8–1.7)	**1.2**	(0.6–2.2)
Currently married	**1.0**		**1.0**		**1.0**		**1.0**		**1.0**	
Marital status difference[d]	$\chi^2_2 = 10.7^*, P = 0.005$		$\chi^2_2 = 7.4^*, P = 0.025$		$\chi^2_2 = 30.7^*, P < 0.001$		$\chi^2_2 = 2.4, P = 0.295$		$\chi^2_2 = 0.2, P = 0.898$	

(cont.)

Table 12.3 (*cont.*)

Correlates	30-day adult SEPAD[a]		Lifetime adult and child SEPAD[b]		Lifetime adult SEPAD[b]		12-month adult SEPAD among lifetime cases[c]		30-day adult SEPAD among 12-month cases[c]	
	OR	(95% CI)	OR	(95% CI)	OR	(95% CI)	OR	(95% CI)	OR	(95% CI)
Education level										
No education	**4.1***	(1.2–14.3)	**2.1**	(0.8–5.2)	**2.3**	(0.9–6.0)	**2.6**	(0.8–8.5)	**1.6**	(0.3–8.3)
Some primary	**2.3**	(0.9–5.8)	**1.5***	(1.1–1.9)	**2.0***	(1.5–2.5)	**1.6**	(0.9–3.0)	**0.9**	(0.3–2.3)
Finished primary	**2.0**	(0.8–4.8)	**1.6***	(1.2–2.2)	**2.0***	(1.5–2.6)	**1.5**	(0.8–2.6)	**0.8**	(0.3–2.0)
Some secondary	**3.9***	(1.9–8.1)	**1.7***	(1.3–2.1)	**2.4***	(1.9–3.0)	**1.7***	(1.0–2.9)	**1.6**	(0.7–3.7)
Finished secondary	**2.0***	(1.1–3.8)	**1.3***	(1.1–1.6)	**1.7***	(1.4–2.0)	**1.4**	(0.8–2.2)	**1.5**	(0.7–3.2)
Some college	**2.4***	(1.2–4.9)	**1.2**	(0.9–1.4)	**1.3***	(1.1–1.6)	**1.5**	(0.9–2.5)	**2.3**	(0.9–5.6)
Finished college	**1.0**		**1.0**		**1.0**		**1.0**		**1.0**	
Education level difference[d]	$\chi^2_6 = 14.9^*, P = 0.021$		$\chi^2_6 = 24.1^*, P = 0.001$		$\chi^2_6 = 68.0^*, P < 0.001$		$\chi^2_6 = 5.5, P = 0.483$		$\chi^2_6 = 6.3, P = 0.393$	
Household income										
Low	**1.5**	(0.9–2.5)	**1.2**	(1.0–1.5)	**1.2***	(1.0–1.4)	**1.9***	(1.3–2.8)	**0.9**	(0.5–1.6)
Low-average	**1.5**	(0.9–2.3)	**1.3***	(1.1–1.6)	**1.3***	(1.1–1.5)	**1.2**	(0.8–1.8)	**1.0**	(0.6–1.8)
High-average	**1.1**	(0.7–1.6)	**1.1**	(1.0–1.3)	**1.0**	(0.9–1.2)	**1.1**	(0.8–1.5)	**1.2**	(0.6–2.3)
High	**1.0**		**1.0**		**1.0**		**1.0**	–	**1.0**	
Household income difference[d]	$\chi^2_3 = 4.2, P = 0.241$		$\chi^2_3 = 9.3^*, P = 0.025$		$\chi^2_3 = 11.5^*, P = 0.009$		$\chi^2_3 = 13.5^*, P = 0.004$		$\chi^2_3 = 0.6, P = 0.909$	
N[e]	**41,974**		**1,618,746**		**1,669,321**		**1,993**		**616**	

*Significant at the 0.05 level, two-sided test.
[a]These estimates are based on logistic regression models adjusted for age, gender, and country.
[b]These estimates are based on survival models adjusted for age-cohorts, gender, person-years, and country.
[c]These estimates are based on logistic regression models adjusted for time since SEPAD onset, age of SEPAD onset, gender, and country.
[d]Chi-square test of significant differences between blocks of socio-demographic variables.
[e]Denominator N: 41,974 = total sample; 1,618,746 and 1,669,321 = number of person-years in the survival models; 1,993 = number of lifetime SEPAD cases; 616 = number of 12-month SEPAD cases.

example, education is more strongly associated with SEPAD onset in low/lower-middle-income countries whereas household income is only associated with SEPAD onset in high-income countries. Another notable difference is that being unmarried is associated with both onset and persistence of adult SEPAD in high-income countries, but these associations are not apparent in the other two country income groups (data not shown).

Comorbidity

As shown in Table 12.4, the majority (78.5%) of respondents with lifetime SEPAD meet criteria for at least one other lifetime disorder, a pattern that is consistent with most other anxiety disorder subtypes. Not surprisingly, anxiety disorders are the most common class of comorbid disorder (58.1% of those with SEPAD have a comorbid anxiety disorder at some stage in their lives) and mood disorders are the next most common comorbidity (52% have a lifetime comorbid mood disorder). Lifetime comorbidity for adult SEPAD is much lower with disruptive behaviour/impulse-control disorders (19.1%) and substance-use disorders (25.9%), consistent with SEPAD's categorization as an internalizing disorder. Patterns of 12-month comorbidity are similar to lifetime comorbidity, with nearly three-quarters (72.3%) of respondents with 12-month SEPAD meeting criteria for at least one other disorder at the same time.

As might be expected, adult and childhood SEPAD differ in the pattern of onset of comorbid disorders. Lifetime comorbid disorders usually precede onset of adult SEPAD, with only 17.7% of adult SEPAD occurring prior to the comorbid disorder. In contrast, childhood onset SEPAD precedes the onset of most comorbid disorders, the exceptions being specific phobia and social anxiety disorder.

Treatment

Only a fairly small proportion of those with 12-month adult SEPAD report seeking external help, with 27.7% reporting treatment in the health care sector (Appendix Table 12A.1) and 30.9% reporting any kind of help-seeking (from health or non-health care sectors). Those with more severe SEPAD are more likely to seek treatment. Similar proportions of those who seek help report treatment from specialist mental health services as from general medical health care. Help-seeking is lowest in low/lower-middle-income countries, with 17.6% of those with 12-month adult SEPAD in these countries seeking help from either health or non-health care sectors, with the corresponding proportions being 23.8% and 44.5% in upper-middle- and high-income countries, respectively.

Discussion

The findings presented in this chapter have several limitations, including variation in response rates across countries, use of a fully structured diagnostic interview which precludes clinical probing to confirm diagnoses, and the retrospective reporting of childhood SEPAD and its AOO. Although we used the DSM-IV one-month duration requirement rather than the recommended (although not mandated) DSM-5 six-month duration in defining adult SEPAD, overestimation of prevalence in relation to the latter diagnostic system is likely to be slight. Recall bias is a more serious concern, as this might have led to an underestimation of lifetime prevalence among remitted cases and an overestimation of persistence, even though the WMH surveys used special probing strategies designed to improve accuracy of recall (see Chapter 3) and in some countries limited the duration of recall by assessing SEPAD only among respondents younger than age 45. If biases exist, SEPAD is a more prevalent lifetime disorder with a lower persistence than suggested by the WMH results.

The lifetime prevalence of 3.1% makes adult SEPAD a moderately prevalent disorder when compared with the other anxiety and depressive disorders included in this volume. Importantly, half of all total (child+adult) SEPAD cases had first onset in adulthood, in most instances in the twenties and early thirties, and a quarter had onset after 40 years. Two-thirds of adult cases had onset after 18 years of age but there was a pattern of persistence or recurrence from childhood in one-third of adult cases. These findings provide strong endorsement for the DSM-5 reformulation of SEPAD as a disorder that can have its onset and manifestation throughout the life course (Silove *et al.* 2016a). SEPAD has a tendency to remit, possibly because the course of the disorder is strongly related to proximate factors such as threatened or actual separations or losses; it seems possible that in most instances, the relatively rapid resolution of these ruptures or losses, whether via psychological mechanisms

Table 12.4 Comorbidity of adult separation anxiety disorder (SEPAD) with other DSM-IV disorders

	Adult SEPAD cases with comorbid disorders, % (SE)									
	Mood disorder		Anxiety disorder		Disruptive behaviour/ impulse-control disorder		Substance-use disorder		Any mental disorder	
	%	SE	%	SE	%	SE	%	SE	%	SE
Lifetime comorbidity[a]										
Lifetime	**52.0**	1.5	**58.1**	1.6	**19.1**	1.2	**25.9**	1.4	**78.5**	1.6
12-month	**58.3**	2.9	**61.7**	2.8	**19.7**	2.0	**26.3**	2.2	**82.2**	2.8
12-month comorbidity[b]										
12-month	**44.8**	2.7	**53.5**	2.7	**12.8**	1.8	**11.0**	1.5	**72.3**	2.9
Temporal priority of adult SEPAD[c]										
Lifetime	**38.4**	1.8	**14.5**	1.4	**33.2**	3.2	**37.4**	2.7	**17.7**	1.2
12-month	**29.4**	2.9	**11.7**	2.1	**26.2**	4.7	**26.3**	4.3	**13.2**	1.9

[a]Percentage of respondents with either lifetime or 12-month adult SEPAD who also meet lifetime criteria for at least one of the other DSM-IV disorders.
[b]Percentage of respondents with 12-month adult SEPAD who also meet 12-month criteria for at least one of the other disorders.
[c]Percentage of respondents with either lifetime or 12-month adult SEPAD and at least one of the other disorders, whose age-of-onset of adult SEPAD is reported to be younger than the age-of-onset of all comorbid disorders under consideration.

or repair of the interpersonal sphere, may hasten remission of the reaction. Whether these immediate interpersonal issues are responsible for the onset and remission of SEPAD requires closer examination now that an extensive array of background risk factors have been identified, including female gender, heredity, early family dysfunction including parental overprotection, exposure to multiple traumatic losses and other traumas, socio-economic disadvantage and pre-existing insecure attachment styles, amongst others (Battaglia *et al.* 2009; Manicavasagar *et al.* 2009; Silove *et al.* 2015, 2016b). A fruitful direction of research is the pursuit of biomarkers for SEPAD, with early evidence suggesting that abnormal oxytocin functioning may characterize the disorder, consistent with accumulating knowledge that this neuropeptide plays a key role in the attachment process (Costa *et al.* 2009; Eapen *et al.* 2014).

The degree of role impairment associated with 12-month SEPAD differed markedly across country income groups, the disorder being much more disabling in the high- and upper-middle-income countries than in the low/lower-middle-income countries. It may be that there is a greater tolerance or acceptance of the more extreme forms of SA behaviours in traditional, collectivist societies more typical of low-income countries, whereas that pattern is more likely to be regarded as dysfunctional in the individualistic cultures of high-income countries where independence is a highly valued characteristic. In the WMH data there was a somewhat greater proportion of severe impairment associated with SEPAD in the social (25.4%) and relationship (24.8%) domains compared with the work (20.0%) and home domains (18.7%), a finding that is consistent with the formulation of the disorder, which emphasizes difficulties that relate primarily to the interpersonal sphere. Although this was a general finding across WMH countries, the distinction between the social/relationship domains and the work/home spheres of functioning was particularly accentuated in high-income countries, further emphasizing the potential differences between societies that are more individualistic than collective in their customs. Nevertheless, further research is needed to examine directly whether collectivist cultures are more accepting of a higher level of SEPAD symptoms amongst adults.

The finding that women across all country income groups had greater likelihood of SEPAD is consistent with past observations in clinic samples (Pini *et al.* 2010; Silove *et al.* 2010). This observation may simply reflect the general tendency for women to experience a higher prevalence of the full range of internalizing disorders than men. In addition, however, it may be that women's propensity to manifest SA symptoms relates to their traditional role as carers and protectors of children and other vulnerable members of the group (the elderly, the infirm) (Silove *et al.* 1995b). More generally, the data suggest that persons with SEPAD show high levels of socio-economic vulnerability, including being divorced or separated (or single in high-income countries) and having low levels of education and increased rates of unemployment. Of interest is that in a study in Canada, children showing a pattern of high and worsening SA symptoms as they advanced into adolescence came from families where there was high parental unemployment (Battaglia *et al.* 2016). Nevertheless, the general relationship of socio-economic factors and SEPAD is likely to be complex, conditions of insecurity contributing to provoking and perpetuating symptoms and the functional impairment integral to the disorder adding to socio-economic difficulties, thereby generating a vicious cycle.

More than three-quarters of those with SEPAD experienced comorbid disorders, anxiety disorders being the most common associated disorders, followed by mood disorders, a pattern that is consistent with findings from clinic studies (Pini *et al.* 2010; Silove *et al.* 2010). In general, adult SEPAD showed much greater comorbidity with the internalizing than the externalizing disorders, consistent with the notion that the category belongs within the former broad spectrum. SEPAD in childhood is more likely to precede comorbid disorders, the reverse pattern being evident for adult SEPAD. The overall pattern therefore suggests a complex interplay between SEPAD and other disorders across the life course. As suggested by developmental theory, early onset SEPAD may be an important mediator of childhood adversity, such as exposure to trauma, abuse, and family dysfunction, thereby creating risk for a wider range of anxiety and depressive disorders in childhood and adulthood (Milrod *et al.* 2014). A refinement of this model would take into account more explicitly the possibility that adult SEPAD is a key factor in the pathway, either as a precursor to or a concomitant of other anxiety and depressive disorders (Silove *et al.* 2016a).

Only a small proportion of respondents with 12-month adult SEPAD sought help during the prior year, those experiencing greater impairment being more likely to seek assistance. The propensity to seek help and the availability of services are likely to account for the much increased rate of help-seeking amongst persons with SEPAD in high income countries. The relatively lower overall proportion of adults seeking help for SEPAD as compared to other common anxiety and depressive disorders (see Chapter 22) may be attributable to several factors. First, the boundary between adaptive SA and SEPAD remains indistinct, particularly because the tendency to seek support from others is a universal in relation to typical human responses to threat or insecurity (Manicavasagar *et al.* 2016). Families and the wider social network therefore may tolerate a high level of SEPAD symptoms in one member, the system adapting and in some cases even reinforcing the individual's symptoms (Manicavasagar *et al.* 2016). The difference in impairment observed across country income groups illustrates how powerful cultural factors may be in setting the threshold of tolerance of SEPAD symptoms. Even within high-income countries, there may be distinctive relationship patterns that discourage help-seeking amongst persons with SEPAD. For example, a dominant male may accommodate or even tacitly encourage SA symptoms in his female partner, covertly benefiting from her constrained, largely home-bound lifestyle and thereby maintaining the power imbalance in the relationship. In addition, there is a risk that clinicians who adhere to the custom of restricting SEPAD to childhood may overlook the diagnosis in an adult, instead making an alternative, more conventional diagnosis, such as of panic disorder, agoraphobia, or generalized anxiety disorder (Manicavasagar *et al.* 2016). Such an oversight may have adverse consequences in relation to treatment outcomes. There is some evidence, for example, that the use of conventional pharmacological treatments for other anxiety disorders may be less effective where comorbid adult SEPAD is present (Miniati *et al.* 2012).

In conclusion, the present data add substantially to cumulative evidence that SEPAD is a disorder that commonly manifests beyond childhood and can have its onset beyond the age of 18 years. In that regard, the findings support the changes made to the definition of SEPAD in DSM-5. It therefore is important to raise the awareness of clinicians to recognize the importance of identifying the disorder whenever it occurs across the life span. Further work is needed to devise and test treatments that are specific to SEPAD, particularly amongst adults.

References

Battaglia, M. (2015). Separation anxiety: at the neurobiological crossroads of adaptation and illness. *Dialogues in Clinical Neuroscience*, 17, 277.

Battaglia, M., Pesenti-Gritti, P., Medland, S. E., *et al.* (2009). A genetically informed study of the association between childhood separation anxiety, sensitivity to CO2, panic disorder, and the effect of childhood parental loss. *Archives of General Psychiatry*, 66, 64–71.

Battaglia, M., Touchette, É., Garon-Carrier, G., *et al.* (2016). Distinct trajectories of separation anxiety in the preschool years: persistence at school entry and early-life associated factors. *Journal of Child Psychology and Psychiatry*, 57, 39–46.

Bowlby, J. (1960). Separation anxiety: a critical review of the literature. *Journal of Child Psychology and Psychiatry*, 1, 251–69.

Costa, B., Pini, S., Gabelloni, P., *et al.* (2009). Oxytocin receptor polymorphisms and adult attachment style in patients with depression. *Psychoneuroendocrinology*, 34, 1506–14.

Eapen, V., Dadds, M., Barnett, B., *et al.* (2014). Separation anxiety, attachment and inter-personal representations: disentangling the role of oxytocin in the perinatal period. *PLoS One*, 9:e107745.

Klein, D. F. (1964). Delineation of two drug-responsive anxiety syndromes. *Psychopharmacology*, 5:397–408.

Klein, R. G. (1995). Is panic disorder associated with childhood separation anxiety disorder? *Clinical Neuropharmacology*, 18, S7–14.

Kossowsky, J., Pfaltz, M. C., & Schneider, S. (2013). The Separation Anxiety Hypothesis of Panic Disorder revisited: a meta-analysis. *Am J Psychiatry*, 170, 768–81.

Last, C. G., Strauss, C. C., & Francis, G. (1987). Comorbidity among childhood anxiety disorders. *The Journal of Nervous and Mental Disease*, 175, 726–30.

Manicavasagar, V. & Silove, D. (2016). Why are we still missing adult separation anxiety disorder in clinical practice? *Australian and New Zealand Journal of Psychiatry*, 50, 807–8.

Manicavasagar, V., Silove, D., Curtis, J., & Wagner, R. (2000). Continuities of separation anxiety from early life into adulthood. *Journal of Anxiety Disorders*, 14:1–8.

Manicavasagar, V., Silove, D., Marnane, C., *et al.* (2009). Adult attachment styles in panic disorder with and without comorbid adult separation anxiety disorder. *Australian and New Zealand Journal of Psychiatry*, 43, 167–72.

Manicavasagar, V., Silove, D., Wagner, R., & Drobny, J. (2003). A self-report questionnaire for measuring separation anxiety in adulthood. *Comprehensive Psychiatry*, 30, 146–53.

Milrod, B., Markowitz, J. C., Gerber, A. J., *et al.* (2014). Childhood separation anxiety and the pathogenesis and treatment of adult anxiety. *American Journal of Psychiatry*, 171, 34–43.

Miniati, M., Calugi, S., Rucci, P., *et al.* (2012). Predictors of response among patients with panic disorder treated with medications in a naturalistic follow-up: the role of adult separation anxiety. *Journal of Affective Disorder*, 136, 675–9.

Pini, S., Abelli, M., Shear, K., *et al.* (2010). Frequency and clinical correlates of adult separation anxiety in a sample of 508 outpatients with mood and anxiety disorders. *Acta Psychiatrica Scandinavica*, 122, 40–6.

Roberson-Nay, R., Klein, D. F., Klein, R. G., *et al.* (2010). Carbon dioxide hypersensitivity in separation-anxious offspring of parents with panic disorder. *Biological Psychiatry*, 67, 1171–7.

Roberson-Nay, R., Moruzzi, S., Ogliari, A., *et al.* (2013). Evidence for distinct genetic effects associated with response to 35% CO2. *Depression and Anxiety*, 30, 259–66.

Shear, K., Jin, R., Ruscio, A. M., *et al.* (2006). Prevalence and correlates of estimated DSM-IV child and adult separation anxiety disorder in the National Comorbidity Survey Replication (NCS-R). *American Journal of Psychiatry*, 163, 1074–83.

Silove, D., Alonso, J., Bromet, E., *et al.* (2015). Pediatric-onset and adult-onset separation anxiety disorder across countries in the World Mental Health Survey. *American Journal of Psychiatry*, 172, 647–56.

Silove, D., Harris, M., Morgan, A., *et al.* (1995a). Is early separation anxiety a specific precursor of panic disorder-agoraphobia? A community study. *Psychological Medicine*, 25, 405–11.

Silove, D., Manicavasagar, V., O'Connell, D., *et al.* (1995b). Genetic factors in early separation anxiety: implications for the genesis of adult anxiety disorders. *Acta Psychiatrica Scandinavica*, 92, 17–24.

Silove, D., Manicavasagar, V., & Pini, S. (2016a). Can separation anxiety disorder escape its attachment to childhood? *World Psychiatry*, 15, 113–5.

Silove, D. M., Marnane, C. L., Wagner, R., *et al.* (2010). The prevalence and correlates of adult separation anxiety disorder in an anxiety clinic. *BMC Psychiatry*, 10, 21.

Silove, D. M., Tay, A. K., Tol, W. A., *et al.* (2016b). Patterns of separation anxiety symptoms amongst pregnant women in conflict-affected Timor-Leste: associations with traumatic loss, family conflict, and intimate partner violence. *Journal of Affective Disorders*, 205, 292–300.

Chapter

13 Intermittent Explosive Disorder

Kate M. Scott, Carmen C. W. Lim, Ali Al-Hamzawi, Jordi Alonso

Introduction

Anger has been linked with psychopathology since classical times (Novaco 2010), a tie that remains embedded in the English language with the word 'mad' being a colloquial term for both anger and insanity. Anger and its behavioural expression (e.g., irritability, hostility, and aggression) may accompany the clinical presentation of many mental disorders. It is for this reason that it has been long debated as to whether aggression is just a correlate of other mental disorders, or whether it might, under some circumstances, constitute a mental disorder in its own right.

It is not just aggression ('anger turned outwards') that has been linked with psychopathology; psychodynamic theory has long focused on 'anger turned inwards' (repression) as a central feature of depression (Busch 2009). But it is interesting to note that although the idea that repression of anger is bad for health (physical and mental) has had enormous influence on popular views of anger and health (Tavris 1989; Lilienfeld *et al.* 2011), repression of anger does not feature in current classifications of mental disorders. Aggression though, does, with impulsive aggression being the central feature of the diagnosis of intermittent explosive disorder (IED).

There has been much less research on the epidemiology of IED compared with other psychiatric disorders, principally due to significant problems with diagnostic criteria in earlier versions of DSM (Coccaro *et al.* 1998). These problems revolved around the difficulty of determining the frequency and type of aggressive outbursts that would warrant classification as a mental disorder, as well as the problem of how to differentiate the disorder from personality styles characterized by recurrent aggressive behaviour. Although debated (Coccaro 2012), DSM-IV criteria are sufficiently well operationalized to have allowed research into the epidemiology of IED. IED was included in DSM-IV as a subsidiary disorder (not elsewhere classified) but it is classified in DSM-5 within the category of disruptive, impulse-control, and conduct disorders.

Aggression can be classified as defensive, premeditated, or impulsive; defensive aggression falls within the bounds of normal behaviour, while premeditated and impulsive aggression are both considered pathological (Coccaro 2012). Impulsive aggression can be thought of as a spontaneous aggressive response to provocation with loss of behavioural control, while premeditated aggression is considered a more planned or intentional form of aggression. Premeditated aggression is viewed as falling within the personality disorder spectrum, so only impulsive aggression is currently potentially classifiable as a mental disorder. Coccaro and colleagues have collected a large body of evidence indicating that impulsive aggression can be distinguished from premeditated aggression on a range of social and biological factors and in terms of responsiveness to treatment (Coccaro 2012). It is this kind evidence that has been crucial to the case for the inclusion of IED in the DSM classification of mental disorders.

The essential feature of IED as defined in DSM-IV is the occurrence of repeated episodes of impulsive aggression resulting in verbal or physical assaults or property destruction. The impulsive outbursts that characterize IED have rapid onset with little or no prodromal period and usually last fewer than 30 minutes. To meet criteria for the disorder these outbursts need to be greatly out of proportion to any precipitating stressor and to not be better accounted for by another mental disorder. Although not conclusive, there is some evidence that IED is not simply the pathological end of the continuum of impulsive aggression that occurs in the general population, but rather a distinct clinical entity with distinguishing characteristics such as early onset, family history, and help-seeking (Ahmed *et al.* 2010).

The first large population based studies of DSM-IV IED occurred in the United States as part of the World Mental Health (WMH) Surveys Initiative. The National Comorbidity Survey Replication (NCS-R) found a lifetime prevalence of 5.4% (Kessler *et al.*

2006), and the adolescent supplement found a lifetime prevalence of 5.3% (McLaughlin *et al.* 2012). Because extensive research has linked prior exposure to violence with subsequent perpetration of violence (Song *et al.* 1998; McKinney *et al.* 2009), and some studies have also linked prior trauma exposure with IED diagnosis (Fincham *et al.* 2009; Nickerson *et al.* 2012), it has been hypothesized that IED might be more prevalent in countries with higher rates of violence, trauma exposure, or civil conflict (Fincham *et al.* 2009; Al-Hamzawi *et al.* 2012; Axinn *et al.* 2013; Rees *et al.* 2013). In apparent support of this hypothesis a high 12-month prevalence of IED (9.5%) was found in Timor Leste where it was interpreted by the researchers as 'a reaction to extreme forms of injustice' (Rees *et al.* 2013). A high rate of IED was also observed in an earlier study in South Africa (Fincham *et al.* 2009) that has been widely cited as supportive of the hypothesis that war and civil conflict could elevate prevalence of IED. However, the high estimate in the South African study has turned out to be erroneous[1] and the study in Timor Leste used a very different assessment instrument from the Composite International Diagnostic Interview (CIDI) used in the NCS-R and other WMH surveys, making comparison difficult. Moreover, 12-month IED was only 1.5% in the Iraq WMH survey (Al-Hamzawi *et al.* 2012), inconsistent with the hypothesis. As noted, interpretation of variation in IED prevalence across existing studies is difficult given differences in measurement of IED and application of diagnostic hierarchy rules. The WMH Surveys Initiative, in which DSM-IV IED was assessed in 16 countries, therefore provides an important opportunity to examine the epidemiology of IED in a range of countries using consistent methods and diagnostic criteria.

In this chapter we provide information on the cross-national epidemiology of IED examining prevalence, age-of-onset, socio-demographic correlates, comorbidity, associated impairment, and treatment. The analyses have been undertaken in a way that is consistent with the other mental disorders in this book, except that we provide a more detailed breakdown of IED comorbidity with specific mental disorders due to the limited information on this in general population samples in the published literature on IED. We also include two IED-specific tables. One of these provides information on the number and type of aggressive episodes during the worst week of the 12-month prior to interview among those meeting 12-month criteria. The other table is of associations between lifetime traumatic event exposure and subsequent IED onset: we include this due to the strong research interest in the relationship between prior trauma exposure and IED and limited data on it from other sources.

Method

This chapter includes the data from all 16 of the 26 countries included in this volume that assessed IED. These countries include six low/lower-middle-income countries (Colombia, Iraq, Nigeria, Peru, People's Republic of China, Ukraine), five upper-middle-income countries (Brazil, Bulgaria, Lebanon, Romania, South Africa) and five high-income countries (Japan, Northern Ireland, Poland, Portugal, the United States).

DSM-IV Criterion A for IED requires 'several discrete episodes of failure to resist aggressive impulses that result in serious assaultive acts or destruction of property'. This was operationalized in the CIDI by requiring the respondent to report at least three attacks in the same year of at least one of three types of anger attacks: (i) 'when all of a sudden you lost control and broke or smashed something worth more than a few dollars'; (ii) 'when all of a sudden you lost control and hit or tried to hurt someone'; and (iii) 'when all of a sudden you lost control and threatened to hit or hurt someone'. Twelve-month diagnosis was assigned if those meeting lifetime criteria reported at least three attacks in the past 12-months, and 30-day diagnosis was assigned if those meeting 12-month criteria reported an anger attack in the past 30 days.

DSM-IV criterion B for IED requires that the aggressiveness is 'grossly out of proportion to any precipitating psychosocial stressor'. This criterion was operationalized in the CIDI by requiring the respondent to report either that they 'got a lot more angry than most people would have been in the same situation' or that the attack occurred 'without good reason' or that the attack occurred 'in situations where most people would not have had an anger attack'.

DSM-IV criterion C for IED requires that the 'aggressive episodes are not better accounted for by another mental disorder and are not due to the direct physiological effects of a substance or a general medical condition'. This was assessed through a series of questions (see Kessler *et al.* 2006 for details) that ruled IED diagnosis out if anger attacks occurred exclusively

[1] https://www.hcp.med.harvard.edu/wmh/ftpdir/Fincham_et_al_2009_erratum.pdf

when respondents had been drinking or using drugs, when they were in a depressive or manic episode, or as a consequence of an organic cause such as epilepsy, head injury, or use of medications.

This classification of IED is based on the 'narrow' definition of IED reported in the NCS-R (Kessler *et al.* 2006), but for the data presented here we have applied an additional impairment criterion that required respondents to report that their anger attacks caused at least some degree of interference with their work, social life, or relationships (Scott *et al.* 2016). This makes the diagnosis of IED in this chapter more conservative than in earlier reports based on WMH surveys data (Kessler *et al.* 2006, 2012; Yoshimasu & Kawakami 2011; Al-Hamzawi *et al.* 2012), but this inclusion of an impairment criterion is consistent with the diagnostic criteria for other DSM-IV disorders.

How does this definition of IED compare to DSM-5 criteria? DSM-5 IED criteria recognize two different patterns of aggressive outburst: high frequency/low intensity (criterion A1: *non-destructive* verbal or physical aggression occurring at least twice weekly for at least three months) or low frequency/high intensity (criterion A2: at least three *destructive* outbursts within a year-long period) (Coccaro *et al.* 2014b). DSM-5 criteria also require that the outbursts cause functional impairment, consistent with the algorithm used here. But although our diagnostic algorithm requires three aggressive outbursts within one year there was insufficient information in the CIDI on the lifetime frequency of specific types of aggressive outburst to develop an algorithm consistent with DSM-5's specification of criterion A1 and A2.

Results

Prevalence and Age-of-Onset

There is quite substantial variation in the prevalence of IED across countries (Table 13.1). Lifetime prevalence is 0.8% in all countries combined and ranges from a low of less than 0.1% in Nigeria to a high of 2.7% in the United States. The average 12-month prevalence in all countries combined is 0.4%, with 0.3% meeting criteria for 30-day prevalence. A little over half (53.6%) of those with lifetime disorders report symptoms in the past 12-months and a substantial proportion (61.9%) of the 12-month cases report symptoms in the past 30 days; these results indicate that IED can be moderately persistent. Lifetime prevalence of IED varies significantly ($F = 19.1$, $P < 0.001$) across country income groups showing a gradient from lower prevalence in low/lower-middle-income countries to higher prevalence in the high-income countries. However, the higher average prevalence in high-income countries is strongly influenced by the high prevalence in the United States, with none of the other high-income countries having prevalence approaching that of the United States. By contrast, the indirect indictors of disorder persistence (12-month/lifetime) and episode persistence (30-day/12-month) are higher in the low/lower-middle-income countries than in the high-income countries, with a significant inverse gradient across country income groups for episode persistence ($F = 4.3$, $P = 0.014$)

IED is one of the earlier onset disorders, typically beginning in late adolescence, with a median age-of-onset in all countries combined of 17 (16 in high-income countries; 18 in low/lower-middle-income countries and 19 in upper-middle-income countries), with a fairly narrow inter-quartile range across countries of 13–23 (Appendix Table 13A.1). Projected lifetime risk of IED is 0.9 for all countries combined, only slightly higher than the lifetime prevalence estimate of 0.8; this reflects the young age-of-onset.

Type of Anger Attacks in the Past 12 Months

Respondents reporting IED symptoms in the prior 12 months were asked to think about the week during the 12 months when they had their most violent aggressive outburst, and to indicate the number and type of angry outbursts they experienced during that week. Respondents could report more than one type of attack. As the results indicate, the most commonly reported attacks (by 235/357) are the less destructive types involving slamming a door, kicking a chair, or throwing clothes. But a substantial number report that they broke something or several things during the angry outburst and 42% (51+100/357) report hurting someone. It is evident that in each category of attack the means are higher than the median, indicating that a small group of individuals report multiple experiences of each type of attack anger, with some individuals reporting more than one instance of arson, torturing an animal or hurting someone during the specified week.

Role Impairment

The proportion of those with 12-month IED who report severe impairment in at least one domain is 38.9% in all countries combined, varying (non-significantly) from 26.7% in upper-middle-income countries to 36.5%

Table 13.1 Prevalence of DSM-IV intermittent explosive disorder (IED) in the World Mental Health surveys

Country	Lifetime prevalence[a]		12-month prevalence[b]		30-day prevalence[c]		12-month prevalence of IED among lifetime cases		30-day prevalence of IED among 12-month cases		Sample size used
	%	SE	%	SE	%	SE	%	SE	%	SE	
Low/lower-middle-income countries	**0.6**	**0.1**	**0.4**	**0.0**	**0.3**	**0.0**	**60.1**	**3.8**	**70.4**	**5.0**	**36,498**
Colombia	1.2	0.2	0.5	0.1	0.4	0.1	41.9	6.1	75.7	10.0	4,426
Iraq	0.4	0.2	0.4	0.2	0.3	0.1	93.9	6.1	86.6	10.9	4,332
Nigeria	0.0	0.0	0.0	0.0	0.0	0.0	79.6	20.7	25.9	27.2	6,752
Peru	0.6	0.2	0.2	0.1	0.2	0.1	37.7	10.3	72.1	13.6	3,930
PRC (Beijing/Shanghai)	0.5	0.1	0.3	0.1	0.2	0.1	52.8	13.9	71.5	13.5	5,201
PRC (Shenzhen)	0.7	0.1	0.6	0.1	0.4	0.1	83.9	5.7	63.7	10.8	7,132
Ukraine	1.1	0.2	0.6	0.1	0.4	0.1	56.3	7.9	69.7	9.9	4,725
Upper-middle-income countries	**0.7**	**0.1**	**0.3**	**0.1**	**0.2**	**0.0**	**48.3**	**5.6**	**71.6**	**6.7**	**19,884**
Brazil	0.7	0.1	0.4	0.1	0.2	0.1	53.0	10.8	49.5	14.2	5,037
Bulgaria	0.2	0.1	0.2	0.1	0.1	0.1	68.8	17.2	84.6	11.4	5,318
Lebanon	0.6	0.1	0.3	0.1	0.2	0.1	44.4	12.6	89.9	10.9	2,857
Romania	0.5	0.2	0.3	0.2	0.3	0.2	66.0	18.7	93.1	7.3	2,357
South Africa	1.2	0.3	0.5	0.2	0.3	0.1	37.9	9.6	70.9	9.0	4,315
High-income countries	**1.1**	**0.1**	**0.6**	**0.1**	**0.3**	**0.0**	**51.4**	**3.8**	**52.2**	**4.4**	**31,681**
Japan	0.4	0.1	0.2	0.1	0.1	0.0	66.6	11.8	39.5	16.2	4,129
Northern Ireland	1.1	0.2	0.4	0.1	0.3	0.1	31.7	7.5	76.2	12.2	4,340
Poland	0.2	0.0	0.1	0.0	0.0	0.0	49.4	13.2	36.0	16.4	10,081
Portugal	0.5	0.1	0.3	0.1	0.1	0.1	45.9	11.7	46.3	24.0	3,849
United States	2.7	0.2	1.5	0.2	0.8	0.1	55.0	4.8	51.9	5.0	9,282
All countries combined	**0.8**	**0.0**	**0.4**	**0.0**	**0.3**	**0.0**	**53.6**	**2.5**	**61.9**	**3.2**	**88,063**
WHO regions[d]											
Region of the Americas	1.6	0.1	0.8	**0.1**	0.5	0.1	51.7	3.7	55.4	4.4	22,675
African region	0.5	0.1	0.2	0.1	0.1	0.1	40.1	9.1	66.1	9.8	11,067
Western Pacific region	0.6	0.1	0.4	0.1	0.3	0.1	72.5	6.0	61.7	8.1	16,462
Eastern Mediterranean region	0.5	0.1	0.3	0.1	0.3	0.1	69.0	9.8	87.7	8.2	7,189
Western European region	0.9	0.1	0.3	0.1	0.2	0.1	35.9	6.3	64.8	13.0	8,189
Eastern European region	0.4	0.0	0.2	0.0	0.2	0.0	57.8	6.1	69.6	7.0	22,481
Comparison between countries[e]	$F_{16,v} = 21.9^*, P < 0.001$		$F_{16,v} = 7.9^*, P < 0.001$		$F_{16,v} = 8.3^*, P < 0.001$		$F_{16,v} = 2.4^*, P = 0.002$		$F_{16,v} = 1.4, P = 0.153$		
Comparison between low-, middle- and high-income country groups[e]	$F_{2,v} = 19.1^*, P < 0.001$		$F_{2,v} = 5.5^*, P = 0.044$		$F_{2,v} = 0.9, P = 0.405$		$F_{2,v} = 2.0, P = 0.133$		$F_{2,v} = 4.3^*, P = 0.014$		
Comparison between WHO regions[e]	$F_{5,v} = 26.1^*, P < 0.001$		$F_{5,v} = 8.3^*, P < 0.001$		$F_{5,v} = 5.4^*, P < 0.001$		$F_{5,v} = 4.1^*, P = 0.001$		$F_{5,v} = 1.5, P = 0.186$		

*Significant at the 0.05 level, two-sided test.

[a]Lifetime narrow IED: lifetime IED with hierarchy and required three or more anger attacks in at least one year of life.

[b]Twelve-month narrow IED: 12-month IED with hierarchy and required three or more anger attacks in the past 12 months.

[c]Thirty-day narrow IED: 30-day IED with hierarchy and required three or more anger attacks in the past 12 months.

[d]**Region of the Americas** (Colombia, Brazil, Peru, United States); **African region** (South Africa, Nigeria); **Western Pacific region** (PRC (Shenzhen), PRC (Beijing and Shanghai), Japan); **Eastern Mediterranean region** (Iraq, Lebanon); **Western European region** (Northern Ireland, Portugal); **Eastern European region** (Romania, Poland, Bulgaria, Ukraine).

[e]Wald design-corrected F-tests were used to determine if there is variation in prevalence estimates across countries. The denominator degree of freedom, v, is 770.

PRC: People's Republic of China.

Table 13.2 Type and number of anger attacks during the week of the past year containing the most violent attack, among those with 12-month IED (n = 357)

Type of anger attack	Number of attacks in the week				
	n	Mean	SE	Median	(IQR)
Slam a door, kick a chair, or throw clothes in anger	235	5.5	0.6	2	(1–5)
Break something in anger	170	3.2	0.3	1	(1–2)
Break several things in anger	104	2.7	0.3	1	(1–3)
Purposely set fire or destroy someone else's property	29	1.8	0.4	1	(1–2)
Purposely injure or torture an animal	16	2.1	0.3	1	(1–4)
Threaten someone	178	4.3	0.5	1	(1–3)
Hurt someone so badly that they needed medical attention	51	1.4	0.1	1	(1–2)
Hurt someone badly, but not enough to need medical attention	100	2.7	0.3	1	(1–3)

in low/lower-middle-income countries and 44.7% in high-income countries (Appendix Table 13A.2). In all countries combined, severe impairment is reported more frequently in the social and relationship domains than in the work and home domains, although this pattern of stronger impairment in the social domains is less evident in the upper-middle-income countries. The highest levels of impairment are in the Ukraine, with 56.6% reporting severe impairment, followed by 50.1% of those with IED in the United States reporting severe impairment.

Socio-demographic Correlates

The likelihood of having the disorder at all (lifetime IED column) is significantly greater among males, the young, the unemployed, those with less education, and those who are divorced or separated (Table 13.3), with young age and low education being the strongest correlates. The correlates of current (30-day) burden of IED are for the most part similar to those of lifetime IED, indicating that the onset profile largely drives the current burden profile. One exception to that, however, is household income; high-average household income, relative to high household income, is associated with decreased likelihood of both current burden of IED and episode persistence, although this pattern is only significant for current burden (OR 0.5).

No socio-demographic correlates are significantly associated with odds of IED persistence (12-month/lifetime). One correlate that is notable by its absence of association with persistence is gender. As mentioned above, being male is associated with both lifetime IED and current burden, but the likelihood of disorder or episode persistence is just as high among women as among men.

Comorbidity

As evident in Table 13.4, more than three-quarters (81.7%) of respondents with lifetime IED meet criteria for at least one other lifetime disorder. Alcohol abuse is the single most common comorbid disorder (36.5% have lifetime comorbid alcohol abuse) closely followed by depression (35.2%). The most common class of comorbid disorders is anxiety disorders (58.5%), reflecting the large number of anxiety disorders. It may seem as if there is not especially high comorbidity with the childhood disruptive behaviour disorders (conduct disorder and oppositional defiance disorder) with which IED might have been thought to have most in common, with only around 16% of those with IED having lifetime comorbidity with one of these disorders. However, it is not possible to draw any conclusions about the relative strength of associations between IED and specific types of comorbid disorders from this table as it only provides a descriptive picture of the comorbidity burden in IED. The disruptive behaviour disorders are not very common, and this has to be taken into account in evaluating associations between IED and specific comorbidities. Bivariate associations between all of the mental disorders are presented in Chapter 20, and they show that IED is somewhat more strongly associated with conduct disorder and oppositional defiant disorder than with other disorders.

As expected from the adolescent median age-of-onset, IED onset precedes onset of comorbid mood disorders in 66.9% of cases, but only precedes comorbid anxiety disorders in 26.7% of cases due to the earlier onset of the two most prevalent anxiety disorders, specific phobia, and social anxiety disorder. IED onset also typically precedes substance-use disorders onset (74.0% of lifetime cases), but does not precede most disruptive behaviour disorders – although it does precede conduct disorder in a substantial minority of cases (45%).

Associations of Traumatic Events with Onset of IED

This next set of results examines associations between lifetime traumatic events and the likelihood of developing IED, due to strong theoretical interest in these relationships. From discrete-time survival analyses that examined traumatic events as predictors of first onset of IED (see Scott *et al.* 2016 for details on the analysis), including control for demographic variables (age, gender, education, marital status, employment status) and country, we find that most types of lifetime traumas are associated with subsequent first onset of IED (Table 13.5). The traumas with the strongest associations with IED onset are being physically abused as a child (OR 3.6) and witnessing family violence as a child (OR 3.5). The next column of data in Table 13.5 shows results from models that included all traumatic events together, in addition to the controls mentioned above. In this model several individual traumatic events lose significance as predictors, indicating that their significance in the bivariate models is due to their co-occurrence with childhood physical abuse and other traumatic events. Childhood physical abuse remains the strongest predictor of IED both in terms of the experience of physical abuse as a child (OR 2.2) and the witnessing of it (OR 2.3). Non-combat war experience, intimate or sexual violence, and other (private) events are also associated with odds of IED in the multivariate model with ORs all <2.0. Combat experience is protective in the multivariate model (OR 0.3). The final column of data shows that odds of IED onset increase substantially with the experience of an increasing number of different types of traumatic events, ranging from OR of 3.1 for one type of event to 8.0 for four or more types of events.

Treatment

Few with IED receive treatment, with only 25% of those with 12-month IED (of any severity) reporting some kind of treatment in the health care sector (Appendix Table 13A.3). Treatment in the non-health care sector is rare. Treatment is especially low in the low/lower-middle-income countries with 12% reporting treatment in the health care sector, compared with 28.4% reporting treatment in the upper-middle-income countries and 33.5% reporting treatment in the high-income countries (Appendix Table 13A.3). In all countries combined, treatment rates are similar for IED cases with mild versus moderate impairment (17.9% and 18.6%, respectively), but a higher proportion (30.5%) of those in the severe impairment category report treatment.

Discussion

As with all the mental disorders considered in this volume, it should be borne in mind that their retrospective assessment may quite substantially underestimate lifetime prevalence (Moffitt *et al.* 2010; Takayanagi *et al.* 2014) so the prevalence estimates provided here should be considered conservative. In addition, despite methodological improvement in age-of-onset recall accuracy as detailed in Chapter 3, it is likely that some inaccuracies in age-of-onset timing remain and this limitation may have affected time-lagged associations between traumatic events and IED onset as well as the estimates of temporal priority in the comorbidity analyses. It should also be noted that IED was not included in the clinical reappraisal studies that helped confirm the clinical validity of the CIDI diagnoses in the WMH surveys (Haro *et al.* 2006) and this is an important area for future research.

Within the context of those limitations, we found the lifetime prevalence of conservatively defined DSM-IV IED to be 0.8% averaged across all countries, indicating that it is one of the rarer disorders measured in the WMH surveys. Although prevalence varied considerably across countries, it is interesting to note that we did not find higher prevalence rates in countries characterized by war, terrorism, and conflict, as has been hypothesized (Fincham *et al.* 2009; Al-Hamzawi *et al.* 2012; Rees *et al.* 2013). The variation in IED prevalence across countries may in part reflect variation in willingness to disclose mental health symptoms or the performance of the diagnostic interview (Kessler & Üstün 2008; Yoshimasu & Kawakami 2011). That said, the pattern we see of prevalence being positively

Table 13.3 **Bivariate associations between socio-demographic correlates and DSM-IV intermittent explosive disorder (IED), all countries combined**

Correlates	30-day IED[a]		Lifetime IED[b]		12-month IED among lifetime cases[c]		30-day IED among 12-month cases[c]	
	OR	(95% CI)	OR	(95% CI)	OR	(95% CI)	OR	(95% CI)
Age-cohort								
18–29	**5.0***	(2.0–12.6)	**10.4***	(6.8–16.0)				
30–44	**4.1***	(1.7–10.0)	**5.5***	(3.7–8.2)				
45–59	**3.1***	(1.2–8.0)	**3.4***	(2.3–5.2)				
60+	1.0		1.0					
Age-cohort difference[d]	$\chi^2_3 = 13.9^*$, P = 0.003		$\chi^2_3 = 144.0^*$, P < 0.001					
Age-of-onset								
Early					**2.2***	(1.3–3.8)	**0.4***	(0.2–1.0)
Early-average					**1.7***	(1.0–2.8)	0.8	(0.3–1.8)
Late-average					**1.8***	(1.1–3.0)	0.6	(0.2–1.4)
Late					1.0		1.0	
Age-of-onset difference[d]					$\chi^2_3 = 8.9^*$, P = 0.031		$\chi^2_3 = 5.5$, P = 0.140	
Time since onset (continuous)					**0.99***	(0.97–1.00)	**1.03***	(1.01–1.06)
Gender								
Female	**0.7***	(0.5–0.9)	**0.7***	(0.6–0.8)	1.0	(0.7–1.5)	1.1	(0.6–2.0)
Male	1.0		1.0		1.0		1.0	
Gender difference[d]	$\chi^2_1 = 6.6^*$, P = 0.010		$\chi^2_1 = 21.6^*$, P < 0.001		$\chi^2_1 = 0.0$, P = 0.940		$\chi^2_1 = 0.2$, P = 0.650	
Employment status								
Student	0.6	(0.3–1.5)	0.9	(0.5–1.5)	0.6	(0.2–1.8)	0.5	(0.1–1.9)
Homemaker	1.1	(0.6–2.0)	0.8	(0.6–1.2)	1.0	(0.5–2.1)	1.9	(0.6–6.3)
Retired	**0.3***	(0.1–0.7)	0.6	(0.4–1.2)	0.7	(0.3–1.6)	0.3	(0.1–1.1)
Other	**1.8***	(1.2–2.9)	**1.5***	(1.1–1.9)	1.0	(0.6–1.6)	**2.3***	(1.1–4.6)
Employed	1.0		1.0		1.0		1.0	

Table 13.3 (*cont.*)

Correlates	30-day IED[a]		Lifetime IED[b]		12-month IED among lifetime cases[c]		30-day IED among 12-month cases[c]	
	OR	(95% CI)	OR	(95% CI)	OR	(95% CI)	OR	(95% CI)
Employment status difference[d]	$\chi^2_4 = 17.2^*$, P = 0.002		$\chi^2_4 = 12.5^*$, P = 0.014		$\chi^2_4 = 1.7$, P = 0.783		$\chi^2_4 = 12.4^*$, P = 0.015	
Marital status								
Never married	**0.6***	(0.4–0.9)	**1.0**	(0.8–1.3)	**0.8**	(0.5–1.3)	**0.5***	(0.3–0.9)
Divorced/separated/widowed	**1.4**	(0.9–2.2)	**1.3***	(1.0–1.8)	**1.5**	(0.8–2.5)	**0.7**	(0.3–1.4)
Currently married	**1.0**		**1.0**		**1.0**		**1.0**	
Marital status difference[d]	$\chi^2_2 = 9.6^*$, P = 0.008		$\chi^2_2 = 4.0$, P = 0.132		$\chi^2_2 = 3.9$, P = 0.144		$\chi^2_2 = 6.0$, P = 0.050	
Education level								
No education	–	–	–	–	–	–	–	–
Some primary	**2.5***	(1.2–5.0)	**2.3***	(1.6–3.3)	**1.3**	(0.5–3.6)	**1.5**	(0.3–8.6)
Finished primary	**1.3**	(0.6–3.0)	**1.7***	(1.1–2.7)	**1.2**	(0.5–3.1)	**0.4**	(0.1–1.8)
Some secondary	**2.5***	(1.4–4.4)	**2.3***	(1.7–3.3)	**1.6**	(0.8–2.9)	**1.2**	(0.5–2.7)
Finished secondary	**1.5**	(0.8–2.8)	**1.7***	(1.3–2.4)	**1.1**	(0.6–1.9)	**0.6**	(0.2–1.5)
Some college	**1.3**	(0.7–2.2)	**1.5***	(1.1–2.1)	**0.9**	(0.5–1.6)	**0.7**	(0.3–1.6)
Finished college	**1.0**		**1.0**		**1.0**		**1.0**	
Education level difference[d]	$\chi^2_6 = 14.6^*$, P = 0.024		$\chi^2_6 = 31.7^*$, P < 0.001		$\chi^2_6 = 8.5$, P = 0.201		$\chi^2_6 = 5.7$, P = 0.459	
Household income								
Low	**1.0**	(0.6–1.6)	**1.3**	(1.0–1.7)	**1.1**	(0.6–1.8)	**0.6**	(0.3–1.4)
Low-average	**0.9**	(0.5–1.4)	**1.0**	(0.7–1.3)	**1.2**	(0.6–2.3)	**0.7**	(0.3–1.7)
High-average	**0.5***	(0.3–0.8)	**0.9**	(0.7–1.2)	**0.9**	(0.5–1.5)	**0.4***	(0.2–0.9)
High	**1.0**		**1.0**		**1.0**		**1.0**	
Household income difference[d]	$\chi^2_3 = 10.1^*$, P = 0.018		$\chi^2_3 = 9.5^*$, P = 0.023		$\chi^2_3 = 1.6$, P = 0.649		$\chi^2_3 = 5.4$, P = 0.148	
N[e]	**88,063**		**3,731,811**		**674**		**357**	

*Significant at the 0.05 level, two-sided test.
[a]These estimates are based on logistic regression models adjusted for age, gender and country.
[b]These estimates are based on survival models adjusted for age-cohorts, gender, person-years, and country.
[c]These estimates are based on logistic regression models adjusted for time since IED onset, age of IED onset, gender, and country.
[d]Chi-square test of significant differences between blocks of socio-demographic variables.
[e]Denominator N: 88,063 = total sample; 3,731,811 = number of person-years in the survival models; 674 = number of lifetime IED cases; 357 = number of 12-month IED cases.

Table 13.4 Comorbidity of intermittent explosive disorder (IED) with other DSM-IV disorders, all countries combined

	IED cases with comorbid disorders					
	Lifetime comorbidity[a]		12-month comorbidity[b]		Temporal priority of IED[c]	
	%	SE	%	SE	%	SE
I. Mood disorders						
Major depressive episode	**35.2**	2.5	**25.2**	2.9	**68.1**	3.2
Bipolar disorder	**14.1**	1.6	**13.1**	2.2	**79.2**	6.3
Any mood disorder	**40.8**	2.6	**29.4**	3.0	**67.2**	3.3
II. Anxiety disorders						
Panic disorder	**9.5**	1.2	**8.3**	1.5	**54.9**	5.9
Generalized anxiety disorder	**20.8**	2.1	**19.1**	2.8	**62.6**	5.6
Social phobia	**23.1**	1.9	**18.8**	2.5	**28.1**	4.4
Specific phobia	**21.8**	1.8	**19.4**	2.4	**5.5**	1.9
Agoraphobia	**8.7**	1.2	**6.5**	1.5	**38.3**	7.1
Post-traumatic stress disorder	**15.5**	1.5	**11.0**	1.7	**54.9**	5.8
Separation anxiety disorder	**6.0**	1.0	–	–	**21.7**	9.6
Adult separation anxiety disorder	**15.6**	1.6	**4.9**	1.4	**74.3**	4.7
Any anxiety disorder	**58.5**	2.4	**49.4**	3.2	**26.7**	3.0
III. Disruptive behaviour/ impulse-control disorders						
Attention deficit disorder	**12.0**	1.9	**11.2**	2.3	**14.1**	5.0
Conduct disorder	**16.6**	2.1	**3.4**	1.2	**44.9**	6.3
Oppositional defiant disorder	**16.5**	1.9	**4.3**	1.3	**24.5**	5.5
Binge-eating disorder with hierarchy	**2.5**	0.7	**1.0**	0.5	**50.3**	13.6
Bulimia with hierarchy	**1.7**	0.6	**1.2**	0.7	**49.5**	16.9
Any impulse-control disorder	**30.9**	2.5	**16.6**	2.6	**27.1**	4.6
IV. Substance-use disorders						
Alcohol abuse	**36.5**	2.3	**17.2**	2.4	**78.3**	3.3
Alcohol dependence	**17.2**	2.0	**10.0**	2.1	**92.4**	2.7
Drug abuse	**15.7**	1.8	**5.5**	1.5	**72.9**	5.4
Drug dependence	**8.0**	1.2	**3.1**	1.1	**94.3**	4.2
Any substance-use disorder	**39.6**	2.4	**20.6**	2.8	**74.0**	3.5
V. Any mental disorder	**81.7**	2.2	**68.2**	3.5	**28.8**	2.5

[a]Percentage of respondents with lifetime IED who also meet lifetime criteria for at least one of the other DSM-IV disorders.
[b]Percentage of respondents with 12-month IED who also meet 12-month criteria for at least one of the other disorders.
[c]Percentage of respondents with either lifetime IED and at least one of the other disorders, whose age-of-onset of IED is reported to be younger than the age-of-onset of all comorbid disorders under consideration.

related to country income level is consistent with the pattern we see for most of the mental disorders and this pattern is discussed further in Chapter 22.

We found that lifetime prevalence of IED was higher among males, the young, the unemployed, and those with lower educational attainment, consistent with prior clinical and community studies (Coccaro *et al.* 2005; Kessler *et al.* 2006; Ortega *et al.* 2008; Kessler *et al.* 2012). Marital separation/divorce was also weakly associated with increased likelihood of lifetime IED and although the direction of that association is unclear, other WMH data suggests that IED is associated with increased likelihood of divorce, although not once comorbid disorders are taken into account (Breslau *et al.* 2011). Relative to being married, being never married was associated with decreased episode persistence and thereby also with decreased current burden of IED. These varied associations with marital status, together with the reported greater functional impairment in the social domains, suggest that turbulent intimate relationships both contribute to and are consequences of IED.

Within countries, we saw the expected associations between lower socio-economic status (household income and education) and higher likelihood of having IED at all. But we also found that current prevalence of IED at time of interview was higher among those in the highest household income category relative to the second-to-highest household income category. This latter finding will take some further research to understand but it may reflect either the stresses associated with higher occupational status, or that aggressive traits increase the likelihood of higher income as some research has suggested (Judge *et al.* 2012).

Table 13.5 Associations (odds ratios) between lifetime traumatic events and the subsequent onset of DSM-IV intermittent explosive disorder[a]

Type of lifetime traumatic event	Bivariate model[b]		Multivariate type model[c]		Multivariate number model[d]	
	OR	(95% CI)	OR	(95% CI)	OR	(95% CI)
I. War events						
Combat experience	**0.5**	(0.2–1.3)	**0.3***	(0.1–0.7)	–	–
Other war experience	**2.3***	(1.4–3.6)	**1.8***	(1.1–2.8)	–	–
II. Other interpersonal violence						
Physically abused as a child	**3.6***	(2.8–4.8)	**2.2***	(1.6–3.1)	–	–
Physically assaulted or threatened	**1.6***	(1.1–2.4)	**1.0**	(0.6–1.6)	–	–
III. Intimate or sexual violence						
Physically abused or threatened by spouse or romantic partner	**3.1***	(2.1–4.6)	**1.7***	(1.0–2.8)	–	–
Sexually assaulted	**2.9***	(2.1–4.2)	**1.6***	(1.0–2.4)	–	–
IV. Accident						
Automobile accident	**1.1**	(0.7–1.8)	**0.8**	(0.5–1.3)	–	–
Other life-threatening accident	**1.4**	(1.0–2.1)	**0.9**	(0.6–1.5)	–	–
Natural disaster	**1.2**	(0.8–1.9)	**0.8**	(0.5–1.3)	–	–
Life-threatening illness	**2.0***	(1.2–3.3)	**1.5**	(0.9–2.6)	–	–
V. Death						
Unexpected death of a loved one	**1.7***	(1.2–2.4)	**1.3**	(0.9–1.8)	–	–
VI. Network events						
Other LTE to a loved one	**1.5**	(0.8–2.5)	**0.8**	(0.5–1.5)	–	–
Witnessed a traumatic injury or death	**1.8***	(1.2–2.7)	**1.3**	(0.8–2.0)	–	–
Witnessed family violence as a child	**3.5***	(2.8–4.4)	**2.3***	(1.8–3.0)	–	–
VII. Other						
Other events	**2.4***	(1.6–3.7)	**1.5***	(1.0–2.4)	–	–
Joint significance of all types of traumatic events χ^2_{15} [P-value]	–	–	**χ^2_{15} = 339.2*, P < 0.001**		–	–
VIII. Number of traumatic events						
Exactly one type	–	–	–	–	**3.1***	(2.4–4.0)
Exactly two types	–	–	–	–	**4.5***	(3.1–6.5)
Exactly three types	–	–	–	–	**5.6***	(3.7–8.7)
Four or more types	–	–	–	–	**8.0***	(5.3–11.9)
Joint significance of all numbers of traumatic events χ^2_4 [P-value]	–	–	–	–	**χ^2_4 = 130.4*, P < 0.001**	

*Significant at the 0.05 level, two-sided test.
[a]Analysis for this table was performed on 14 out of 17 surveys due to restriction of data on lifetime traumatic events, and on the Part 2 subsamples in those surveys (n = 33,970).
[b]Bivariate models: each trauma type was estimated as a predictor of IED onset in a separate discrete-time survival model controlling for age-cohorts, gender, person-year, education, marriage, employment status, and country.
[c]Model was estimated with dummy variables for all trauma types entered simultaneously as predictors of IED onset, including the controls specified in (b).
[d]Model was estimated with dummy variables for number of traumas (without any information about type of trauma) as predictors of IED onset including the controls specified in (b).

We found IED to have a median age-of-onset of 17, which is in the mid-range of estimates from prior studies (Coccaro 2012). This estimate makes it one of the earlier onset disorders included in this volume. Also consistent with prior studies is the finding of a high degree of comorbidity with other mental disorders (Coccaro *et al.* 2005; Kessler *et al.* 2006) and in particular the high comorbidity with substance-use, anxiety, and mood disorders. Chapter 20 provides further indication that the comorbidity patterns of IED do not place it exclusively in the category of externalizing disorders, compared with other typical externalizing disorders (e.g., substance-use disorders or conduct disorder).

From the information respondents provided on the type and frequency of anger attacks during the week of their most violent attack it appears that many anger attacks are non-destructive, although individuals engaging in these less destructive attacks might also have engaged in the more destructive attacks. Anger attacks that cause harm to others are also common, with 43% per cent of those meeting 12-month criteria for IED reporting that they had hurt someone badly during their most violent anger attack. Moreover, a small proportion reported purposely torturing or injuring an animal, or arson. Our data do not allow us to determine whether some of these acts might have been premeditated rather than reactive. A recent study of a predominantly clinical population found that 5.9% of those meeting criteria for DSM-5 IED were also classified as 'highly likely' to meet criteria for psychopathic personality (Coccaro *et al.* 2014a).

Although the WMH findings suggest that a substantial minority of individuals with IED (39%) are significantly disabled by their disorder, especially in terms of social and relationship functioning, the majority only reported mild-moderate impairment. This finding conflicts with a recent study that found participants meeting DSM-5 criteria for IED reported much greater impairment across all domains (occupational, social, legal) compared with participants meeting criteria for other mental disorders (Kulper *et al.* 2015). However, the IED group in that study was a self-selected sample that were characterized by substantially higher levels of lifetime mental disorder comorbidity than the mental disorder control group; this suggests that the IED group were more clinically severe. The WMH data on impairment are important because they are more representative of IED in the general population. In this respect we note that the 38.9% with severe impairment places IED in the bottom third of disorders ranked by proportion with severe impairment (see Chapter 22). This may be because some individuals with IED may not be fully aware of, or may partly deny, the full ramifications of their aggressive outbursts either for themselves or for those on the receiving end of the outbursts. The sporadic/intermittent nature of the aggressive outbursts may also be a factor that reduces associated impairment.

Our results indicate that a wide range of traumatic events are associated with risk of IED, but after controlling for the clustering of traumatic events in peoples' lives it is the experience (direct or witnessing) of physical violence in childhood that most strongly predicts IED onset. One other recent study that considered multiple forms of child maltreatment found that only physical abuse was independently associated with IED (Fanning *et al.* 2014). Finding an association between physical abuse in childhood and IED in adolescence and adulthood is not surprising given the large amount of research on the intergenerational transmission of violence mediated by a range of neurobiological, emotional, cognitive, and behavioural mechanisms (Van Goozen *et al.* 2007). It is interesting, though, that we found witnessing of family violence to be associated with IED onset even after controlling for the direct experience of violence. Prior research has found that the witnessing of family violence is generally a less potent risk factor compared to direct experience of physical abuse but that it is nonetheless a reliable and independent predictor risk factor for youth involvement in violence (Yexley *et al.* 2002). We also found that prior experiences of intimate partner violence and sexual assault were independently associated with IED onset. Other studies have found IED to be associated with reports of intimate partner violence (O'Leary *et al.* 2008; Murray-Close *et al.* 2010) and although it is not surprising that IED would increase risk of perpetration of intimate partner violence, our time-lagged analyses suggest that experience of intimate partner violence may be a risk factor for the onset of IED. Prospective studies will be required to confirm this direction of association but it underscores the comment made earlier that relationship difficulties may precede as well as follow IED. Finally, the experience of non-combat violence emerged as a risk factor for IED onset, but by contrast, combat experience was protective. This latter finding may reflect military selection procedures or aspects of military training.

In summary, IED prevalence varies substantially across countries with an average of 0.8% in this group of 16 countries, and shows a positive gradient of increasing prevalence with increasing country income level. IED is more common in males, the young and the socially disadvantaged. It is one of the earlier onset disorders and is highly comorbid with a wide range of other disorders. Traumatic lifetime experiences involving violence, especially those occurring early in life, are predictively associated with lifetime odds of IED. A substantial minority of those with IED report significant functional impairment but this likely underestimates the true societal costs of IED in terms of the effects of explosive anger attacks on families and relationships.

Acknowledgements

Portions of the results appearing in this chapter appeared previously in: Scott, K. M, Lim, C. C. W., Hwang, I., Adamowski, T., Al-Hamzawi, A., Bromet, E., Bunting, B., Ferrand, M., Florescu, S., Gureje, O., Hinkov, H., Karam, E., Lee, S., Posada-Villa, J., Stein, D. J., Tachimori, H., Viana, M. C., Xavier, M., Kessler, R. C. (2016). The cross-national epidemiology of DSM-IV intermittent explosive disorder. *Psychological Medicine,* 46, 3161–3172, used with permission from Cambridge University Press, 2016.

References

Ahmed, A. O., Green, B. A., McCloskey, M. S., *et al.* (2010). Latent structure of intermittent explosive disorder in an epidemiological sample. *Journal of Psychiatric Research,* 44, 663–72.

Al-Hamzawi, A., Al-Diwan, J., Al-Hasnawi, S., *et al.* (2012). The prevalence and correlates of intermittent explosive disorder in Iraq. *Acta Psychiatrica Scandinavica*, 126, 219–28.

Axinn, W. G., Ghimire, D. J., Williams, N. E., *et al.* (2013). Gender, traumatic events, and mental health disorders in a rural Asian setting. *Journal of Health and Social Behavior*, 54, 444–61.

Breslau, J., Miller, E., Jin, R., *et al.* (2011). A multinational study of mental disorders, marriage, and divorce. *Acta Psychiatrica Scandinavica*, 124, 474–86.

Busch, F. N. (2009). Anger and depression. *Advances in Psychiatric Treatment*, 15, 271.

Coccaro, E. F. (2012). Intermittent explosive disorder as a disorder of impulsive aggression for DSM-5. *American Journal of Psychiatry*, 169, 577–88.

Coccaro, E. F., Kavoussi, R. J., Berman, M. E., *et al.* (1998). Intermittent explosive disorder-revised: development, reliability, and validity of research criteria. *Comprehensive Psychiatry*, 39, 368–76.

Coccaro, E. F., Lee, R., McCloskey, M. S. (2014a). Relationship between psychopathy, aggression, anger, impulsivity, and intermittent explosive disorder. *Aggressive Behavior*, 40, 526–36.

(2014b). Validity of the new A 1 and A 2 criteria for DSM-5 intermittent explosive disorder. *Comprehensive Psychiatry*, 55, 260–7.

Coccaro, E. F., Posternak, M. A., Zimmerman, M. (2005). Prevalence and features of intermittent explosive disorder in a clinical setting. *The Journal of Clinical Psychiatry*, 66, 1478–227.

Fanning, J. R., Meyerhoff, J. J., Lee, R., *et al.* (2014). History of childhood maltreatment in intermittent explosive disorder and suicidal behavior. *Journal of Psychiatric Research*, 56, 10–17.

Fincham, D., Grimsrud, A., Corrigall, J., *et al.* (2009). Intermittent explosive disorder in South Africa: prevalence, correlates and the role of traumatic exposures. *Psychopathology*, 42, 92–8.

Haro, J. M., Arbabzadeh-Bouchez, S., Brugha, T. S., *et al.* (2006). Concordance of the Composite International Diagnostic Interview Version 3.0 (CIDI 3.0) with standardized clinical assessments in the WHO World Mental Health Surveys. *International Journal of Methods in Psychiatric Research*, 15, 167–80.

Judge, T. A., Livingston, B. A., Hurst, C. (2012). Do nice guys – and gals – really finish last? The joint effects of sex and agreeableness on income. *Journal of Personality and Social Psychology*, 102, 390.

Kessler, R. C., Coccaro, E. F., Fava, M., *et al.* (2006). The prevalence and correlates of DSM-IV intermittent explosive disorder in the National Comorbidity Survey Replication. *Archives of General Psychiatry*, 63, 669–78.

Kessler, R. C., Coccaro, E. F., Fava, M.,*et al.* (2012). The phenomenology and epidemiology of intermittent explosive disorder. In *The Oxford Handbook of Impulse Control Disorders* (eds. J. E. Grant and M. N. Potenza), pp. 149–64. Oxford: Oxford University Press.

Kessler, R. C., Üstün, T. B. eds. (2008). *The WHO World Mental Health Surveys: Global Perspectives on the Epidemiology of Mental Disorders*. New York, NY: Cambridge University Press.

Kulper, D. A., Kleiman, E. M., McCloskey, M. S., *et al.* (2015). The experience of aggressive outbursts in intermittent explosive disorder. *Psychiatry Research*, 225, 710–15.

Lilienfeld, S. O., Lynn, S. J., Ruscio, J., *et al.* (2011). *50 Great Myths of Popular Psychology: Shattering Widespread Misconceptions about Human Behavior*. Chichester: John Wiley & Sons.

McKinney, C. M., Caetano, R., Ramisetty-Mikler, S., *et al.* (2009). Childhood family violence and perpetration and victimization of intimate partner violence: findings from a national population-based study of couples. *Annals of Epidemiology*, 19, 25–32.

McLaughlin, K. A., Green, J. G., Hwang, I., *et al.* (2012). Intermittent explosive disorder in the National Comorbidity Survey Replication Adolescent Supplement. *Archives of General Psychiatry*, 69, 1131–9.

Moffitt, T., Caspi, A., Taylor, A., *et al.* (2010). How common are common mental disorders? Evidence that lifetime prevalence rates are doubled by prospective versus retrospective ascertainment. *Psychological Medicine*, 40, 899.

Murray-Close, D., Ostrov, J. M., Nelson, D. A., *et al.* (2010). Proactive, reactive, and romantic relational aggression in adulthood: measurement, predictive validity, gender differences, and association with Intermittent Explosive Disorder. *Journal of Psychiatric Research*, 44, 393–404.

Nickerson, A., Aderka, I. M., Bryant, R. A., *et al.* (2012). The relationship between childhood exposure to trauma and intermittent explosive disorder. *Psychiatry Research*, 197, 128–34.

Novaco, R. W. (2010). Anger and psychopathology. In *International Handbook of Anger: Constituent and*

Concomitant Biological, Psychological, and Social Processes (eds. M. Potegal, G. Stemmler, and C. Spielberger), pp. 465–97. New York: Springer.

O'Leary, K. D., Tintle, N., Bromet, E. J., *et al.* (2008). Descriptive epidemiology of intimate partner aggression in Ukraine. *Social Psychiatry & Psychiatric Epidemiology*, 43, 619–26.

Ortega, A. N., Canino, G., Alegria, M. (2008). Lifetime and 12-month intermittent explosive disorder in Latinos. *American Journal of Orthopsychiatry*, 78, 133–9.

Rees, S., Silove, D., Verdial, T., *et al.* (2013). Intermittent explosive disorder amongst women in conflict affected Timor-Leste: associations with human rights trauma, ongoing violence, poverty, and injustice. *PLoS One*, 8, e69207.

Scott, K. M., Lim, C. C. W., Hwang, I., *et al.* (2016). The cross-national epidemiology of DSM-IV intermittent explosive disorder. *Psychological Medicine*, 46, 3161–72.

Song, L., Singer, M. I., Anglin, T. M. (1998). Violence exposure and emotional trauma as contributors to adolescents' violent behaviors. *Archives of Pediatrics and Adolescent Medicine*, 152, 531–6.

Takayanagi, Y., Spira, A. P., Roth, K. B., *et al.* (2014). Accuracy of reports of lifetime mental and physical disorders: results from the Baltimore Epidemiological Catchment Area Study. *JAMA Psychiatry*, 71, 273–80.

Tavris, C. (1989). *Anger: The Misunderstood Emotion.* New York: Simon and Schuster.

Van Goozen, S. H., Fairchild, G., Snoek, H., *et al.* (2007). The evidence for a neurobiological model of childhood antisocial behavior. *Psychological Bulletin*, 133, 149.

Yexley, M., Borowsky, I., Ireland, M. (2002). Correlation between different experiences of intrafamilial physical violence and violent adolescent behavior. *Journal of Interpersonal Violence*, 17, 707–20.

Yoshimasu, K., Kawakami, N. (2011). Epidemiological aspects of intermittent explosive disorder in Japan; prevalence and psychosocial comorbidity: findings from the World Mental Health Japan Survey 2002–2006. *Psychiatry Research*, 186, 384–9.

Chapter 14

Attention-Deficit Hyperactivity Disorder

John Fayyad, Josep Maria Haro, Sergio Aguilar-Gaxiola, Ronald C. Kessler

Introduction

Although most epidemiological studies of the prevalence and correlates of childhood and adult Attention-Deficit Hyperactivity Disorder (ADHD) have taken place in the United States (US), Australia, and Western Europe, there has been a recent increase in comparable studies in other parts of the world and the publication of several comprehensive reviews (Polanczyk *et al.* 2007, 2014; Polanczyk & Jensen 2008; Alhraiwil *et al.* 2015; Thomas *et al.* 2015). Taken together, these reports make it clear that ADHD is an important disorder throughout the world given its early age-of-onset, strong associations with the subsequent onset and persistence of secondary disorders, persistence into adulthood, and strong associations with impaired role functioning throughout the lifespan. A challenge in comparing cross-national results, though, is that existing epidemiological studies vary widely in measures, classification systems, and data collection procedures. The World Mental Health (WMH) Surveys Initiative has been the largest and most systematic effort to address these methodological problems to date based on retrospective reports being obtained from adult WMH respondents about childhood ADHD and separate questions being asked about adult ADHD.

Previous WMH reports presented data from the first 10 national samples to assess ADHD in terms of prevalence and correlates regarding both childhood and adult ADHD (Fayyad *et al.* 2007), the associations of childhood ADHD with subsequent secondary comorbid disorders (Kessler *et al.* 2011), the predictors of ADHD persistence into adulthood (Lara *et al.* 2009), and the role impairments associated with adult ADHD (de Graaf *et al.* 2008). The current chapter presents an update on these results based on the most recent WMH data, which come from the 20 WMH surveys out of the 29 included in this volume that assessed ADHD (Fayyad *et al.* 2017).

Methods

Diagnostic Assessment

As with other diagnoses, lifetime prevalence of DSM-IV ADHD was assessed with the WHO Composite International Diagnostic Interview (CIDI) Version 3.0 (Kessler & Üstün 2004), but in the case of childhood ADHD the CIDI retrospective assessment was based on the Diagnostic Interview Schedule (DIS) (Robins & Helzer 1985). Included here were questions about the nine DSM-IV symptoms of inattention (AD) and the nine symptoms of hyperactivity-impulsivity (HD) (at least six of nine in one or both sets required for a diagnosis), age-of-onset of these symptoms (at last some of which had to start before age seven), and impairments caused by these symptoms (which had to occur in at least two role domains).

Although our original intent was to assess only childhood ADHD in the WMH surveys, we included questions in the ADHD section to parallel those in other diagnostic sections asking respondents whether they still had problems with inattention or impulsivity-hyperactivity and, if so, how much these symptoms caused impairments in their daily functioning. When we began analysis of the data for the earliest WMH surveys, we were struck by the high proportions of respondents with diagnoses of childhood ADHD who reported still having symptoms that interfered with their current functioning. Based on this observation, we became familiar with a nascent literature suggesting that a substantial proportion of cases of childhood ADHD persist into adulthood (Faraone *et al.* 2000; Weiss *et al.* 2000), but this claim was at the time controversial (Wolf & Wasserstein 2001).

Multiple Imputation Strategy to Arrive at Adult ADHD Prevalence Estimates

We conducted a small (n = 154) follow-up study of respondents with childhood ADHD in the US sample.

The follow-up survey was carried out by telephone with trained clinical interviewers administering the Adult ADHD Clinical Diagnostic Scale (ACDS) Version 1.2 (Adler & Cohen 2004; Adler & Spencer 2004). As reported elsewhere (Kessler *et al.* 2006), a substantial number of respondents met criteria for DSM-IV adult ADHD, and a number of others had subthreshold adult ADHD with significant role impairment. Based on these results, we developed an imputation scheme using information available in all WMH surveys. Diagnostic classification accuracy based on this approach was quite good in the clinical reappraisal sample, with area under the receiver operating characteristic curve (AUC) of 0.86. Based on this result, Multiple Imputation (MI; Rubin 1987) was used to assign imputed clinical diagnoses of adult ADHD to respondents in all WMH surveys based on the coefficients in the prediction equation in the US clinical reappraisal sample. Importantly, this approach assumes that the association between CIDI responses and clinical diagnoses is constant across countries. The statistical details of the MI method are discussed elsewhere (Kessler *et al.* 2006). The important points to emphasize here are that MI generates unbiased prevalence estimates under the model, that individual-level estimates have good accuracy when, as in this case, AUC is high, and that a simulation adjusts standard errors for the effects of classification error due to imperfect imputation. The imputation equation used here was somewhat less refined than in the earlier US study because not all countries included all predictors used in the US imputation equation.

Results

ADHD Prevalence in Childhood and Persistence into Adulthood

Estimated prevalence of ADHD in childhood averages 2.2% across the surveys, but varies strongly across samples (0.1–8.1%) resulting in a wide inter-quartile (IQR) range (0.9–2.9%) (Table 14.1). Prevalence is significantly related to country income level, with prevalence of 3.3% in high-, 2.2% in upper-middle-, and 0.6% in low/lower-middle-income countries (χ^2_2 = 113.3, P < 0.001). Subthreshold childhood ADHD (4–5 rather than 6+ AD and/or HD symptoms in addition to other required criteria) is even more prevalent (3.7% across countries; 4.7% in high-, 4.0% in upper-middle-, and 2.2% in low/lower-middle-income countries; χ^2_2 = 48.9, P < 0.001). Conditional prevalence of current (at the time of interview) adult ADHD averages 57.0% across surveys among respondents with a history of childhood ADHD (56.2% in high-, 54.1% in upper-middle-, and 71.7% in low/lower-middle-income countries; χ^2_2 = 2.4, P = 0.30) and 41.1% among respondents with a history of subthreshold childhood ADHD (36.9% in high-, 46.8% in upper-middle-, and 45.9% in low/lower-middle-income countries; χ^2_2 = 3.9, P = 0.14).

Current prevalence of adult ADHD in the total sample averages 2.8% across surveys, again varying strongly across samples (0.6–7.3%) resulting in a wide IQR (1.8–4.1%) and with a higher prevalence in high-income countries (3.6%) and upper-middle-income countries (3.0%) than in low/lower-middle income (1.4%) countries (χ^2_2 = 40.5, P < 0.001). Adult ADHD is thus more prevalent than childhood ADHD and this pattern is consistent in high- (3.6% versus 3.3%), upper-middle- (3.0% versus 2.2%), and low/lower-middle- (2.8% versus 2.2%) income countries.

Socio-demographic Correlates

Pooled across surveys, childhood ADHD is significantly more common among men than women (OR 1.6) and significantly but non-monotonically associated with educational attainment (χ^2_1 = 21.1, P < 0.001) (Table 14.2). Childhood ADHD is not significantly associated with respondent age at the time of interview (which, as noted above, was 18–44), current (at time of interview) employment status, current marital status, or current income. The same basic socio-demographic patterns are found with subthreshold childhood ADHD. Persistence of childhood ADHD into adulthood (i.e., current prevalence) among childhood cases, in comparison, is significantly associated with respondent employment status (employed versus all others; χ^2_1 = 11.3, P = 0.001) due to comparatively low persistence among the currently employed. None of the socio-demographic variables are significantly related to adult ADHD among subthreshold childhood cases.

The strength of associations between socio-demographic variables and adult ADHD is, in effect, a weighted combination of the associations with childhood ADHD in the total sample and adult persistence among childhood threshold and subthreshold cases. Adult ADHD prevalence is significantly higher among men than women (OR 1.6) and significantly associated with young age (χ^2_1 = 12.4, P < 0.001), less than college educational attainment (χ^2_1 = 16.1, P< 0.001), and being unmarried (χ^2_1 = 8.4, P = 0.004). The higher

Table 14.1 Multiply imputed prevalence estimates of DSM-IV attention-deficit hyperactivity disorder (ADHD) in each WMH sample[a]

	Childhood ADHD				Adult ADHD among childhood cases of ...				Adult ADHD in the total sample		(N)[b]
	Threshold		Subthreshold		Threshold		Subthreshold				
	%	(SE)	%	(SE)	%	(SE)	%	(SE)	%	(SE)	
Low/lower-middle-income countries											
Colombia	1.2	(0.3)	2.9	(0.5)	84.9	(10.2)	51.5	(8.8)	2.5	(0.5)	(1,731)
Iraq	0.1	(0.1)	1.0	(0.2)	77.0	(19.2)	47.9	(14.6)	0.6	(0.2)	(3,227)
Peru	0.8	(0.2)	2.5	(0.5)	58.4	(14.1)	35.4	(12.4)	1.4	(0.5)	(1,287)
PRC[c] (Shenzhen)	0.7	(0.2)	3.0	(0.6)	62.8	(21.4)	46.1	(8.2)	1.8	(0.4)	(2,190)
Total	**0.6**	**(0.1)**	**2.2**	**(0.2)**	**71.7**	**(9.5)**	**45.9**	**(5.5)**	**1.4**	**(0.2)**	**(8,435)**
Upper-middle-income countries											
Brazil (São Paulo)	2.5	(0.4)	7.0	(1.0)	76.2	(14.5)	58.2	(10.7)	5.9	(1.2)	(1,824)
Colombia (Medellin)	2.5	(0.5)	3.0	(0.7)	59.2	(10.7)	51.5	(12.5)	3.0	(0.7)	(970)
Lebanon	1.5	(0.4)	3.3	(1.2)	52.4	(15.0)	29.9	(17.1)	1.8	(0.7)	(595)
Mexico	3.0	(0.4)	3.7	(0.7)	32.8	(7.3)	25.8	(8.6)	1.9	(0.4)	(1,736)
Romania	0.4	(0.3)	0.7	(0.4)	45.7	(40.8)	54.7	(24.3)	0.6	(0.4)	(940)
Total	**2.2**	**(0.2)**	**4.0**	**(0.4)**	**54.1**	**(7.0)**	**46.8**	**(7.6)**	**3.0**	**(0.5)**	**(6,065)**
High-income countries											
Belgium	2.9	(1.1)	8.6	(2.1)	71.9	(16.5)	22.7	(10.0)	4.1	(1.5)	(486)
France	4.7	(1.2)	8.9	(1.4)	58.8	(14.0)	50.9	(10.5)	7.3	(1.8)	(727)
Germany	1.8	(0.7)	5.6	(1.5)	67.9	(16.1)	33.7	(8.5)	3.1	(0.8)	(621)
Italy	0.9	(0.2)	3.7	(0.7)	84.1	(11.1)	55.1	(11.2)	2.8	(0.6)	(853)
Netherlands	2.9	(0.9)	9.2	(1.6)	82.3	(14.4)	28.4	(9.3)	5.0	(1.6)	(516)
Northern Ireland	3.2	(0.8)	4.5	(0.7)	98.8	(2.0)	64.0	(8.2)	6.0	(0.8)	(907)
Poland	0.3	(0.1)	0.8	(0.2)	69.7	(9.4)	62.6	(14.5)	0.8	(0.2)	(2,276)
Portugal	1.5	(0.4)	4.0	(0.7)	56.3	(15.3)	54.0	(11.1)	3.0	(0.7)	(1,070)
Spain	1.8	(0.8)	1.9	(0.5)	33.6	(20.6)	29.2	(12.3)	1.2	(0.6)	(960)
Spain (Murcia)	2.0	(0.5)	4.2	(0.7)	72.9	(21.6)	44.3	(17.5)	3.3	(1.1)	(631)
United States	8.1	(0.6)	6.6	(0.5)	46.0	(4.9)	22.5	(4.6)	5.2	(0.6)	(3,197)
Total	**3.3**	**(0.2)**	**4.7**	**(0.3)**	**56.2**	**(4.8)**	**36.9**	**(4.3)**	**3.6**	**(0.4)**	**(12,244)**
All countries combined	**2.2**	**(0.1)**	**3.7**	**(0.2)**	**57.0**	**(4.4)**	**41.1**	**(4.3)**	**2.8**	**(0.3)**	**(26,744)**
χ^2	113.3*		48.9*		2.4		3.9		40.5*		

*Significant at the 0.05 level, two-sided test.
[a]Sample restricted to respondents ages 18–44 at interview and Part II sample.
[b]These are denominator N's; that is, the number of people assessed rather than the number with ADHD.
[c]People's Republic of China.

Table 14.2 Socio-demographic correlates of multiply imputed DSM-IV attention-deficit hyperactivity disorder (ADHD) in all WMH countries combined (n = 26,744)[a]

	Childhood ADHD				Adult ADHD among childhood cases of ...				Adult ADHD in the total sample		(N)[b]
	Threshold		Subthreshold		Threshold		Subthreshold				
	%	(SE)	%	(SE)	%	(SE)	%	(SE)	%	(SE)	
Gender											
Male	2.7	(0.2)	4.3	(0.2)	57.5	(4.9)	42.0	(4.4)	3.4	(0.3)	(11,491)
Female	1.7	(0.1)	3.2	(0.2)	56.2	(5.2)	39.8	(5.2)	2.2	(0.2)	(15,253)
χ^{2c}	24.0*		18.4*		0.0		0.3		26.8*		
Age											
18–24	2.4	(0.2)	4.3	(0.3)	60.9	(6.0)	43.5	(5.0)	3.3	(0.4)	(6,632)
25–34	1.9	(0.2)	3.7	(0.2)	57.2	(6.0)	43.8	(5.3)	2.7	(0.3)	(10,112)
35–44	2.3	(0.2)	3.3	(0.3)	53.2	(5.6)	34.7	(5.4)	2.4	(0.3)	(10,000)
χ^{2c}	1.3		12.3*		2.8		1.4		12.4*		
Education											
No education	0.8	(0.5)	1.9	(0.9)	26.9	(23.4)	61.8	(20.3)	1.4	(0.8)	(570)
Some primary	2.3	(0.4)	4.1	(0.6)	75.2	(8.2)	47.1	(8.2)	3.6	(0.6)	(1,690)
Finished primary	1.4	(0.2)	4.4	(0.8)	71.2	(8.4)	37.8	(11.8)	2.7	(0.7)	(2,137)
Some secondary	2.5	(0.3)	3.7	(0.4)	54.5	(8.3)	35.5	(5.6)	2.6	(0.4)	(5,027)
Finished secondary	2.3	(0.2)	3.9	(0.3)	58.0	(5.9)	44.0	(5.2)	3.1	(0.3)	(8,244)
Some college	2.8	(0.3)	4.3	(0.4)	54.9	(5.2)	41.6	(6.3)	3.4	(0.4)	(4,662)
Finished college	1.6	(0.2)	2.6	(0.3)	50.1	(7.5)	38.1	(6.7)	1.8	(0.3)	(4,414)
χ^{2c}	21.1*		16.1*		1.6		0.4		16.1*		
Employment status											
Employed	2.3	(0.1)	4.1	(0.2)	52.7	(4.7)	41.4	(4.5)	2.9	(0.3)	(17,660)
Student	1.7	(0.3)	2.5	(0.4)	74.1	(9.2)	41.2	(8.9)	2.3	(0.4)	(1,669)
Homemaker	1.1	(0.2)	2.3	(0.3)	61.7	(9.3)	44.4	(7.9)	1.7	(0.3)	(4,020)
Retired	3.2	(2.2)	1.2	(0.8)	52.0	(16.2)	39.8	(29.4)	2.2	(1.5)	(78)
Unemployed	2.9	(0.4)	4.3	(0.5)	68.1	(7.5)	37.4	(8.0)	3.6	(0.6)	(3,317)
χ^{2c}	0.5		0.2		11.3*		0.1		1.4		
Marital status											
Married/cohabitating	2.0	(0.1)	3.5	(0.2)	53.6	(5.1)	38.8	(4.9)	2.4	(0.3)	(16,000)
Previously married	4.2	(0.5)	4.2	(0.8)	54.8	(7.4)	43.8	(11.8)	4.1	(0.8)	(1,862)
Never married	2.3	(0.2)	4.1	(0.3)	61.8	(5.8)	43.5	(4.5)	3.2	(0.3)	(8,882)
χ^{2c}	2.8		3.2		3.2		1.2		8.4*		
Household Income[d]											
Low	2.1	(0.2)	3.6	(0.3)	65.3	(5.1)	43.1	(5.2)	3.0	(0.3)	(7,528)
Low-average	2.6	(0.3)	4.0	(0.3)	51.2	(6.6)	42.0	(5.8)	3.0	(0.4)	(6,263)
High-average	2.4	(0.2)	3.8	(0.4)	58.0	(5.8)	37.3	(5.6)	2.8	(0.4)	(6,719)
High	1.7	(0.2)	3.5	(0.3)	51.7	(7.1)	41.9	(6.0)	2.4	(0.3)	(6,234)
χ^{2c}	1.1		0.9		0.0		0.5		1.6		

*Significant at the 0.05 level, two-sided design-based multiply-imputed test.

[a]Based on multivariate logistic regression equations in which all predictors were included simultaneously. All models include dummy variable controls for surveys.

[b]These are denominator N's; that is, numbers of respondents in the total sample with the socio-demographic characteristic defined by the row heading.

[c]Each χ^2 test has one degree of freedom. Tests for age, education, and income are based on continuous versions of those predictors. The test for employment status compares employed to all others. The test for marital status compares married/cohabiting to all others.

[d]Income is defined as the ratio of pre-tax family income to number of household members. Households with ratios half the median within-survey value or lower were categorized as 'low' income; those with ratios between half the median and the median were categorized as 'low-average'; those with ratios greater than the median up to three times the median as 'high-average'; and those greater than three times the median as 'high'.

prevalence among men than women is due to the significantly elevated odds of childhood ADHD noted above. The significant inverse association of age with current adult ADHD is due to a significant inverse association of age with subthreshold childhood ADHD, an insignificant inverse association of age with childhood threshold ADHD, and a significant inverse association of age with adult persistence of ADHD among childhood cases. The significant association of current adult ADHD with being unmarried is due to significantly elevated odds of childhood threshold ADHD with being previously married at the time of interview, in addition to insignificant trend associations of being previously married and never married with persistence among childhood threshold and subthreshold cases.

Comorbidity

Twelve-month adult ADHD is significantly and positively comorbid with 12-month prevalence of other mental disorders considered in the WMH surveys (Table 14.3). ORs are in the range between 2.5 (major depressive disorder) and 15.0 (oppositional defiant disorder) with individual comorbid disorders, 4.4 with a summary variable of having any comorbid disorder, and increasing ORs with number of comorbid disorders (3.0 with exactly one comorbid disorder, 6.2 with exactly two, and 9.6 with three or more; $\chi^2_2 = 66.7$, $P < 0.001$). Retrospective age-of-onset reports were used to date temporal priorities between onset ages of ADHD and comorbid disorders. Given the early age-of-onset of ADHD required in DSM-IV, it is not surprising that we find ADHD to be the temporally primary disorder in the vast majority of cases of comorbidities involving mood disorders (86.0–94.0%), anxiety disorders other than specific phobia (70.5–90.2%), and substance-use disorders (94.8–99.1 %). Specific phobia is the only comorbid disorder that was more likely to be temporally primary than ADHD (specific phobia first in 53.1% of cases, ADHD first in 29.1%, and same year in the remaining 17.8%).

Given the strong temporal priority of ADHD over the vast majority of comorbid disorders, we examined the extent to which ADHD predicted the subsequent first onset of the other disorders assessed in the surveys. We distinguished between respondents who had (i) AD-only versus HD (with or without AD) childhood symptom profiles in order to see if those profiles are differentially associated with the subsequent onset of temporally secondary disorders. Also, we distinguished between active and remitted ADHD cases in order to determine if the ORs of secondary disorders occurring decrease significantly with the remission of ADHD. In initial models, we also evaluated the significance of the difference between active and remitted ADHD depending on whether the childhood ADHD had an AD-only or HD symptom profile. However, as this interaction was not significant in all models ($\chi^2_1 = 0.0–3.4$, $P = 0.88–0.07$), we focused on the coefficients in the additive model (Table 14.4). Three broad patterns of results are noteworthy. First, all but one of the ORs for secondary disorders associated with *remitted* ADHD are elevated (ORs = 1.1–2.7, with a median of 1.6 and IQR of 1.2–2.0) and nearly half are statistically significant ($\chi^2_1 = 4.4–37.3$, $P = 0.036$ to <0.001). Second, the odds of secondary disorders associated with *active* ADHD are consistently elevated relative to those associated with remitted ADHD (ORs = 1.2–4.6) and nearly two-thirds of these ORs are statistically significant ($\chi^2_1 = 4.3–15.9$, $P = 0.041$ to <0.001). Third, the ORs associated with the AD-only subtype do not differ meaningfully from those associated with the HD subtype, with each of the two having the same median (1.6) and very similar IQRs (1.1–2.0 for AD-only; 1.2–2.2 for HD).

Disability

Unlike most other chapters in this volume, functioning in the prior 30 days was examined with the WHO Disability Assessment Schedule (WHO-DAS; Üstün et al. 2010) rather than the SDS because WHO-DAS, unlike SDS, contains a scale for impairments in cognition. The latter are believed to be of special importance for adult ADHD. We found that respondents with adult ADHD are more likely to have disability in cognition (21.8%) than in any other WHO-DAS dimensions, although respondents with adult ADHD have significantly elevated odds of all these outcomes (Table 14.5). Respondents with current ADHD are also significantly more likely than others to report at least one day out of role in the 30 days before interview due to health problems (OR 2.6). However, further analysis showed that these significant associations are to some extent due to comorbid disorders, as indicated by the ORs attenuating when controls are introduced for 12-month comorbid disorders.

Table 14.3 Bivariate 12-month co-occurrence and lifetime age-of-onset temporal priority of multiply imputed DSM-IV adult attention-deficit hyperactivity disorder (ADHD) with other DSM IV disorders (n = 26,744)[a]

	Conditional prevalence estimates				Age-of-onset temporal priority								
	ADHD/Co[b]		Co/ADHD[c]		ADHD first		Other disorder first		Both in the same year				
	%	(SE)	%	(SE)	%	(SE)	%	(SE)	%	(SE)	OR	(95% CI)	(N)[d]s
I. Mood disorders													
Major depressive disorder	8.1	(0.8)	15.0	(1.5)	86.0	(2.7)	8.9	(2.3)	5.1	(2.1)	2.5*	(2.0–3.2)	(199)
Bipolar spectrum disorder	15.2	(1.7)	9.4	(1.3)	94.0	(2.7)	3.1	(2.1)	2.8	(1.9)	5.4*	(4.0–7.2)	(92)
Any mood disorder	9.3	(0.8)	21.9	(1.9)	86.4	(2.2)	8.3	(1.8)	5.3	(1.6)	3.2*	(2.6–4.1)	(287)
II. Anxiety disorders													
Generalized anxiety disorder	8.3	(1.5)	3.8	(0.7)	83.9	(7.4)	9.3	(6.2)	6.8	(4.5)	2.6*	(1.7–3.9)	(47)
Panic disorder	14.4	(2.3)	5.7	(1.0)	90.2	(3.9)	3.9	(2.0)	5.9	(3.7)	4.5*	(3.0–6.6)	(70)
Specific phobia	8.9	(0.9)	20.9	(1.9)	29.1	(4.4)	53.1	(4.6)	17.8	(3.0)	3.4*	(2.6–4.3)	(250)
Social phobia	12.0	(1.4)	12.6	(1.4)	70.5	(4.7)	16.5	(3.8)	13.0	(2.7)	3.9*	(2.9–5.1)	(152)
Any anxiety disorder	8.8	(0.7)	34.2	(2.4)	48.0	(3.4)	37.9	(3.5)	14.2	(2.1)	3.7*	(3.0–4.6)	(400)
III. Substance-use disorders													
Alcohol abuse without dependence	9.4	(1.7)	5.1	(1.0)	98.0	(2.0)	2.1	(2.0)	0.0	(0.0)	3.0*	(1.9–4.6)	(49)
Drug abuse without dependence	16.1	(5.1)	2.7	(0.9)	94.8	(5.3)	0.0	(0.0)	5.2	(5.3)	4.8*	(2.3–10.1)	(16)
Any substance-use disorder	11.5	(1.5)	11.4	(1.6)	99.1	(0.9)	0.9	(0.9)	0.0	(0.0)	3.8*	(2.8–5.2)	(100)
IV. Disruptive Behaviour disorders													
Intermittent explosive disorder	10.9	(1.4)	12.8	(1.6)	78.7	(5.1)	12.6	(4.5)	8.7	(3.2)	3.8*	(2.7–5.2)	(101)
Oppositional defiant disorder	35.5	(4.5)	8.3	(1.4)	49.8	(7.6)	25.7	(6.9)	24.5	(7.9)	15.0*	(9.7–23.2)	(83)
Any disruptive behaviour disorder	15.6	(1.6)	15.2	(1.7)	64.5	(5.3)	19.0	(4.1)	16.5	(4.5)	6.2*	(4.6–8.4)	(169)
V. Total													
Exactly one[e]	5.5	(0.6)	23.0	(1.9)	73.8	(3.8)	18.1	(3.3)	8.1	(2.3)	3.0*	(2.3–3.9)	(242)
Exactly two[e]	11.2	(1.3)	14.3	(1.7)	90.6	(3.1)	5.6	(2.6)	3.8	(1.7)	6.2*	(4.4–8.8)	(163)
Three or more[e]	17.7	(1.7)	14.4	(1.6)	90.2	(2.6)	3.2	(1.2)	6.6	(2.1)	9.6*	(6.9–13.3)	(180)
Any	8.3	(0.6)	51.7	(3.1)	55.6	(2.8)	31.2	(2.8)	13.2	(2.0)	4.4*	(3.4–5.7)	(585)

*Significant at the 0.05 level, two-sided test.

[a]All models assessed with Part II weight (except Iraq and Romania) and control for countries. ADHD is the outcome variable in the models. Countries without the row disorder are dropped from the % calculations and the models. ESEMeD countries (Belgium, Germany, Italy, Netherlands, Spain, France) do not have dysthymia, bipolar, drug-use, and intermittent explosive disorder. PRC (Shenzhen) does not have posttraumatic stress disorder, any of the substance-use disorders, oppositional defiant disorder or adult antisocial behaviour disorder. Portugal does not have drug-use disorders. Iraq does not have oppositional defiant disorder or adult antisocial behaviour disorder. Mexico, Spain (Murcia), and Colombia (Medellin) all do not have intermittent explosive disorder.

[b]Conditional prevalence estimates of adult ADHD in the subsamples of respondents with the comorbid disorders.

[c]Conditional prevalence estimates of the comorbid disorders in the subsample of respondents with adult ADHD.

[d]Denominator N is the number of people with both ADHD and the row disorder.

[e]Onset of 'Exactly two' disorders takes the age-of-onset of the second earliest disorder the respondent was assessed with. Onset of 'Three or more' disorders takes the third earliest disorder the respondent was assessed with.

Table 14.4 Associations of childhood ADHD subtypes and comorbid lifetime DSM-IV disorders, in all countries combined (N = 26,744)[a]

	Active versus remitted ADHD		Remitted childhood AD-only		Remitted childhood HD	
	OR	(95% CI)	OR	(95% CI)	OR	(95% CI)
I. Mood disorders						
Major depressive disorder	1.2	(1.0–1.6)	2.0*	(1.6–2.5)	1.7*	(1.3–2.2)
Bipolar spectrum disorder	2.0*	(1.3–2.9)	1.7*	(1.0–2.8)	2.3*	(1.5–3.6)
II. Anxiety disorders						
Panic disorder/agoraphobia	1.5	(1.0–2.1)	1.9*	(1.2–2.9)	1.6*	(1.1–2.6)
Generalized anxiety disorder	1.6	(1.0–2.7)	1.4	(0.8–2.5)	1.9*	(1.1–3.4)
Specific phobia	1.9*	(1.1–3.3)	1.3	(0.7–2.2)	1.2	(0.7–2.2)
Social phobia	1.7*	(1.0–2.7)	1.6	(1.0–2.7)	1.3	(0.8–2.3)
III. Substance-use disorders						
Alcohol abuse with or without dependence	1.3	(0.9–1.7)	2.0*	(1.5–2.8)	2.2*	(1.6–2.9)
Drug abuse with or without dependence	1.4*	(1.1–2.0)	2.0*	(1.4–3.0)	2.7*	(1.8–4.0)
IV. Disruptive Behaviour disorders						
Intermittent explosive disorder	2.7*	(1.7–4.4)	1.1	(0.7–1.8)	1.2	(0.7–2.1)
Oppositional defiant disorder	4.6*	(1.7–12.1)	0.8	(0.3–2.3)	1.1	(0.4–2.8)

*Significant at the 0.05 level, two-sided test.
[a]All models are person-year models assessed with Part II weight (except Iraq and Romania), controlling for time-invariant dummies for country, gender, dummy for threshold childhood ADHD, time-varying continuous age, age-squared, and dummy active (time-varying dummy for whether the person-year is less than or equal to the age of recency of ADHD).

Table 14.5 Disability in 30-day functioning associated with DSM-IV adult attention-deficit hyperactivity disorder (n = 26,744)

Disability domain	Prevalence of disability		With controls for socio-demographics[b]		With controls for socio-demographics and comorbid 12-month DSM-IV disorders[c]	
	%[a]	(SE)	OR	(95% CI)	OR	(95% CI)
Cognition	21.8	(2.0)	3.8*	(2.9–4.8)	2.1*	(1.6–2.8)
Social interaction	10.8	(1.4)	3.3*	(2.4–4.4)	1.5*	(1.1–2.1)
Self-care	4.8	(0.9)	2.1*	(1.4–3.3)	1.2	(0.8–1.8)
Mobility	15.5	(1.6)	2.5*	(1.9–3.3)	1.6*	(1.2–2.0)
Days-out-of-role	29.3	(2.2)	2.6*	(2.1–3.3)	1.6*	(1.3–2.1)

*Significant at the 0.05 level, two-sided test.
[a]% with disability among those with ADHD.
[b]Based on logistic regression equations controlling for country, gender, age, education, employment, marital status, and income. Twelve-month disability is the outcome variable in the models. The ORs presented are for ADHD as the predictor.
[c]Based on logistic regression equations controlling for country, gender, age, education, employment, marital status, income, any 12-month mood disorder, any 12-month anxiety disorder, any 12-month substance-use disorder. Thirty-Day disability is the outcome variable in the models. The ORs presented are for ADHD as the predictor.

Treatment

Roughly one-fifth (21.8%) of respondents with 12-month ADHD received some treatment for mental health problems in the 12 months before interview (Table 14.6). This treatment rate is significantly related to country income level (28.8% in high, 15.5% in upper-middle-, and 6.8% in low/lower-middle-income countries; $\chi^2_2 = 35.8$, $P < 0.001$). In high-income countries, the majority of these patients were treated either

Table 14.6 Twelve-month treatment among respondents with multiply imputed DSM-IV adult attention-deficit hyperactivity disorder (ADHD) (N = 26,744)

	General medical		Any mental health		Human services		CAM[b]		Any professional		Any treatment for ADHD	
	%[a]	(SE)	%[a]	(SE)	%[a]	(SE)	%[a]	(SE)	%[a]	(SE)	%[a]	(SE)
Low/lower-middle-income countries												
Colombia	0.6	(0.4)	6.4	(3.3)	0.4	(0.4)	0.8	(0.8)	7.2	(3.4)	0.0	(0.0)
Iraq	0.0	(0.0)	0.0	(0.0)	0.7	(1.2)	0.0	(0.0)	0.7	(1.2)	0.0	(0.0)
Peru	0.0	(0.0)	12.9	(4.9)	0.0	(0.0)	3.6	(3.5)	15.7	(5.7)	0.0	(0.0)
PRC[c] (Shenzhen)	1.0	(0.8)	2.3	(2.3)	0.0	(0.0)	2.4	(1.3)	5.4	(2.8)	0.0	(0.0)
Total	**0.6**	**(0.3)**	**5.0**	**(1.6)**	**0.3**	**(0.2)**	**1.6**	**(0.8)**	**6.8**	**(1.8)**	**0.0**	**(0.0)**
Upper-middle-income countries												
Brazil (São Paulo)	7.2	(2.4)	12.3	(3.3)	1.1	(1.0)	4.8	(2.1)	20.4	(4.2)	1.9	(1.1)
Colombia (Medellin)	1.3	(1.3)	7.7	(3.7)	0.0	(0.0)	0.0	(0.0)	9.0	(4.4)	0.0	(0.0)
Lebanon	0.3	(1.5)	0.8	(0.9)	0.0	(0.0)	0.0	(0.0)	1.1	(1.7)	0.0	(0.0)
Mexico	2.9	(1.9)	8.2	(4.9)	0.0	(0.0)	2.1	(1.4)	12.4	(5.1)	1.9	(1.9)
Romania	0.0	(0.0)	0.0	(0.0)	0.0	(0.0)	0.0	(0.0)	0.0	(0.0)	0.0	(0.0)
Total	**4.9**	**(1.5)**	**9.8**	**(2.2)**	**0.7**	**(0.6)**	**3.1**	**(1.3)**	**15.5**	**(2.8)**	**1.4**	**(0.7)**
High-income countries												
Belgium	10.5	(10.5)	13.8	(7.8)	0.0	(0.0)	0.0	(0.0)	21.5	(11.1)	0.0	(0.0)
France	7.4	(2.7)	5.6	(3.3)	0.0	(0.0)	0.0	(0.0)	9.6	(3.6)	0.0	(0.0)
Germany	0.0	(0.0)	6.9	(5.8)	2.7	(2.8)	0.0	(0.0)	9.7	(6.0)	0.0	(0.0)
Italy	10.6	(4.2)	4.4	(2.8)	0.0	(0.0)	1.3	(1.3)	11.9	(4.5)	0.0	(0.0)
Netherlands	18.6	(9.1)	18.8	(10.5)	2.2	(2.2)	12.3	(8.6)	23.8	(10.8)	1.9	(1.7)
Northern Ireland	18.9	(6.7)	13.9	(6.2)	0.6	(0.6)	2.6	(2.6)	25.5	(9.1)	0.6	(0.6)
Poland	7.2	(5.9)	3.5	(2.6)	4.2	(3.1)	0.0	(0.0)	12.9	(6.9)	5.8	(5.7)
Portugal	20.4	(8.0)	4.9	(3.3)	1.8	(1.8)	0.0	(0.0)	22.4	(8.1)	0.0	(0.0)
Spain	10.2	(5.6)	13.9	(6.9)	0.0	(0.0)	0.0	(0.0)	19.9	(8.9)	3.2	(3.4)
Spain (Murcia)	10.4	(5.8)	4.2	(6.0)	0.0	(0.0)	0.0	(0.0)	14.6	(5.2)	0.0	(0.0)
United States	27.9	(4.3)	28.6	(3.8)	12.5	(2.5)	9.3	(2.3)	49.7	(4.1)	13.2	(2.9)
Total	**17.9**	**(2.2)**	**15.9**	**(2.0)**	**4.9**	**(1.0)**	**4.4**	**(1.1)**	**28.8**	**(2.6)**	**5.1**	**(1.1)**
All countries combined	**11.8**	**(1.4)**	**12.6**	**(1.4)**	**3.1**	**(0.7)**	**3.7**	**(0.7)**	**21.8**	**(1.9)**	**3.3**	**(0.7)**
χ^2	51.7*		13.7*		1.5*		3.6		35.8*		3.6	

*Significant at the 0.05 level, two-sided test.
[a]% with 12-month treatment among those with ADHD.
[b]Complimentary and alternative medicine.
[c]People's Republic of China.

in the mental health specialty sector (15.9% of all cases) or the general medical sector (17.9%). In upper-middle and low/lower-middle-income countries, in comparison, patients were considerably more likely to be treated in the mental health specialty sector (9.8% in upper-middle- and 5.0% in low/lower-middle-income countries) than the general medical sector (4.9% in upper-middle- and 0.6% in low/lower-middle-income countries).

Two other observations about the 12-month treatment data are noteworthy. First, the sum of the proportions of cases treated in each of the four service sectors considered in the WMH surveys is roughly 50% higher in high-income countries (43.1% [i.e., 17.9% + 15.9% + 4.9% + 4.4%]) than the proportion of cases with any treatment in one or more of those sectors (28.8%). This means that the average person with 12-month ADHD in high-income countries who received treatment for mental health problems in the past 12 months was seen in 1.5 service sectors. This average is considerably lower in upper-middle- (1.2 service sectors) and low/lower-middle- (1.1 service sectors) income countries. Previous WMH analyses have shown that this pattern of obtaining care for emotional problems in multiple service sectors in high-income countries is typical of people with a wide range of other DSM-IV disorders and is not unique to ADHD (Wang et al. 2007).

Second, 12-month treatment *specifically for ADHD* among respondents with 12-month ADHD (shown in the last column of the table) is dramatically lower than 12-month treatment for any emotional problems among the same respondents (3.3% vs. 21.8%). This same pattern is found in high- (5.1% vs. 28.8%), upper-middle- (1.4% vs. 15.5%), and low/lower-middle- (0.0% vs. 6.8%) income countries. This is consistent with the finding that a substantial part of the impairment of adult ADHD is associated with comorbid disorders. A question can be raised as to how often the treating clinicians are aware that these patients have comorbid ADHD.

Discussion

Several limitations of the analysis are noteworthy. The most obvious one is that childhood ADHD was assessed retrospectively and adult ADHD was estimated from an imputation model rather than directly. Retrospective assessment could be problematic because people with ADHD often lack insight into their conditions, leading to under-reports of prevalence (Murphy & Adler 2004) and considerably higher prevalence estimates when information is also provided by informants (Alexander & Liljequist 2016; Breda *et al.* 2016). Another limitation is that MI calibration was carried out only in the US which was an outlier in terms of prevalence, raising questions about the accuracy of the diagnostic threshold in other countries. A third limitation is that estimates of associations with outcomes are attenuated in MI models due to the inclusion of imputation error. A final noteworthy limitation is that the population to which imputation was made was restricted to WMH respondents who met full criteria for childhood ADHD.

Within the context of these limitations, the results reported here build on previous evidence about the cross-national epidemiology of ADHD in a number of ways. The most basic of these involves prevalence estimates. Population prevalence estimates for childhood ADHD have varied widely in previous epidemiological surveys, from less than 1% to over 20%, but with a central tendency of 4–6%. A recent quantitative analysis of worldwide studies reported pooled current prevalence estimates of 6.5% for children and 2.7% for adolescents (Polanczyk et al. 2007). The WMH retrospective estimate of 3.3% in high-income countries is intermediate between these two estimates, while the estimate of 2.2% in upper-middle-income countries is lower and the estimate of 0.6% in low/lower-middle-income countries is substantially lower than the lower bounds of these estimates.

Much less evidence exists on the population prevalence of adult ADHD. Early studies suggested that prevalence is low based on evidence of low adult persistence in studies that followed patients who were treated for ADHD as children into adulthood (Hill & Schoener 1996; Faraone *et al.* 2006), but there are a number of obvious methodological flaws with such studies (Sawilowsky & Musial 1988; Mannuzza *et al.* 2003). General population screening studies subsequently carried out found much higher prevalence estimates, with a meta-analysis estimating average prevalence to be 2.5% (Simon *et al.* 2009) and subsequent community surveys reporting results generally consistent with this estimate: 5.8% in Brazil (Polanczyk *et al.* 2010), 3.0% in France (Caci *et al.* 2014), 4.7% in Germany (de Zwaan *et al.* 2012), 1.3–4.6% (threshold-subthreshold) in Hungary (Bitter *et al.* 2010), and 1.1% in South Korea (Park *et al.* 2011). The WMH prevalence estimate of 2.8% is very similar to the average estimate in the meta-analysis (which, importantly, did not include any of the WMH surveys in the review), although the WMH series includes a much wider range of countries and, as with childhood ADHD, finds a strong association between country income level and prevalence.

One striking result of our prevalence analysis is that the estimated prevalence of adult ADHD is higher than that of childhood ADHD. This is true because a substantial proportion of adult threshold cases were subthreshold childhood cases according to retrospective reports. As one might expect, transition probabilities for becoming an adult case were higher for childhood threshold than subthreshold cases, but the fact that there were so many childhood subthreshold cases and that the transition probabilities to adult caseness were substantial for subthreshold childhood cases combine to result in a substantial proportion of adults with ADHD reporting subthreshold ADHD in childhood.

Previous prospective studies that focused on follow-up of childhood cases into adulthood are unable to evaluate the possibility that many adults with ADHD had subthreshold symptoms in childhood, as the denominator population for these studies consisted of patients who had threshold ADHD in childhood. It would be valuable for prospective community-based research to investigate this issue by following epidemiological samples of children who were classified as having either threshold or subthreshold ADHD in community surveys or school surveys (e.g., Green *et al.* 2010) into adulthood to determine whether or not the retrospective WMH results hold up prospectively. Another possibility is that this pattern in the WMH data might be due to downward recall bias about the severity of childhood symptoms among adults with threshold ADHD. It is noteworthy, though, that another related issue is that a higher proportion of subthreshold childhood cases will become threshold cases in adulthood when DSM-5 diagnostics are used, as DSM-5 requires only five symptoms of either AD or HD for a diagnosis of adult ADHD compared to six in DSM-IV and six for childhood cases in both DSM-IV and DSM-5.

By combining retrospectively recalled threshold and subthreshold childhood ADHD in the total sample (2.2% and 3.7%, respectively), the current rate of 2.8% of adult ADHD reflects a persistence rate of 47.4%. Since we did not measure subthreshold adult ADHD, this persistence rate is likely to be an underestimate of the true persistence of ADHD from childhood into adulthood. As noted above, recent community cohort studies have suggested that there may be later-onset cases of ADHD, including adult onset cases that have no history of ADHD in childhood (Moffitt *et al.* 2015; Agnew-Blais *et al.* 2016; Caye *et al.* 2016a). As noted above, the CIDI did not inquire about new onset ADHD in adulthood among respondents who did report at least subthreshold ADHD in childhood. As a result, our reported prevalence excludes these individuals from consideration.

It is unclear whether the association of ADHD prevalence with country income level reflects differences in true prevalence, differential recall, differential validity of the CIDI questions across countries, or some combination of these factors. One strong possibility is that objectively assessed inattention and hyperactivity-impulsivity might be less impairing in lower-income than higher-income countries given that these symptoms might interfere less with the role demands of people in the former than latter countries. Given the very strong cross-national gradient and the plausibility of this possibility, it would be valuable to carry out a cross-national comparative analysis that used objective performance-based neurocognitive tests to evaluate prevalence of the cognitive deficits underlying adult ADHD rather than relying only on self-report assessments. It is noteworthy in this regard that performance-based neurocognitive tests have been used in a number of recent studies of adult ADHD (e.g., Dehili *et al.* 2013; Surman *et al.* 2015; Micoulaud-Franchi *et al.* 2016) and could be used in parallel in community surveys using recently-developed technology for administering such tests in web-based surveys (www.manybrains.net). It is important to note, though, that the neurocognitive tests studied in adult ADHD up to now have been heterogeneous, in many cases only weakly correlated with each other, and non-specific for adult ADHD, making it unclear whether this line of research has yet progressed sufficiently to warrant implementing such tests in large-scale cross-national community epidemiological surveys.

Previous research has also studied socio-demographic correlates of ADHD. Perhaps the most consistently documented correlate is gender, with prevalence consistently higher among boys than girls and a higher relative prevalence of the predominantly inattentive subtype among girls than boys (Rucklidge 2010). Although earlier estimates indicated a male-to-female ratio of 9:1, a subsequent meta-analysis concluded that the true prevalence ratio is closer to 2.45:1 in non-referred community samples (Polanczyk & Jensen 2008). This finding suggests that previously reported higher ratios may have been a function of referral or treatment bias, as it is known that a higher proportion of boys than girls with ADHD receive treatment (Derks *et al.* 2007). The WMH OR of 1.6 for childhood ADHD among boys:girls is somewhat lower than that average. We also found the same OR for adult ADHD due to the absence of a significant gender difference in persistence of childhood ADHD into adulthood. This finding is consistent with a recent meta-analysis (which, it should be noted, included the results of an early WMH analysis of the predictors of persistence of childhood ADHD into adulthood based on our first 10 surveys (Lara *et al.* 2009)), which failed to find a significant gender difference in persistence of ADHD into adulthood (Caye *et al.* 2016b).

Age is a second socio-demographic characteristic that has been examined in studies of ADHD prevalence. Meta-analysis finds that this association is negative (Simon *et al.* 2009), a result that we replicate in the WMH surveys despite the fact that the age range of our sample was truncated (18–44). Other commonly studied correlates are various indicators of socio-economic status (SES). Although the associations of childhood ADHD with these correlates are confounded in treatment samples by selection bias, we would expect an inverse association with parental SES by virtue of the high heritability of childhood ADHD (Posthuma & Polderman 2013) along with an association of ADHD with low socio-economic attainment (Polderman *et al.* 2010). Meta-analysis shows, consistent with this expectation, that parental SES is inversely related to childhood ADHD, with children from low-SES families having an ADHD prevalence close to twice that of other children (Russell *et al.* 2016).

The WMH data focused on respondent SES rather than parental SES. We found that while both threshold and subthreshold childhood ADHD were associated with significant reductions in odds of completing college, persistence of childhood ADHD into adulthood was not associated with educational attainment. The significant association of childhood ADHD with reduced educational attainment is consistent with the results of a meta-analysis (Polderman *et al.* 2010), but we are unaware of any previous research on educational attainment and persistence of childhood ADHD into adulthood. It is conceivable that low educational attainment is influenced by childhood but not adult ADHD, while level of educational attainment among individuals who have completed their education has no influence on the course of ADHD. A more perplexing finding is that we failed to find a significant association between respondent household income per family member and adult ADHD. This result is inconsistent with other evidence suggesting that adult ADHD is associated with low household income (Martel 2013). The reason for this discrepancy between the WMH results and the results of earlier studies is unclear.

Finally, we found that respondents with adult ADHD were significantly less likely than other respondents to be currently married due to elevated odds of being previously married. This finding is consistent with previous research showing that adult attention deficits are elevated among people who are divorced (Bouchard & Saint-Aubin 2014). Our finding of high comorbidity in ADHD is consistent with much previous research (Babcock & Ornstein 2009; Mao & Findling 2014; Karlsdotter *et al.* 2016), although it is unclear from these data whether ADHD is a causal risk factor or a noncausal risk marker. Our finding that respondents with remitted ADHD continue to have elevated risk of subsequent first onset of several other disorders argues indirectly for ADHD being a noncausal risk marker, but the even more consistently significant elevated odds of secondary disorders associated with active than remitted ADHD raises the possibility that ADHD might also be a causal risk factor for secondary disorders. This issue is becoming one of increasing public health importance, as interest grows in focusing on treatment of childhood ADHD as a secondary prevention strategy for downstream disorders. Research in this area is coming to recognize that a number of mediators and moderators of the presumed effects of ADHD on secondary disorders might exist that represent alternative targets for preventive intervention (Molina & Pelham 2014). Our retrospective finding that individuals with remitted ADHD have the same significantly elevated risk of some subsequent secondary disorders such as alcohol-use disorder as those with active ADHD could be of value here in leading a recognition that *history* of childhood ADHD (i.e., whether or not still active) is a risk marker for subsequent onset of alcohol abuse (Tuithof *et al.* 2012).

Our results regarding role impairments in adult ADHD are also consistent with much previous research (Ivanchak *et al.* 2012; Kupper *et al.* 2012; Bouchard & Saint-Aubin 2014). However, we also showed that substantial proportions of these associations are more proximally due to comorbid mental disorders. Given the evidence that remitted ADHD often predicts subsequent onset of secondary disorders, a question can be raised whether some unmeasured biological and/or environmental determinants of both ADHD and later-onset disorders might account for the impairments associated with ADHD. An investigation of this possibility is beyond the scope of this chapter. However, we know from experimental research on the effects of ADHD treatment on objective performance data that some part of the association between adult ADHD and role performance is due to a direct and modifiable causal effect of ADHD (Biederman *et al.* 2012), implying that if role impairments played a part in predicting subsequent onset of temporally secondary disorders we would expect that risk of these disorders would return to their level in the general population with the remission of ADHD. That the WMH results suggest that this risk does not return to the population level after ADHD remission consequently implies that factors other than the impairment caused by ADHD account for the associations of remitted ADHD with subsequent onset of temporally secondary disorders.

Our results regarding 12-month adult ADHD treatment, finally, are broadly consistent with much other research in showing that only a minority of people with mental disorders obtain treatment and that this treatment rate is lower in less developed than developed countries (Wang *et al.* 2007). Other WMH research on treatment seeking for mental disorders has shown that the most important barrier is failure to recognize that the symptoms of the disorder constitute evidence of an 'illness' that could profit from treatment (Andrade *et al.* 2014). Not only ADHD but also other disorders with symptoms that are, in effect, extreme versions of normal experiences that either begin in childhood (e.g., extreme shyness in social phobia) or develop slowly over time (e.g., extreme worry in generalized anxiety disorder) have this profile of low treatment seeking for the disorder (ten Have *et al.* 2013), and the majority of patients are in treatment for a comorbid disorder that is more readily recognized as a condition needing treatment (e.g., depression, alcohol abuse). This lack of awareness has been noted in the past and has led to calls for increased public and professional training on how to diagnose adult ADHD (Asherson *et al.* 2012). Our results suggest strongly that training programmes of this sort are needed.

Acknowledgements

An earlier version of this chapter was published in: Fayyad, J., Sampson, N. A., Hwang, I., Adamowski, T., Aguilar-Gaxiola, S., Al-Hamzawi, A., Andrade, L. H., Borges, G., de Girolamo, G., Florescu, S., Gureje, O., Haro, J. M., Hu, C., Karam, E. G., Lee, S., Navarro-Mateu, F., O'Neill, S., Pennell, B. E., Piazza, M., Posada-Villa, J., ten Have, M., Torres, Y., Xavier, M., Zaslavsky, A. M., Kessler, R. C., WHO World Mental Health Survey Collaborators. (2017). The descriptive epidemiology of DSM-IV adult ADHD in the World Health Organization World Mental Health Surveys. *Attention Deficit and Hyperactivity Disorders*, 9(1), 47–65.

References

Adler, L., & Cohen, J. (2004). Diagnosis and evaluation of adults with attention-deficit/hyperactivity disorder. *The Psychiatric Clinics of North America* 27, 187–201.

Adler, L., & Spencer, T. (2004). *The Adult ADHD Clinical Diagnostic Scale (ACDS), version 1.2.* New York: New York University School of Medicine.

Agnew-Blais, J. C., Polanczyk, G., Danese, A., *et al.* (2016). Persistence, remission & emergence of ADHD in young adulthood: results from a longitudinal, prospective population-based cohort. *JAMA Psychiatry*, 73, 713–20.

Alexander, L., & Liljequist, L. (2016). Determining the accuracy of self-report versus informant-report using the Conners' Adult ADHD Rating Scale. *Journal of Attention Disorders* 20, 346–52.

Alhraiwil, N. J., Ali, A., Househ, M. S., Al-Shehri, A. M., & El-Metwally, A. A. (2015). Systematic review of the epidemiology of attention deficit hyperactivity disorder in Arab countries. *Neurosciences (Riyadh)* 20, 137–44.

Andrade, L. H., Alonso, J., Mneimneh, Z., *et al.* (2014). Barriers to mental health treatment: results from the WHO World Mental Health (WMH) surveys. *Psychological Medicine* 44, 1303–17.

Asherson, P., Akehurst, R., Kooij, J. J., *et al.* (2012). Under diagnosis of adult ADHD: cultural influences and societal burden. *Journal of Attention Disorders* 16(Suppl 5), 20S–38S.

Babcock, T., & Ornstein, C. S. (2009). Comorbidity and its impact in adult patients with attention-deficit/hyperactivity disorder: a primary care perspective. *Postgraduate Medicine* 121, 73–82.

Biederman, J., Fried, R., Hammerness, P., *et al.* (2012). The effects of lisdexamfetamine dimesylate on the driving performance of young adults with ADHD: a randomized, double-blind, placebo-controlled study using a validated driving simulator paradigm. *Journal of Psychiatric Research* 46, 484–91.

Bitter, I., Simon, V., Balint, S., *et al.* (2010). How do different diagnostic criteria, age and gender affect the prevalence of attention deficit hyperactivity disorder in adults? An epidemiological study in a Hungarian community sample. *European Archives of Psychiatry and Clinical Neuroscience* 260, 287–96.

Bouchard, G., & Saint-Aubin, J. (2014). Attention deficits and divorce. *Canadian Journal of Psychiatry* 59, 480–6.

Breda, V., Rovaris, D. L., Vitola, E. S., *et al.* (2016). Does collateral retrospective information about childhood attention-deficit/hyperactivity disorder symptoms assist in the diagnosis of attention-deficit/hyperactivity disorder in adults? Findings from a large clinical sample. *The Australian and New Zealand Journal of Psychiatry* 50, 557–65.

Caci, H. M., Morin, A. J., & Tran, A. (2014). Prevalence and correlates of attention deficit hyperactivity disorder in adults from a French community sample. *The Journal of Nervous and Mental Disease* 202, 324–32.

Caye, A., Rocha, T. B.-M., Anselmi, L., *et al.* (2016a). Attention-deficit/hyperactivity disorder trajectories from childhood to young adulthood: evidence from a birth cohort supporting a late-onset syndrome. *JAMA Psychiatry* 73, 705–12.

Caye, A., Spadini, A. V., Karam, R. G., *et al.* (2016b). Predictors of persistence of ADHD into adulthood: a systematic review of the literature and meta-analysis. *European Child & Adolescent Psychiatry*, 25, 1151–9.

de Graaf, R., Kessler, R. C., Fayyad, J., *et al.* (2008). The prevalence and effects of adult attention-deficit/hyperactivity disorder (ADHD) on the performance of workers: results from the WHO World Mental Health Survey Initiative. *Occupational and Environmental Medicine* 65, 835–42.

de Zwaan, M., Gruss, B., Müller, A., *et al.* (2012). The estimated prevalence and correlates of adult ADHD in a German community sample. *European Archives of Psychiatry and Clinical Neuroscience* 262, 79–86.

Dehili, V. M., Prevatt, F., & Coffman, T. P. (2017). An analysis of the Barkley Deficits in Executive Functioning Scale in a college population: does it predict symptoms of ADHD better than a visual-search task? *Journal of Attention Disorders*, 21, 567–74.

Derks, E. M., Hudziak, J. J., & Boomsma, D. I. (2007). Why more boys than girls with ADHD receive treatment: a study of Dutch twins. *Twin Research Human Genetics* 10(5), 765–70.

Faraone, S. V., Biederman, J., & Mick, E. (2006). The age-dependent decline of attention deficit hyperactivity disorder: a meta-analysis of follow-up studies. *Psychological Medicine* 36, 159–65.

Faraone, S.V., Biederman, J., Spencer, T., *et al.* (2000). Attention-deficit/hyperactivity disorder in adults: an overview. *Biological Psychiatry* 48, 9–20.

Fayyad, J., de Graaf, R., Kessler, R., *et al.* (2007). Cross-national prevalence and correlates of adult attention-deficit hyperactivity disorder. *The British Journal of Psychiatry* 190, 402–9.

Fayyad, J., Sampson, N. A., Hwang, I., *et al.* (2017). The descriptive epidemiology of DSM-IV adult ADHD in the World Health Organization World Mental Health Surveys. *Attention Deficit and Hyperactivity Disorders* 9, 47–65.

Green, J. G., Avenevoli, S., Finkelman, M., *et al.* (2010). Attention deficit hyperactivity disorder: concordance of the adolescent version of the Composite International Diagnostic Interview Version 3.0 (CIDI) with the K-SADS in the US National Comorbidity Survey Replication Adolescent (NCS-A) supplement. *International Journal of Methods in Psychiatric Research* 19, 34–49.

Hill, J. C., & Schoener, E. P. (1996). Age-dependent decline of attention deficit hyperactivity disorder. *American Journal of Psychiatry* 153, 1143–6.

Ivanchak, N., Fletcher, K., & Jicha, G.A. (2012). Attention-deficit/hyperactivity disorder in older adults: prevalence and possible connections to mild cognitive impairment. *Current Psychiatry Reports* 14, 552–60.

Karlsdotter, K., Bushe, C., Hakkaart, L., *et al.* (2016). Burden of illness and health care resource utilization in adult psychiatric outpatients with attention-deficit/hyperactivity disorder in Europe. *Current Medical Research and Opinion* 32, 1547–56.

Kessler, R. C., Adler, L., Barkley, R., *et al.* (2006). The prevalence and correlates of adult ADHD in the United States: results from the National Comorbidity Survey Replication. *The American Journal of Psychiatry* 163, 716–23.

Kessler, R. C., Ormel, J., Petukhova, M., *et al.* (2011). Development of lifetime comorbidity in the World Health Organization world mental health surveys. *Archives of General Psychiatry* 68, 90–100.

Kessler, R. C., & Üstün, T. B. (2004). The World Mental Health (WMH) Survey Initiative version of the World Health Organization (WHO) Composite International Diagnostic Interview (CIDI). *International Journal of Methods in Psychiatric Research* 13, 93–121.

Kessler, R. C., & Üstün, T. B. (Eds). (2008). *The WHO World Mental Health Surveys: Global Perspectives on the Epidemiology of Mental Disorders*. Cambridge, UK: Cambridge University Press.

Knäuper, B., Cannell, C. F., Schwarz, N., *et al.* (1999). Improving accuracy of major depression age-of-onset reports in the US National Comorbidity Survey. *International Journal of Methods in Psychiatric Research* 8, 39–48.

Kupper, T., Haavik, J., Drexler, H., *et al.* (2012). The negative impact of attention-deficit/hyperactivity disorder on occupational health in adults and adolescents. *International Archives of Occupational and Environmental Health* 85, 837–47.

Lara, C., Fayyad, J., de Graaf, R., *et al.* (2009). Childhood predictors of adult attention-deficit/hyperactivity disorder: results from the World Health Organization World Mental Health Survey Initiative. *Biological Psychiatry* 65, 46–54.

Mannuzza, S., Klein, R. G., & Moulton, J. (2003). Persistence of Attention-Deficit/Hyperactivity Disorder into adulthood: what have we learned from the prospective follow-up studies? *Journal of Attention Disorders* 7, 93–100.

Mao, A. R., & Findling, R. L. (2014). Comorbidities in adult attention-deficit/hyperactivity disorder: a practical guide to diagnosis in primary care. *Postgraduate Medicine* 126, 42–51.

Martel, M. M. (2013). Individual differences in attention deficit hyperactivity disorder symptoms and associated executive dysfunction and traits: sex, ethnicity, and family income. *American Journal of Orthopsychiatry* 83, 165–75.

Micoulaud-Franchi, J. A., Lopez, R., Cermolacce, M., *et al.* (2016). Sensory gating capacity and attentional function in adults with ADHD: a preliminary neurophysiological and neuropsychological study. *Journal of Attention Disorders*. DOI: 10.1177/1087054716629716 [Epub ahead of print].

Moffitt, T. E., Houts, R., Asherson, P., *et al.* (2015). Is adult ADHD a childhood-onset neurodevelopmental disorder? Evidence from a four-decade longitudinal cohort study. *American Journal of Psychiatry* 172, 967–77.

Molina, B. S., & Pelham, W. E., Jr. (2014). Attention-deficit/hyperactivity disorder and risk of substance use disorder: developmental considerations, potential pathways, and opportunities for research. *Annual Review of Clinical Psychology* 10, 607–39.

Murphy, K. R., & Adler, L. A. (2004). Assessing attention-deficit/hyperactivity disorder in adults: focus on rating scales. *The Journal of Clinical Psychiatry* 65(Suppl 3), 12–17.

Park, S., Cho, M. J., Chang, S. M., *et al.* (2011). Prevalence, correlates, and comorbidities of adult ADHD symptoms in Korea: results of the Korean epidemiologic catchment area study. *Psychiatry Research* 186, 378–83.

Polanczyk, G., de Lima, M. S., Horta, B. L., Biederman, J., & Rohde, L. A. (2007). The worldwide prevalence of ADHD: a systematic review and metaregression analysis. *The American Journal of Psychiatry* 164, 942–8.

Polanczyk, G., & Jensen, P. (2008). Epidemiologic considerations in attention deficit hyperactivity disorder: a review and update. *Child and Adolescent Psychiatric Clinics of North America* 17, 245–60.

Polanczyk, G., Laranjeira, R., Zaleski, M., *et al.* (2010). ADHD in a representative sample of the Brazilian population: estimated prevalence and comparative adequacy of criteria between adolescents and adults according to the item response theory. *International Journal of Methods in Psychiatric Research* 19, 177–84.

Polanczyk, G. V., Willcutt, E. G., Salum, G. A., *et al.* (2014). ADHD prevalence estimates across three decades: an updated systematic review and meta-regression analysis. *International Journal of Epidemiology* 43, 434–42.

Polderman, T. J., Boomsma, D. I., Bartels, M., *et al.* (2010). A systematic review of prospective studies on attention problems and academic achievement. *Acta Psychiatrica Scandinavica* 122, 271–84.

Posthuma, D., & Polderman, T. J. (2013). What have we learned from recent twin studies about the etiology of neurodevelopmental disorders? *Current Opinion in Neurology* 26, 111–21.

Robins, L., & Helzer, J. (1985). *Diagnostic Interview Schedule (DIS Version III-A)*. St. Louis, MO: Washington University, Department of Psychiatry.

Rubin, D. (1987). *Multiple Imputation for Nonresponse in Surveys*. New York: John Wiley & Sons.

Rucklidge, J. J. (2010). Gender differences in attention-deficit/hyperactivity disorder. *The Psychiatric Clinics of North America* 33, 357–73.

Russell, A. E., Ford, T., Williams, R., *et al.* (2016). The association between socioeconomic disadvantage and Attention Deficit/Hyperactivity Disorder (ADHD): a systematic review. *Child Psychiatry and Human Development* 47, 440–58.

Sawilowsky, S., Musial, J.L. (1988) Modeling ADHD exponential decay. *The ADHD Report 1988* 6(1),10–11.

Simon, V., Czobor, P., Balint, S., *et al.* (2009). Prevalence and correlates of adult attention-deficit hyperactivity disorder: meta-analysis. *The British Journal of Psychiatry* 194, 204–11.

Surman, C. B., Biederman, J., Spencer, T., *et al.* (2015). Neuropsychological deficits are not predictive of deficient emotional self-regulation in adults with ADHD. *Journal of Attention Disorders* 19, 1046–53.

ten Have, M., de Graaf, R., van Dorsselaer, S., *et al.* (2013). Lifetime treatment contact and delay in treatment seeking after first onset of a mental disorder. *Psychiatric Services* 64, 981–9.

Thomas, R., Sanders, S., Doust, J., *et al.* (2015). Prevalence of attention-deficit/hyperactivity disorder: a systematic review and meta-analysis. *Pediatrics* 135, e994–1001.

Tuithof, M., ten Have, M., van den Brink, W., *et al.* (2012). The role of conduct disorder in the association between ADHD and alcohol use (disorder). Results from the Netherlands Mental Health Survey and Incidence Study-2. *Drug and Alcohol Dependence* 123, 115–21.

Üstün, T. B., Chatterji, S., Kostanjsek, N., *et al.* (2010). Developing the World Health Organization Disability Assessment Schedule 2.0. *Bulletin of the World Health Organization* 88, 815–23.

Wang, P. S., Aguilar-Gaxiola, S., Alonso, J., *et al.* (2007). Use of mental health services for anxiety, mood, and substance disorders in 17 countries in the WHO World Mental Health surveys. *Lancet* 370, 841–50.

Weiss, M., Hechtman, L., & Weiss, G. (2000). ADHD in parents. *Journal of the American Academy of Child and Adolescent Psychiatry* 39, 1059–61.

Wolf, L. E., & Wasserstein, J. (2001). Adult ADHD. Concluding thoughts. *Annals of the New York Academy of Sciences* 931, 396–408.

Chapter 15

Oppositional Defiant Disorder and Conduct Disorder

Brianna J. Turner, Chiyi Hu, José Posada Villa, Matthew K. Nock

Introduction

Oppositional defiant disorder (ODD) and conduct disorder (CD) involve recurrent and persistent patterns of disruptive behaviours (World Health Organization [WHO] 1992; American Psychiatric Association [APA] 2013). To meet criteria for diagnosis, this pattern of behaviour must be sufficiently severe that it is developmentally atypical and results in impairment. ODD is defined by the presence of defiant, disobedient, and hostile behaviours, whereas CD is defined by the presence of serious violations of the rights of others or of societal norms (APA 2013). These disorders are frequently comorbid, overlapping in approximately 60% of community youth with CD (Rowe *et al.* 2002; Maughan *et al.* 2004) and 96% of clinically referred youth with CD (Frick *et al.* 1992). The highly overlapping nature of these disorders is acknowledged in current diagnostic systems, although within slightly different models: whereas the ICD-10 conceptualizes ODD as a potential precursor to more severe CD behaviours (WHO 1992), the DSM-5 treats ODD and CD as independent disorders while recognizing the correlated nature of their symptoms and risk factors (APA 2013).

Empirical support exists for each conceptualization. ODD symptoms typically precede the development of CD (Loeber *et al.* 1992; Burke *et al.* 2005; Nock *et al.* 2007; Rowe *et al.* 2010), and predict elevated risk for subsequent CD (Rowe *et al.* 2002; Burke *et al.* 2010; Diamantopoulou *et al.* 2010). However, many youth with ODD (68%) do not go on to develop CD (Biederman *et al.* 1996), and approximately 44% of youth with CD did not have preceding ODD (Rowe *et al.* 2010). Moreover, although the disorders share numerous risk factors (see Loeber *et al.* 2000 for a review), nearly 50% of the genetic variance in CD appears to be unique to this disorder (Lahey & Waldman 2012). For the purposes of this chapter, we adopt a conceptualization that is consistent with the DSM, and treat ODD and CD as distinct but related disorders.

ODD and CD typically emerge during childhood (Maughan *et al.* 2004; Nock *et al.* 2006, 2007) and are relatively stable through childhood and adolescence (Offord *et al.* 1992; Cohen *et al.* 1993; Caspi & Moffitt 1995; Lahey *et al.* 1995; Nock *et al.* 2006, 2007). Because of the widespread impairments that typically result from these disorders, ODD and CD constitute some of the most common reasons for referral to child and adolescent mental health services (Robins 1991; Kazdin 1995; Loeber *et al.* 2000). Indeed, most adolescents (45% to 80%) with symptoms of ODD and CD exhibit impairment related to these disorders (West *et al.* 2003; Leung *et al.* 2008; Ravens-Sieberer *et al.* 2008) and approximately one in four youth are identified as needing treatment (Ravens-Sieberer *et al.* 2008). Persistence into adulthood, however, appears to be rare: the majority (70%) of youth with ODD no longer meet diagnostic criteria for the disorder by age 18 (Nock *et al.* 2007) and only approximately 10% of youth with CD continue to exhibit serious and persistent antisocial behaviours into adulthood (Moffitt *et al.* 2002). Even when ODD and CD remit, however, these disorders are associated with a variety of negative outcomes later in life, including financial and work problems, poor educational attainment, and substance use (Zoccolillo *et al.* 1992; Kessler & Frank 1997; Maughan & Rutter 2001; Moffitt *et al.* 2002; Nock *et al.* 2006; Breslau *et al.* 2008). Moreover, longitudinal studies consistently show that ODD and CD are associated with substantial heterotypic continuity, predicting elevated risk of subsequent anxiety, mood, eating, and substance disorders (Lavigne *et al.* 2001; Rowe *et al.* 2002, 2010; Kim-Cohen *et al.* 2003; Burke *et al.* 2005; Nock *et al.* 2006, 2007; Copeland *et al.* 2009).

Although substantial research has examined the prevalence, course, and correlates of ODD and CD, much of the extant literature is restricted to samples of clinically referred or high-risk youth, limiting our ability to understand the true burden these disorders exert in the broader population. Put another way, to the extent that individuals in child and adolescent mental health clinics and juvenile justice departments represent a more highly impaired or disruptive segment of the total affected population, estimates of the prevalence and severity of these disorders based on these samples may skew our understanding of how prevalent and debilitating these conditions really are. Studies using sampling techniques designed to more accurately represent the general population are crucial in addressing this gap.

Epidemiological studies of ODD and CD remain relatively rare, and those that have been undertaken have predominantly occurred in Europe, North America, Australia, and New Zealand (see Canino *et al.* 2010 for a review). A recent meta-regression of 25 epidemiological studies suggested a pooled prevalence of 3.3% for ODD and 3.2% for CD (Canino *et al.* 2010). Despite the authors' expectation that the prevalence of ODD and CD would vary across regions, this study did not find geographic differences by continent in lifetime prevalence estimates of ODD or CD. Instead, results suggested that methodological differences between studies, including differing diagnostic criteria (see also Lahey *et al.* 1990; Boyle *et al.* 1996), assessment methods, and sampling strategies, contributed to variability in prevalence estimates. Although this review included prevalence estimates of ODD and CD from several epidemiological studies conducted in non-Western countries (e.g., Sugawara *et al.* 1999; Ashenafi *et al.* 2001; Wacharasindhu & Panyyayong 2002; Leung *et al.* 2008), the authors note that data regarding the course and consequences of these disorders in middle and low-income countries is sparse. This recent review thus revealed three critical gaps that must be addressed to advance our understanding of the cross-national prevalence and burden of ODD and CD: (1) a broader representation of countries, especially developing and non-Western nations, is needed in cross-national comparisons; (2) comparable sampling and assessment strategies across countries is required to facilitate meaningful regional comparisons; and (3) data regarding the developmental course, comorbidity, and consequences of these disorders is needed to expand our understanding of the burden associated with ODD and CD. This chapter addresses each of these gaps.

Methods

With respect to ODD, 15 countries provided data for a total of 74,034 people, 35,152 of whom received the more detailed interviews (Part II). Twelve of the 15 countries restricted the administration of Part II surveys to respondents aged 18 and 44, resulting in a final sample of 25,615 adults for results describing the prevalence, course, comorbidity, and consequences of ODD. Diagnostic criteria for ODD require that an individual exhibit a clinically significant pattern of angry or irritable mood (e.g., frequently losing one's temper; being easily annoyed), argumentative or defiant behaviour (e.g., frequently arguing or refusing to comply with authority figures; disobeying rules) or vindictiveness (e.g., often feeling taken advantage of or treated unfairly; acting vengefully to 'get people back' for perceived wrongs) lasting at least six months. At least four of the eight core symptoms must be endorsed to meet the threshold for diagnosis; in addition, symptoms must result in functional impairment (i.e., significant problems at work or school, or in social relationships) and must not be better accounted for by other medical or psychiatric conditions. Although the DSM-IV and ICD-10 included diagnostic decision rules that ODD could not be diagnosed in the presence of more severe conduct problems, in this chapter we focus on describing ODD without the diagnostic hierarchy. This is consistent with the revisions to the diagnostic criteria for ODD in the DSM-5, and we believe better captures the burden of ODD in the population. Instances where results differ depending on whether or not the DSM-IV diagnostic hierarchy is applied are noted in the text.

With respect to CD, 19 countries provided data for a total of 91,214 people; three countries restricted the administration of Part II surveys to respondents aged 18 to 39, and 12 countries administered Part II surveys only to respondents between the ages of 18 and 44, resulting in a final sample of 30,028 adults for results describing the prevalence, course, comorbidity, and consequences of CD. Diagnostic criteria for CD assess symptoms in four core domains: aggression to people and animals (e.g., repeated physical fights; use of a weapon against another person), destruction of property (e.g., breaking windows, slashing tires, vandalizing, or writing graffiti on buildings), deceitfulness or theft (e.g., frequent lying; shoplifting), and serious rule violations (e.g., frequent truancy or curfew violations; running away from home). At least three of the 15 symptoms must be endorsed to meet the diagnostic threshold; like ODD, these symptoms must be sufficiently disruptive so as to result in functional impairment and must not be better accounted for by other disorders.

Results

Prevalence of ODD and CD

The cross-national lifetime prevalence of ODD is 3.1%. Lifetime prevalence estimates for ODD vary considerably between countries (see Table 15.1), ranging from 0.5% (Germany) to 10.1% (United States). Similarly, 12-month prevalence estimates for ODD range from < 0.1% (Spain) to 1.1% (United States), with an overall 12-month prevalence of 0.5%. Variability in prevalence appears to be partially accounted for by geographic differences: there is significantly higher lifetime and 12-month prevalence of ODD in the Americas (4.1% and 0.7%, respectively), compared to Western European (1.8% and 0.3%, respectively) or Eastern European countries (2.0% and 0.1%, respectively). Moreover, there is a higher lifetime prevalence of ODD in high-income countries (3.6%) compared to upper-middle- (2.4%) and low/lower-middle-income countries (2.9%).

The cross-national lifetime prevalence of CD is 2.3%, although country-specific rates vary widely,

Table 15.1 Prevalence of DSM-IV oppositional defiant disorder (ODD) in the World Mental Health surveys

Country	Lifetime prevalence		12-month prevalence		12-month prevalence of ODD among lifetime cases		Sample size used
	%	SE	%	SE	%	SE	
Low/lower-middle-income countries	**2.9**	0.4	**0.4**	0.1	**14.7**	3.6	**3,018**
Colombia	3.4	0.5	0.5	0.2	16.0	4.4	1,731
Peru	2.2	0.5	0.3	0.2	12.3	6.2	1,287
Upper-middle-income countries	**2.4**	0.2	**0.6**	0.1	**24.6**	3.8	**8,446**
Brazil	1.6	0.2	0.5	0.2	33.3	7.1	5,037
Colombia (Medellin)	4.1	0.6	0.7	0.2	16.9	4.5	1,673
Mexico	2.8	0.4	**0.6**	0.2	21.1	5.1	1,736
High-income countries	**3.6**	0.2	**0.5**	0.1	**13.2**	1.7	**14,151**
Belgium	1.2	0.5	0.4	0.3	34.4	18.6	486
France	3.4	1.0	0.7	0.3	22.0	10.2	727
Germany	0.5	0.3	0.3	0.2	61.4	21.7	621
Italy	0.8	0.3	0.1	0.1	9.7	7.2	853
Northern Ireland	3.0	0.4	0.6	0.3	18.7	7.6	1,986
Poland	2.0	0.4	0.1	0.1	6.2	2.6	2,276
Portugal	2.0	0.4	0.4	0.2	18.2	6.8	1,070
Spain	0.6	0.2	<0.1	0.0	5.3	5.2	960
Spain (Murcia)	1.1	0.3	<0.1	0.0	1.0	1.1	1,459
Netherlands	2.7	1.0	0.9	0.6	33.7	17.2	516
United States	10.1	0.8	1.1	0.2	11.1	1.7	3,197
All countries combined	**3.1**	0.2	**0.5**	0.1	**16.2**	1.5	**25,615**
WHO regions[a]							
Region of the Americas	4.1	0.2	0.7	0.1	16.2	1.8	14,661
Western European region	1.8	0.2	0.3	0.1	19.3	4.0	8,678
Eastern European region	2.0	0.4	0.1	0.1	6.2	2.6	2,276
Comparison between countries[b]	**$F_{15,v} = 11.3$*, $P < 0.001$**		**$F_{15,v} = 5.2$*, $P < 0.001$**		**$F_{15,v} = 1.7$*, $P = 0.049$**		
Comparison between low-, middle-, and high-income country groups[b]	**$F_{2,v} = 7.8$*, $P < 0.001$**		**$F_{2,v} = 0.5$, $P = 0.587$**		**$F_{2,v} = 3.5$*, $P = 0.032$**		
Comparison between WHO regions[b]	**$F_{5,v} = 30.7$*, $P < 0.001$**		**$F_{5,v} = 16.3$*, $P < 0.001$**		**$F_{5,v} = 4.0$*, $P = 0.018$**		

*Significant at the 0.05 level, two-sided test.

[a]**Region of the Americas** (Colombia, Mexico, Brazil, Peru, United States, Colombia (Medellin)); **Western European region** (Belgium, France, Germany, Netherlands, Spain, Northern Ireland, Portugal, Spain (Murcia)); **Eastern European region** (Poland)

[b]Wald design-corrected F-tests were used to determine if there is variation in prevalence estimates across countries. The denominator degree of freedom, v, is 813.

Table 15.2 Prevalence of DSM-IV conduct disorder (CD) in the World Mental Health surveys

Country	Lifetime prevalence		12-month prevalence		12-month prevalence of CD among lifetime cases		Sample size used
	%	SE	%	SE	%	SE	
Low/lower-middle-income countries	**1.5**	0.2	**0.3**	0.1	**21.9**	5.0	**5,332**
Colombia	2.1	0.4	0.5	0.2	22.2	7.2	1,731
Nigeria	0.3	0.2	–	–	–	–	1,203
Peru	1.7	0.3	0.3	0.1	14.7	7.6	1,287
PRC (Beijing/Shanghai)	0.5	0.2	0.1	0.1	16.9	15.9	570
Ukraine	3.6	0.9	1.2	0.6	32.8	11.8	541
Upper-middle-income countries	**1.5**	0.1	**0.3**	0.1	**19.3**	3.9	**11,398**
Brazil	2.1	0.2	0.5	0.1	22.9	6.0	5,037
Colombia (Medellin)	2.1	0.4	0.3	0.1	14.5	5.5	1,673
Lebanon	1.0	0.4	0.2	0.2	20.9	15.3	595
Mexico	1.3	0.3	0.2	0.1	17.3	10.0	1,736
Romania	0.4	0.2	–	–	–	–	2,357
High-income countries	**3.2**	0.2	**0.3**	0.1	**10.8**	1.8	**13,298**
Belgium	3.1	1.3	0.7	0.6	23.9	13.4	486
France	2.5	1.0	0.3	0.2	11.9	7.9	727
Germany	1.3	0.6	–	–	–	–	621
Northern Ireland	2.0	0.3	0.1	0.1	5.7	4.1	1,986
Poland	0.5	0.1	0.1	0.1	22.6	12.5	2,276
Portugal	2.2	0.5	0.1	0.1	5.5	4.2	1,070
Spain	0.5	0.2	<0.1	0.0	7.9	7.8	960
Spain (Murcia)	0.7	0.3	<0.1	0.0	1.4	1.6	1,459
Netherlands	1.3	0.5	0.4	0.3	32.0	17.7	516
United States	9.5	0.8	1.0	0.2	10.9	2.2	3,197
All countries combined	**2.3**	0.1	**0.3**	0.0	**14.5**	1.6	**30,028**
WHO regions[a]							
Region of the Americas	**3.5**	0.2	**0.5**	0.1	**14.9**	1.9	14,661
African region	0.3	0.2	–	–	–	–	1,203
Western Pacific region	0.5	0.2	0.1	0.1	16.9	15.9	570
Eastern Mediterranean region	1.0	0.4	0.2	0.2	20.9	15.3	595
Western European region	1.6	0.2	0.2	0.1	9.8	3.2	7,825
Eastern European region	0.8	0.2	0.2	0.1	23.5	8.2	5,174
Comparison between countries[b]	$F_{19,v}=11.5^*$, $P<0.001$		$F_{19,v}=4.3^*$, $P<0.001$		$F_{19,v}=1.3$, $P=0.158$		
Comparison between low-, middle-, and high-income country groups[b]	$F_{2,v}=21.7^*$, $P<0.001$		$F_{2,v}=0.2$, $P=0.838$		$F_{2,v}=3.6^*$, $P=0.028$		
Comparison between WHO regions[b]	$F_{5,v}=31.9^*$, $P<0.001$		$F_{5,v}=14.2^*$, $P<0.001$		$F_{5,v}=1.3$, $P=0.245$		

*Significant at the 0.05 level, two-sided test.

[a] **Region of the Americas** (Colombia, Mexico, Brazil, Peru, United States, Colombia (Medellin)); **African region** (Nigeria); **Western Pacific region** (PRC: Beijing and Shanghai); **Eastern Mediterranean region** (Lebanon); **Western European region** (Belgium, France, Germany, Netherlands, Spain, Northern Ireland, Portugal, Spain (Murcia)); **Eastern European region** (Romania, Poland, Ukraine).

[b] Wald design-corrected F-tests were used to determine if there is variation in prevalence estimates across countries. The denominator degree of freedom, v, is 972.

from 0.3% (Nigeria) to 9.5% (United States; see Table 15.2). The 12-month prevalence of CD ranges from <0.1% (Spain) to 1.2% (Ukraine). As with ODD, variability in prevalence of CD is related to regional and income level differences. There is a significantly higher lifetime (3.5%) and 12-month (0.5%) prevalence of CD in the Americas, compared to other geographic regions (0.5% to 1.6% lifetime prevalence, 0.1% to 0.2% 12-month prevalence). Moreover, lifetime CD is more prevalent in high-income countries (3.2%) compared to upper-middle- (1.5%) and low/lower-middle-income countries (1.5%).

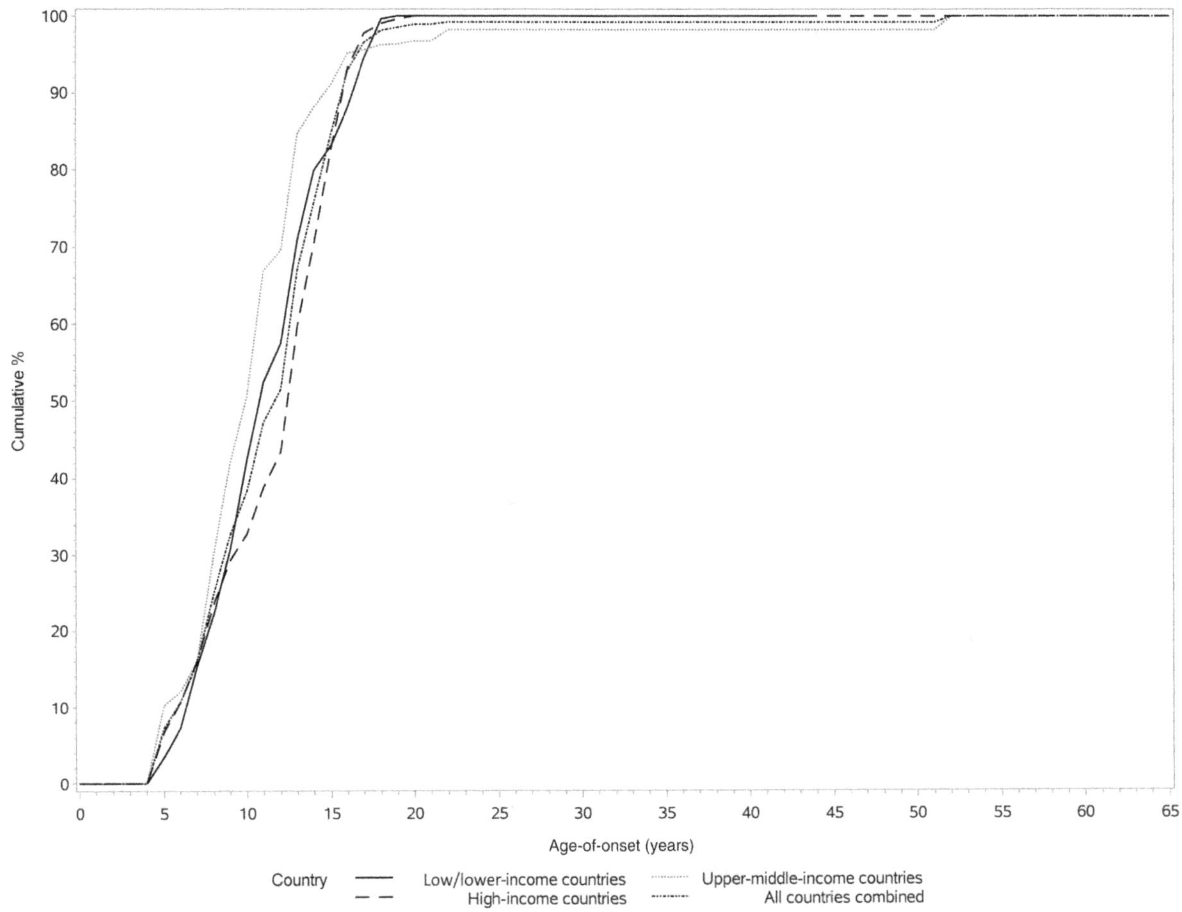

Figure 15.1 Cumulative age-of-onset distributions of DSM-IV oppositional defiant disorder by country income groups and in all countries combined.

Age-of-Onset of ODD and CD

Figure 15.1 displays the distribution of ages-of-onset for ODD by country income group. As shown in this figure, the onset of ODD begins in early childhood, around age five, and increases through childhood and adolescence until age 20. The majority of respondents who develop ODD do so between ages 8 and 14, with a median age-of-onset of 12. Country income group comparisons suggest a slightly later onset in high-income versus upper-middle-income countries. Regional comparisons reveal a younger median age-of-onset in the Americas (age 11) compared to Western Europe (age 13) and Eastern Europe (age 15). Additionally, there are some country-level differences: ODD has a notably earlier onset in Belgium, where 90% of lifetime cases exhibited the disorder by age 11, whereas the onset of ODD persists later in Brazil, where the last 5% of lifetime cases did not experience the onset of ODD until age 22 or later (detailed data not shown).

Figure 15.2 displays the distribution of ages-of-onset for CD by country income group. CD has a later onset than ODD, with new onsets beginning around age 7 and increasing through adolescence until age 19. The majority of individuals develop CD between the ages of 10 and 15, with a median age-of-onset of 13. Although CD onset has a similar pattern across country income groups and regions, there are country-level differences. Onset of CD begins later in Spain (5th percentile for onset = 12 years old) and Romania (5th percentile for onset = 13 years old), and extends into early adulthood in the Netherlands (75th percentile for onset = 29 years old; detailed data not shown).

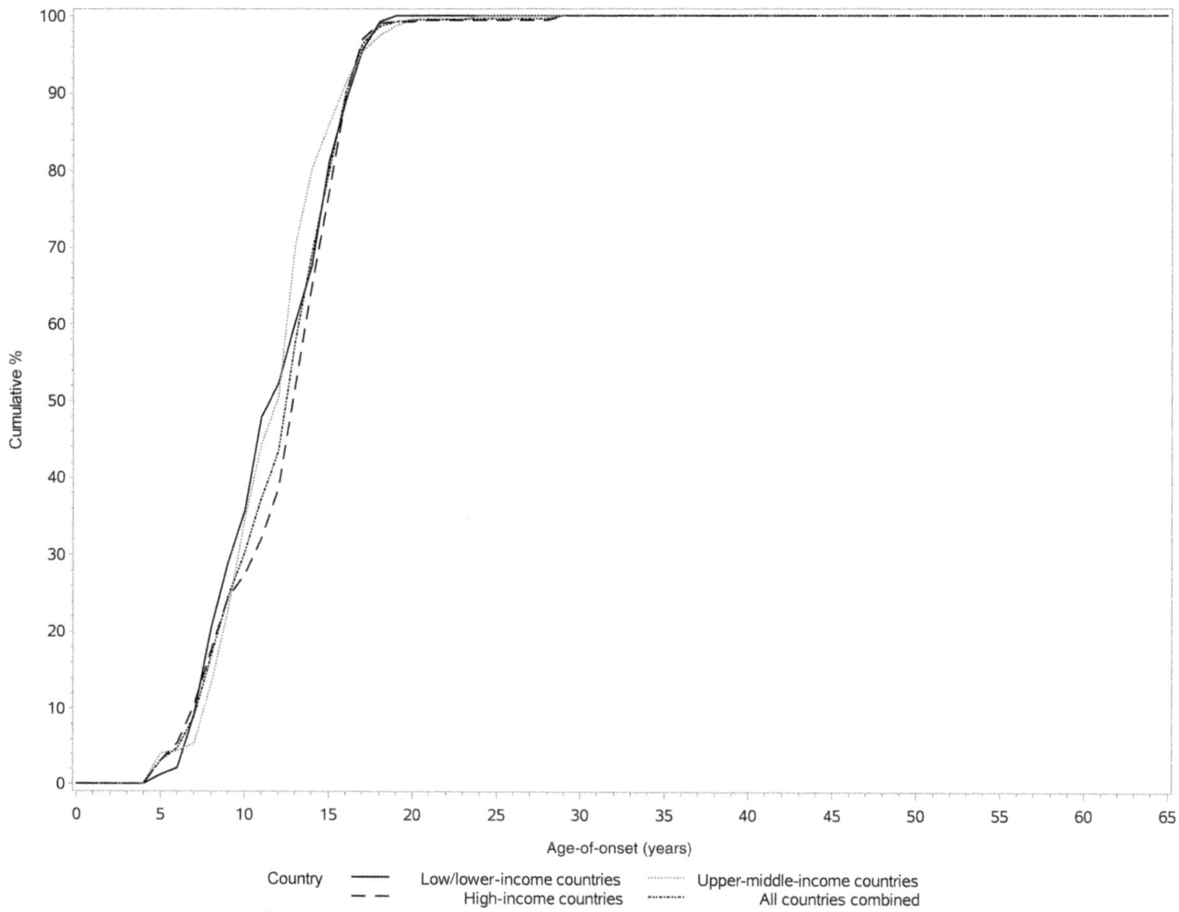

Figure 15.2 Cumulative age-of-onset distributions of DSM-IV conduct disorder by country income groups and in all countries combined.

Persistence of ODD and CD

Examining the number of respondents with a lifetime history of ODD or CD who also meet diagnostic criteria in the past 12 months can provide an indication of the persistence of these disorders within the population. Particularly for disorders like ODD and CD, which begin early in life, examining the 12-month/lifetime ratio in adult respondents can illuminate how likely these conditions are to persist into adulthood.

The overall rate of persistence of ODD is 16.2% (see Table 15.1). There is significant variability in persistence estimates across countries, which range from 1.0% (Murcia region of Spain) to 61.4% (Germany). This variability is related to both regional and income level differences. ODD is more persistent in Western European countries (19.3%) and the Americas (16.2%), compared to Eastern European countries (6.2%). Moreover, ODD is more persistent in upper-middle-income countries (24.6%), compared to high- (13.2%), and low/lower-middle-income countries (14.7%). An early onset of ODD is associated with significantly greater likelihood of persistence into adulthood in upper-middle- and high-income countries (country income group-specific data not shown), whereas in low/lower-middle-income countries more remote ODD onset is associated with lower likelihood of persistence.

The overall rate of persistence of CD is 14.5% (see Table 15.2). Persistence estimates again vary considerably across countries, from 1.4% (Murcia region of Spain) to 32.8% (Ukraine). Although persistence of CD does not differ by geographic region, CD is significantly less persistent in high-income countries (10.8%), compared to upper-middle- (19.3%) and low/lower middle-income countries (21.9%). Persistence of CD does not differ based on age of CD onset (see Table 15.4); however, more remote CD onset is associated with lower rates of CD persistence in low/lower middle- and upper-middle income countries, but not in high-income countries (country income group comparisons not shown).

Socio-demographic Correlates

Considering the total sample, younger cohorts (people <35 years old) are more likely to report a lifetime history of ODD and CD (see Tables 15.3 and 15.4). Examining these effects cross-nationally reveals that the higher odds of ODD among younger respondents, particularly for the cohort between ages 18 and 24, are observed across high-, upper-middle-, and low/lower-middle-income countries (see Appendix Tables 15A.1–15A.3). Younger cohorts also have higher odds of CD in upper-middle- and high-income countries, but not in low/lower-middle-income countries (cross-national comparisons for socio-demographic correlates of CD are not shown).

Women are significantly less likely to report a lifetime history of ODD and CD, but once ODD or CD begins these disorders are equally persist (i.e., 12-month/lifetime rate) in men and women. Comparing country income groups reveals that the lower odds of ODD in women are uniquely observed in low/lower-middle-income countries, whereas the lower odds of CD in women are consistently observed across all three country income groups.

Having an 'other' employment status (i.e., being disabled and unable to work, or being unemployed) is associated with significantly elevated lifetime odds of ODD and CD and with greater persistence (12-month/lifetime) of lifetime ODD. Comparing country income groups reveals that 'other' employment status is associated with a higher likelihood of lifetime ODD in low/lower-middle- and high-income, but not upper-middle-income countries, whereas this association is present across all country income groups for CD. Additionally, being retired confers a lower likelihood of ODD and CD in high-income countries only.

Being divorced, separated, or widowed is significantly associated with lifetime reports of ODD and CD, relative to respondents who are currently married or have never been married. Comparing country income groups, however, reveals that the elevated rate of ODD and CD among divorced, separated or widowed respondents is observed only in high-income countries. Never having been married is also associated with greater persistence of CD among respondents in high-income countries.

Having fewer years of education is significantly associated with reported lifetime history, as well as with greater persistence of ODD and CD. Relative to respondents who have finished college, those with fewer years of education are significantly more likely to report lifetime ODD. Among respondents with a lifetime history of ODD, those who have not completed secondary school are more likely to experience persistent ODD (i.e., ODD in the last 12 months). Relative to respondents with some college education, those who have completed secondary school or less are more likely to report lifetime CD. Country income group comparisons suggest this pattern is consistent across countries, although overall odds of lifetime ODD did not significantly differ by education category in upper-middle-income countries.

Household income category is not associated with reported lifetime history of ODD or CD. Country income group comparisons reveal that ODD is more persistent among respondents in high-income countries with low to low-average household incomes. No other household income category differences were observed.

Comorbidity

In the total sample, 89.3% of respondents with lifetime ODD report at least one other lifetime mental disorder. Among respondents with ODD in the past 12 months, 96.1% have at least one other lifetime disorder and 89.8% have had another mental disorder within the past 12 months. The most commonly comorbid disorders with ODD are anxiety disorders (60.4% co-occurrence for lifetime history, 71.1% co-occurrence within the past 12 months), followed by impulse-control disorders (56.1% lifetime co-occurrence, 51.4% 12-month co-occurrence), mood disorders (43.0% lifetime co-occurrence, 42.2% 12-month co-occurrence), and substance-use disorders (45.0% lifetime co-occurrence, 22.2% 12-month co-occurrence). Examining the temporal priority of disorders reveals that ODD typically emerges prior to mood and substance-use disorders (in 79.0% and 87.9% of respondents with lifetime ODD, respectively), whereas the temporal priority of ODD compared to anxiety and impulse-control disorders is more mixed, with ODD emerging first in 40.9% and 30.7% of lifetime ODD cases, respectively (detailed data not shown).

Table 15.3 Bivariate associations between socio-demographic correlates and DSM-IV oppositional defiant disorder (ODD), all countries combined

Correlates	Lifetime ODD[a]		12-month ODD among lifetime cases[b]	
	OR	(95% CI)	OR	(95% CI)
Age-cohort				
18–24	**2.3***	(1.8–2.8)		
25–34	**1.3***	(1.1–1.6)		
35+	**1.0**			
Age-cohort difference[c]	$\chi^2_2 = 64.4^*, P < 0.001$			
Age-of-onset				
Early			**3.8***	(1.9–7.6)
Early-average			**1.8**	(0.9–3.5)
Late-average			**1.6**	(0.8–3.0)
Late			**1.0**	
Age-of-onset difference[c]			$\chi^2_3 = 17.8^*, P = 0.001$	
Time since onset (continuous)			**1.00**	(0.97–1.02)
Gender				
Female	**0.8***	(0.7–0.9)	**1.2**	(0.8–1.8)
Male	**1.0**		**1.0**	
Gender difference[c]	$\chi^2_1 = 11.7^*, P = 0.001$		$\chi^2_1 = 0.9, P = 0.334$	
Employment status				
Student	**1.1**	(0.8–1.6)	**1.5**	(0.6–3.8)
Homemaker	**1.0**	(0.7–1.3)	**1.2**	(0.6–2.3)
Retired	**0.7**	(0.3–1.9)	–	–
Other	**1.7***	(1.4–2.1)	**2.2***	(1.3–3.6)
Employed	**1.0**		**1.0**	
Employment status difference[c]	$\chi^2_4 = 28.6^*, P < 0.001$		$\chi^2_4 = 10.3^*, P = 0.036$	
Marital status				
Never married	**1.0**	(0.8–1.3)	**1.5***	(1.0–2.3)
Divorced/separated/widowed	**1.5***	(1.1–2.1)	**1.5**	(0.8–2.9)
Currently married	**1.0**		**1.0**	
Marital status difference[c]	$\chi^2_2 = 7.4^*, P = 0.025$		$\chi^2_2 = 4.5, P = 0.103$	
Education level				
Some primary	**1.7***	(1.1–2.6)	**3.0***	(1.3–6.9)
Finished primary	**1.8***	(1.2–2.7)	**4.5***	(1.9–10.8)
Some secondary	**2.2***	(1.6–3.1)	**2.6***	(1.2–5.7)
Finished secondary	**1.6***	(1.2–2.0)	**1.7**	(0.9–3.5)
Some college	**1.5***	(1.1–2.0)	**1.9**	(0.8–4.6)
Finished college	**1.0**		**1.0**	
Education level difference[c]	$\chi^2_6 = 30.4^*, P < 0.001$		$\chi^2_6 = 16.3^*, P = 0.012$	
Household income				
Low	**1.0**	(0.8–1.2)	**2.0***	(1.2–3.5)
Low-average	**1.0**	(0.8–1.2)	**1.8***	(1.0–3.5)
High-average	**1.0**	(0.8–1.3)	**1.4**	(0.7–2.8)
High	**1.0**		**1.0**	
Household income difference[c]	$\chi^2_3 = 0.1, P = 0.992$		$\chi^2_3 = 7.2, P = 0.067$	
N[d]	**902,842**		**1,113**	

*Significant at the 0.05 level, two-sided test.
[a]These estimates are based on survival models adjusted for age-cohorts, gender, person-years, and country.
[b]These estimates are based on logistic regression models adjusted for time since ODD onset, age of ODD onset, gender, and country.
[c]Chi-square test of significant differences between blocks of socio-demographic variables.
[d]Denominator N: 902,842 = number of person-years in the survival models; 1,113 = number of lifetime ODD cases.

Table 15.4 Bivariate associations between socio-demographic correlates and DSM-IV conduct disorder (CD), all countries combined

Correlates	Lifetime CD[a]		12-month CD among lifetime cases[b]	
	OR	(95% CI)	OR	(95% CI)
Age-cohort				
18–24	**2.4***	(1.9–3.0)		
25–34	**1.9***	(1.5–2.3)		
35+	**1.0**			
Age-cohort difference[c]	$\chi^2_2 = 59.8^*, P < 0.001$			
Age-of-onset				
Early			**2.1**	(0.9–4.6)
Early-average			**1.5**	(0.7–3.4)
Late-average			**0.9**	(0.3–2.1)
Late			**1.0**	
Age-of-onset difference[c]			$\chi^2_3 = 5.8, P = 0.123$	
Time since onset (continuous)			**0.95***	(0.92–0.98)
Gender				
Female	**0.5***	(0.4–0.5)	**0.6**	(0.3–1.0)
Male	**1.0**		**1.0**	
Gender difference[c]	$\chi^2_1 = 78.6^*, P < 0.001$		$\chi^2_1 = 3.7, P = 0.054$	
Employment status				
Student	**0.7**	(0.5–1.1)	**0.8**	(0.3–2.6)
Homemaker	**0.9**	(0.6–1.4)	**0.7**	(0.3–1.7)
Retired	**0.3***	(0.2–0.6)	–	–
Other	**1.9***	(1.4–2.5)	**0.9**	(0.5–1.8)
Employed	**1.0**		**1.0**	
Employment status difference[c]	$\chi^2_4 = 38.2^*, P < 0.001$		$\chi^2_4 = 1.4, P = 0.852$	
Marital status				
Never married	**0.8**	(0.6–1.1)	**2.0***	(1.1–3.6)
Divorced/separated/widowed	**1.4***	(1.1–1.9)	**4.0***	(1.4–11.1)
Currently married	**1.0**		**1.0**	
Marital status difference[c]	$\chi^2_2 = 10.3^*, P = 0.006$		$\chi^2_2 = 9.7^*, P = 0.008$	
Education level				
Some primary	**2.9***	(1.8–4.5)	**2.3**	(0.5–9.7)
Finished primary	**2.9***	(1.7–4.7)	**1.3**	(0.3–5.4)
Some secondary	**3.3***	(2.4–4.6)	**0.7**	(0.2–2.6)
Finished secondary	**1.8***	(1.3–2.5)	**1.3**	(0.3–5.4)
Some college	**1.3**	(0.9–1.8)	**1.0**	(0.2–3.9)
Finished college	**1.0**		**1.0**	
Education level difference[c]	$\chi^2_6 = 65.9^*, P < 0.001$		$\chi^2_6 = 212.2^*, P < 0.001$	
Household income				
Low	**1.3**	(1.0–1.6)	**0.5**	(0.3–1.2)
Low-average	**1.2**	(0.9–1.6)	**0.5**	(0.2–1.0)
High-average	**1.0**	(0.8–1.4)	**0.4***	(0.2–1.0)
High	**1.0**		**1.0**	
Household income difference[c]	$\chi^2_3 = 4.0, P = 0.265$		$\chi^2_3 = 5.8, P = 0.121$	
N[d]	**1,084,925**		**888**	

*Significant at the 0.05 level, two-sided test.
[a]These estimates are based on survival models adjusted for age-cohorts, gender, person-years, and country.
[b]These estimates are based on logistic regression models adjusted for time since CD onset, age of CD onset, gender, and country.
[c]Chi-square test of significant differences between blocks of socio-demographic variables.
[d]Denominator N: 1,084,925 = number of person-years in the survival models; 888 = number of lifetime CD cases.

In the total sample, 87.3% of respondents with lifetime CD have at least one other lifetime mental disorder, and 85.2% of respondents with 12-month CD have at least one other lifetime mental disorder. The rate of 12-month co-occurrence of CD with another disorder is 73.2%. The most commonly comorbid disorders are impulse-control disorders (56.2% co-occurrence for lifetime history, 42.1% co-occurrence within the past 12 months), followed by anxiety disorders (53.4% lifetime co-occurrence, 41.5% 12-month co-occurrence), substance-use disorders (52.8% lifetime co-occurrence, 31.7% 12-month co-occurrence), and mood disorders (40.6% lifetime co-occurrence, 29.8% 12-month co-occurrence). Age-of-onset comparisons reveal that CD typically emerges prior to mood and substance-use disorders (in 74.8% and 86.3% of respondents with lifetime CD, respectively). Similar to the pattern for ODD, the temporal priority of CD relative to anxiety and impulse-control disorders is mixed, with CD emerging first in 34.4% and 27.0% of lifetime CD cases, respectively (detailed data not shown).

Role Impairment and Treatment

Respondents with 12-month ODD commonly report functional impairment related to their ODD symptoms. In the total sample, 42.7% of respondents report severe role impairment in at least one domain. Severe impairment is reported across social (31.3%), relationship (31.2%), occupational (29.8%), and home (26.1%) domains (detailed data not shown). Respondents who report the most severe impairment spend on average 106.7 days-out-of-role due to ODD, whereas those with the least severe impairment spend an average of 8.9 days-out-of-role due to ODD. Rates of severe impairment related to ODD do not differ by geographic region or by country income group (data not shown). Information regarding CD-related functional impairment was not collected in the CIDI interviews.

With respect to treatment, 44.2% of respondents in the total sample with 12-month ODD report seeking treatment. Treatment is most commonly received in the health care sector (38.6%), which includes specialty mental health (26.2%) and general medical services (22.8%). Receiving treatment in other sectors, such as complementary alternative medicine (9.2%) and human services (8.1%), is less often reported. Cross-national comparisons reveal that respondents in high-income countries are significantly more likely to have received treatment, particularly in the health care and human services sectors, compared to respondents in upper-middle-income countries (income group comparisons not shown).

Treatment of CD is less common but occurs in similar settings. In respondents with 12-month CD, 29.9% have received services in connection with their mental health. The most common treatment setting is health care services (23.5%), including specialty mental health (13.7%) and general medical services (12.4%). The human services sector (5.5%) and complementary alternative medicine (4.2%) are less often engaged. Examining these rates cross-nationally does not reveal significant differences in treatment utilization across country income groups (income group comparisons not shown).

Discussion

This chapter describes three major advances to our current understanding of ODD and CD. First, it reveals the cross-national lifetime prevalences of ODD and CD, which are 3.1% and 2.3%, respectively. Second, it highlights the consistent age-of-onset and sequencing of ODD and CD relative to comorbid psychiatric disorders across countries. Third, it underscores that despite the severity and persistence of ODD and CD, as well as their comorbidities with other psychiatric conditions, most people with these disorders do not receive treatment. These insights can guide policy, prevention, and treatment efforts, directing investments that are likely to have the greatest impact in reducing the burden associated with these disorders.

The cross-national lifetime prevalence estimates of ODD and CD in the WMH surveys are similar to those reported in a recent meta-regression of epidemiological studies (Canino *et al.* 2010). Unlike the meta-regression, however, we found significant regional differences in ODD and CD prevalence. Specifically, the WHM surveys suggest that ODD and CD are more prevalent in the Americas and in high-income countries, compared to other regions and country income groups. Although the uniform assessment strategies utilized in the WMH surveys addresses a methodological limitation of previous literature (see Canino *et al.* 2010), the present cross-national comparisons nonetheless remain vulnerable to various sources of error (e.g., norms regarding the acceptability and desirability of reporting various behaviours; culturally bound interpretations of screening items; differences in survey response rates; etc.).

To our knowledge, the WMH surveys are the first epidemiological studies to report cross-national data regarding the 12-month prevalence of ODD and CD, in addition to lifetime prevalence. The 12-month rates are substantial (roughly 1 in 200 for ODD, and 1 in 330 for CD), particularly given the serious impairment that results from these disorders. Thus, the 12-month prevalence helps to document the substantial costs to individuals and society exerted by these disorders at any given time.

These results also provide important information about the remarkable cross-national consistency in the developmental course of ODD and CD. ODD and CD emerge in late childhood to early adolescence, with median onsets at ages 12 and 13, respectively. Consistent with established developmental trends in the onset of different psychiatric conditions, ODD and CD are shown to follow the onset of the phobias and some impulse-control disorders, but emerge prior to most anxiety, mood and substance-use disorders. Whereas there are some regional differences in the age-of-onset of ODD, with younger onset in the Americas versus Europe, the onset of CD appears relatively uniform across geographic regions. Although the higher lifetime rates of ODD and CD in younger versus older cohorts could suggest increasing prevalence of these disorders, it is important to keep in mind that retrospective methods such as those employed in the WMH studies can produce biased estimates of disorders that occur early in life (see Loeber *et al.* 2000). Nonetheless, our results suggest that ODD symptoms persist into adulthood in roughly one out of every six individuals who have ever had the disorder. Persistence of CD into adulthood occurs in approximately one in seven people who ever met criteria for this disorder. Country income level appears to have contrary effects on the persistence of each disorder: whereas ODD is more persistent in high-income countries, CD is significantly less likely to persist in high-income countries.

Study results also inform about subpopulations that are at higher risk of developing ODD and CD. Results corroborate previously identified at-risk groups: males, people who are unmarried, and those with lower educational attainment (Burke *et al.* 2002). Cross-national comparisons of these relationships represent an important advancement. Specifically, results suggest that marital status and household income may be particularly relevant risk factors in high-income countries. Socio-demographic factors have somewhat limited utility in guiding intervention and prevention efforts, however, as they are often either static (e.g., impossible or unlikely to be modified), or represent the consequences rather than causes of the disorder.

Despite documenting substantial impairment and alarming rates of comorbidity (up to 89%) with other psychiatric conditions, these results suggest that only 30–45% of people with ODD or CD receive treatment for these disorders. Even when ODD and CD remit, comorbid conditions likely contribute to ongoing impairment, underscoring the potential utility of early screening and treatment. Managing these demands in countries with scarcer resources and less developed healthcare infrastructures will likely remain a significant challenge, however, given the intensity of many efficacious treatments that reduce such behavioural problems (e.g., Henggeler 2012). Given that most people who receive care do so outside of specialty mental health settings, establishing screening and referral services within primary care, general medical, and human service settings may have considerable benefit. Fortunately, a number of evidence-based treatments for children and families affected by ODD or CD have been developed (see Kazdin 1997; Steiner & Remsing 2007; Henggeler 2012), and previous research examining societal risk factors, such as rates of childhood poverty and unemployment (Guerra *et al.* 1995; Fergusson *et al.* 1997), can guide policies and prevention programs to reduce these disorders (see, for example, the guidelines developed by the Conduct Problems Prevention Research Group 2002a,b). These results therefore underscore the urgent need to develop portable and scalable interventions to reduce ODD and CD.

These results are limited in several important ways. First, the WMH data are based on retrospective self-reports, which are limited by recall biases, forgetting, and other inaccuracies. For childhood-onset disorders such as ODD and CD, the use of multiple informants (e.g., parent reports) often reveals higher prevalence estimates than self-report alone and may improve accuracy (Loeber *et al.* 1989; Angold & Costello 1996). In addition, there may be cross-national differences in willingness to endorse ODD and CD-relevant behaviours, particularly given varying cultural attitudes towards oppositional and rule-breaking behaviours. Although interview methods were carefully translated and back-translated to ensure their accuracy, attenuation of endorsement remains a possibility. Additional limitations arise due to the limited representation of some regions (e.g., Asia, Africa) among countries participating in the WMH surveys. Moreover, although countries are continuing to enrol, at the time of writing this chapter the sample included only a few lower-income countries, limiting some cross-national comparisons and the conclusions we can draw about the prevalence, course, and impact of ODD and CD in lower-income regions. Finally, while identifying high-risk groups by examining socio-demographic correlates of ODD and CD is an important task, the cross-sectional nature of the WMH surveys does not permit exploration of causal relationships or dynamic patterns of risk. Future studies should examine cross-national differences in the role of putative causal factors for ODD and CD (e.g., parental psychopathology; childhood adversity; neuropsychological impairment) to guide intervention and prevention efforts.

These limitations notwithstanding, this chapter presents a comprehensive, cross-national examination of the prevalence, course, and consequences of ODD and CD. The results highlight important directions for future research. First, longitudinal research is necessary to validate the relatively uniform pattern of onset and course in ODD and CD across countries and regions. It is useful to note that our findings correspond well with existing longitudinal studies examining the emergence, persistence, and comorbidity of ODD and CD (Biederman *et al.* 1996; Burke *et al.* 2010; Rowe *et al.* 2010; Reef *et al.* 2011). Second, whereas results of this study underscore the burden these disorders exert on individuals and communities, they do not directly inform how to optimally mitigate this burden. As mentioned previously, development of portable and efficient screening, treatment, and prevention strategies is an essential step in reducing the global burden of mental health problems.

References

Angold, A. & Costello, E. J. (1996). The relative diagnostic utility of child and parent reports of oppositional defiant behaviors. *International Journal of Methods in Psychiatric Research*, 6(4), 253–9.

Ashenafi, Y., Kebede, D., Desta, M., *et al.* (2001). Prevalence of mental and behavioural disorders in Ethiopian children. *East African Medical Journal*, 78(6), 308–11.

American Psychiatric Association (2013). *Diagnostic and Statistical Manual of Mental Disorders, Fifth Edition (DSM-5)* (5th ed.). Washington, DC: American Psychiatric Association.

Biederman, J., Faraone, S. V., Milberger, S., *et al.* (1996). Is childhood oppositional defiant disorder a precursor to adolescent conduct disorder? Findings from a four-year follow-up study of children with ADHD. *Journal of the American Academy of Child and Adolescent Psychiatry*, 35(9), 1193–204. doi: 10.1097/00004583-199609000-00017.

Boyle, M. H., Offord, D. R., Racine, Y., *et al.* (1996). Identifying thresholds for classifying childhood psychiatric disorder: issues and prospects. *Journal of the American Academy of Child and Adolescent Psychiatry*, 35(11), 1440–8. doi: 10.1097/00004583-199611000-00012.

Breslau, J., Lane, M., Sampson, N., *et al.* (2008). Mental disorders and subsequent educational attainment in a US national sample. *Journal of Psychiatric Research*, 42(9), 708–16. doi: 10.1016/j.jpsychires.2008.01.016.

Burke, J. D., Hipwell, A. E., & Loeber, R. (2010). Dimensions of oppositional defiant disorder as predictors of depression and conduct disorder in preadolescent girls. *Journal of the American Academy of Child and Adolescent Psychiatry*, 49(5), 484–92.

Burke, J. D., Loeber, R., & Birmaher, B. (2002). Oppositional defiant disorder and conduct disorder: a review of the past 10 years, part II. *Journal of the American Academy of Child and Adolescent Psychiatry*, 41(11), 1275–93. doi: 10.1097/00004583-200211000-00009.

Burke, J. D., Loeber, R., Lahey, B. B., *et al.* (2005). Developmental transitions among affective and behavioral disorders in adolescent boys. *Journal of Child Psychology and Psychiatry, and Allied Disciplines*, 46(11), 1200–10. doi: 10.1111/j.1469-7610.2005.00422.x.

Canino, G., Polanczyk, G., Bauermeister, J. J., *et al.* (2010). Does the prevalence of CD and ODD vary across cultures? *Social Psychiatry and Psychiatric Epidemiology*, 45(7), 695–704. doi:10.1007/s00127-010-0242-y.

Caspi, A., & Moffitt, T. E. (1995). The continuity of maladaptive behavior: From description to understanding in the study of antisocial behavior. In D. Cicchetti & D. J. Cohen (Eds.), *Developmental psychopathology, Vol. 2: Risk, disorder, and adaptation* (pp. 472–511). Oxford, England: John Wiley & Sons.

Cohen, P., Cohen, J., Kasen, S., *et al.* (1993). An epidemiological study of disorders in late childhood and adolescence? I. Age- and gender-specific prevalence. *Journal of Child Psychology and Psychiatry*, 34(6), 851–67. doi: 10.1111/j.1469-7610.1993.tb01094.x.

Copeland, W. E., Shanahan, L., Costello, E. J., *et al.* (2009). Childhood and adolescent psychiatric disorders as predictors of young adult disorders. *Archives of General Psychiatry*, 66(7), 764–72. doi: 10.1001/archgenpsychiatry.2009.85.

Diamantopoulou, S., Verhulst, F. C., & van der Ende, J. (2010). Testing developmental pathways to antisocial personality problems. *Journal of Abnormal Child Psychology*, 38(1), 91–103. doi: 10.1007/s10802-009-9348-7.

Fergusson, D. M., Horwood, L. J., & Lynskey, M. T. (1997). The effects of unemployment on psychiatric illness during young adulthood. *Psychological Medicine*, 27(2), 371–81.

Frick, P. J., Lahey, B. B., Loeber, R., *et al.* (1992). Familial risk factors to oppositional defiant disorder and conduct disorder: parental psychopathology and maternal parenting. *Journal of Consulting and Clinical Psychology*, 60(1), 49–55.

Conduct Problems Prevention Research Group (2002a). Evaluation of the first 3 years of the Fast Track prevention trial with children at high risk for adolescent conduct problems. *Journal of Abnormal Child Psychology*, 30(1), 19–35.

(2002b). The implementation of the Fast Track program: an example of a large-scale prevention science efficacy trial. *Journal of Abnormal Child Psychology*, 30(1), 1–17.

Guerra, N. G., Huesmann, L. R., Tolan, P. H., *et al.* (1995). Stressful events and individual beliefs as correlates of economic disadvantage and aggression among urban children. *Journal of Consulting and Clinical Psychology*, 63(4), 518–28.

Henggeler, S. W. (2012). Multisystemic therapy: clinical foundations and research outcomes. *Psychosocial Intervention*, 21(2), 181–193. doi: 10.5093/in2012a12.

Kazdin, A. E. (1995). Child, parent and family dysfunction as predictors of outcome in cognitive-behavioral treatment of antisocial children. *Behaviour Research and Therapy*, 33(3), 271–81.

(1997). Parent management training: evidence, outcomes, and issues. *Journal of the American Academy of Child and Adolescent Psychiatry*, 36(10), 1349–56. doi: 10.1097/00004583-199710000-00016.

Kessler, R. C., & Frank, R. G. (1997). The impact of psychiatric disorders on work loss days. *Psychological Medicine*, 27(4), 861–73. doi: 10.1017/S0033291797004807.

Kim-Cohen, J., Caspi, A., Moffitt, T. E., *et al.* (2003). Prior juvenile diagnoses in adults with mental disorder: developmental follow-back of a prospective-longitudinal cohort. *Archives of General Psychiatry*, 60(7), 709–17. doi: 10.1001/archpsyc.60.7.709.

Lahey, B. B., Loeber, R., Hart, E. L., *et al.* (1995). Four-year longitudinal study of conduct disorder in boys: patterns and predictors of persistence. *Journal of Abnormal Psychology*, 104(1), 83–93.

Lahey, B. B., Loeber, R., Stouthamer-Loeber, M., *et al.* (1990). Comparison of DSM-III and DSM-III-R diagnoses for prepubertal children: changes in prevalence and validity. *Journal of the American Academy of Child and Adolescent Psychiatry*, 29(4), 620–6. doi: 10.1097/00004583-199007000-00017.

Lahey, B. B., & Waldman, I. D. (2012). Annual research review: phenotypic and causal structure of conduct disorder in the broader context of prevalent forms of psychopathology. *Journal of Child Psychology and Psychiatry, and Allied Disciplines*, 53(5), 536–57. doi: 10.1111/j.1469-7610.2011.02509.x.

Lavigne, J. V., Cicchetti, C., Gibbons, R. D., *et al.* (2001). Oppositional defiant disorder with onset in preschool years: longitudinal stability and pathways to other disorders. *Journal of the American Academy of Child and Adolescent Psychiatry*, 40(12), 1393–400. doi: 10.1097/00004583-200112000-00009.

Leung, P. W. L., Hung, S., Ho, T., *et al.* (2008). Prevalence of DSM-IV disorders in Chinese adolescents and the effects of an impairment criterion: a pilot community study in Hong Kong. *European Child & Adolescent Psychiatry*, 17(7), 452–61. doi: 10.1007/s00787-008-0687-7.

Loeber, R., Burke, J. D., Lahey, B. B., *et al.* (2000). Oppositional defiant and conduct disorder: a review of the past 10 years, part I. *Journal of the American Academy of Child and Adolescent Psychiatry*, 39(12), 1468–84. doi: 10.1097/00004583-200012000-00007.

Loeber, R., Green, S. M., Lahey, B. B., *et al.* (1989). Optimal informants on childhood disruptive behaviors. *Development and Psychopathology*, 1(4), 317–37.

Loeber, R., Green, S. M., Lahey, B. B., *et al.* (1992). Developmental sequences in the age of onset of disruptive child behaviors. *Journal of Child and Family Studies*, 1(1), 21–41. doi: 10.1007/BF01321340.

Maughan, B., Rowe, R., Messer, J., *et al.* (2004). Conduct disorder and oppositional defiant disorder in a national sample: developmental epidemiology. *Journal of Child Psychology and Psychiatry*, 45(3), 609–21. doi: 10.1111/j.1469-7610.2004.00250.x.

Maughan, B., & Rutter, M. (2001). Antisocial children grown up. In J. Hill and B. Maughan (Eds.), *Conduct disorders in childhood and adolescence* (pp. 507–52). New York, NY: Cambridge University Press.

Moffitt, T. E., Caspi, A., Harrington, H., *et al.* (2002). Males on the life-course-persistent and adolescence-limited antisocial pathways: follow-up at age 26 years. *Development and Psychopathology*, 14(1), 179–207.

Nock, M. K., Kazdin, A. E., Hiripi, E., *et al.* (2006). Prevalence, subtypes, and correlates of DSM-IV conduct disorder in the National Comorbidity Survey Replication. *Psychological Medicine*, 36(5), 699–710. doi: 10.1017/S0033291706007082.

Nock, M. K., Kazdin, A. E., Hiripi, E., *et al.* (2007). Lifetime prevalence, correlates, and persistence of oppositional defiant disorder: results from the National Comorbidity Survey Replication. *Journal of Child Psychology and Psychiatry, and Allied Disciplines*, 48(7), 703–13. doi: 10.1111/j.1469-7610.2007.01733.x.

Offord, D. R., Boyle, M. H., Racine, Y. A., *et al.* (1992). Outcome, prognosis, and risk in a longitudinal follow-up study. *Journal of the American Academy of Child & Adolescent Psychiatry*, 31(5), 916–23. doi: 10.1097/00004583-199209000-00021.

Ravens-Sieberer, U., Wille, N., Erhart, M., *et al.* (2008). Prevalence of mental health problems among children and adolescents in Germany: results of the BELLA study within the National Health Interview and Examination Survey. *European Child & Adolescent Psychiatry*, 17, 22–33. doi: 10.1007/s00787-008-1003-2.

Reef, J., Diamantopoulou, S., van Meurs, I., *et al.* (2011). Developmental trajectories of child to adolescent externalizing behavior and adult DSM-IV disorder: results of a 24-year longitudinal study. *Social Psychiatry and Psychiatric Epidemiology*, 46(2), 1233–41. doi: 10.1007/s00127-010-0297-9.

Robins, L. N. (1991). Conduct disorder. *Journal of Child Psychology and Psychiatry, and Allied Disciplines*, 32(1), 193–212.

Rowe, R., Costello, E. J., Angold, A., *et al.* (2010). Developmental pathways in oppositional defiant disorder and conduct disorder. *Journal of Abnormal Psychology*, 119(4), 726–38. doi: 10.1037/a0020798.

Rowe, R., Maughan, B., Pickles, A., *et al.* (2002). The relationship between DSM-IV oppositional defiant disorder and conduct disorder: findings from the Great Smoky Mountains Study. *Journal of Child Psychology and Psychiatry, and Allied Disciplines*, 43(3), 365–73.

Steiner, H., & Remsing, L. (2007). Practice parameter for the assessment and treatment of children and adolescents with oppositional defiant disorder. *Journal of the American Academy of Child and Adolescent Psychiatry*, 46(1), 126–41. doi: 10.1097/01.chi.0000246060.62706.af.

Sugawara, M., Mukai, T., Kitamura, T., *et al.* (1999). Psychiatric disorders among Japanese children. *Journal of the American Academy of Child and Adolescent Psychiatry*, 38(4), 444–52. doi: 10.1097/00004583-199904000-00018.

Wacharasindhu, A., & Panyyayong, B. (2002). Psychiatric disorders in Thai school-aged children: I Prevalence. *Journal of the Medical Association of Thailand = Chotmaihet Thangphaet*, 85, S125–36.

West, P., Sweeting, H., Der, G., *et al.* (2003). Voice-DISC identified DSM-IV disorders among 15-year-olds in the west of Scotland. *Journal of the American Academy of Child and Adolescent Psychiatry*, 42(8), 941–9. doi: 10.1097/01.chi.0000046907.27264.E4.

World Health Organization (1992). *International Statistical Classification of Diseases and Related Health Problems, 10th Revision (ICD-10)* (10th ed.). Geneva: World Health Organization.

Zoccolillo, M., Pickles, A., Quinton, D., *et al.* (1992). The outcome of childhood conduct disorder: implications for defining adult personality disorder and conduct disorder. *Psychological Medicine*, 22(4), 971–86.

Chapter

16 Alcohol-Use Disorders

Meyer D. Glantz, Jacek Moskalewicz, José Miguel Caldas-de-Almeida, Louisa Degenhardt

Introduction

The category of alcohol-use disorders (AUDs) refers to a pattern of compulsive maladaptive alcohol use despite clinically significant symptoms and problems. While there is no consensually agreed upon phenotype, research has shown that AUDs are serious psychiatric conditions with cognitive, behavioural, and physiological symptoms leading to potentially major adverse consequences.

According to the World Health Organization's (WHO) 2014 Global Status Report on Alcohol and Health, harmful use of alcohol caused approximately 3.3 million deaths in 2012 (or 5.9% of all deaths) and 17.1% of these deaths were attributable to neuropsychiatric disorders, primarily AUDs. The report estimates that 5.1% of the global burden of disease and injury, equivalent to 139 million disability-adjusted life years (DALYs), was caused by alcohol use, with 24.6% of those DALYs attributable to neuropsychiatric disorders, primarily AUDs (WHO 2014). Heavy alcohol use is a risk factor for non-psychiatric health disorders including malignant neoplasms, liver cirrhosis, cardiovascular deaths, as well as unintentional and intentional injuries which contribute to the burden of harm associated with alcohol use (Rehm & Shield 2013). The economic burden of alcohol use has not been measured consistently across studies but is estimated to be more than 1% of the gross national product in high-income and middle-income countries (Rehm *et al.* 2009). Alcohol consumption and disease burden are increasing worldwide (Degenhardt *et al.* 2013).

The *Diagnostic and Statistical Manual* (DSM-IV-TR, American Psychiatric Association 2000) distinguishes two categories of AUDs, alcohol abuse (ALA) and alcohol dependence (ALD). Both diagnoses are defined as maladaptive patterns of alcohol use leading to clinically significant impairment or distress identifiable by manifested polythetic sets of symptoms. DSM-IV diagnoses are based on polythetic classifications, meaning that diagnoses are based on meeting the criteria for a subset of shared characteristics, none of which are individually required. In DSM-IV, a diagnosis of ALA is preempted by a diagnosis of ALD if the individual has ever met the criteria for ALD.

ALA is defined as recurrent or continued alcohol use despite one or more of the following occurring within a 12-month period: alcohol use resulting in a failure to fulfil major role obligations at work, school, or home; alcohol use in situations in which it is physically hazardous; alcohol use-related legal problems; alcohol use despite having persistent or recurrent social or interpersonal problems caused or exacerbated by the effects of alcohol use.

ALD is defined as a cluster of three or more of the following symptoms occurring at any time in the same 12-month period: tolerance; withdrawal; alcohol use in larger amounts or over a longer period than intended; persistent desire or unsuccessful efforts to cut down or control alcohol use; a great deal of time spent on activities necessary to obtain alcohol, use of alcohol, or use to recover from its effects; important social, occupational, or recreational activities given up or reduced because of alcohol use; continued alcohol use despite knowledge of having a persistent or recurrent physical or psychological problem that is likely to have been caused or exacerbated by alcohol use.

When single country, regional, or multi-country studies of alcohol use issues have been conducted they have typically focused on measurement of consumption, physical harm, or mortality rather than mental disorder. Prior to the World Mental Health (WMH) Surveys Initiative most of the available adult population data on the epidemiology of AUDs has come from single country studies, such as reports from the United States (Hasin *et al.* 2007), Australia (Andrews *et al.* 2001), Great Britain (Jenkins *et al.* 1997), Mexico (Medina-Mora *et al.* 2001), and Canada (Adlaf *et al.* 2005). It is difficult to compare findings in these different studies as they generally have not used equivalent assessments, administrations, diagnostic systems, sampling, and analysis approaches. A few multi-country or regional studies using a standardized assessment have been conducted. One early notable effort used the Diagnostic Interview Schedule (Robins *et al.* 1981), which includes an assessment of DSM-III (American Psychiatric Association 1980) ALA and ALD to assess samples in coordinated studies in 10 different cultural regions (Helzer & Canino 1992). There was wide variation in the lifetime prevalence rates of DSM-III ALA and/or ALD ranging from 0.45% in Shanghai to 22% in Korea and 23% in United States native Mexican Americans, although there was similarity in a number of associated variables. The WMH surveys standardize methodological factors, which facilitates the cross-national comparison of the prevalence and associated factors of AUDs in a large number of participating countries, making it almost uniquely able to address certain questions and controversies about AUDs.

There are two other major concerns related to cross-national comparisons of AUDs. The first relates to the psychiatric significance and consistency of the symptoms across countries.

There is relatively little dispute about the cross-national comparability of the ALD criteria. However, some have questioned the psychiatric significance of the three social consequences-related ALA criteria, maintaining that they are essentially socially determined potential or actual consequences (Sher *et al.* 2009), that they confound the distinction between the disorder itself and societal responses (Rounsaville *et al.* 1986), and that due to the varying social and cultural environmental factors they are not reliable and consistent diagnostic criteria appropriate for use in worldwide assessments and comparisons across countries (Rounsaville 2002; Room 2006). Further, a study in the United States found that more than 83.6% of those diagnosed with ALA met the diagnosis based on the hazardous-use criterion and that 69.3% did so solely through repeated instances of drinking and driving (Keyes & Hasin 2008), suggesting that the hazardous-use criterion and ALA diagnoses based on it are culturally and socially biased and sensitive to socio-economic status, variations in the enforcement of drinking and driving laws, and access to cars (Babor & Caetano 2008). If valid, these concerns suggest that variations in country prevalences of ALA are likely to reflect varying social, cultural, and economic factors rather than differing occurrences of ALA psychiatric disorder. However, there is evidence that despite cross-national socio-cultural variability the ALA criteria identify significant psychiatric disorder in both developed and developing countries in the WMH surveys (Glantz *et al.* 2014).

The second major concern is that environmental and social factors that are necessary, conducive, or deterrent of ALA and ALD and their development may vary across countries and might strongly influence the prevalence of AUDs. These limiting factors include alcohol availability, regulation and cost, abstention rates, social tolerance and consequences for impaired function or public intoxication, legal sanctions and enforcement, common alcohol-use patterns, mores and contexts of drinking, etc. For example, the WHO found that worldwide in 2010, individuals 15 years and older drank an average of 6.2 litres of pure alcohol per year. However, the per capita pure alcohol consumption ranged from 0.7 litres in the WHO Eastern Mediterranean region to 10.9 litres in the WHO European region. Further, although 48% of the global adult population had never drunk any alcohol, the prevalence of lifetime alcohol abstinence varied from 18.9% in the WHO region of the Americas to 89.8% in the Eastern Mediterranean region (WHO 2014).

It is likely that these limiting environmental factors account for and possibly reflect some of the cross-national variation in prevalence of AUDs. The possible influence of these factors is important to interpretation of the country AUD prevalences and to inferences about explanations for the varying AUD prevalences. However, interpretations should not assume simple causality and speculations must be cautious regarding how prevalences might change if different environmental and social conditions were instituted. It is worth noting that contextual influence may be more the case with AUDs than with other psychiatric disorders. For example, limited alcohol availability and high rates of lifetime abstention in a country probably limit possible AUDs prevalence but there are no counterpart variables for most other mental disorders such as schizophrenia or bipolar disorder. While varying socio-cultural environments may affect the development of AUDs and their prevalence, this does not negate the reality of the alcohol-use psychopathologies when they do develop or the validity of the estimates of the extant AUD prevalences and correlates in the participating countries at the time of assessment. The WMH surveys data provide an opportunity to compare the cross-national prevalences of ALA and ALD and consider the consistencies of patterns of associations of AUDs and correlates.

Methods

Data analysed for this chapter come from 28 of the 29 WMH surveys included in this volume (AUDs were not assessed in Shenzhen): see Table 16.1 for country listing.

As described in Chapter 3 the CIDI interview was divided into two parts. Part I assessed lifetime presence of core mental disorders. Respondents in Australia, Belgium, Brazil (São Paulo), Bulgaria, Colombia, France, Germany, Italy, Lebanon, Mexico, New Zealand, Nigeria, Peru, PRC Beijing/Shanghai, Spain, the Netherlands, and Ukraine were administered the AUDs and drug-use disorders (DUDs) assessment as part of their Part I interview. Additional disorders and correlates and information about service use were fully assessed in Part II. All respondents who met criteria for any of the core mental disorders were administered Part II. In addition, a probability subsample of approximately 25% of other Part I respondents who did not meet criteria for any core or substance-use disorder were administered Part II. The subsample was weighted to be representative of the populations from which they were selected and to account for the under-representation of non-cases.

Respondents in Colombia (Medellin), Japan, Northern Ireland, Poland, Portugal, Spain (Murcia), and the United States were administered a version of Part I that assessed lifetime presence of core mental disorders and a screen for substance-use disorders (SUDS, i.e. AUDs and/or DUDs). In these countries the full assessments for SUDs were included in Part II of the interview. All respondents who met criteria for any of the core mental disorders or the screen for SUDs were administered Part II, as were a weighted probability subsample of approximately 25% of other Part I respondents who did not meet criteria for any core disorder or the SUD screen. All participants in Iraq, Israel, Romania, and South Africa were administered both parts of the interview. Combining participants from all 28 surveys, of the 140,132 respondents who completed Part I, 77,226 completed Part II and 121,121 comprised the weighted subsample assessed for AUDs and described here. Not all of the 121,121 respondents who were fully assessed for AUDs were assessed for all of the correlates discussed here as some correlates were assessed in Part II.

In the earliest 13 WMH surveys (Colombia, Nigeria, Peru, PRC Beijing/Shanghai, Ukraine, Bulgaria, Lebanon, Mexico, South Africa, Japan, Israel, New Zealand, and the United States), if a respondent did not endorse any of the ALA criteria, they were not asked questions related to ALD. Although symptoms of abuse often precede dependence, it is possible for dependence to occur without prior symptoms of abuse. In order to evaluate the prevalence of such cases, the skip logic was revised for later WMH surveys to assess ALD among respondents who had not endorsed any symptoms of abuse. For the purpose of improving cross-national comparability of survey data collected before and after this revision to the CIDI, regression-based imputation models were developed and validated from random half-samples of the new WMH surveys and applied to the earlier WMH surveys. This imputation adjusted for the absence of information relating to ALD without abuse in the earlier WMH surveys and allows for improved estimates of lifetime dependence prevalence. Further details of the methodology are described elsewhere (Lago *et al.* 2017). Adjusted data were used in the analyses presented here.

The CIDI 3.0 survey instrument includes a series of 16 questions that operationalize the DSM-IV symptom criteria for ALA and ALD. Respondents met criteria for diagnosis of ALA by endorsing at least one of the four abuse symptoms and met criteria for diagnosis of ALD by endorsing at least three of the seven dependence symptoms. Respondents who met criteria for either ALA or ALD were considered to have an AUD. The DSM-IV hierarchy rule was followed so that respondents could not be diagnosed with both ALA and ALD and any respondents who met criteria for both AUD disorders were diagnosed as ALD. The 12-month and 30-day prevalence of ALA or ALD was defined as respondents having reported symptoms of the specific AUD in the associated timeframe. For respondents diagnosed with both AUD and for whom the hierarchy rule was employed, only symptoms of the hierarchical disorder, ALD, were considered in determining 12-month and 30-day prevalence.

Results

Prevalence

Tables 16.1–16.3 show the prevalences of ALA, ALD, and AUDs for each of the 28 WMH surveys, the countries combined, the countries grouped by World Bank income levels, and the WHO regions. The average lifetime prevalence of ALA in all countries combined is 6.2% ranging from 0.5% in Iraq to 18.7% in Australia.

Table 16.1 Prevalence of DSM-IV alcohol abuse (ALA) in the World Mental Health surveys

Country	Lifetime prevalence		12-month prevalence		30-day prevalence		12-month prevalence of ALA among lifetime cases		30-day prevalence of ALA among 12-month cases		Sample size used
	%	SE	%	SE	%	SE	%	SE	%	SE	
Low/lower-middle-income countries	**4.4**	**0.2**	**1.2**	**0.1**	**0.4**	**0.0**	**27.4**	**1.6**	**33.5**	**3.2**	**29,366**
Colombia	6.9	0.5	1.3	0.2	0.2	0.1	19.1	3.2	17.4	5.5	4,426
Iraq	0.5	0.2	0.1	0.1	0.1	0.1	21.6	11.9	85.4	17.6	4,332
Nigeria	1.9	0.2	0.4	0.1	0.1	0.0	23.1	2.9	30.1	7.7	6,752
Peru	4.3	0.3	1.0	0.2	0.2	0.1	24.2	3.5	21.3	6.2	3,930
PRC (Beijing/Shanghai)	3.7	0.3	0.8	0.2	0.3	0.1	22.8	3.4	37.2	9.6	5,201
Ukraine	10.0	0.7	3.7	0.4	1.5	0.2	37.1	2.8	40.0	4.8	4,725
Upper-middle-income countries	**4.7**	**0.2**	**1.4**	**0.1**	**0.5**	**0.1**	**29.3**	**1.7**	**33.3**	**3.6**	**27,339**
Brazil	6.6	0.5	1.7	0.3	0.9	0.2	26.6	3.1	48.9	7.4	5,037
Bulgaria	2.2	0.2	0.8	0.2	0.3	0.1	35.4	5.4	38.3	10.3	5,318
Colombia (Medellin)	8.0	1.2	1.5	0.3	0.4	0.2	18.7	4.2	26.7	9.0	1,673
Lebanon	1.2	0.3	0.3	0.2	0.2	0.2	25.4	9.7	83.0	13.8	2,857
Mexico	4.2	0.3	1.0	0.2	0.1	0.1	23.6	4.4	15.0	5.2	5,782
Romania	2.4	0.3	0.4	0.2	0.2	0.2	17.6	6.6	56.1	21.0	2,357
South Africa	8.8	0.7	3.5	0.4	0.9	0.2	39.4	3.3	26.5	6.2	4,315
High-income countries	**7.7**	**0.1**	**1.4**	**0.1**	**0.4**	**0.0**	**17.7**	**0.7**	**31.1**	**2.1**	**64,416**
Australia	18.7	0.6	2.6	0.2	0.7	0.1	14.1	1.2	27.9	4.1	8,463
Belgium	6.6	0.8	1.4	0.4	0.6	0.2	20.7	4.2	47.8	11.6	2,419
France	5.5	0.5	0.7	0.2	0.1	0.1	13.4	3.0	15.6	7.8	2,894
Germany	4.9	0.4	0.8	0.2	0.2	0.1	15.4	3.1	23.9	8.7	3,555
Israel	3.9	0.3	1.0	0.1	0.3	0.1	25.9	3.2	27.1	6.1	4,859
Italy	0.9	0.1	0.1	0.0	< 0.1	0.0	8.7	5.0	33.0	27.1	4,712
Japan	6.5	0.7	0.5	0.2	0.1	0.1	7.6	2.8	30.5	14.3	1,682
New Zealand	7.5	0.3	1.5	0.1	0.5	0.1	19.7	1.8	33.2	5.2	12,790
Northern Ireland	10.7	0.9	2.3	0.4	0.7	0.2	21.7	3.8	29.8	8.4	1,986
Poland	8.8	0.4	2.2	0.3	0.6	0.1	24.5	2.8	27.8	5.2	4,000
Portugal	8.7	1.0	1.3	0.2	0.6	0.2	15.1	3.3	44.7	10.8	2,060
Spain	3.0	0.4	0.6	0.1	0.2	0.1	19.5	4.0	35.7	13.0	5,473
Spain (Murcia)	4.9	0.7	0.6	0.3	0.2	0.2	13.2	6.9	37.8	23.3	1,459
Netherlands	7.4	0.8	1.5	0.3	0.8	0.3	20.0	3.9	53.0	12.2	2,372
United States	7.8	0.4	1.6	0.1	0.4	0.1	20.9	1.6	25.8	3.6	5,692

Table 16.1 *(cont.)*

Country	Lifetime prevalence		12-month prevalence		30-day prevalence		12-month prevalence of ALA among lifetime cases		30-day prevalence of ALA among 12-month cases		Sample size used
	%	SE	%	SE	%	SE	%	SE	%	SE	
All countries combined	**6.2**	**0.1**	**1.3**	**0.0**	**0.4**	**0.0**	**21.4**	**0.6**	**32.2**	**1.6**	**121,121**
WHO regions[a]											
Region of the Americas	6.1	0.2	1.4	0.1	0.4	0.0	22.3	1.3	27.9	2.8	26,540
African region	4.6	0.3	1.6	0.2	0.4	0.1	35.3	2.6	27.1	5.3	11,067
Western Pacific region	10.1	0.3	1.6	0.1	0.5	0.1	16.3	1.0	31.0	3.1	28,136
Eastern Mediterranean region	2.0	0.2	0.5	0.1	0.2	0.1	25.4	3.0	39.3	7.7	12,048
Western European region	5.0	0.2	0.9	0.1	0.3	0.0	17.5	1.3	36.7	4.2	26,930
Eastern European region	6.1	0.2	1.9	0.1	0.7	0.1	31.3	1.9	36.9	3.5	16,400
Comparison between countries[b]	$F_{27,v} = 74.4^*$, $P < 0.001$		$F_{27,v} = 20.7^*$, $P < 0.001$		$F_{27,v} = 6.6^*$, $P < 0.001$		$F_{27,v} = 4.6^*$, $P < 0.001$		$F_{27,v} = 1.4$, $P = 0.088$		
Comparison between low-, middle-, and high-income country groups[b]	$F_{2,v} = 139.4^*$, $P < 0.001$		$F_{2,v} = 1.6$, $P = 0.207$		$F_{2,v} = 0.3$, $P = 0.746$		$F_{2,v} = 28.8^*$, $P < 0.001$		$F_{2,v} = 0.3$, $P = 0.761$		
Comparison between WHO regions[b]	$F_{5,v} = 148.9^*$, $P < 0.001$		$F_{5,v} = 28.7^*$, $P < 0.001$		$F_{5,v} = 6.2^*$, $P < 0.001$		$F_{5,v} = 16.7^*$, $P < 0.001$		$F_{5,v} = 1.4$, $P = 0.217$		

*Significant at the 0.05 level, two-sided test.
[a]**Region of the Americas** (Colombia, Mexico, Brazil, Peru, United States, Colombia (Medellin)); **African region** (South Africa, Nigeria); **Western Pacific region** (PRC: Beijing and Shanghai, Japan, Australia, New Zealand); **Eastern Mediterranean region** (Israel, Iraq, Lebanon); **Western European region** (Belgium, France, Germany, Italy, Netherlands, Spain, Northern Ireland, Portugal, Spain (Murcia)); **Eastern European region** (Romania, Poland, Bulgaria, Ukraine).
[b]Wald design-corrected F-tests were used to determine if there is variation in prevalence estimates across countries. The denominator degree of freedom, v, is 5331.
PRC: People's Republic of China.

Table 16.2 Prevalence of DSM-IV alcohol dependence (ALD) in the World Mental Health surveys

Country	Lifetime prevalence		12-month prevalence		30-day prevalence		12-month prevalence of ALD among lifetime cases		30-day prevalence of ALD among 12-month cases		Sample size used
	%	SE	%	SE	%	SE	%	SE	%	SE	
Low/lower-middle-income countries	**1.5**	**0.1**	**0.8**	**0.1**	**0.4**	**0.1**	**53.3**	**2.8**	**54.6**	**4.4**	**29,366**
Colombia	2.5	0.4	1.2	0.3	0.6	0.2	48.7	6.3	45.9	8.4	4,426
Iraq	0.2	0.1	<0.1	0.0	<0.1	0.0	6.1	5.2	55.9	34.9	4,332
Nigeria	0.3	0.1	0.2	0.1	0.1	0.0	67.4	10.7	49.5	15.9	6,752
Peru	1.5	0.2	0.6	0.1	0.3	0.1	37.5	6.2	53.4	12.0	3,930
PRC (Beijing/Shanghai)	1.1	0.2	0.6	0.2	0.3	0.1	60.1	8.3	49.8	13.0	5,201
Ukraine	3.7	0.4	2.2	0.2	1.4	0.2	60.0	4.1	61.7	6.2	4,725
Upper-middle-income countries	**2.4**	**0.1**	**0.9**	**0.1**	**0.4**	**0.1**	**38.2**	**2.7**	**46.6**	**4.8**	**27,339**
Brazil	3.3	0.3	1.3	0.2	0.7	0.1	41.2	3.4	52.8	8.8	5,037
Bulgaria	0.9	0.1	0.3	0.1	0.1	0.1	31.9	7.3	39.7	18.7	5,318
Colombia (Medellin)	4.8	0.8	1.7	0.4	0.7	0.3	36.5	7.5	41.6	11.2	1,673
Lebanon	0.4	0.2	0.3	0.1	0.2	0.1	71.0	10.9	72.4	20.8	2,857
Mexico	3.8	0.4	1.2	0.3	0.5	0.2	31.5	5.7	41.9	11.4	5,782
Romania	0.7	0.2	0.3	0.1	0.3	0.1	50.3	13.1	73.9	15.1	2,357
South Africa	2.7	0.4	1.2	0.2	0.5	0.1	45.4	6.6	41.7	8.4	4,315
High-income countries	**2.7**	**0.1**	**0.8**	**0.0**	**0.3**	**0.0**	**31.3**	**1.3**	**40.7**	**2.4**	**64,416**
Australia	4.0	0.3	1.4	0.2	0.6	0.1	36.2	3.5	43.6	5.8	8,463
Belgium	1.7	0.5	0.3	0.1	0.1	0.1	17.1	3.8	36.8	22.4	2,419
France	1.6	0.3	0.5	0.2	0.2	0.1	33.8	8.7	36.3	16.6	2,894
Germany	1.5	0.3	0.3	0.1	0.1	0.0	21.2	6.7	20.6	11.8	3,555
Israel	0.4	0.1	0.1	0.1	0.1	0.0	31.6	10.7	48.0	20.9	4,859
Italy	0.3	0.1	0.1	0.0	<0.1	0.0	26.2	9.0	48.6	25.1	4,712
Japan	0.9	0.2	0.2	0.1	–	–	27.8	8.6	–	–	1,682
New Zealand	4.7	0.2	1.4	0.1	0.6	0.1	30.7	2.0	43.2	3.9	12,790
Northern Ireland	2.5	0.4	0.7	0.2	0.4	0.2	29.6	7.1	47.0	14.9	1,986
Poland	2.2	0.2	1.2	0.2	0.4	0.1	56.0	5.8	35.6	6.4	4,000
Portugal	1.3	0.3	0.3	0.1	0.2	0.1	19.5	7.9	73.2	17.5	2,060
Spain	0.6	0.1	0.1	0.1	0.1	0.1	17.5	9.9	70.9	22.2	5,473
Spain (Murcia)	1.5	0.5	0.3	0.2	<0.1	0.0	20.6	13.5	13.5	14.9	1,459
Netherlands	1.5	0.3	0.4	0.1	0.1	0.1	28.2	8.1	24.2	13.4	2,372
United States	6.0	0.4	1.7	0.2	0.6	0.1	27.7	2.5	37.5	4.7	5,692

Table 16.2 (*cont.*)

Country	Lifetime prevalence		12-month prevalence		30-day prevalence		12-month prevalence of ALD among lifetime cases		30-day prevalence of ALD among 12-month cases		Sample size used
	%	SE	%	SE	%	SE	%	SE	%	SE	
All countries combined	**2.3**	**0.1**	**0.8**	**0.0**	**0.4**	**0.0**	**36.3**	**1.1**	**45.3**	**2.0**	**121,121**
WHO regions[a]											
Region of the Americas	3.7	0.2	1.3	0.1	0.6	0.1	34.6	2.0	44.2	3.8	26,540
African region	1.3	0.1	0.6	0.1	0.3	0.1	48.9	5.9	43.4	7.4	11,067
Western Pacific region	3.6	0.1	1.2	0.1	0.5	0.1	34.1	1.8	43.4	3.2	28,136
Eastern Mediterranean region	0.3	0.1	0.1	0.0	0.1	0.0	36.8	9.1	61.1	15.3	12,048
Western European region	1.2	0.1	0.3	0.0	0.1	0.0	24.2	2.8	38.9	6.9	26,930
Eastern European region	2.0	0.1	1.1	0.1	0.6	0.1	54.2	3.1	53.0	4.7	16,400
Comparison between countries[b]	$F_{27,v} = 36.2^*$, $P < 0.001$		$F_{27,v} = 20.6^*$, $P < 0.001$		$F_{27,v} = 11.1^*$, $P < 0.001$		$F_{27,v} = 4.0^*$, $P < 0.001$		$F_{27,v} = 1.0$, $P = 0.421$		
Comparison between low-, middle-, and high-income country groups[b]	$F_{2,v} = 49.1^*$, $P < 0.001$		$F_{2,v} = 0.9$, $P = 0.407$		$F_{2,v} = 1.8$, $P = 0.163$		$F_{2,v} = 22.2^*$, $P < 0.001$		$F_{2,v} = 3.9^*$, $P = 0.020$		
Comparison between WHO regions[b]	$F_{5,v} = 130.4^*$, $P < 0.001$		$F_{5,v} = 59.6^*$, $P < 0.001$		$F_{5,v} = 24.2^*$, $P < 0.001$		$F_{5,v} = 11.2^*$, $P < 0.001$		$F_{5,v} = 1.0$, $P = 0.444$		

*Significant at the 0.05 level, two-sided test.

[a] **Region of the Americas** (Colombia, Mexico, Brazil, Peru, United States, Colombia (Medellin)); **African region** (South Africa, Nigeria); **Western Pacific region** (PRC: Beijing and Shanghai, Japan, Australia, New Zealand); **Eastern Mediterranean region** (Israel, Iraq, Lebanon); **Western European region** (Belgium, France, Germany, Italy, Netherlands, Spain, Northern Ireland, Portugal, Spain (Murcia)); **Eastern European region** (Romania, Poland, Bulgaria, Ukraine).

[b] Wald design-corrected F-tests were used to determine if there is variation in prevalence estimates across countries. The denominator degree of freedom, v, is 5331.

PRC: People's Republic of China.

Table 16.3 Prevalence of DSM-IV alcohol-use disorder (AUD) in the World Mental Health surveys

Country	Lifetime prevalence		12-month prevalence		30-day prevalence		12-month prevalence of AUD among lifetime cases		30-day prevalence of AUD among 12-month cases		Sample size used
	%	SE	%	SE	%	SE	%	SE	%	SE	
Low/lower-middle-income countries	**5.9**	**0.2**	**2.0**	**0.1**	**0.8**	**0.1**	**33.9**	**1.4**	**41.9**	**2.5**	**29,366**
Colombia	9.4	0.6	2.6	0.3	0.8	0.2	27.1	3.1	31.2	5.3	4,426
Iraq	0.7	0.2	0.1	0.1	0.1	0.1	17.2	9.8	82.4	17.7	4,332
Nigeria	2.2	0.2	0.7	0.1	0.2	0.1	29.6	3.0	36.6	7.9	6,752
Peru	5.7	0.4	1.6	0.2	0.5	0.1	27.6	2.3	32.5	6.9	3,930
PRC (Beijing/Shanghai)	4.7	0.4	1.5	0.2	0.6	0.1	31.1	3.7	42.7	8.1	5,201
Ukraine	13.7	0.8	5.9	0.5	2.9	0.3	43.3	2.3	48.1	3.6	4,725
Upper-middle-income countries	**7.2**	**0.2**	**2.3**	**0.1**	**0.9**	**0.1**	**32.3**	**1.5**	**38.6**	**2.9**	**27,339**
Brazil	9.8	0.6	3.1	0.4	1.6	0.2	31.5	2.4	50.6	4.3	5,037
Bulgaria	3.2	0.3	1.1	0.2	0.4	0.1	34.3	4.0	38.7	9.1	5,318
Colombia (Medellin)	12.8	1.4	3.2	0.5	1.1	0.3	25.4	3.8	34.7	7.7	1,673
Lebanon	1.6	0.3	0.6	0.2	0.5	0.2	36.7	9.5	77.9	12.4	2,857
Mexico	8.0	0.6	2.2	0.4	0.6	0.2	27.3	3.9	29.6	6.5	5,782
Romania	3.1	0.3	0.8	0.3	0.5	0.3	24.8	7.3	64.1	13.2	2,357
South Africa	11.5	0.8	4.7	0.4	1.4	0.3	40.8	3.0	30.5	5.8	4,315
High-income countries	**10.4**	**0.2**	**2.2**	**0.1**	**0.8**	**0.0**	**21.2**	**0.7**	**34.7**	**1.6**	**64,416**
Australia	22.7	0.6	4.1	0.3	1.4	0.2	18.0	1.3	33.5	3.5	8,463
Belgium	8.3	0.9	1.6	0.4	0.8	0.3	20.0	3.6	45.8	11.4	2,419
France	7.1	0.5	1.3	0.3	0.3	0.1	17.9	3.6	24.2	8.8	2,894
Germany	6.5	0.6	1.1	0.2	0.2	0.1	16.8	3.2	22.9	6.9	3,555
Israel	4.3	0.3	1.1	0.2	0.3	0.1	26.5	3.0	29.6	6.0	4,859
Italy	1.3	0.2	0.2	0.1	0.1	0.0	13.6	4.5	41.4	18.6	4,712
Japan	7.3	0.7	0.7	0.2	0.1	0.1	10.0	2.7	20.3	9.3	1,682
New Zealand	12.1	0.4	2.9	0.2	1.1	0.1	24.0	1.4	38.1	3.4	12,790
Northern Ireland	13.2	1.0	3.1	0.5	1.0	0.3	23.2	3.5	34.0	8.6	1,986
Poland	11.1	0.5	3.4	0.3	1.0	0.1	30.8	2.3	30.6	4.0	4,000
Portugal	10.0	1.0	1.6	0.3	0.8	0.2	15.7	3.1	49.4	10.0	2,060
Spain	3.6	0.4	0.7	0.2	0.3	0.1	19.2	3.9	40.8	12.0	5,473
Spain (Murcia)	6.4	0.6	0.9	0.4	0.3	0.2	14.8	5.7	30.2	15.2	1,459
Netherlands	8.9	0.9	1.9	0.3	0.9	0.3	21.3	3.4	46.6	10.7	2,372
United States	13.8	0.6	3.3	0.3	1.0	0.1	23.9	1.6	31.7	3.3	5,692

Table 16.3 (*cont.*)

Country	Lifetime prevalence		12-month prevalence		30-day prevalence		12-month prevalence of AUD among lifetime cases		30-day prevalence of AUD among 12-month cases		Sample size used
	%	SE	%	SE	%	SE	%	SE	%	SE	
All countries combined	**8.6**	**0.1**	**2.2**	**0.1**	**0.8**	**0.0**	**25.4**	**0.6**	**37.2**	**1.3**	**121,121**
WHO regions[a]											
Region of the Americas	9.8	0.3	2.6	0.1	0.9	0.1	26.9	1.2	35.7	2.2	26,540
African region	5.9	0.3	2.2	0.2	0.7	0.1	38.2	2.4	31.6	5.0	11,067
Western Pacific region	13.7	0.3	2.9	0.1	1.0	0.1	21.0	0.9	36.3	2.3	28,136
Eastern Mediterranean region	2.4	0.2	0.6	0.1	0.3	0.1	27.1	2.9	43.6	6.8	12,048
Western European region	6.2	0.2	1.2	0.1	0.4	0.1	18.8	1.3	37.2	3.7	26,930
Eastern European region	8.1	0.3	3.0	0.2	1.3	0.1	37.0	1.6	42.8	2.7	16,400
Comparison between countries[b]	**$F_{27,v} = 100.1$*, $P < 0.001$**		**$F_{27,v} = 32.8$*, $P < 0.001$**		**$F_{27,v} = 12.7$*, $P < 0.001$**		**$F_{27,v} = 6.4$*, $P < 0.001$**		**$F_{27,v} = 1.7$*, $P = 0.012$**		
Comparison between low-, middle-, and high-income country groups[b]	**$F_{2,v} = 163.2$*, $P < 0.001$**		**$F_{2,v} = 2.1$, $P = 0.126$**		**$F_{2,v} = 1.0$, $P = 0.382$**		**$F_{2,v} = 45.8$*, $P < 0.001$**		**$F_{2,v} = 2.9$, $P = 0.054$**		
Comparison between WHO regions[b]	**$F_{5,v} = 253.0$*, $P < 0.001$**		**$F_{5,v} = 72.2$*, $P < 0.001$**		**$F_{5,v} = 23.5$*, $P < 0.001$**		**$F_{5,v} = 24.9$*, $P < 0.001$**		**$F_{5,v} = 1.3$, $P = 0.241$**		

*Significant at the 0.05 level, two-sided test.

[a]**Region of the Americas** (Colombia, Mexico, Brazil, Peru, United States, Colombia (Medellin)); **African region** (South Africa, Nigeria); **Western Pacific region** (PRC: Beijing and Shanghai, Japan, Australia, New Zealand); **Eastern Mediterranean region** (Israel, Iraq, Lebanon); **Western European region** (Belgium, France, Germany, Italy, Netherlands, Spain, Northern Ireland, Portugal, Spain (Murcia)); **Eastern European region** (Romania, Poland, Bulgaria, Ukraine).

[b]Wald design-corrected F-tests were used to determine if there is variation in prevalence estimates across countries. The denominator degree of freedom, v, is 5331.

PRC: People's Republic of China.

The average 12-month prevalence of ALA for all countries is 1.3%, ranging from 0.1% in Iraq to 3.7% in the Ukraine. The average 30-day prevalence of ALA for all countries is 0.4% ranging from less than 0.1% in Italy to 1.5% in the Ukraine. The average lifetime prevalence of ALD in all countries combined is 2.3% ranging from 0.2% in Iraq to 6% in the United States. The average 12-month prevalence of ALD for all countries is 0.8% ranging from less than 0.1% in Iraq to 2.2% in the Ukraine. The average 30-day prevalence of ALD for all countries is 0.4% ranging from less than 0.1% in Iraq, Italy, and Spain-Murcia to 0.7% in Brazil and Colombia-Medellin. For AUDs the average lifetime prevalence in all countries combined is 8.6%.

The average lifetime prevalence rate of ALA, ALD, and AUD is significantly higher in the high-income countries and lower in the low/lower-middle-income countries, however, this pattern is not found for 12-month or 30-day prevalence. There are also significant differences in the lifetime, 12-month, and 30-day prevalences of ALA, ALD, and AUDs among the WHO regions. Given that of the WHO regions, the WHO Eastern Mediterranean region has the highest prevalence of alcohol abstinence and the lowest per capita alcohol consumption, it is not surprising that the Eastern Mediterranean region has the lowest prevalences of lifetime and 12-month ALA, ALD, and AUDs. Although prevalences vary across countries, in all countries the lifetime prevalence of ALA is larger than the lifetime prevalence of ALD. The 12-month prevalence of ALA is larger than the 12-month prevalence of ALD in 24 of the 28 surveys while there is no clear pattern for 30-day prevalence.

Age-of-Onset

Previous research has shown that in the WMH surveys the median age-of-onset (AOO) for alcohol use is between 16 and 20 years for all countries with the earliest use being in European countries and the latest being in the Middle East and Africa (Degenhardt *et al.* 2008). Globally, not only does alcohol use often begin in adolescence but so do AUDs (Table 16.4). Across all countries, the earliest 5% of lifetime AUD cases have onsets by age 16 with the youngest onset being age 10 in Romania and the oldest being age 19 in Japan. The earliest 10% of lifetime AUDs cases across all countries combined have onset by 17 years which means that of those individuals who will at some point develop an AUD in their lifetime, 10% will have done so by the age of 17.

When considering ages-of-onset for higher percentages of AUD cases, AOO of AUD is generally lower at higher levels of country income. The earliest quarter of lifetime cases across all countries have onsets by age 19 with onsets by age 21 in low/lower-middle-income countries, by age 20 in upper-middle-income countries, and by age 19 in high-income countries where the greatest variation is found, ranging between 17 years in New Zealand and 22 years in Japan. The median AOO of AUDs across all countries is 23 years of age, with a median of 27 years in low/lower-middle-income countries, 26 years in upper-middle-income countries, and 21 years in high-income countries. Considering that the median age of first alcohol use is between 16 and 20 years for all countries it is noteworthy that half of all cases of AUDs begin by age 23 in all countries combined and in the relatively narrow range in individual countries from age 20 in New Zealand to age 29 in Nigeria.

Of all lifetime cases across all countries, 75% have onsets by age 31 with onsets by age 36 in low/lower-middle-income countries, by age 33 in upper-middle-income countries, and by age 31 in high-income countries, with variation in all three country income levels. Risk for onset continues at older ages. Based on projections shown in Table 16.4, 90% of lifetime cases across all countries have onsets by age 44 and 95% by age 51. Although there is great variation among countries, projected risk at age 75 across all countries is 10.9%, with 8.4% in low/lower-middle-income countries, 9.6% in upper-middle-income countries, and 12.7% in high-income countries.

Persistence

Two indirect measures of disorder and symptom persistence were computed (Tables 16.1–16.3). The 12-month AUD among lifetime cases measure can be considered an indicator of disorder persistence. For all countries combined, the rates are 21.4% for ALA, 36.3% for ALD, and 25.4% for AUD. There is significant variation across countries ranging from 7.6% to 39.4% for ALA, 6.1% to 71% for ALD, and 10% to 43.3% for AUD. The 30-day AUD among 12-month cases measure can be considered an indirect indicator of symptom persistence. For all countries combined, the rates are 32.2% for ALA, and 45.3% for ALD, with neither significantly different across countries, and 37.2% for AUD which is significantly different across countries ranging from 20.3% to 82.4%. The 12-month/lifetime

Table 16.4 Age at selected percentiles on the standardized age-of-onset distributions of DSM-IV alcohol-use disorder (AUD) with projected lifetime risk at age 75

Country	Ages at selected percentiles								Lifetime prevalence of AUD		Projected risk at age 75	
	5	10	25	50	75	90	95	99	%	SE	%	SE
Low/lower-middle-income countries	**17**	**18**	**21**	**27**	**36**	**46**	**51**	**66**	**5.9**	**0.2**	**8.4**	**0.3**
Colombia[a]	15	18	20	26	35	41	49	53	9.4	0.6	12.7	1.0
Iraq	17	17	21	23	44	44	47	47	0.7	0.2	1.1	0.5
Nigeria	16	17	21	29	41	52	57	61	2.2	0.2	3.8	0.3
Peru[a]	17	18	21	26	34	44	46	49	5.7	0.4	7.9	0.6
PRC (Beijing/Shanghai)	18	19	21	26	32	41	46	53	4.7	0.4	6.0	0.5
Ukraine	17	19	21	27	34	42	50	58	13.7	0.8	17.6	1.1
Upper-middle-income countries	**16**	**18**	**20**	**26**	**33**	**46**	**51**	**57**	**7.2**	**0.2**	**9.6**	**0.3**
Brazil	16	18	20	25	37	49	53	57	9.8	0.6	13.7	0.8
Bulgaria	18	18	21	23	31	38	46	51	3.2	0.3	3.8	0.3
Colombia (Medellin)[a]	13	16	20	26	36	49	49	54	12.8	1.4	16.3	2.2
Lebanon	16	18	20	23	41	43	58	58	1.6	0.3	2.2	0.4
Mexico[a]	17	18	21	27	38	52	54	62	8.0	0.6	12.3	1.0
Romania	10	17	21	28	36	41	46	53	3.1	0.3	4.3	0.3
South Africa	17	19	21	26	32	46	52	59	11.5	0.8	16.0	1.1
High-income countries	**16**	**17**	**19**	**21**	**31**	**41**	**50**	**64**	**10.4**	**0.2**	**12.7**	**0.2**
Australia	16	17	19	21	28	41	51	69	22.7	0.6	26.7	0.9
Belgium	17	18	20	23	31	44	51	56	8.3	0.9	10.5	1.1
France	17	18	19	23	32	41	51	56	7.1	0.5	8.8	0.6
Germany	16	17	19	26	36	51	68	73	6.5	0.6	8.7	0.9
Israel	18	19	20	24	29	41	48	63	4.3	0.3	5.3	0.4
Italy	17	19	20	28	35	41	48	55	1.3	0.2	1.6	0.3
Japan	19	20	22	26	37	46	51	57	7.3	0.7	9.5	0.9
New Zealand	15	16	17	20	26	41	47	62	12.1	0.4	14.6	0.5
Northern Ireland	16	17	19	21	30	43	50	69	13.2	1.0	16.8	1.5
Poland[b]	17	19	21	21	31	41	41	49	11.1	0.5	13.4	0.6
Portugal	17	18	20	23	37	61	61	61	10.0	1.0	11.5	1.2
Spain	17	18	20	23	35	41	43	56	3.6	0.4	4.6	0.5
Spain (Murcia)	16	17	19	22	31	41	41	46	6.4	0.6	7.8	0.9
Netherlands	16	17	19	21	36	47	52	64	8.9	0.9	11.4	1.2
United States	15	16	18	21	29	39	45	54	13.8	0.6	16.8	0.7
All countries combined	**16**	**17**	**19**	**23**	**31**	**44**	**51**	**64**	**8.6**	**0.1**	**10.9**	**0.2**
WHO regions												
Region of the Americas	16	17	20	25	34	46	50	57	9.8	0.3	13.2	0.4
African region	17	18	21	26	35	46	53	60	5.9	0.3	8.8	0.5
Western Pacific region	16	17	19	21	29	41	49	65	13.7	0.3	16.4	0.4
Eastern Mediterranean region	17	18	21	24	31	44	49	63	2.4	0.2	3.2	0.3
Western European region	17	17	19	23	34	46	53	68	6.2	0.2	7.8	0.3
Eastern European region	17	19	21	26	33	41	46	56	8.1	0.3	10.3	0.4

[a]The projected risk for these countries is at age 65 because the age range of these surveys is between 18 and 65.
[b]The projected risk for this country is at age 64 because the age range of this survey is between 18 and 64.
PRC: People's Republic of China.

and the 30-day/12-month rates for ALA and ALD are somewhat low compared to many other mental disorders (see Chapter 22), especially given the generally attributed chronic and relapsing nature of AUDs. As indicated by both measures, although less prevalent, ALD is more persistent than ALA.

Socio-demographic Correlates

Consistent with previous studies, men are significantly more likely than women to have a lifetime (χ^2_1 = 2,526.1, P < 0.001) or 30-day (χ^2_1 = 212.1, P < 0.001) AUD (Table 16.5). The odds for men having a lifetime AUD is more than five times the odds for that of women, and the odds for men having a 30-day AUD is more than three times the odds for women. There are indications from other research that in younger cohorts, the prevalence of women's use of alcohol (Degenhardt *et al.* 2008), binge drinking, and AUDs (Keyes *et al.* 2008) is becoming more similar to men's prevalences. It is notable that the gender difference is less pronounced for the indicator of disorder persistence and not evident at all for symptom persistence.

Earlier AOO is associated with greater likelihood of 12-month AUD among lifetime cases (χ^2_3 = 104.9, P < 0.001) indicating that younger AOO of lifetime AUD is associated with a higher probability of disorder persistence. There is a significant difference in the odds of respondents having a lifetime (χ^2_3 = 1,603.5, P < 0.001) or 30-day (χ^2_3 = 161.9, P < 0.001) AUD depending on their age at the time of interview, with younger people more likely to both ever and currently meet criteria for an AUD. Marital status is significantly associated with lifetime (χ^2_2 = 162.5, P < 0.001) and 30-day (χ^2_2 = 29.0, P < 0.001) AUDs, with respondents who were married at the time of interview having the lowest odds of having an AUD followed in probability by those who were never married, and with those who were divorced, separated, or widowed having the greatest likelihood. There is a significant association of education level with 30-day AUD (χ^2_6 = 47.6, P < 0.001), with decreased likelihood of 30-day AUD with increasing educational attainment. This higher 30-day prevalence among those with less education seems to be largely driven by the associations of lower education with disorder and symptom persistence, rather than an association between lower education and lifetime odds of AUDs.

Comorbidity

It is well established that AUDs are highly comorbid with other mental disorders (Merikangas *et al.* 1998; Stinson *et al.* 2005; Pani *et al.* 2010; Lai *et al.* 2015) and high comorbidity is also found in the WMH data. As shown in Table 16.6, of those respondents with a 12-month AUD, 58.8% have at least one other DSM-IV mental disorder in their lifetime and 42.9% meet criteria for at least one other mental disorder within the same 12 months. For those respondents with a lifetime AUD and at least one other mental disorder, the onset of the AUD was at a younger age than the lifetime comorbid disorders in 44.4% of the cases of comorbid mood disorders, in 21.3% of comorbid anxiety disorder cases, in 20.8% of the comorbid disruptive behaviour/impulse-control disorder cases, in 41.9% of the other SUD cases, and in 24.9% of the cases of any comorbid disorders. Inferences about temporal priority and causal influence should be tempered by the likelihood of there being multiple patterns of comorbidity, some including bi-direction of influence, that onset of disorder symptoms is often not a discrete event occurring at a single point in time, and that symptom development is likely to be transactional, meaning that as symptoms progress over time they reciprocally facilitate and exacerbate each other (Glantz & Leshner 2000). Further, research suggests that AUDs and mood, anxiety and other impulse-control-related mental disorders may share common underlying influences or pathways (Hasin *et al.* 2007; Kessler *et al.* 2011).

Role Impairment

The Sheehan Disability Scale (SDS) (Leon *et al.* 1997) was incorporated into the CIDI modules for AUDs for a subset of countries. As shown in Table 16.7, 30.8% of those with 12-month AUD in all countries combined report having at least one area of their life where they experienced severe impairment associated with their AUD. While this is a considerable level of role impairment and higher than that of some other mental disorders included in this volume, AUD is not among the most impairing disorders. This is consistent with the WMH findings on days-out-of-role associated with AUD and other mental and physical disorders (Alonso *et al.* 2011). Further research is needed to explicate the impact of AUDs on impairment and role function.

Treatment

Only a small proportion of those with 12-month AUD report treatment in the 12 months prior to the

Table 16.5 Bivariate associations between socio-demographic correlates and DSM-IV alcohol-use disorder (AUD) (all countries combined)

Correlates	30-day AUD[a]		Lifetime AUD[b]		12-month AUD among lifetime cases[c]		30-day AUD among 12-month cases[c]	
	OR	(95% CI)	OR	(95% CI)	OR	(95% CI)	OR	(95% CI)
Age-cohort								
18–29	**9.4***	(6.5–13.5)	**10.2***	(9.1–11.5)				
30–44	**6.1***	(4.2–8.9)	**6.0***	(5.4–6.6)				
45–59	**4.3***	(2.9–6.3)	**3.4***	(3.1–3.8)				
60+	**1.0**		**1.0**					
Age-cohort difference[d]	$\chi^2_3 = 161.9^*$, $P < 0.001$		$\chi^2_3 = 1{,}603.5^*$, $P < 0.001$					
Age-of-onset								
Early					**2.2***	(1.9–2.6)	**1.5***	(1.2–2.0)
Early-average					**1.7***	(1.4–2.1)	**1.5***	(1.1–2.1)
Late-average					**1.3***	(1.1–1.5)	**1.4***	(1.0–1.9)
Late					**1.0**		**1.0**	
Age-of-onset difference[d]					$\chi^2_3 = 104.9^*$, $P < 0.001$		$\chi^2_3 = 10.4^*$, $P = 0.015$	
Time since onset (continuous)					**0.94***	(0.94–0.95)	**1.02***	(1.01–1.03)
Gender								
Female	**0.3***	(0.2–0.3)	**0.2***	(0.2–0.2)	**0.8***	(0.7–1.0)	**1.2**	(1.0–1.6)
Male	**1.0**		**1.0**		**1.0**		**1.0**	
Gender difference[d]	$\chi^2_1 = 212.1^*$, $P < 0.001$		$\chi^2_1 = 2{,}526.1^*$, $P < 0.001$		$\chi^2_1 = 6.6^*$, $P = 0.010$		$\chi^2_1 = 2.9$, $P = 0.088$	
Employment status								
Student	**0.7**	(0.4–1.1)	**0.8***	(0.7–1.0)	**1.3**	(0.9–1.8)	**1.0**	(0.6–1.7)
Homemaker	**1.1**	(0.7–1.6)	**0.9***	(0.8–1.0)	**1.0**	(0.8–1.4)	**1.4**	(0.9–2.4)
Retired	**0.8**	(0.5–1.2)	**0.8***	(0.7–0.9)	**1.3**	(0.9–1.7)	**1.2**	(0.7–2.2)
Other	**1.6***	(1.3–2.1)	**1.5***	(1.4–1.6)	**1.4***	(1.2–1.6)	**1.0**	(0.8–1.4)
Employed	**1.0**		**1.0**		**1.0**		**1.0**	
Employment status difference[d]	$\chi^2_4 = 22.4^*$, $P < 0.001$		$\chi^2_4 = 143.4^*$, $P < 0.001$		$\chi^2_4 = 16.5^*$, $P = 0.002$		$\chi^2_4 = 2.3$, $P = 0.678$	
Marital status								
Never married	**1.4***	(1.2–1.7)	**1.3***	(1.2–1.4)	**1.7***	(1.4–1.9)	**1.1**	(0.9–1.5)
Divorced/separated/widowed	**1.9***	(1.4–2.5)	**1.6***	(1.5–1.7)	**1.2**	(1.0–1.4)	**1.1**	(0.8–1.6)
Currently married	**1.0**		**1.0**		**1.0**		**1.0**	
Marital status difference[d]	$\chi^2_2 = 29.0^*$, $P < 0.001$		$\chi^2_2 = 162.5^*$, $P < 0.001$		$\chi^2_2 = 47.2^*$, $P < 0.001$		$\chi^2_2 = 1.0$, $P = 0.595$	

(cont.)

Table 16.5 (*cont.*)

Correlates	30-day AUD[a]		Lifetime AUD[b]		12-month AUD among lifetime cases[c]		30-day AUD among 12-month cases[c]	
	OR	(95% CI)	OR	(95% CI)	OR	(95% CI)	OR	(95% CI)
Education level								
No education	**5.3***	(2.4–12.1)	**1.3**	(1.0–1.6)	**3.5***	(1.8–6.7)	**3.8***	(1.5–9.6)
Some primary	**3.3***	(2.1–5.3)	**1.7***	(1.5–2.0)	**1.5***	(1.1–2.1)	**1.7**	(0.9–3.1)
Finished primary	**2.8***	(1.8–4.3)	**1.7***	(1.5–2.0)	**1.5***	(1.1–2.1)	**1.2**	(0.7–2.0)
Some secondary	**2.6***	(1.9–3.7)	**1.8***	(1.6–2.0)	**1.4***	(1.1–1.7)	**1.4**	(0.9–2.0)
Finished secondary	**1.8***	(1.3–2.6)	**1.4***	(1.3–1.5)	**1.2***	(1.0–1.5)	**1.2**	(0.9–1.8)
Some college	**1.7***	(1.2–2.4)	**1.4***	(1.3–1.6)	**1.3***	(1.1–1.6)	**1.1**	(0.7–1.6)
Finished college	**1.0**		**1.0**		**1.0**		**1.0**	
Education level difference[d]	$\chi^2_6 = 47.6^*$, $P < 0.001$		$\chi^2_6 = 165.5^*$, $P < 0.001$		$\chi^2_6 = 22.3^*$, $P = 0.001$		$\chi^2_6 = 10.7$, $P = 0.099$	
Household income								
Low	**1.3**	(1.0–1.6)	**1.2***	(1.2–1.3)	**1.2***	(1.0–1.5)	**1.0**	(0.7–1.4)
Low-average	**1.3***	(1.0–1.7)	**1.2***	(1.1–1.2)	**1.1**	(0.9–1.3)	**1.2**	(0.9–1.7)
High-average	**1.0**	(0.8–1.3)	**1.0**	(1.0–1.1)	**1.1**	(0.9–1.3)	**0.9**	(0.7–1.3)
High	**1.0**		**1.0**		**1.0**		**1.0**	
Household income difference[d]	$\chi^2_3 = 7.4$, $P = 0.060$		$\chi^2_3 = 40.5^*$, $P < 0.001$		$\chi^2_3 = 6.3$, $P = 0.096$		$\chi^2_3 = 3.0$, $P = 0.393$	
N[e]	**121,121**		**5,179,126**		**10,495**		**2,578**	

*Significant at the 0.05 level, two-sided test.
[a]These estimates are based on logistic regression models adjusted for age, gender, and country.
[b]These estimates are based on survival models adjusted for age-cohorts, gender, person-years, and country.
[c]These estimates are based on logistic regression models adjusted for time since AUD onset, age of AUD onset, gender, and country.
[d]Chi-square test of significant differences between blocks of socio-demographic variables.
[e]Denominator N: 121,121 = total sample; 5,179,126 = number of person-years in the survival models; 10,495 = number of lifetime AUD cases; 2,578 = number of 12-month AUD cases.

Table 16.6 Comorbidity of alcohol-use disorder (AUD) with other DSM-IV disorders

	AUD cases with comorbid disorders									
	Mood disorder		Anxiety disorder		Disruptive behaviour/ impulse-control disorder		Other substance-use disorder		Any disorder	
	%	SE	%	SE	%	SE	%	SE	%	SE
Lifetime comorbidity[a]										
Lifetime	**26.3**	0.6	**30.6**	0.7	**14.3**	0.7	**21.4**	0.6	**51.7**	0.8
12-month	**28.0**	1.3	**33.4**	1.3	**18.2**	1.5	**26.2**	1.3	**58.8**	1.6
12-month comorbidity[b]										
12-month	**18.5**	1.1	**25.5**	1.1	**14.3**	1.3	**10.9**	0.8	**42.9**	1.4
Temporal priority of AUD[c]										
Lifetime	**44.4**	1.2	**21.3**	1.0	**20.8**	2.1	**41.9**	1.7	**24.9**	0.9
12-month	**33.5**	2.2	**16.7**	1.8	**13.7**	2.4	**39.8**	2.9	**20.5**	1.5

[a]Percentage of respondents with either lifetime or 12-month AUD who also meet lifetime criteria for at least one of the other DSM-IV disorders.
[b]Percentage of respondents with 12-month AUD who also meet 12-month criteria for at least one of the other disorders.
[c]Percentage of respondents with either lifetime or 12-month AUD and at least one of the other disorders, whose AOO of AUD is reported to be younger than the AOO of all comorbid disorders under consideration.

Table 16.7 Severity of role impairment (Sheehan Disability Scale) associated with 12-month alcohol-use disorder (AUD), by country

Country	Proportion with severe role impairment (SDS score: 7–10)										Number of 12-month AUD cases
	Home		Work		Relationship		Social		Any[a]		
	%	SE	%	SE	%	SE	%	SE	%	SE	
Brazil	22.5	6.6	31.8	5.7	28.9	6.2	34.0	5.4	44.6	6.6	143
Colombia (Medellin)	26.1	9.6	31.6	9.9	11.3	5.2	14.4	5.8	38.2	10.3	66
Romania	42.4	17.9	12.9	9.1	–	–	15.1	10.5	51.2	17.9	17
Australia	14.1	4.4	9.0	3.8	14.3	4.1	11.7	3.8	20.0	4.3	308
Northern Ireland	21.1	10.9	26.9	12.5	8.8	5.7	9.5	5.3	26.9	12.5	60
Poland	32.7	5.2	25.8	5.5	25.3	6.6	19.7	3.4	40.0	6.7	166
Portugal	3.3	3.3	–	–	5.2	3.6	1.8	1.7	8.4	4.8	39
All countries combined	**21.4**	**2.6**	**18.7**	**2.4**	**18.1**	**2.6**	**17.2**	**2.0**	**30.8**	**2.9**	**818**
Comparison between countries[b]	**$F_{7,v} = 2.6$*, P = 0.009**		**$F_{7,v} = 4.1$*, P < 0.001**		**$F_{7,v} = 2.4$*, P = 0.014**		**$F_{7,v} = 3.4$*, P < 0.001**		**$F_{7,v} = 2.9$*, P = 0.003**		

*Significant at the 0.05 level, two-sided test.
A dash indicates low cell count (<5 cases).
[a]People with severe impairment across any of the four domains met criteria for 'any' severe impairment.
[b]Wald design-corrected F-tests were used to determine if there is variation in impairment severity across countries. The denominator degree of freedom, v, is 581.

interview. As shown in Table 16.8, among respondents with a 12-month AUD, for all countries combined, 20.3% report having had some intervention in any of the treatment sectors in the previous year. Any treatment for 12-month AUD ranges from 9.3% in low/lower-middle-income countries, to 16.8% in upper-middle-income countries, and to 26.3% in high-income countries. For all countries combined, 18% of 12-month AUD respondents report treatment-seeking in either the mental health specialist sector or the general medical sector, while only 5.7% report intervention in either the human services sector or the

Table 16.8 Among those with 12-month alcohol-use disorder, percent reporting treatment in the past 12 months

Sector of treatment	%	SE	Comparison between country income groups[a]
Specialty mental health[b]			
Low/lower-income countries	3.9	0.8	$F_{2,v} = 26.7^*$, $P < 0.001$
Upper-middle-income countries	9.1	1.6	
High-income countries	15.8	1.2	
All countries combined	**11.6**	**0.8**	
General medical[c]			
Low/lower-income countries	4.1	1.0	$F_{2,v} = 31.4^*$, $P < 0.001$
Upper-middle-income countries	6.0	1.4	
High-income countries	16.1	1.1	
All countries combined	**11.1**	**0.8**	
Any health care[d]			
Low/lower-income countries	7.6	1.3	$F_{2,v} = 32.2^*$, $P < 0.001$
Upper-middle-income countries	13.6	2.0	
High-income countries	24.2	1.5	
All countries combined	**18.0**	**1.0**	
Human services[e]			
Low/lower-income countries	–	–	$F_{2,v} = 8.8^*$, $P < 0.001$
Upper-middle-income countries	2.2	0.8	
High-income countries	3.8	0.7	
All countries combined	**2.7**	**0.4**	
CAM[f]			
Low/lower-income countries	1.2	0.5	$F_{2,v} = 7.0^*$, $P < 0.001$
Upper-middle-income countries	3.1	0.9	
High-income countries	4.5	0.7	
All countries combined	**3.4**	**0.5**	
Any non-health care[g]			
Low/lower-income countries	1.8	0.6	$F_{2,v} = 12.8^*$, $P < 0.001$
Upper-middle-income countries	5.3	1.2	
High-income countries	7.4	0.9	
All countries combined	**5.7**	**0.6**	
Any treatment[h]			
Low/lower-income countries	9.3	1.4	$F_{2,v} = 29.7^*$, $P < 0.001$
Upper-middle-income countries	16.8	2.2	
High-income countries	26.3	1.5	
All countries combined	**20.3**	**1.0**	

*Significant at the 0.05 level, two-sided test.

[a] Wald design-corrected F-tests were used to determine if there is variation in treatment estimates across country income groups. The denominator degree of freedom, v, is 5331.

[b] The mental health specialist sector, which includes psychiatrist and non-psychiatrist mental health specialists (psychiatrist, psychologist, or other non-psychiatrist mental health professional; social worker or counsellor in a mental health specialty setting; use of a mental health helpline; or overnight admissions for a mental health or drug or alcohol problems, with a presumption of daily contact with a psychiatrist).

[c] The general medical sector (general practitioner, other medical doctor, nurse, occupational therapist, or any healthcare professional).

[d] The mental health specialist sector or the general medical sector.

[e] The human services sector (religious or spiritual advisor or social worker or counsellor in any setting other than a specialty mental health setting).

[f] The CAM (complementary and alternative medicine) sector (any other type of healer such as herbalist or homeopath, participation in an internet support group, or participation in a self-help group).

[g] The human services sector or CAM.

[h] Any treatment listed above.

complementary and alternative medicine (CAM) sector. This is notable as the CAM sector includes self-help groups including Alcoholics Anonymous and other 12-step programmes, which are often assumed to be major interventions for AUDs in at least some countries. In addition, at all country income levels, a higher proportion of 12-month AUD respondents seek treatment in the more resource intensive health care sector than the less costly non-health care sector. Across all treatment sectors, country income level is positively associated with the percentage seeking treatment with about 2–4 times as many respondents in high-income countries reporting treatment in each of the treatment sectors compared to those in low/lower-middle-income countries. It is likely that some 12-month AUD respondents had received treatment at some previous point longer ago than the prior year. However, this would mean that these respondents had relapsed.

Discussion

The average lifetime prevalence of AUDs in all countries combined was 8.6% ranging from 0.7% in Iraq to 22.7% in Australia. This is a high level of disorder prevalence especially considering the high level of health and economic burden associated with AUDs. The combined average 12-month AUD prevalence was 2.2% ranging from 0.1% in Iraq to 5.9% in the Ukraine while the average 30-day prevalence of AUDs was 0.9% ranging from 0.1% in Iraq, Italy, and Japan to 2.9% in the Ukraine. This wide range of AUD prevalences is what would be expected based on findings from other country and regional studies (e.g. Cochrane *et al.* 2003; Mathers & Ayuso-Mateos 2003; Lukassen, & Beaudet 2005; Rehm *et al.* 2005; Wittchen & Jacobi 2005; Hasin *et al.* 2007; Pan American Health Organization 2007; Chen & Yin 2008) and the range found in the WMH surveys overlaps with those estimates.

Despite the range of prevalences, the WMH results confirm a number of well-documented clinical and epidemiological findings. AUD prevalences are much higher for men than women. Risk for onset of AUD begins in adolescence with half of all lifetime cases beginning by age 23, although new onsets continue through later life. Being married and more educated is associated with lower risk for AUD. Comorbidity with other mental disorders is common and despite the harms and impairments associated with AUDs, there is a low prevalence of treatment. The consistency of these patterns across countries despite the varying socio-cultural environments provides an informative perspective on the nature of AUDs.

The AUD prevalences found in the WMH surveys vary widely but they reflect the varying extent and burden of AUDs in the different countries. If AUDs were considered only for people who had consumed at least some alcohol, it is possible that the range of prevalences would be reduced (Rehm *et al.* 2003). Future WMH analyses will compare population AUD prevalences with AUDs among drinkers and examine possible differences in the patterns and associations.

There were significant differences in AUD prevalences across the WHO Regions. The Eastern Mediterranean region, which has the lowest per capita alcohol consumption and lowest proportion of drinkers, had the lowest AUD prevalences. It seems reasonable to assume that low consumption and high abstention are limiting factors on the development of AUDs. However, this effect may exert more influence at lower levels of alcohol consumption. For example, while the annual per capita alcohol consumption of both France and Australia is 12.2 litres of pure alcohol, which is a relatively high level, the lifetime prevalence of AUDs is 7.1% for France and 22.7% for Australia. While there may be a number of contributors to this difference, one possible factor might be a difference in the prevalence of heavy episodic or binge drinking which may have relatively more severe consequences and association with AUDs than more temperate patterns (Rehm *et al.* 2003). France has been shown to have the lowest level of binge drinking in Europe (Leifman 2002) while Australia has comparatively high rates (Toumbourou *et al.* 2005; Yang, Zhao & Srivastava 2016). Unfortunately, there are some indications that higher risk patterns of drinking are becoming more common among young people in Europe (Hibell *et al.* 2000). When considering environmental influences on AUDs it should be noted that AUD is approximately 50% heritable (Verhulst *et al.* 2015) although environmental influences are important moderators of genetic effects (Dick & Kendler 2012).

It is important to note the limitations of the WMH survey findings. Given that 26 countries participated in the WMH surveys, there is not full representation of all regions, income levels and other country characteristics. There was variation in response rates across countries and possibly cross-national differences in willingness to disclose personal information about alcohol use and problems. Respondent information is subject to the limitations of recall inherent in retrospective reporting. The WMH Surveys Initiative is based on household surveys, and therefore the homeless, people in jails, prisons, hospitals, homeless shelters, halfway houses and sober living group homes, SUD inpatient treatment facilities, or living on military bases were not part of the sampling frame. Within the context of these limitations, the WMH results provide new and useful data about the prevalences and associations of AUDs across countries.

The concept and diagnostic criteria for AUDs were significantly revised in the DSM-5 (American Psychiatric Association 2013). The distinction between abuse and dependence was removed, conceptualizing AUD as a single disorder. The legal problems symptom criteria was removed and a craving criteria was added. Lastly, DSM-5 uses numbers of symptom criteria to distinguish three levels of AUD severity. The WMH surveys assessed the symptoms required for AUD diagnoses according to both DSM-IV and DSM-5 classifications. Comparison of DSM-IV and DSM-5 diagnoses in the WMH surveys found that while the lifetime prevalences of AUD were similar when using the two systems, a large number of people were not consistently identified by both classifications (Slade *et al.* 2016).

Although further work is needed, the WMH findings on AUDs provide important information and demonstrate not only the feasibility but the benefits of studying AUDs in a cross-national programme of research.

Acknowledgements

The views and opinions expressed in this publication are those of the authors only and do not necessarily represent the views, official policy, or position of the US Department of Health and Human Services or any of its affiliated institutions or agencies. Dr. Glantz's role on this study is through his involvement as a Science Officer on U01-MH60220. He had no involvement in the other cited grants.

References

Adlaf, E. M., Begin, P., & Sawka, E. (2005). *Canadian Addiction Survey (CAS): A National Survey of Canadians' Use of Alcohol and Other Drugs: Prevalence of Use and Related Harms: Detailed Report*. Ottawa: Canadian Centre on Substance Abuse.

Alonso, J., Petukhova, M., Vilagut, G., *et al.* (2011). Days out of role due to common physical and mental conditions: results from the WHO World Mental Health surveys. *Molecular Psychiatry*, 16(12), 1234–46.

American Psychiatric Association (1980). *Diagnostic and Statistical Manual, 3rd ed. (DSM-III)*. Washington, DC: American Psychiatric Association.

(2000). *Diagnostic and Statistical Manual of Mental Disorders, 4th ed. (text revision) (DSM-IV-TR)*. Washington, DC: American Psychiatric Association.

(2013). *Diagnostic and Statistical Manual of Mental Disorders, 5th ed. (DSM-5)*. Washington, DC: American Psychiatric Association.

Andrews, G., Henderson, S., & Hall, W. (2001). Prevalence, comorbidity, disability and service utilization. Overview of the Australian National Mental Health Survey. *The British Journal of Psychiatry*, 178(2), 145–53.

Babor, T. F., & Caetano, R. (2008). The trouble with alcohol abuse: what are we trying to measure, diagnose, count and prevent? *Addiction*, 103(7), 1057–9.

Chen, C. C., & Yin, S. J. (2008). Alcohol abuse and related factors in Asia. *International Review of Psychiatry*, 20(5), 425–33.

Cochrane, J., Chen, H., Conigrave, K. M., *et al.* (2003). W. Alcohol use in China. *Alcohol and Alcoholism*, 38(6), 537–42.

Degenhardt, L., Chiu, W. T., Sampson, N., *et al.* (2008). Toward a global view of alcohol, tobacco, cannabis, and cocaine use: findings from the WHO World Mental Health Surveys. *PLoS Medicine*, 5(7), e141.

Degenhardt, L., Whiteford, H. A., Ferrari, A. J., *et al.* (2013). Global burden of disease attributable to illicit drug use and dependence: findings from the Global Burden of Disease Study 2010. *The Lancet*, 382(9904), 1564–74.

Dick, D. M., & Kendler, K. S. (2012). The impact of gene–environment interaction on alcohol use disorders. *Alcohol Research: Current Reviews*, 34(3), 318.

Glantz, M. D., & Leshner, A. I. (2000). Drug abuse and developmental psychopathology. *Development and Psychopathology*, 12(04), 795–814.

Glantz, M. D., Medina-Mora, M. E., Petukhova, M., *et al.* (2014). Alcohol abuse in developed and developing countries in the World Mental Health surveys: socially defined consequences or psychiatric disorder? *The American Journal on Addictions*, 23(2), 145–55.

Hasin, D. S., Stinson, F. S., Ogburn, E., *et al.* (2007). Prevalence, correlates, disability, and comorbidity of DSM-IV alcohol abuse and dependence in the United States: results from the National Epidemiologic Survey on Alcohol and Related Conditions. *Archives of General Psychiatry*, 64(7), 830–42.

Helzer, J. E., & Canino, G. J. (1992). *Alcoholism in North America, Europe, and Asia*. New York: Oxford University Press.

Hibell, B., Andersson, B., Ahlström, S., *et al.* (2000). The 1999 ESPAD Report. *Alcohol and Other Drug Use among Students in 30 European Countries*. Stockholm: Pompidou Group, Council of Europe.

Jenkins, R., Bebbington, P., Brugha, T., *et al.* (1997) The national psychiatric morbidity surveys of Great Britain – initial findings from the household survey. *Psychological Medicine*, 27, 775–89.
Kessler, R. C., Ormel, J., Petukhova, M., *et al.* (2011). Development of lifetime comorbidity in the WHO World Mental Health (WMH) surveys. *Archives of General Psychiatry*, 68(1), 90–100.
Keyes, K. M., Grant, B. F., & Hasin, D. S. (2008). Evidence for a closing gender gap in alcohol use, abuse, and dependence in the United States population. *Drug and Alcohol Dependence*, 93(1), 21–9.
Keyes, K. M., & Hasin, D. S. (2008). Socio-economic status and problem alcohol use: the positive relationship between income and the DSM-IV alcohol abuse diagnosis. *Addiction*, 103(7), 1120–30.
Lago, L., Glantz, M., Kessler, R., *et al.* (2017). Substance dependence among those without symptoms of substance abuse in the World Mental Health Survey. *International Journal of Methods in Psychiatric Research*, e1557.
Lai, H. M. X., Cleary, M., Sitharthan, T., *et al.* (2015). Prevalence of comorbid substance use, anxiety and mood disorders in epidemiological surveys, 1990–2014: a systematic review and meta-analysis. *Drug and Alcohol Dependence*, 154, 1–13.
Leifman, H. (2002). A comparative analysis of drinking patterns in six EU countries in the year 2000. *Contemporary Drug Problems*, 29(3), 501–48.
Leon, A. C., Olfson, M., Portera, L., *et al.* (1997). Assessing psychiatric impairment in primary care with the Sheehan disability scale. *International Journal of Psychiatry in Medicine*, 27, 93–105.
Lukassen, J., & Beaudet, M. P. (2005). Alcohol dependence and depression among heavy drinkers in Canada. *Social Science and Medicine*, 61(8), 1658–67.
Mathers, C. D., & Ayuso-Mateos, J. L. (2003). *Global Burden of Alcohol Use Disorders in the Year 2000: Summary of Methods and Data Sources*. Geneva: World Health Organization, www.who.int/healthinfo/statistics/bod_alcohol.pdf (accessed 25 December 2016).
Medina-Mora, M., Villatoro, J., Caraveo, J., *et al.* (2001). Patterns of alcohol consumption and related problems in Mexico: results from two general population surveys. *Surveys of Drinking Patterns and Problems in Seven Developing Countries*. Geneva: World Health Organization, 14–31.
Merikangas, K. R., Mehta, R. L., Molnar, B. E., *et al.* (1998). Comorbidity of substance use disorders with mood and anxiety disorders: results of the International Consortium in Psychiatric Epidemiology. *Addictive Behaviors*, 23(6), 893–907.
Pan American Health Organization (2007). *Alcohol, Gender, Culture and Harms in the Americas: PAHO Multicentric Study Final Report*. Washington, DC: OPS.
Pani, P. P., Maremmani, I., Trogu, E., *et al.* (2010). Delineating the psychic structure of substance abuse and addictions: should anxiety, mood and impulse-control dysregulation be included? *Journal of Affective Disorders*, 122(3), 185–97.
Rehm, J., Mathers, C., Popova, S., *et al.* (2009). Global burden of disease and injury and economic cost attributable to alcohol use and alcohol-use disorders. *The Lancet*, 373(9682), 2223–33.
Rehm, J. U. R., Rehn, N., Room, R., *et al.* (2003). The global distribution of average volume of alcohol consumption and patterns of drinking. *European Addiction Research*, 9(4), 147–56.
Rehm, J., Room, R., van den Brink, W., *et al.* (2005). Alcohol use disorders in EU countries and Norway: an overview of the epidemiology. *European Neuropsychopharmacology*, 15(4), 377–88.
Rehm, J., & Shield, K. D. (2013). Alcohol and mortality: global alcohol-attributable deaths from cancer, liver cirrhosis, and injury in 2010. *Alcohol Research*, 35, 174–83.
Robins, L. N., Helzer, J. E., Croughan, J. L., *et al.* (1981). National Institute of Mental Health Diagnostic Interview Schedule: its history, characteristics and validity. *Archives of General Psychiatry*, 38, 381–9.
Room, R. (2006). Taking account of cultural and societal influences on substance use diagnoses and criteria. *Addiction*, 101(s1), 31–9.
Rounsaville, B. J. (2002). Experience with ICD-10/DSM-IV substance use disorders. *Psychopathology*, 35(2–3), 82–88.
Rounsaville, B. J., Spitzer, R. L., & Williams, J. B. (1986). Proposed changes in DSM-III substance use disorders: description and rationale. *American Journal of Psychiatry*, 143, 463–8.
Sher, K. J., Wolf, S. T., & Martinez, J. A. (2009). How can etiological research inform the distinction between normal drinking and disordered drinking. *Handbook of Drug Use Etiology*, 225–46.
Slade, T., Chiu, W. T., Glantz, M., *et al.* (2016). A cross-national examination of differences in classification of lifetime alcohol use disorder between DSM-IV and DSM-5: findings from the World Mental Health Survey. *Alcoholism: Clinical and Experimental Research*, 40(8), 1728–36.
Stinson, F. S., Grant, B. F., Dawson, D. A., *et al.* (2005). Comorbidity between DSM-IV alcohol and specific drug use disorders in the United States: results from the National Epidemiologic Survey on alcohol and related conditions. *Drug and Alcohol Dependence*, 80(1), 105–16.
Toumbourou, J. W., Beyers, J. M., Catalano, R. F., *et al.* (2005). Youth alcohol and other drug use in the United States and Australia: a cross-national comparison of three state-wide samples. *Drug and Alcohol Review*, 24(6), 515–23.
Verhulst, B., Neale, M. C., & Kendler, K. S. (2015). The heritability of alcohol use disorders: a meta-analysis

of twin and adoption studies. *Psychological Medicine*, 45(5), 1061–72.
Wittchen, H. U., & Jacobi, F. (2005). Size and burden of mental disorders in Europe – a critical review and appraisal of 27 studies. *European Neuropsychopharmacology*, 15(4), 357–76.
World Bank Group (Ed.). (2012). *World Development Indicators 2012*. Washington: World Bank Publications.
World Health Organization (2014). *Global Status Report on Alcohol and Health*. Geneva: World Health Organization.
Yang, O., Zhao, X., & Srivastava, P. (2016). Binge drinking and antisocial and unlawful behaviours in Australia. *Economic Record*, 92(297), 222–40.

Chapter 17

Drug-Use Disorders

Louisa Degenhardt, Yolanda Torres, Hristo Hinkov, Margreet ten Have, Meyer D. Glantz

Introduction

Illicit drugs are those whose extra-medical use has been prohibited under international and national control systems. They include (but are not limited to) heroin, cannabis, amphetamines, and cocaine. A range of pharmaceutical drugs that are strictly controlled may also be used outside the bounds of a doctor's prescription, including opioids and benzodiazepines.

The illicit use of drugs has been documented in many countries, but large gaps remain in our knowledge of the extent of the use of these drugs, and especially the extent of problem or dependent use (UNODC 2015). The problematic use of illicit drugs is associated with considerable mortality and morbidity, of which drug-use disorder (DUD) is one potential consequence. DUDs can cause considerable harm to the individual, the community, and have important implications for public health and social policy (Greater London Alcohol and Drug Alliance 2004; United Nations Office on Drugs and Crime 2008, 2009).

The *Diagnostic and Statistical Manual* DSM-IV-TR (American Psychiatric Association 2000) distinguishes two categories of DUDs, drug abuse (DRA) and drug dependence (DRD). Both diagnoses are defined as maladaptive patterns of drug use leading to clinically significant impairment or distress. DRA is defined as recurrent or continued drug use despite one or more of the following occurring within a 12-month period: drug use resulting in a failure to fulfil major role obligations at work, school, or home; drug use in situations in which it is physically hazardous; drug use-related legal problems; drug use despite having persistent or recurrent social or interpersonal problems caused or exacerbated by the effects of drug use.

DRD is defined as a cluster of three or more of the following symptoms occurring at any time in the same 12-month period: tolerance; withdrawal; drug use in larger amounts or over a longer period than intended; persistent desire or unsuccessful efforts to cut down or control drug use; a great deal of time spent on activities necessary to obtain drugs, use drugs, or use to recover from their effects; important social, occupational, or recreational activities are given up or reduced because of drug use; continued drug use despite knowledge of having a persistent or recurrent physical or psychological problem that is likely to have been caused or exacerbated by drug use.

Illicit drug use and associated disease burden are estimated to have increased over the past few decades (Degenhardt & Hall 2012; Degenhardt *et al.* 2013, 2016b). The Global Burden of Disease (GBD) study has estimated that there have been significant increases in the number of people with DUDs since 1990, with the modelled prevalence varying dramatically across substances and countries. Yet certainty around these modelled estimates is limited by the fact that there are substantial gaps in existing data.

The World Drug Report (WDR), which is produced annually by the United Nations Office on Drugs and Crime (UNODC), is an annual global review of drug use, seizures, trafficking and cultivation of illicit drugs (UNODC 2015). The WDR relies on each member state completing an Annual Reports Questionnaire, and depends upon a wide range of data of varying quality. In many cases, the evidence on which these estimates are based is not reported by member states. There are large gaps in reporting, particularly in Africa, Asia, and Oceania.

A review of published data on illicit drug use and dependence found that although illicit drug use had been identified in most countries around the globe, data on the prevalence of illicit drug use and dependence was patchy and variable in quality and methods used to derive the estimates (Degenhardt *et al.* 2011a), making it difficult to directly compare estimates. Most data involving representative samples of adults came from studies in single countries or regions within countries (Degenhardt *et al.* 2011a).

The World Mental Health (WMH) Surveys Initiative standardizes methodological factors, which facilitates the cross-national comparison of the prevalence and associated factors of DUDs in a large number of participating countries. This makes it almost uniquely able to address certain questions and controversies about DUDs.

As was discussed in greater detail in Chapter 16 on alcohol-use disorders (AUDs), there are two concerns related to cross-national comparisons of DUDs. The first relates to the psychiatric significance and consistency of the symptoms across countries, particularly for DRA, whose criteria focus in large part upon consequences of substance use that are affected by social, legal, and societal responses to substance use rather than being an inherent consequence of use (Rounsaville *et al.* 1986; Babor & Caetano 2008; Sher *et al.* 2009). In the context of the WMH surveys, variations in prevalence across countries could be a reflection of these variations in responses to use.

The second issue is that environmental and social factors that increase (or decrease) risks for drug use may vary across countries, affecting the prevalence of DUDs. These include drug availability, cost, social tolerance, and social consequences for drug use, legal sanctions and enforcement, and the contexts of drug use and ways in which drugs are taken that may affect risk of developing problematic use (e.g., via injection versus smoked). It is likely that these factors account for some of the cross-national variation in prevalence of DUDs, but it is difficult to know which, if any, might have affected the development and prevalence of DUDs. They also do not discount the importance of the condition once it has developed within an individual. The WMH data provide an opportunity to compare the cross-national prevalence of DRA and DRD and consider the consistencies of patterns of associations of DUDs and correlates.

Methods

DUDs were assessed in 26/29 of the WMH surveys included in this volume (the three exclusions were Shenzhen and Portugal which did not assess these disorders, and Romania, which did assess DUD but had too few cases for it to be included in this chapter). See Table 17.2 for country listing. As described in Chapter 3, the WHO Composite International Diagnostic Interview (CIDI) interview was divided into two parts. Part I assessed lifetime presence of core mental disorders. Respondents in Australia, Belgium, Brazil (São Paulo), Bulgaria, Colombia (urban areas), France, Germany, Italy, Lebanon, Mexico (urban areas), New Zealand, Nigeria, Peru, PRC Beijing/Shanghai, Spain, the Netherlands, and Ukraine were administered the AUD and DUD assessment as part of their Part I interview. Respondents in Colombia (Medellin), Japan, Northern Ireland, Poland, Spain (Murcia), and the United States were administered a version of Part I that assessed lifetime presence of core mental disorders and a screen for substance-use disorders (SUDs, i.e., AUDs and/or DUDs). In these countries the full assessments for SUDs were included in Part II of the interview. All respondents who met criteria for any of the core mental disorders or the screen for SUDs were administered Part II as were a weighted probability subsample of approximately 25% of other Part I respondents who did not meet criteria for any core disorder or the SUD screen. All participants in Iraq, Israel, Romania, and South Africa were administered both parts of the interview. Combining participants from all 26 surveys, of the 133,926 respondents who completed Part I, 72,810 completed Part II and 87,977 comprised the weighted subsample assessed for DUDs and described here. Not all of the 87,977 respondents who were fully assessed for DUDs were assessed for all of the correlates discussed here as some correlates were assessed in Part II.

Within the CIDI drug use section used in the earliest 13 WMH surveys (Colombia, Nigeria, Peru, PRC Beijing/Shanghai, Ukraine, Bulgaria, Lebanon, Mexico, South Africa, Japan, Israel, New Zealand, and the United States), if a respondent did not endorse any of the drug-abuse criteria, they were not asked questions related to DRD. Although symptoms of abuse often preempt dependence, it is possible for dependence to occur without prior symptoms of abuse. In order to evaluate the prevalence of such cases, the skip logic was revised for later WMH surveys to assess DRD among respondents who had not endorsed any symptoms of abuse. For the purpose of improving cross-national comparability of survey data collected before and after this revision to the CIDI, regression-based imputation models were developed and validated from random half-samples of the new WMH surveys and applied to the earlier WMH surveys. This imputation adjusted for the absence of information relating to DRD without abuse in the 13 earlier WMH surveys and allows for improved estimates of lifetime dependence prevalence. Further details of the methodology are described elsewhere (Lago *et al.* 2017).

The interview included a series of 16 questions that operationalize the DSM-IV symptom criteria for DRA and DRD. Respondents met criteria for diagnosis of

DRA by endorsing at least one of the four abuse symptoms and met criteria for diagnosis of DRD by endorsing at least three of the seven dependence symptoms. Respondents who met criteria for either DRA or DRD were considered to have a DUD. The DSM-IV hierarchy rule was followed so that respondents could not be diagnosed with both DRA and DRD and any respondents who met criteria for both DUD disorders were diagnosed as DRD. The 12-month and 30-day prevalence of DRA or DRD was defined as respondents having reported symptoms of the specific DUD in the associated timeframe. For respondents diagnosed with both DUD and for whom the hierarchy rule was employed, only symptoms of the hierarchical disorder, DRD, were considered in determining 12-month and 30-day prevalence.

Regional adaptions to the source instrument meant the type of drugs assessed in the illicit drug-use section varied considerably between WMH surveys. A selection of drugs was assessed universally, including cannabis, cocaine, and prescription drugs. The category of prescription drugs was considered either as a singular broad category or as a combination of questions relating to sedatives, stimulants, and analgesics/painkillers; the illegal use of which was defined as having used without the recommendation of a health professional or for any reason other than a health professional said they should be used. All other drugs considered by each survey are summarized in Table 17.1. Most surveys assessed DRA and DRD at the general illicit drug level, with only Australia, New Zealand, and Poland having asked diagnosis questions at the drug-specific level. To increase cross-national comparability, a DUD was assigned if the appropriate criteria were met either for a specific drug or a combination of drugs.

Results

Prevalence

The prevalence of DRA, DRD, and DUDs is shown in Tables 17.2–17.4 for individual countries, country income groups and WHO regions. There are significant differences in lifetime, 12-month, and 30-day DRA, DRD, and DUD prevalence across countries and regions. The average lifetime prevalence of DRA in all countries combined is 2.2%, ranging from 0.1% in Iraq to 4.9% in the United States (Table 17.2). DRA lifetime prevalence shows a clear gradient of increasing prevalence with increasing country income level, ranging from 0.6% in the low/lower-middle-income countries to 3.0% in the high-income countries. The average 12-month prevalence of DRA for all countries is 0.4%, ranging from <0.1% in Japan, Spain (Murcia), Peru, Lebanon, and Bulgaria, to 1.3% in South Africa. The average 30-day prevalence of DRA for all countries is 0.1%, with multiple countries having no cases of DRA in the past month, ranging up to 0.3% in Northern Ireland and Colombia (Medellin).

As would be expected with a more severe disorder, the rates of DRD are lower than the rates of DRA. The average lifetime prevalence of DRD in all countries combined is 1.2%, ranging from <0.1% in Iraq, Nigeria, PRC, and Japan, to 3.5% in the United States (Table 17.3). As observed for DRA, DRD lifetime prevalence is significantly higher among higher-income countries, increasing from 0.3% in low/lower-middle-income countries to 1.7% in high-income countries. The average 12-month prevalence of DRD for all countries is 0.3%. The highest levels of 12-month DRD are in New Zealand

Table 17.1 Drugs assessed in the World Mental Health Surveys

Survey	Cannabis	Cocaine	Prescription drugs	Other drugs assessed
Australia	✓	✓	✓	amphetamine, methamphetamine, speed, ice, base, ecstasy, heroin, opium, peyote
Poland[a]	✓	✓	✓	club drugs, hallucinogens, opioids, inhalants/solvents
Ukraine	✓	✓	✓	heroin, shirka, LSD, ecstasy
ESEMeD[b]	✓	✓	✓	heroin, opium, ecstasy, inhalants, hallucinogens
Israel[c]	✓	✓	✓	LSD, ecstasy, glue, heroin, opium, methadone
All others	✓	✓	✓	heroin, opium, glue, LSD, peyote

[a]Poland also gave respondents the opportunity to volunteer the name of any other illegal drug they had used, if not already listed.
[b]The ESEMeD surveys are: Belgium, France, Italy, Spain, Netherlands, and Germany.
[c]Use of kaat and datura was assessed, however, DUD questions were not asked in relation to these drugs.

Table 17.2 Prevalence of DSM-IV drug abuse (DRA) in the World Mental Health surveys

Country	Lifetime prevalence		12-month prevalence		30-day prevalence		12-month prevalence of DRA among lifetime cases		30-day prevalence of DRA among 12-month cases		Sample size used
	%	SE	%	SE	%	SE	%	SE	%	SE	
Low/lower-middle-income countries	**0.6**	**0.1**	**0.1**	**0.0**	**<0.1**	**0.0**	**23.4**	**5.3**	**29.7**	**10.5**	**18,179**
Colombia	0.9	0.2	0.2	0.1	0.1	0.1	26.0	8.2	37.3	17.7	4,426
Iraq	0.1	0.1	0.1	0.1	<0.1	0.0	85.0	16.3	18.0	20.3	4,332
Nigeria	1.0	0.2	0.2	0.1	0.1	0.1	23.4	9.4	38.3	21.0	2,143
Peru	0.8	0.1	<0.1	0.0	<0.1	0.0	6.1	5.3	20.0	22.6	3,930
PRC (Beijing/Shanghai)	0.4	0.2	0.1	0.0	<0.1	0.0	12.6	9.4	81.8	16.3	1,628
Ukraine	0.4	0.2	0.2	0.2	–	–	40.4	27.4	–	–	1,720
Upper-middle-income countries	**1.7**	**0.1**	**0.4**	**0.1**	**0.1**	**0.0**	**26.5**	**2.9**	**21.7**	**6.0**	**20,071**
Brazil	1.5	0.2	0.3	0.1	0.1	0.1	17.4	5.2	30.0	16.8	5,037
Bulgaria	0.2	0.1	<0.1	0.0	–	–	2.9	3.2	–	–	2,233
Colombia (Medellin)	3.4	0.5	0.5	0.2	0.3	0.1	16.0	4.8	49.9	15.4	1,673
Lebanon	0.3	0.3	<0.1	0.0	–	–	6.7	8.3	–	–	1,031
Mexico	0.9	0.2	0.2	0.1	<0.1	0.0	23.4	6.6	20.3	11.7	5,782
South Africa	3.4	0.3	1.3	0.2	0.2	0.1	37.5	5.1	15.5	7.9	4,315
High-income countries	**3.0**	**0.1**	**0.5**	**0.0**	**0.2**	**0.0**	**15.9**	**1.1**	**31.9**	**3.5**	**49,727**
Australia	4.6	0.2	0.7	0.1	0.2	0.1	14.1	1.8	38.3	7.7	8,463
Belgium	3.4	0.7	1.0	0.5	0.1	0.1	30.0	12.6	7.9	7.1	1,043
France	2.6	0.3	0.4	0.1	0.2	0.1	17.0	3.1	37.5	16.1	1,436
Germany	2.4	0.5	0.2	0.2	<0.1	0.0	10.0	6.1	10.9	11.9	1,323
Israel	1.4	0.2	0.3	0.1	0.1	0.0	18.6	4.8	32.9	12.9	4,859
Italy	2.1	0.4	0.2	0.1	0.1	0.0	11.7	5.8	28.1	18.5	1,779
Japan	0.2	0.1	<0.1	0.0	–	–	9.2	8.3	–	–	1,682
New Zealand	3.1	0.2	0.6	0.1	0.1	0.0	17.7	2.3	26.4	6.8	12,790
Northern Ireland	2.7	0.4	0.3	0.2	0.3	0.2	12.7	5.5	77.1	14.3	1,986
Poland	1.2	0.2	0.1	0.1	0.1	0.0	11.9	5.0	68.3	21.0	4,000
Spain	3.8	0.5	0.8	0.3	0.2	0.1	21.3	7.7	29.1	13.2	2,121
Spain (Murcia)	2.4	0.7	<0.1	0.0	–	–	0.8	0.7	–	–	1,459
Netherlands	1.0	0.3	0.1	0.1	0.1	0.1	10.9	7.6	60.2	29.8	1,094
United States	4.9	0.3	0.8	0.1	0.2	0.1	16.6	1.9	28.7	6.1	5,692

Table 17.2 (*cont.*)

Country	Lifetime prevalence		12-month prevalence		30-day prevalence		12-month prevalence of DRA among lifetime cases		30-day prevalence of DRA among 12-month cases		Sample size used
	%	SE	%	SE	%	SE	%	SE	%	SE	
All countries combined	**2.2**	**0.1**	**0.4**	**0.0**	**0.1**	**0.0**	**18.2**	**1.0**	**29.2**	**2.9**	**87,977**
WHO regions[a]											
Region of the Americas	2.0	0.1	0.3	0.0	0.1	0.0	17.4	1.7	30.6	5.0	26,540
African region	2.6	0.2	0.9	0.1	0.2	0.1	35.7	4.6	17.5	7.5	6,458
Western Pacific region	3.3	0.1	0.5	0.1	0.2	0.0	15.9	1.5	31.9	5.1	24,563
Eastern Mediterranean region	0.8	0.1	0.2	0.1	<0.1	0.0	23.4	6.0	28.1	11.6	10,222
Western European region	2.6	0.2	0.4	0.1	0.1	0.0	15.5	2.9	31.6	8.0	12,241
Eastern European region	0.7	0.1	0.1	0.0	<0.1	0.0	14.8	5.9	44.4	20.2	7,953
Comparison between countries[b]	$F_{25,v} = 34.9^*$, $P < 0.001$		$F_{25,v} = 9.7^*$, $P < 0.001$		$F_{25,v} = 3.9^*$, $P < 0.001$		$F_{25,v} = 1.6^*$, $P = 0.023$		$F_{25,v} = 0.9$, $P = 0.662$		
Comparison between low-, middle-, and high-income country groups[b]	$F_{2,v} = 225.3^*$, $P < 0.001$		$F_{2,v} = 22.7^*$, $P < 0.001$		$F_{2,v} = 10.8^*$, $P < 0.001$		$F_{2,v} = 6.5^*$, $P = 0.001$		$F_{2,v} = 1.0$, $P = 0.356$		
Comparison between WHO regions[b]	$F_{5,v} = 69.9^*$, $P < 0.001$		$F_{5,v} = 12.1^*$, $P < 0.001$		$F_{5,v} = 3.4^*$, $P = 0.004$		$F_{5,v} = 3.5^*$, $P = 0.003$		$F_{5,v} = 0.7$, $P = 0.648$		

*Significant at the 0.05 level, two-sided test.
A dash indicates low cell count (<5 cases).
[a]**Region of the Americas** (Colombia, Mexico, Brazil, Peru, United States, Colombia (Medellin)); **African region** (South Africa, Nigeria); **Western Pacific region** (PRC: Beijing and Shanghai, Japan, Australia, New Zealand); **Eastern Mediterranean region** (Israel, Iraq, Lebanon); **Western European region** (Belgium, France, Germany, Italy, Netherlands, Spain, Northern Ireland, Spain (Murcia)); **Eastern European region** (Poland, Bulgaria, Ukraine).
[b]Wald design-corrected F-tests were used to determine if there is variation in prevalence estimates across countries. The denominator degree of freedom, v, is 5269.
PRC: People's Republic of China.

Table 17.3 Prevalence of DSM-IV drug dependence (DRD) in the World Mental Health surveys

Country	Lifetime prevalence		12-month prevalence		30-day prevalence		12-month prevalence of DRD among lifetime cases		30-day prevalence of DRD among 12-month cases		Sample size used
	%	SE	%	SE	%	SE	%	SE	%	SE	
Low/lower-middle-income countries	**0.3**	**0.0**	**0.1**	**0.0**	**0.1**	**0.0**	**34.2**	**6.4**	**53.9**	**15.1**	**18,179**
Colombia	0.8	0.2	0.2	0.1	0.1	0.1	30.2	7.1	56.9	22.2	4,426
Iraq	<0.1	0.0	–	–	–	–	–	–	–	–	4,332
Nigeria	<0.1	0.0	–	–	–	–	–	–	–	–	2,143
Peru	0.3	0.1	0.1	0.1	0.1	0.1	51.4	19.7	66.1	24.4	3,930
PRC (Beijing/Shanghai)	<0.1	0.0	–	–	–	–	–	–	–	–	1,628
Ukraine	0.6	0.2	0.2	0.1	<0.1	0.0	32.9	12.9	21.7	16.6	1,720
Upper-middle-income countries	**0.8**	**0.1**	**0.2**	**0.0**	**0.1**	**0.0**	**30.9**	**4.1**	**49.1**	**9.4**	**20,071**
Brazil	1.4	0.3	0.5	0.1	0.3	0.1	37.6	6.3	55.6	14.5	5,037
Bulgaria	–	–	–	–	–	–	–	–	–	–	2,233
Colombia (Medellin)	1.9	0.4	0.5	0.2	0.2	0.1	26.4	8.2	41.9	17.4	1,673
Lebanon	0.1	0.1	0.1	0.1	0.1	0.1	100.0	0.0	53.4	30.5	1,031
Mexico	0.5	0.1	0.1	0.0	<0.1	0.0	23.0	9.9	32.2	17.9	5,782
South Africa	0.6	0.2	0.1	0.1	0.1	0.0	23.1	8.4	48.0	22.2	4,315
High-income countries	**1.7**	**0.1**	**0.5**	**0.0**	**0.2**	**0.0**	**26.0**	**2.0**	**39.4**	**4.1**	**49,727**
Australia	2.9	0.3	0.7	0.1	0.2	0.1	23.1	4.0	29.9	7.1	8,463
Belgium	1.1	0.6	0.7	0.5	0.7	0.5	63.4	13.8	100.0	0.0	1,043
France	0.9	0.3	0.4	0.2	0.2	0.1	39.9	18.1	53.5	23.3	1,436
Germany	0.5	0.3	0.3	0.3	0.1	0.0	69.3	18.6	24.8	20.9	1,323
Israel	0.3	0.1	0.1	0.0	<0.1	0.0	22.1	11.4	24.4	22.6	4,859
Italy	0.4	0.1	0.1	0.1	<0.1	0.0	30.2	11.7	33.8	20.5	1,779
Japan	<0.1	0.0	<0.1	0.0	–	–	39.0	33.6	–	–	1,682
New Zealand	2.5	0.2	0.8	0.1	0.4	0.1	33.2	3.5	43.1	6.4	12,790
Northern Ireland	0.6	0.2	0.2	0.1	<0.1	0.0	34.9	13.9	18.4	13.6	1,986

Table 17.3 ***(cont.)***

Country	Lifetime prevalence		12-month prevalence		30-day prevalence		12-month prevalence of DRD among lifetime cases		30-day prevalence of DRD among 12-month cases		Sample size used
	%	SE	%	SE	%	SE	%	SE	%	SE	
Poland	0.2	0.1	0.2	0.1	0.1	0.0	69.0	13.0	37.1	20.5	4,000
Spain	0.3	0.1	<0.1	0.0	<0.1	0.0	2.6	2.7	100.0	0.0	2,121
Spain (Murcia)	1.2	0.4	0.1	0.1	–	–	7.6	6.3	–	–	1,459
Netherlands	1.1	0.6	0.1	0.0	<0.1	0.0	5.7	4.2	28.3	25.6	1,094
United States	3.5	0.2	0.5	0.1	0.2	0.1	14.8	2.6	37.2	8.2	5,692
All countries combined	**1.2**	**0.1**	**0.3**	**0.0**	**0.1**	**0.0**	**27.2**	**1.7**	**42.0**	**3.7**	**87,977**
WHO regions[a]											
Region of the Americas	1.4	0.1	0.3	0.0	0.2	0.0	23.2	2.4	47.2	6.8	26,540
African region	0.4	0.1	0.1	0.0	<0.1	0.0	22.8	8.3	48.0	22.2	6,458
Western Pacific region	2.3	0.1	0.7	0.1	0.3	0.0	28.8	2.7	38.4	4.9	24,563
Eastern Mediterranean region	0.2	0.0	<0.1	0.0	<0.1	0.0	28.5	10.8	33.6	19.0	10,222
Western European region	0.7	0.1	0.2	0.1	0.1	0.0	29.6	7.0	50.6	14.1	12,241
Eastern European region	0.2	0.1	0.1	0.0	<0.1	0.0	50.9	11.3	32.1	15.0	7,953
Comparison between countries[b]	**$F_{25,v}=21.9$*, $P<0.001$**		**$F_{25,v}=7.8$*, $P<0.001$**		**$F_{25,v}=3.9$*, $P<0.001$**		**$F_{24,v}=2.1$*, $P=0.002$**		**$F_{21,v}=0.6$, $P=0.898$**		
Comparison between low-, middle-, and high-income country groups[b]	**$F_{2,v}=109.5$*, $P<0.001$**		**$F_{2,v}=25.6$*, $P<0.001$**		**$F_{2,v}=6.6$*, $P=0.001$**		**$F_{2,v}=1.1$, $P=0.333$**		**$F_{2,v}=0.7$, $P=0.472$**		
Comparison between WHO regions[b]	**$F_{5,v}=66.7$*, $P<0.001$**		**$F_{5,v}=21.0$*, $P<0.001$**		**$F_{5,v}=11.2$*, $P<0.001$**		**$F_{5,v}=1.3$, $P=0.250$**		**$F_{5,v}=0.4$, $P=0.842$**		

*Significant at the 0.05 level, two-sided test.
A dash indicates low cell count (<5 cases).
[a]**Region of the Americas** (Colombia, Mexico, Brazil, Peru, United States, Colombia (Medellin)); **African region** (South Africa, Nigeria); **Western Pacific region** (PRC: Beijing and Shanghai, Japan, Australia, New Zealand); **Eastern Mediterranean region** (Israel, Iraq, Lebanon); **Western European region** (Belgium, France, Germany, Italy, Netherlands, Spain, Northern Ireland, Spain (Murcia)); **Eastern European region** (Poland, Bulgaria, Ukraine).
[b]Wald design-corrected F-tests were used to determine if there is variation in prevalence estimates across countries. The denominator degree of freedom, v, is 5269. Comparisons between countries for 12 months/LT and 30 days/12 months did not include surveys with zero number of cases in (lifetime and 12 months) or (12 months and 30 days).
PRC: People's Republic of China.

(0.8%), Australia, and Belgium (0.7%). Multiple countries do not have any 30-day cases of DRD, and the average 30-day prevalence of DRD for all countries is 0.1%.

For any DUDs, the category that includes either DRA or DRD, the average lifetime prevalence in all countries combined is 3.5% (Table 17.4). The highest levels are observed in the United States (8.4%), Australia (7.5%), and New Zealand (5.6%). The average 12-month prevalence of DUDs for all countries is 0.7%, ranging from less than 0.1% (Bulgaria and Japan) up to 1.7% (Belgium). The average 30-day prevalence of DUDs for all countries is 0.3%.

The prevalences of DRA, DRD, and DUD are significantly higher in the high-income countries than in the low/lower-middle-income countries for all time periods (lifetime, past year, and 30-day). There are also significant differences in prevalence of DRA, DRD, and DUDs among the WHO regions. The Western Pacific region (which contains Australia and New Zealand) has the highest levels of DUDs in all timeframes, with lower levels in the Eastern European and Eastern Mediterranean countries.

Although there is a wide range in the differences across countries, in all countries the lifetime prevalence of DRA is higher than the lifetime prevalence of DRD. The 12-month prevalences of DRA and DRD are much more similar across countries.

Persistence

Two indirect indicators of disorder and episode persistence were computed (Tables 17.2–17.4). The proportion of lifetime cases of DUD who had a DUD in the past 12 months (data column 4) is the indicator of disorder persistence. For all countries combined, the rates are 18.2% for DRA, 27.2% for DRD, and 21.4% for DUD, equating to around one in four or five lifetime cases having an active disorder in the previous year. There is significant variation across countries, but in many instances these estimates are based upon small numbers of cases. In contrast to the prevalence estimates, there is no significant variation in these disorder persistence estimates when the countries are grouped by income or WHO region.

The estimates for the indicator of episode persistence (30-day DUD/12-month cases; data column 5), are 29.2% for DRA, 42.0% for DRD, and 35.0% for DUD. None of these estimates vary significantly across countries, but again the very small numbers of cases involved limited power to detect differences.

Both of these indicators of persistence suggest that, although it is less prevalent, DRD is more persistent than DRA. Additionally, the persistence rates for DRA and DRD are somewhat low compared to many of the other mental disorders included in this volume (see Chapter 22), especially given the generally attributed chronic and relapsing nature of DUDs. This may potentially reflect the fact that population-based surveys are likely to capture less severe cases of DUDs, and additionally that many people with active DUDs may not be in the sampling frame of these surveys (which exclude inpatient treatment facilities, homeless shelters, refuges, and correctional facilities).

Age-of-Onset

In earlier WMH reports, we found that the median age-of-onset (AOO) for drug use was between 16 and 20 years for all countries, with the earliest use being in European countries and the latest being in the Middle East and Africa (Degenhardt *et al.* 2008). In this chapter, we show that not only does drug use often begin in adolescence but so do DUDs (Table 17.5). Across all countries, the earliest 5% of lifetime DUD cases have onsets by age 15; 50% of cases have onset by age 20. Across countries, there is variation in the AOO of DUDs. Lower-income countries tend to have older median AOO than higher-income countries. Of all lifetime cases across all countries, 75% have onsets by age 25. This also varies across countries and by country income level: 75% of cases have onset by age 27 in low/lower-middle- and upper-middle-income countries, compared to 24 years in high-income countries. Based on projections, 90% of lifetime cases across all countries have onsets by age 35 and 95% by age 45. Although there is great variation among countries, projected risk at age 75 across all countries is 4.1%, with 1.1% in low/lower-middle-income countries, 3.0% in upper-middle-income countries, and 5.5% in high-income countries.

Role Impairment

Only six countries assessed the severity of DUDs using the Sheehan Disability Scale and only four of these had sufficient 12 month cases to analyse (Brazil, Colombia (Medellin), Northern Ireland, and Poland), so the findings of this analysis must be interpreted with caution. As shown in Table 17.6, across these four countries almost half (45.8%) of those with 12-month DUD report having at least one area of their life where they experience severe impairment associated with their DUD; this proportion did not differ across countries. This is higher than is seen for

Table 17.4 Prevalence of DSM-IV drug-use disorder (DRD) in the World Mental Health surveys

Country	Lifetime prevalence		12-month prevalence		30-day prevalence		12-month prevalence of DUD among lifetime cases		30-day prevalence of DUD among 12-month cases		Sample size used
	%	SE	%	SE	%	SE	%	SE	%	SE	
Low/lower-middle-income countries	**0.9**	**0.1**	**0.3**	**0.0**	**0.1**	**0.0**	**27.1**	**4.1**	**40.1**	**9.9**	**18,179**
Colombia	1.7	0.3	0.5	0.1	0.2	0.1	28.1	5.1	47.5	15.7	4,426
Iraq	0.2	0.1	0.1	0.1	<0.1	0.0	78.7	18.2	18.0	20.3	4,332
Nigeria	1.0	0.2	0.2	0.1	0.1	0.1	23.0	9.2	38.3	21.0	2,143
Peru	1.1	0.1	0.2	0.1	0.1	0.1	18.2	8.4	54.8	23.3	3,930
PRC (Beijing/Shanghai)	0.5	0.2	0.1	0.0	<0.1	0.0	12.3	9.1	81.8	16.3	1,628
Ukraine	1.0	0.3	0.4	0.2	<0.1	0.0	36.1	13.7	11.3	9.7	1,720
Upper-middle-income countries	**2.5**	**0.1**	**0.7**	**0.1**	**0.2**	**0.0**	**27.9**	**2.3**	**31.4**	**5.3**	**20,071**
Brazil	2.9	0.4	0.8	0.2	0.4	0.1	27.1	4.3	47.1	11.3	5,037
Bulgaria	0.2	0.1	<0.1	0.0	–	–	2.9	3.2	–	–	2,233
Colombia (Medellin)	5.2	0.7	1.0	0.2	0.5	0.2	19.7	4.2	46.1	11.2	1,673
Lebanon	0.5	0.2	0.2	0.1	0.1	0.1	33.7	29.7	45.9	26.2	1,031
Mexico	1.4	0.2	0.3	0.1	0.1	0.0	23.3	4.9	24.4	9.4	5,782
South Africa	4.0	0.4	1.4	0.2	0.3	0.1	35.3	4.5	18.9	7.6	4,315
High-income countries	**4.8**	**0.1**	**0.9**	**0.1**	**0.3**	**0.0**	**19.6**	**1.0**	**35.6**	**2.8**	**49,727**
Australia	7.5	0.4	1.3	0.1	0.4	0.1	17.6	1.8	34.1	5.8	8,463
Belgium	4.5	0.9	1.7	0.7	0.8	0.5	38.2	11.2	45.6	22.5	1,043
France	3.5	0.4	0.8	0.2	0.4	0.2	22.8	4.8	44.5	13.7	1,436
Germany	2.9	0.5	0.6	0.3	0.1	0.1	20.1	9.2	19.1	9.1	1,323
Israel	1.7	0.2	0.3	0.1	0.1	0.0	19.2	4.4	31.2	11.3	4,859
Italy	2.5	0.4	0.4	0.1	0.1	0.0	14.8	4.7	30.1	13.3	1,779
Japan	0.3	0.1	<0.1	0.0	–	–	14.7	9.6	–	–	1,682
New Zealand	5.6	0.3	1.4	0.1	0.5	0.1	24.6	2.0	36.4	5.0	12,790
Northern Ireland	3.3	0.5	0.6	0.2	0.3	0.2	17.0	5.6	53.8	14.8	1,986
Poland	1.4	0.2	0.3	0.1	0.2	0.1	21.6	6.3	51.3	17.0	4,000
Spain	4.1	0.5	0.8	0.3	0.2	0.1	19.9	7.1	29.8	13.3	2,121
Spain (Murcia)	3.7	0.8	0.1	0.1	–	–	3.1	2.4	–	–	1,459
Netherlands	2.1	0.7	0.2	0.1	0.1	0.1	8.3	4.6	49.0	26.1	1,094
United States	8.4	0.4	1.3	0.1	0.4	0.1	15.8	1.4	32.0	5.0	5,692
All countries combined	**3.5**	**0.1**	**0.7**	**0.0**	**0.3**	**0.0**	**21.4**	**0.9**	**35.0**	**2.4**	**87,977**

(cont.)

Table 17.4 (*cont.*)

Country	Lifetime prevalence		12-month prevalence		30-day prevalence		12-month prevalence of DUD among lifetime cases		30-day prevalence of DUD among 12-month cases		Sample size used
	%	SE	%	SE	%	SE	%	SE	%	SE	
WHO regions[a]											
Region of the Americas	3.4	0.1	0.7	0.1	0.3	0.0	19.8	1.3	38.6	4.3	26,540
African region	3.0	0.3	1.0	0.1	0.2	0.1	33.9	4.2	20.4	7.2	6,458
Western Pacific region	5.5	0.2	1.2	0.1	0.4	0.0	21.2	1.3	35.5	3.8	24,563
Eastern Mediterranean region	0.9	0.1	0.2	0.1	0.1	0.0	24.3	5.4	29.2	10.1	10,222
Western European region	3.3	0.2	0.6	0.1	0.2	0.1	18.5	2.8	38.1	7.7	12,241
Eastern European region	1.0	0.1	0.2	0.1	0.1	0.0	23.8	5.6	37.8	12.6	7,953
Comparison between countries[b]	**$F_{25,v} = 45.5^*$, $P < 0.001$**		**$F_{25,v} = 15.4^*$, $P < 0.001$**		**$F_{25,v} = 6.9^*$, $P < 0.001$**		**$F_{25,v} = 2.1^*$, $P = 0.001$**		**$F_{25,v} = 0.8$, $P = 0.741$**		
Comparison between low-, middle-, and high-income country groups[b]	**$F_{2,v} = 300.8^*$, $P < 0.001$**		**$F_{2,v} = 47.4^*$, $P < 0.001$**		**$F_{2,v} = 15.9^*$, $P < 0.001$**		**$F_{2,v} = 6.4^*$, $P = 0.002$**		**$F_{2,v} = 0.4$, $P = 0.684$**		
Comparison between WHO regions[b]	**$F_{5,v} = 122.9^*$, $P < 0.001$**		**$F_{5,v} = 25.5^*$, $P < 0.001$**		**$F_{5,v} = 12.3^*$, $P < 0.001$**		**$F_{5,v} = 2.4^*$, $P = 0.034$**		**$F_{5,v} = 1.0$, $P = 0.437$**		

*Significant at the 0.05 level, two-sided test.
A dash indicates low cell count (<5 cases).
[a]**Region of the Americas** (Colombia, Mexico, Brazil, Peru, United States, Colombia (Medellin)); **African region** (South Africa, Nigeria); **Western Pacific region** (PRC: Beijing and Shanghai, Japan, Australia, New Zealand); **Eastern Mediterranean region** (Israel, Iraq, Lebanon); **Western European region** (Belgium, France, Germany, Italy, Netherlands, Spain, Northern Ireland, Spain (Murcia)); **Eastern European region** (Poland, Bulgaria, Ukraine).
[b]Wald design-corrected F-tests were used to determine if there is variation in prevalence estimates across countries. The denominator degree of freedom, v, is 5269.
PRC: People's Republic of China.

Table 17.5 Age at selected percentiles on the standardized age-of-onset distributions of DSM-IV drug-use disorder (DUD) with projected lifetime risk at age 75

Country	Ages at selected percentiles								Lifetime prevalence of DUD		Projected risk at age 75	
	5	10	25	50	75	90	95	99	%	SE	%	SE
Low/lower-middle-income countries	**15**	**16**	**18**	**21**	**27**	**31**	**36**	**51**	**0.9**	**0.1**	**1.1**	**0.1**
Colombia[a]	15	15	18	21	25	29	30	39	1.7	0.3	1.9	0.3
Iraq	20	20	27	27	27	31	41	41	0.2	0.1	0.2	0.1
Nigeria	17	17	20	24	28	31	31	41	1.0	0.2	1.3	0.3
Peru[a]	13	16	17	19	24	28	31	31	1.1	0.1	1.2	0.2
PRC (Beijing/Shanghai)	20	20	20	22	36	51	51	53	0.5	0.2	0.6	0.3
Ukraine	17	17	17	20	21	43	43	43	1.0	0.3	1.1	0.3
Upper-middle-income countries	**15**	**16**	**18**	**21**	**27**	**38**	**42**	**54**	**2.5**	**0.1**	**3.0**	**0.2**
Brazil	15	16	19	21	27	34	39	51	2.9	0.4	3.4	0.5
Bulgaria	16	16	21	21	34	34	34	34	0.2	0.1	0.2	0.1
Colombia (Medellin)[a]	13	15	16	20	24	36	41	54	5.2	0.7	5.8	0.8
Lebanon	20	21	21	26	26	26	26	26	0.5	0.2	0.6	0.3
Mexico[a]	15	17	18	20	28	52	52	52	1.4	0.2	1.7	0.3
South Africa	15	17	19	22	30	41	43	54	4.0	0.4	5.1	0.5
High-income countries	**15**	**16**	**17**	**20**	**24**	**33**	**43**	**59**	**4.8**	**0.1**	**5.5**	**0.1**
Australia	15	16	18	19	22	30	34	41	7.5	0.4	8.4	0.4
Belgium	15	16	19	21	34	38	59	59	4.5	0.9	5.3	1.1
France	17	17	19	24	37	57	57	68	3.5	0.4	4.7	0.7
Germany	5	15	16	20	59	59	59	59	2.9	0.5	4.1	0.9
Israel	18	19	21	23	25	31	35	35	1.7	0.2	1.9	0.2
Italy	15	15	18	21	31	53	59	59	2.5	0.4	3.0	0.5
Japan	5	18	20	24	27	36	36	36	0.3	0.1	0.3	0.1
New Zealand	14	15	16	19	22	28	31	43	5.6	0.3	6.3	0.3
Northern Ireland	16	16	17	19	21	29	47	51	3.3	0.5	3.8	0.6
Poland[b]	5	17	21	58	59	59	59	59	1.4	0.2	2.7	0.6
Spain	15	17	19	25	37	54	59	59	4.1	0.5	5.5	1.0
Spain (Murcia)	6	6	16	21	21	23	27	35	3.7	0.8	4.0	0.8
Netherlands	14	14	17	21	25	51	51	51	2.1	0.7	2.6	0.8
United States	15	16	17	19	24	29	36	42	8.4	0.4	9.7	0.5
All countries combined	**15**	**16**	**18**	**20**	**25**	**35**	**45**	**59**	**3.5**	**0.1**	**4.1**	**0.1**
WHO regions												
Region of the Americas	15	16	17	20	25	31	39	52	3.4	0.1	3.9	0.2
African region	16	17	19	22	30	40	43	54	3.0	0.3	3.9	0.4
Western Pacific region	15	16	17	19	22	29	34	43	5.5	0.2	6.2	0.2
Eastern Mediterranean region	18	19	21	23	27	31	35	35	0.9	0.1	1.1	0.1
Western European region	15	16	18	21	30	54	59	59	3.3	0.2	4.2	0.3
Eastern European region	5	16	19	21	59	59	59	59	1.0	0.1	1.5	0.2

[a]The projected risk for these countries is at age 65 because the age range of these surveys is between 18 and 65.
[b]The projected risk for this country is at age 64 because the age range of this survey is between 18 and 64.
PRC: People's Republic of China.

Table 17.6 Severity of role impairment (Sheehan Disability Scale) associated with 12-month drug-use disorder (DUD), by country

Country	Proportion with severe role impairment (SDS score: 7–10)										Number of 12-month DUD cases
	Home		Work		Relationship		Social		Any[a]		
	%	SE	%	SE	%	SE	%	SE	%	SE	
Brazil	25.4	13.8	26.6	7.1	28.2	7.8	30.2	7.7	41.8	7.6	35
Colombia (Medellin)	22.4	14.7	41.2	17.8	30.4	15.8	16.0	10.8	49.2	17.0	25
Northern Ireland	23.9	12.0	29.9	14.4	31.3	13.7	15.0	10.2	43.7	16.6	13
Poland	2.7	2.9	21.1	13.8	6.8	5.3	6.8	5.3	21.1	13.8	16
All countries combined	**28.5**	**8.9**	**35.1**	**6.8**	**25.6**	**5.6**	**21.9**	**5.3**	**45.8**	**6.8**	**95**
Comparison between countries[b]	$F_{4,v} = 0.9$, P = 0.454		$F_{4,v} = 0.8$, P = 0.572		$F_{4,v} = 1.0$, P = 0.427		$F_{4,v} = 1.0$, P = 0.400		$F_{4,v} = 0.9$, P = 0.501		

A dash indicates low cell count (<5 cases).
[a]Highest severity category across four SDS role domains.
[b]Wald design-corrected F-tests were used to determine if there is variation in impairment severity across countries. The denominator degree of freedom, v, is 460.

AUDs (Chapter 16), where around one-third (30.8%) of cases report severe impairment in at least one role. This is consistent with the WMH findings on days-out-of-role associated with DUD and other mental and physical disorders (Alonso *et al.* 2011). Although the number of cases was too small to detect differences across role domains, the percent reporting severe impairment in all four countries combined appears highest for the work domain and lowest for the social domain. Further research is needed to examine this issue in other countries.

Socio-demographic Correlates

There is an incredibly strong association between age-at-interview (age-cohort) and lifetime DUDs (Table 17.7). People aged 18–29 years have 69.3 times the odds of those aged 60+ years to meet criteria for a lifetime disorder. There is no association between the age-of-onset of DUD and the likelihood of recent DUD among cases, indicating that AOO is not related to probability of persistence. Consistent with previous studies, men are significantly more likely than women to have a lifetime or 30-day DUD. The odds of men having a lifetime or 30-day DUD are about 2.5 times the odds of women.

Marital status is significantly associated with lifetime and 30-day DUDs, with respondents who are divorced, separated, or widowed having the greatest likelihood of DUDs (compared to those who are married). Interestingly, those who have never married are also at elevated odds of lifetime DUDs, and at elevated odds of persistent DUDs (12-month/lifetime). There is a significant association of education level with DUDs, with increased odds of lifetime and 30-day DUD among those with more limited educational attainment (compared to those who have finished college or university). Low educational attainment is also strongly associated with persistence of DUDs. Those who have the lowest levels of household income compared to others in their country have the highest levels of lifetime and 30-day DUDs, and higher odds of persistent DUDs. Finally, those who are unemployed or disabled (the 'other' category of employment status) are significantly more likely to have lifetime DUDs relative to those in employment, a difference that is also apparent but not significant for 30-day prevalence. By contrast, students are significantly less likely to meet current (30-prevalence) criteria for DUDs than those in employment.

Comorbidity

It is well established that DUDs are highly comorbid with other mental disorders (Hall *et al.* 2009; Pani *et al.* 2010; Lai *et al.* 2015). Consistent with this, extremely

Table 17.7 Bivariate associations between socio-demographic correlates and DSM-IV drug-use disorder (DUD) (all countries combined)

Correlates	30-day DUD[a]		Lifetime DUD[b]		12-month DUD among lifetime cases[c]		30-day DUD among 12-month cases[c]	
	OR	(95% CI)	OR	(95% CI)	OR	(95% CI)	OR	(95% CI)
Age-cohort								
18–29	–	–	**69.3***	(51.2–93.6)				
30–44	–	–	**29.0***	(22.1–37.9)				
45–59	–	–	**8.9***	(6.7–11.6)				
60+	–		**1.0**					
Age-cohort difference[d]	–		$\chi^2_3 = 961.9^*$, $P < 0.001$					
Age-of-onset								
Early					**1.1**	(0.8–1.5)	**0.8**	(0.4–1.3)
Early-average					**0.9**	(0.6–1.3)	**0.7**	(0.4–1.2)
Late-average					**0.9**	(0.7–1.2)	**1.0**	(0.6–1.8)
Late					**1.0**		**1.0**	
Age-of-onset difference[d]					$\chi^2_3 = 2.0$, $P = 0.579$		$\chi^2_3 = 2.9$, $P = 0.415$	
Time since onset (continuous)					**0.93***	(0.92–0.95)	**1.03***	(1.01–1.06)
Gender								
Female	**0.4***	(0.3–0.5)	**0.4***	(0.4–0.4)	**0.9**	(0.7–1.2)	**0.8**	(0.5–1.1)
Male	**1.0**		**1.0**		**1.0**		**1.0**	
Gender difference[d]	$\chi^2_1 = 44.9^*$, $P < 0.001$		$\chi^2_1 = 356.0^*$, $P < 0.001$		$\chi^2_1 = 0.6$, $P = 0.450$		$\chi^2_1 = 1.7$, $P = 0.189$	
Employment status								
Student	**0.2***	(0.1–0.4)	**0.8**	(0.6–1.1)	**0.9**	(0.6–1.6)	**0.2***	(0.1–0.6)
Homemaker	**1.4**	(0.8–2.3)	**1.2**	(1.0–1.4)	**1.0**	(0.7–1.5)	**1.2**	(0.5–2.4)
Retired	**–**	–	**1.0**	(0.7–1.5)	**0.7**	(0.2–2.2)	**–**	–
Other	**1.5**	(1.0–2.3)	**1.9***	(1.7–2.2)	**1.3**	(0.9–1.8)	**0.6**	(0.3–1.0)
Employed	**1.0**		**1.0**		**1.0**		**1.0**	
Employment status difference[d]	$\chi^2_4 = 25.4^*$, $P < 0.001$		$\chi^2_4 = 77.0^*$, $P < 0.001$		$\chi^2_4 = 3.4$, $P = 0.490$		$\chi^2_4 = 11.1^*$, $P = 0.025$	

(cont.)

Table 17.7 *(cont.)*

Correlates	30-day DUD[a]		Lifetime DUD[b]		12-month DUD among lifetime cases[c]		30-day DUD among 12-month cases[c]	
	OR	(95% CI)	OR	(95% CI)	OR	(95% CI)	OR	(95% CI)
Marital status								
Never married	**1.4**	(0.9–2.1)	**1.7***	(1.5–1.9)	**1.5***	(1.2–2.0)	**0.7**	(0.4–1.2)
Divorced/separated/widowed	**2.5***	(1.5–4.2)	**1.9***	(1.6–2.1)	**1.3**	(0.9–2.0)	**1.3**	(0.7–2.4)
Currently married	**1.0**		**1.0**		**1.0**		**1.0**	
Marital status difference[d]	$\chi^2_2 = 14.3^*$, P = 0.001		$\chi^2_2 = 149.1^*$, P < 0.001		$\chi^2_2 = 9.1^*$, P = 0.010		$\chi^2_2 = 2.8$, P = 0.243	
Education level								
No education	–	–	**1.5**	(0.9–2.6)	**7.0***	(2.1–23.8)	–	–
Some primary	**2.8***	(1.2–6.5)	**1.9***	(1.5–2.4)	**1.8**	(0.9–3.6)	**1.1**	(0.4–3.3)
Finished primary	**3.3***	(1.4–7.7)	**1.8***	(1.4–2.3)	**1.7**	(0.8–3.3)	**1.3**	(0.4–3.8)
Some secondary	**2.7***	(1.6–4.7)	**2.0***	(1.7–2.3)	**1.5**	(1.0–2.4)	**1.4**	(0.7–2.9)
Finished secondary	**1.5**	(0.9–2.7)	**1.4***	(1.2–1.6)	**1.4**	(0.9–2.1)	**1.0**	(0.5–2.0)
Some college	**1.2**	(0.7–2.1)	**1.3***	(1.1–1.6)	**1.1**	(0.7–1.7)	**1.1**	(0.5–2.5)
Finished college	**1.0**		**1.0**		**1.0**		**1.0**	
Education level difference[d]	$\chi^2_6 = 23.2^*$, P = 0.001		$\chi^2_6 = 83.1^*$, P < 0.001		$\chi^2_6 = 13.9^*$, P = 0.031		$\chi^2_6 = 1.9$, P = 0.926	
Household income								
Low	**1.7***	(1.1–2.5)	**1.6***	(1.4–1.8)	**1.5***	(1.1–2.1)	**0.7**	(0.4–1.3)
Low-average	**1.0**	(0.6–1.6)	**1.2***	(1.1–1.4)	**1.2**	(0.9–1.8)	**0.6**	(0.3–1.1)
High-average	**1.0**	(0.7–1.6)	**1.1**	(1.0–1.3)	**1.4**	(1.0–2.0)	**0.6**	(0.3–1.2)
High	**1.0**		**1.0**		**1.0**		**1.0**	
Household income difference[d]	$\chi^2_3 = 9.7^*$, P = 0.021		$\chi^2_3 = 57.6^*$, P < 0.001		$\chi^2_3 = 7.0$, P = 0.071		$\chi^2_3 = 3.0$, P = 0.398	
N[e]	**87,977**		**3,774,951**		**3,372**		**695**	

*Significant at the 0.05 level, two-sided test.
A dash indicates low cell count (<5 cases).
[a]These estimates are based on logistic regression models adjusted for age, gender, and country.
[b]These estimates are based on survival models adjusted for age-cohorts, gender, person-years, and country.
[c]These estimates are based on logistic regression models adjusted for time since DUD onset, age of DUD onset, gender, and country.
[d]Chi-square test of significant differences between blocks of socio-demographic variables.
[e]Denominator N: 87,977 = total sample; 3,774,951 = number of person-years in the survival models; 3,372 = number of lifetime DUD cases; 695 = number of 12-month DUD cases.

high levels of comorbidity are found among people with DUDs in the WMH surveys, with almost 9 in 10 people with a 12-month DUD having a lifetime history of at least one mental disorder (Table 17.8). This is most commonly an AUD, with two-thirds (66.5%) having a history of an AUD; half have a history of an anxiety disorder (49.0%).

DUDs are not often the first disorder experienced by people with DUD who have more than one disorder. For lifetime DUD cases, only one in five (21.7%) experienced the onset of DUD before their other disorder(s); this appeared largely driven by the fact that anxiety disorders (the second most commonly occurring disorders among DUD cases) occurred before DUD in 82.2% of cases. It is not possible to draw any conclusions about causality in these patterns of associations in these data, given the complexities surrounding comorbidity between drug use and other disorders including potential bi-directional relationships and increasing evidence that a wide range of genetic, familial, social, and environmental influences confer similar risk across mental and substance use disorders.

Treatment

A minority of those with 12-month DUD received some kind of care for a mental or substance-use problem in the 12 months prior to interview (Table 17.9). One-third (33.4%) report 'any health care' in the previous 12-months (either specialist mental health or general medical health treatment), with 21.7% receiving specialist mental health care and 22.1% receiving general medical care. Around one in nine (11.3%) report seeking some kind of intervention in either the human services sector (which included religious advisors and non-specialist counsellors) or the complementary and alternative medicine (CAM) sector (which includes Narcotics Anonymous and other 12-step programmes). 'Any treatment' in the past year for 12-month DUD is 26.7% in low/lower-middle-income countries, 36.7% in upper-middle-income countries, and 38.6% in high-income countries.

Specialist mental health care varies across countries, and is more common in higher-income countries. By contrast, non-health care is more likely in upper-middle-income countries than high-income countries (none of these services are reported by respondents in low/lower-middle-income countries).

Discussion

Globally, DUDs are not distributed evenly. The United States, Australia, and New Zealand had the highest levels of DUDs; much lower levels were observed in countries in Africa, Latin America, the Middle

Table 17.8 Comorbidity of drug-use disorder (DUD) with other DSM-IV disorders

	DUD cases with comorbid disorders									
	Mood disorder		Anxiety disorder		Disruptive behaviour/Impulse-control disorder		Alcohol-use disorder		Any disorder	
	%	SE	%	SE	%	SE	%	SE	%	SE
Lifetime comorbidity[a]										
Lifetime	**36.8**	1.1	**41.3**	1.1	**20.9**	1.3	**64.9**	1.1	**81.8**	1.0
12-month	**43.5**	2.6	**49.0**	2.5	**24.1**	3.1	**66.5**	2.3	**85.5**	2.0
12-month comorbidity[b]										
12-month	**31.7**	2.5	**39.9**	2.5	**16.9**	2.8	**38.5**	2.4	**69.6**	2.5
Temporal priority of DUD[c]										
Lifetime	**41.1**	1.8	**17.8**	1.3	**26.5**	3.9	**36.5**	1.5	**21.7**	1.1
12-month	**29.9**	3.3	**17.1**	2.8	**20.0**	6.9	**33.3**	2.8	**17.5**	2.2

[a]Percentage of respondents with either lifetime or 12-month DUD who also meet lifetime criteria for at least one of the other DSM-IV disorders.
[b]Percentage of respondents with 12-month DUD who also meet 12-month criteria for at least one of the other disorders.
[c]Percentage of respondents with either lifetime or 12-month DUD and at least one of the other disorders, whose AOO of DUD is reported to be younger than the age-of-onset of all comorbid disorders under consideration.

Table 17.9 Among those with 12-month drug-use disorder, percent reporting treatment in the past 12 months

Sector of treatment	%	SE	Comparison between country income groups[a]
Specialty mental health[b]			
Low/lower-middle-income countries	9.5	4.7	$F_{2,v} = 3.3^*$,
Upper-middle-income countries	17.8	3.7	$P = 0.04$
High-income countries	24.0	2.3	
All countries combined	**21.7**	**1.9**	
General medical[c]			
Low/lower-middle-income countries	20.0	9.4	$F_{2,v} = 3.9^*$,
Upper-middle-income countries	13.1	3.3	$P = 0.02$
High-income countries	25.0	2.5	
All countries combined	**22.1**	**2.1**	
Any health care[d]			
Low/lower-middle-income countries	26.7	9.7	$F_{2,v} = 1.1$,
Upper-middle-income countries	28.4	4.5	$P = 0.33$
High-income countries	35.5	2.8	
All countries combined	**33.4**	**2.3**	
Human services[e]			
Low/lower-middle-income countries	–	–	$F_{2,v} = 6.1^*$,
Upper-middle-income countries	6.0	2.3	$P < 0.001$
High-income countries	4.1	1.1	
All countries combined	**4.2**	**1.0**	
CAM[f]			
Low/lower-middle-income countries	–	–	$F_{2,v} = 9.0^*$,
Upper-middle-income countries	13.1	3.7	$P < 0.001$
High-income countries	7.1	1.3	
All countries combined	**7.9**	**1.2**	
Any non-health care[g]			
Low/lower-middle-income countries	–	–	$F_{2,v} = 10.8^*$,
Upper-middle-income countries	17.7	3.7	$P < 0.001$
High-income countries	10.5	1.8	
All countries combined	**11.3**	**1.5**	
Any treatment or care[h]			
Low/lower-middle-income countries	26.7	9.7	$F_{2,v} = 0.7$,
Upper-middle-income countries	36.7	5.1	$P = 0.49$
High-income countries	38.6	2.8	
All countries combined	**37.4**	**2.4**	

*Significant at the 0.05 level, two-sided test.
[a]Wald design-corrected F-tests were used to determine if there is variation in treatment estimates across country income groups. The denominator degree of freedom, v, is 5269.
[b]The mental health specialist sector, which includes psychiatrist and non-psychiatrist mental health specialists (psychiatrist, psychologist or other non-psychiatrist mental health professional; social worker or counsellor in a mental health specialty setting; use of a mental health helpline; or overnight admissions for a mental health or drug problems, with a presumption of daily contact with a psychiatrist).
[c]The general medical sector (general practitioner, other medical doctor, nurse, occupational therapist or any healthcare professional).
[d]The mental health specialist sector or the general medical sector.
[e]The human services sector (religious or spiritual advisor or social worker or counsellor in any setting other than a specialty mental health setting).
[f]The CAM (complementary and alternative medicine) sector (any other type of healer such as herbalist or homeopath, participation in an internet support group, or participation in a self-help group).
[g]The human services sector or CAM.
[h]Any treatment listed above.

East, and Asia. The average lifetime DUD prevalence across all countries combined was 3.5%, ranging from 0.2% in Iraq and Bulgaria, to 8.4% in the United States. This wide range is consistent with other data on the prevalence of illicit drug use and problems (Hall & Degenhardt 2007; Degenhardt *et al.* 2013; UNODC 2015).

These geographic variations in prevalence cannot be regarded as static. There were greater levels of DUDs among younger than older adults, suggesting that drug-use problems have and may continue to change over historical time. It remains to be seen whether there will be changes in the future in levels of DUDs in countries that had lower levels at the time of conduct of the WMH surveys; as noted previously, data suggest that levels have increased globally over past decades (Degenhardt *et al.* 2013).

In the WMH surveys the period of risk for onset of DUDs began in the mid-teen years, extending into adulthood, with about half of cases beginning by age 20, but incidence continuing into middle age. There continues to be a window of risk of developing problems that persists well beyond the most commonly targeted ages. Being less educated, being on a low income (relative to others in that country), being unemployed, and not currently married were each associated with greater likelihood of DUD. In line with a large body of evidence, gender was also strongly related to DUDs, with men more likely than women to have experienced a DUD. Comorbidity with other mental disorders was extremely common and treatment was obtained by only a minority meeting criteria for DUD. These patterns were all observed across countries.

It is important to note that DUD is one of a range of potential adverse health consequences of heavy drug use. Methamphetamine use, for example, may lead to acute psychotic episodes following heavy or 'binge' use (Segal & Kuczenski 1997; Srisurapanont *et al.* 2003; Batki & Harris 2004); violent or aggressive behaviour during acute intoxication (Wright & Klee 2001; Boles & Miotto 2003; McKetin *et al.* 2006) and elevated mortality risk (Singleton *et al.* 2009). Heavy cannabis use increases the risks of motor vehicle accidents, psychosis, and mood disorders (Degenhardt 2001; Hall & Degenhardt 2007; Calabria *et al.* 2010; World Health Organization 2016). Cocaine use has also been associated with paranoia (Satel *et al.* 1991; Mooney *et al.* 2006), suicide (Marzuk *et al.* 1992; Roy 2001), overdose (Degenhardt *et al.* 2011c), and other poor health outcomes (Cregler 1989; Cornish & O'Brien 1996; Falck *et al.* 2003). Opioid users may struggle with dependence over many years, and suffer from poor health and elevated mortality (Degenhardt *et al.* 2011b), particularly from overdose (Degenhardt *et al.* 2004, 2006). Injection of drugs carries additional risks if non-sterile injecting equipment is used, because of potential exposure to HIV and viral hepatitis and other injection-related injuries and diseases (Degenhardt *et al.* 2016a; Larney *et al.* 2017).

The WMH surveys have several important limitations. Given that 26 countries and country regions participated in the WMH surveys assessing DUDs, there is not full representation of all regions, country income levels, and other country characteristics. There was variation in response rates across countries and possibly cross-national differences in willingness to disclose personal information about drug use and problems. Respondent information is subject to the limitations of recall inherent in retrospective reporting leading to potentially substantial underestimates in lifetime prevalence. Survival bias may also contribute to downward bias in lifetime estimates.

In addition to these general limitations that apply to the assessment of all the disorders considered in this volume there are some limitations that are more specific to the assessment of DUDs. The WMH surveys are household surveys, which face limitations when used to assess less common and more stigmatized behaviours. In this situation, drug use can be a rare occurrence and geographically concentrated, as is often the case for heroin, amphetamines, and cocaine use in some countries. Surveys such as WMH that rely on stratified sampling methods are poorly suited to capturing concentrated geographic 'pockets' of drug use (for example, in some inner city areas where the prevalence of drug use may be many times higher than rural areas). Furthermore, the use of households as the primary sampling unit in general population surveys will fail to capture marginalized groups who do not live in traditional household contexts; they may be in prison or hospital, or not be available during the typical hours when such surveys are conducted. Collectively, these limitations indicate that the prevalence rates presented here should be considered lower-bound estimates and that true lifetime prevalence and lifetime risk of DUDs may be substantially higher.

As noted earlier, a core number of drugs were assessed across countries and there was variation in the range of additional substances assessed across countries. In assessing DUDs, with the exception of countries such as Australia where abuse and dependence were assessed for specific substances (cannabis, sedatives, and stimulants), there was assessment of abuse and dependence symptoms without specification of the substance thought to have induced the symptom. This means that for people who had used multiple drugs, it is not clear which specific drug(s) was considered by the respondent to have caused the symptom. Given that there is debate over whether there are important differences in DUDs associated with different drugs or whether it is one fundamentally homogenous disorder, this is a limitation. Since the levels of use of specific drugs varies across countries in the WMH surveys (Degenhardt *et al.* 2008), to the extent that there is differentiation in risk for abuse and dependence upon different kinds of drugs, differences over DUDs may reflect differences in risk of different substances.

Another issue concerns the diagnostic system used in WMH. The conceptualization of and diagnostic criteria for SUDs were significantly revised in the DSM-5 (American Psychiatric Association 2014). The distinction between abuse and dependence was removed, reframing DUD as a single disorder. The legal problems symptom criterion was removed and a craving criterion added. DSM-5 uses numbers of symptom criteria to distinguish three levels of DUD severity. We compared DSM-IV and DSM-5 diagnoses of AUDs in the WMH surveys, and found that although the lifetime prevalence of AUD were similar when using the two systems, a large number of people were not consistently identified by both classifications (Slade *et al.* 2016). It is unclear what the effect would be in DUDs across countries, but it seems reasonable to assume that the same issues would apply, as was found in an analysis of Australian data from WMH examining cannabis-use disorder (Lago *et al.* 2016). For example, we found that even when restricted to moderate-severe cannabis-use disorder (requiring at least four criteria), DSM-5 use disorder had twice the prevalence of DSM-IV dependence cases (Lago *et al.* 2016). This has significant implications if DSM-5 were to be used to plan treatment programmer scale-up and/or treatment coverage. Future research will be important in further exploring these nosological issues.

In conclusion, the WMH surveys have generated novel data on the occurrence and distribution of DUDs across countries and different subpopulations within each country. There are clearly substantial differences in the extent of DUDs across countries, which no doubt reflect myriad social, environmental, legal, and other factors. Nonetheless, we have documented consistencies across these varied countries in terms of the onset and course of these disorders, and a number of consistent correlates. These findings provide foundational data on country-level comparisons of DUDs but there are important diagnostic issues requiring resolution and methodological challenges to be overcome in future cross-national epidemiological research on DUDs.

Acknowledgement

The views and opinions expressed in this publication are those of the authors only and do not necessarily represent the views, official policy, or position of the US Department of Health and Human Services or any of its affiliated institutions or agencies. Dr Glantz's role on this study is through his involvement as a Science Officer on U01-MH60220. He had no involvement in the other cited grants.

References

Alonso, J., Petukhova, M., Vilagut, G., *et al.* (2011). Days out of role due to common physical and mental conditions: results from the WHO World Mental Health surveys. *Molecular Psychiatry* 16, 1234–46.

American Psychiatric Association (2000). *Diagnostic and Statistical Manual of Mental Disorders (DSM-IV-TR).* Washington, DC: American Psychiatric Association.

(2014). *Diagnostic and Statistical Manual of Mental Disorders (Fifth Edition).* Washington, DC: American Psychiatric Association.

Babor, T. F. & Caetano, R. (2008). The trouble with alcohol abuse: what are we trying to measure, diagnose, count and prevent? *Addiction* 103, 1057–9.

Batki, S. L. & Harris, D. S. (2004). Quantitative drug levels in stimulant psychosis: relationship to symptom severity, catecholamines and hyperkinesia. *American Journal on Addictions* 13, 461–70.

Boles, S. M. & Miotto, K. (2003). Substance abuse and violence: a review of the literature. *Aggression and Violent Behavior* 8, 155–74.

Calabria, B., Degenhardt, L., Hall, W., *et al.* (2010). Does cannabis use increase the risk of death? Systematic review of epidemiological evidence on adverse effects of heavy cannabis use. *Drug and Alcohol Review* 29, 318–30.

Cornish, J. W. & O'Brien, C. P. (1996). Crack cocaine abuse: an epidemic with many public health consequences. *Annual Review of Public Health* 17, 2559–273.

Cregler, L. L. (1989). Adverse health consequences of cocaine abuse. *Journal of the National Medical Association* 81, 27–38.

Degenhardt, L., Bucello, C., Calabria, B., *et al.* (2011a). What data are available on the extent of illicit drug use and dependence globally? Results of four systematic reviews. *Drug & Alcohol Dependence* 117, 85–101.

Degenhardt, L., Bucello, C., Mathers, B., *et al.* (2011b). Mortality among regular or dependent users of heroin and other opioids: a systematic review and meta-analysis of cohort studies. *Addiction* 106, 32–51.

Degenhardt, L., Charlson, F., Stanaway, J., *et al.* (2016a). Estimating the burden of disease attributable to injecting drug use as a risk factor for HIV, hepatitis C, and hepatitis B: findings from the Global Burden of Disease Study 2013. *The Lancet Infectious Diseases* 16, 1385–98.

Degenhardt, L., Chiu, W., Sampson, N., *et al.* (2008). Toward a global view of alcohol, tobacco, cannabis, and cocaine use: findings from the WHO World Mental Health Surveys. *PLoS Medicine* 5, 1053–67.

Degenhardt, L. & Hall, W. (2012). Extent of illicit drug use and dependence, and their contribution to the global burden of disease. *Lancet* 379, 55–70.

Degenhardt, L., Hall, W. & Warner-Smith, M. (2006). Using cohort studies to estimate mortality among injecting drug users that is not attributable to AIDS. *Sexually Transmitted Infections* 82, 56–63.

Degenhardt, L., Hall, W. & Warner-Smith, M. *et al.* (2004). Illicit drug use. In *Comparative Quantification of Health Risk: Global and Regional Burden of Disease Attribution to Selected Major Risk Factors* (ed. M. Ezzati, A. D. Lopez, A. Rodgers, & C. J. L. Murray). Geneva: World Health Organization.

Degenhardt, L., Hall, W. D., & Lynskey, M. (2001). The relationship between cannabis use, depression and anxiety among Australian adults: findings from the National Survey of Mental Health and Well-Being. *Social Psychiatry and Psychiatric Epidemiology* 36, 219–27.

Degenhardt, L., Singleton, J., Calabria, B., *et al.* (2011c). Mortality among cocaine users: a systematic review of cohort studies. *Drug & Alcohol Dependence* 113, 88–95.

Degenhardt, L., Stockings, E., Patton, G., *et al.* (2016b). The increasing global health priority of substance use in young people. *The Lancet Psychiatry* 3, 251–64.

Degenhardt, L., Whiteford, H. A., Ferrari, A. J., *et al.* (2013). Global burden of disease attributable to illicit drug use and dependence: findings from the Global Burden of Disease Study 2010. *Lancet* 382, 1564–74.

Falck, R. S., Wang, J., Siegal, H. A., & Carlson, R. G. (2003). Current physical health problems and their predictors among a community sample of crack-cocaine smokers in Ohio. *Journal of Psychoactive Drugs* 35, 471–78.

Greater London Alcohol and Drug Alliance (2004). *The GLADA Crack Cocaine Strategy 2005–08*. London: Greater London Authority.

Hall, W. & Degenhardt, L. (2007). Prevalence and correlates of cannabis use in developed and developing countries. *Current Opinion in Psychiatry* 20, 393–97.

Hall, W., Degenhardt, L., & Teesson, M. (2009). Understanding comorbidity between substance use, anxiety and affective disorders: broadening the research base. *Addictive Behaviors* 34, 526–30.

Lago, L., Bruno, R., & Degenhardt, L. (2016). Concordance of ICD-11 and DSM-5 definitions of alcohol and cannabis use disorders: a population survey. *The Lancet Psychiatry* 3, 673–84.

Lago, L., Glantz, M., Kessler, R. C., *et al.* (2017). Substance dependence among those without symptoms of substance abuse in the World Mental Health Survey. *International Journal of Methods in Psychiatric Research* e1557. DOI: 10.1002/mpr.1557.

Lai, H. M., Cleary, M., Sitharthan, T., *et al.* (2015). Prevalence of comorbid substance use, anxiety and mood disorders in epidemiological surveys, 1990–2014: a systematic review and meta-analysis. *Drug & Alcohol Dependence* 154, 1–13.

Larney, S., Peacock, A., Mathers, B. M., *et al.* (2017). A systematic review of injecting-related injury and disease among people who inject drugs. *Drug & Alcohol Dependence* 171, 39–49.

Marzuk, P. M., Tardiff, K., Leon, A. C., *et al.* (1992). Prevalence of cocaine use among residents of New York City who committed suicide during a one-year period. *American Journal of Psychiatry* 149, 371–5.

McKetin, R., McLaren, J., Riddell, S., *et al.* (2006). The relationship between methamphetamine use and violent behaviour. *Crime and Justice Bulletin* 97, 1–16.

Mooney, M., Sofuoglu, M., Dudish-Poulsen, S., & Hatsukami, D. K. (2006). Preliminary observations of paranoia in a human laboratory study of cocaine. *Addictive Behaviors* 31, 1245–54.

Pani, P. P., Maremmani, I., Trogu, E., *et al.* (2010). Delineating the psychic structure of substance abuse and addictions: should anxiety, mood and impulse-control dysregulation be included? *Journal of Affective Disorders* 122, 185–97.

Rounsaville, B. J., Spitzer, R. L., & Williams, J. B. (1986). Proposed changes in DSM-III substance use disorders: description and rationale. *American Journal of Psychiatry* 143, 463–8.

Roy, A. (2001). Characteristics of cocaine-dependent patients who attempt suicide. *American Journal of Psychiatry* 158, 1215–19.

Satel, S. L., Southwick, S. M., & Gawin, F. H. (1991). Clinical features of cocaine-induced paranoia. *American Journal of Psychiatry* 148, 495–8.

Segal, D. S. & Kuczenski, R. (1997). Repeated binge exposures to amphetamine and methamphetamine: behavioral and neurochemical characterization[comment]. *Journal of Pharmacology & Experimental Therapeutics* 282, 561–73.

Sher, K., Wolf, S., & Martinez, J. (2009). How can etiological research inform the distinction between normal drinking and disordered drinking. In *Handbook of Drug Use Etiology: Theory, Methods, and Empirical Findings* (ed. L. M. Scheier). Washington: American Psychological Association, 225–46.

Singleton, J., Degenhardt, L., Hall, W., *et al.* (2009). Mortality among amphetamine users: a systematic review of cohort studies. *Drug & Alcohol Dependence* 105, 1–8.

Slade, T., Chiu, W.-T., Glantz, M., *et al.* (2016). A cross-national examination of differences in classification of lifetime alcohol use disorder between DSM-IV and DSM-5: findings from the World Mental Health Survey.

Alcoholism, Clinical and Experimental Research 40, 1728–36.

Srisurapanont, M., Ali, R., Marsden, J., *et al.* (2003). Psychotic symptoms in methamphetamine psychotic in-patients. *International Journal of Neuropsychopharmacology* 6, 347–52.

United Nations Office on Drugs and Crime (2008). *2008 Global ATS Assessment: Amphetamines and Ecstasy*. Vienna: United Nations.

(2009). *World Drug Report 2009*. Vienna: United Nations.

UNODC (2015). *World Drug Report 2015*. Vienna: United Nations.

World Health Organization (2016). *The Health and Social Effects of Nonmedical Cannabis Use*. Geneva: World Health Organization.

Wright, S. & Klee, H. (2001). Violent Crime, aggression and amphetamine: what are the implications for drug treatment services? *Drugs: Education, Prevention and Policy* 8, 70–90.

Chapter 18

Bulimia Nervosa and Binge-Eating Disorder

Ronald C. Kessler, James I. Hudson, Victoria Shahly, Andrzej Kiejna, Graça Cardoso

Introduction

Most epidemiologic data on eating disorders come from Western samples (Striegel-Moore & Franko 2003; Wade *et al.* 2011; Smink *et al.* 2012; Javaras & Hudson 2017). In addition, there have been very few recent population-based studies of the prevalence and correlates of eating disorders. Furthermore, most such studies focus on the two specific eating disorders, anorexia nervosa (AN) and bulimia nervosa (BN), specified in DSM-IV and ignore the provisional DSM-IV diagnosis of binge-eating disorder (BED). The latter diagnosis is characterized by recurrent persistent episodes of uncontrolled binge eating with distress but without the inappropriate compensatory behaviours of BN. DSM-5 subsequently recognized BED as a distinct diagnostic entity on the basis of emerging evidence of its validity and clinical importance (Striegel-Moore & Franko 2008; Wonderlich *et al.* 2009). The initial reports from component World Mental Health (WMH) surveys in the United States (Hudson *et al.* 2007) and Western Europe (Preti *et al.* 2009) were influential in this process because they provided the first large representative population-based data on BED in the United States and Europe, showing that BED had a higher prevalence than BN and AN combined, and that BED was associated with obesity and with impairment in role functioning. Epidemiologic studies of BED continue to be rare.

In this chapter, we review the WMH data on the prevalence and correlates of BED and compare the BED data to data on BN. The results reported here are somewhat different from those in earlier WMH reports on BED vs BN (Kessler *et al.* 2013, 2014) because one more recently completed WMH survey has been added to the results reported here. It should be noted that the WMH surveys also assessed AN but that the number of surveys doing so was small and the prevalence estimates quite low, leading us not to present data on AN in this chapter.

Method

Eating disorders were considered of secondary interest in the WMH surveys. As a result, only 15 surveys included these disorders in their assessments and the majority of them made the assessment with only a random subsample of Part II respondents. Only 14 of these surveys are included in the current chapter. The exception is the survey in Romania, which yielded BN and BED lifetime prevalence estimates of 0.2% and 0.0%, respectively (Kessler *et al.* 2013). The Romanian survey was deleted because of extremely low prevalence. The other 14 surveys include two in low/lower-middle-income-countries (Colombia, Peru), two in upper-middle-income countries (São Paulo Brazil, Mexico), and 10 in high-income countries (Belgium, France, Germany, New Zealand, Northern Ireland, Poland, Portugal, Spain, the Netherlands, and the United States). A total of 25,764 respondents were included in the assessment, representing the entire Part II sample in three surveys (São Paulo Brazil, New Zealand, Poland) and probability subsamples of the Part II sample in the other surveys.

As detailed elsewhere, the Composite International Diagnositic Interview (CIDI) symptom questions for DSM-IV BN and BED closely parallel DSM-IV criteria (Kessler *et al.* 2013). There are only two exceptions to that general statement. First, whereas DSM-IV BED requires six months of regular binge eating, the CIDI asked only about three months. However, this duration is consistent both with DSM-IV BN criteria as well as with DSM-5 BED criteria (American Psychiatric Association 2013). Second, DSM-IV requires loss of control and distress regarding binges. Rather than address these symptoms directly, the CIDI questioned about attitudes and behaviours indicative of loss of control and distress (upset at out-of-control eating; feeling guilty, upset, or depressed after binging; continued eating after full; eating until uncomfortably full; eating alone because of embarrassment about volume eaten), introducing some imprecision into these assessments. DSM-IV diagnostic hierarchy rules do not allow BN or BED diagnoses in the presence of AN, or BED in the presence of BN. These hierarchy rules were implemented with retrospective age-of-onset (AOO) reports.

Given the special importance of body-mass index (BMI) for eating disorders, we also use self-reports of current height and weight data reported in the surveys to calculate BMI and examine the associations of 12-month BED and BN with BMI.

Results

Prevalence

Lifetime prevalence estimates average 1.8% for BED (Table 18.1) and 1.0% for BN (Table 18.2) across surveys. Range and inter-quartile range (IQR; 25th–75th percentiles) of lifetime prevalence estimates across surveys are 0.5–4.7% (0.8–1.9%) for BED and 0.2–2.0% (0.4–1.0%) for BN. Twelve-month prevalence estimates (IQR) average 0.8% (0.3–1.0%) for BED and 0.4% (0.2–0.3%) for BN. Thirty-day prevalence is only about half as high as 12-month prevalence (an average across surveys of 55.5% for BED and 51.3% for BN): 0.5% (0.1–0.5) for BED and 0.2% (0.1–0.2) for BN. Lifetime, 12-month, and 30-day prevalence estimates are all higher for BED than BN in the vast majority of countries.

Age-of-Onset and Persistence

Median (IQR) AOO is consistently earlier for BN [21 (19–24)] than BED [24 (21–31)] (Tables 18.3 and 18.4). Inspection of AOO distributions shows the slope to be less steep for BED than BN and the IQR to be narrower for BN than BED, although country-specific AOO curves show considerable variability around these central tendencies. The later AOO distribution of BED leads to the projected lifetime risk at age 75 [2.5% (1.0–2.6%)] being a good deal higher than lifetime prevalence [1.8% (0.8–1.9)]. Projected lifetime risk of BN [1.2% (0.6–1.2)], in comparison, is much more similar to lifetime prevalence [1.0% (0.4–1.0)].

A direct measure of retrospectively reported persistence examined in our previous report on BED and BN (Kessler *et al.* 2013) was somewhat higher for BN than BED, with median (IQR) years in episode 6.5 (2.2–15.4) for BN and 4.3 (1.0–11.7) for BED. However, the mean (IQR) ratio of 12-month/lifetime prevalence in Tables 18.1 and 18.2, which can be thought of as an indirect measure of persistence, is lower for BN [36.7% (28.3–58.0)] than BED [44.4% (34.3–51.1)], although within-survey differences are inconsistent (eight higher for BN than BED; six higher for BED than BN).

Associations with Body-Mass Index (BMI)

As reported in our original WMH paper on BED and BN (Kessler *et al.* 2013), WMH respondents with BED and BN have significantly higher current BMI than respondents without a history of eating disorders. Lower proportions of respondents with lifetime and 12-month BN and BED are underweight (0.5–1.5% vs 2.8%, $z = 1.4–6.4$, $P = 0.16 < 0.001$) or normal weight (25.0–33.7% vs 47.3%, $t = 4.6–7.7$, $P < 0.001$), and higher proportions are obese (32.8–41.7% vs 15.8%, $t = 4.5–7.5$, $P < 0.001$) than those without lifetime eating disorders. No significant BN vs BED differences exist in proportions underweight, normal weight, overweight, obese, or severely obese ($t = 0.3–1.0$, $P = 0.29–0.78$). Disaggregated results (reported in Kessler *et al.* 2013) found equivalent patterns in the WMH surveys carried out in the United States, Latin America, Europe, and New Zealand.

Impairment in Role Attainment and Role Functioning

An earlier WMH report estimated time-lagged associations between temporally primary eating disorders and subsequent role transitions (Kessler *et al.* 2013). We found there that both BED and BN predicted significantly increased subsequent levels of educational attainment among women but not men and that early-onset BED predicted reduced odds of current (at time of interview) marriage (among females) and reduced odds of current employment (among males). However, these significant associations all disappeared when controls were introduced into the prediction equations for comorbid disorders.

In Tables 18.5 and 18.6 we show associations of 12-month eating disorders with role impairments. Severe role impairment is reported by 21.3% of

Table 18.1 Prevalence of DSM-IV binge-eating disorder (BED) in the World Mental Health surveys

Country	Lifetime prevalence		12-month prevalence		30-day prevalence		12-month prevalence of BED among lifetime cases		30-day prevalence of BED among 12-month cases		Sample size used
	%	SE	%	SE	%	SE	%	SE	%	SE	
Low/lower-middle-income countries	**0.8**	**0.2**	**0.3**	**0.1**	**0.1**	**0.0**	**37.0**	**10.1**	**25.8**	**12.4**	**2,114**
Colombia	0.9	0.2	0.3	0.1	–	–	34.3	13.1	–	–	1,217
Peru	0.8	0.3	0.3	0.2	0.2	0.1	40.8	15.9	56.9	18.0	897
Upper-middle-income countries	**3.8**	**0.3**	**1.4**	**0.2**	**0.9**	**0.2**	**38.0**	**5.9**	**65.8**	**6.3**	**4,178**
Brazil	4.7	0.3	1.8	0.3	1.2	0.2	38.5	6.6	66.8	6.8	2,942
Mexico	1.6	0.4	0.5	0.2	0.3	0.2	33.9	11.8	57.9	19.8	1,236
High-income countries	**1.5**	**0.1**	**0.7**	**0.1**	**0.4**	**0.0**	**48.2**	**3.0**	**52.6**	**4.7**	**19,472**
Belgium	1.2	0.4	0.7	0.4	0.5	0.4	53.0	20.3	74.0	20.5	518
France	1.7	0.8	0.3	0.2	0.3	0.2	20.1	16.4	95.3	5.4	466
Germany	0.5	0.2	0.1	0.1	0.1	0.1	16.6	12.0	100.0	0.0	658
New Zealand	1.9	0.2	1.0	0.1	0.6	0.1	51.1	4.2	62.6	6.3	7,312
Northern Ireland	1.5	0.3	0.8	0.3	0.3	0.2	57.8	13.1	34.6	16.1	1,432
Poland	0.6	0.1	0.3	0.1	0.1	0.0	45.1	10.6	19.5	11.5	4,000
Portugal	2.4	0.6	1.1	0.4	0.8	0.4	44.5	13.9	80.0	15.7	509
Spain	0.8	0.3	0.5	0.3	0.0	0.0	62.7	20.8	8.0	7.2	1,057
Netherlands	0.9	0.5	0.1	0.1	–	–	7.8	8.2	–	–	540
United States	2.6	0.3	1.2	0.2	0.6	0.1	46.5	5.8	47.3	9.9	2,980
All countries combined	**1.8**	**0.1**	**0.8**	**0.1**	**0.5**	**0.0**	**44.4**	**2.8**	**55.5**	**3.7**	**25,764**
WHO regions[a]											
Region of the Americas	2.7	0.2	1.1	0.1	0.6	0.1	40.5	4.2	56.8	5.2	9,272
Western Pacific region	1.9	0.2	1.0	0.1	0.6	0.1	51.1	4.2	62.6	6.3	7,312
Western European region	1.2	0.2	0.6	0.1	0.3	0.1	45.1	7.4	46.9	10.6	5,180
Eastern European region	0.6	0.1	0.3	0.1	0.1	0.0	45.1	10.6	19.5	11.5	4,000
Comparison between countries[b]	**$F_{13,v} = 12.7$*, $P < 0.001$**		**$F_{13,v} = 8.7$*, $P < 0.001$**		**$F_{13,v} = 7.3$*, $P < 0.001$**		**$F_{13,v} = 0.9$, $P = 0.537$**		**$F_{13,v} = 1.9$*, $P = 0.032$**		
Comparison between low-, middle- and high-income country groups[b]	**$F_{2,v} = 38.6$*, $P < 0.001$**		**$F_{2,v} = 13.0$*, $P < 0.001$**		**$F_{2,v} = 20.0$*, $P < 0.001$**		**$F_{2,v} = 1.5$, $P = 0.230$**		**$F_{2,v} = 3.3$*, $P = 0.038$**		
Comparison between WHO regions[b]	**$F_{3,v} = 36.1$*, $P < 0.001$**		**$F_{3,v} = 15.2$*, $P < 0.001$**		**$F_{3,v} = 20.3$*, $P < 0.001$**		**$F_{3,v} = 1.0$, $P = 0.374$**		**$F_{3,v} = 2.2$, $P = 0.088$**		

*Significant at the 0.05 level, two-sided test.

[a]Region of the Americas (Colombia, Mexico, Brazil, Peru, United States); Western Pacific region (New Zealand); Western European region (Belgium, France, Germany, Netherlands, Spain, Northern Ireland, Portugal); Eastern European region (Poland).

[b]Wald design-corrected F-tests were used to determine if there is variation in prevalence estimates across countries. The denominator degree of freedom, v, is 658.

Table 18.2 Prevalence of DSM-IV bulimia nervosa (BN) in the World Mental Health surveys

Country	Lifetime prevalence		12-month prevalence		30-day prevalence		12-month prevalence of BN among lifetime cases		30-day prevalence of BN among 12-month cases		Sample size used
	%	SE	%	SE	%	SE	%	SE	%	SE	
Low/lower-middle-income countries	**0.4**	**0.1**	**0.2**	**0.1**	**0.1**	**0.1**	**66.2**	**14.1**	**30.7**	**20.4**	**2,114**
Colombia	0.4	0.1	0.2	0.1	0.1	0.1	58.0	18.5	43.7	30.1	1,217
Peru	0.4	0.2	0.3	0.2	0.0	0.0	78.3	19.8	16.5	17.6	897
Upper-middle-income countries	**1.6**	**0.2**	**0.7**	**0.2**	**0.4**	**0.1**	**45.3**	**6.2**	**47.7**	**10.7**	**4,178**
Brazil	2.0	0.2	0.9	0.2	0.4	0.1	46.9	6.9	46.2	11.7	2,942
Mexico	0.8	0.2	0.3	0.1	0.2	0.1	35.7	12.2	59.3	19.5	1,236
High-income countries	**0.9**	**0.1**	**0.3**	**0.0**	**0.2**	**0.0**	**32.0**	**3.2**	**55.3**	**5.6**	**19,472**
Belgium	1.1	0.5	0.3	0.3	0.3	0.3	28.3	23.0	100.0	0.0	518
France	0.7	0.4	0.2	0.2	0.2	0.2	26.9	21.4	100.0	0.0	466
Germany	0.4	0.1	0.2	0.1	0.2	0.2	62.8	17.0	63.5	38.0	658
New Zealand	1.3	0.1	0.5	0.1	0.3	0.0	33.8	4.4	55.8	7.4	7,312
Northern Ireland	0.5	0.1	0.2	0.1	0.1	0.0	36.2	14.0	44.5	23.6	1,432
Poland	0.2	0.1	0.1	0.0	0.0	0.0	22.1	9.2	19.6	17.7	4,000
Portugal	0.8	0.3	0.5	0.2	0.1	0.1	60.3	21.7	22.2	17.3	509
Spain	0.7	0.4	0.1	0.1	0.0	0.0	16.5	12.8	23.9	23.2	1,057
Netherlands	0.9	0.5	0.1	0.1	0.1	0.1	13.4	11.0	100.0	0.0	540
United States	1.0	0.2	0.3	0.1	0.2	0.1	30.7	6.8	61.1	10.7	2,980
All countries combined	**1.0**	**0.1**	**0.4**	**0.0**	**0.2**	**0.0**	**36.7**	**3.0**	**51.3**	**5.2**	**25,764**
WHO regions[a]											
Region of the Americas	1.2	0.1	0.5	0.1	0.2	0.1	42.7	4.7	48.5	8.2	9,272
Western Pacific region	1.3	0.1	0.5	0.1	0.3	0.0	33.8	4.4	55.8	7.4	7,312
Western European region	0.7	0.1	0.2	0.1	0.1	0.0	31.1	7.3	55.8	13.9	5,180
Eastern European region	0.2	0.1	0.1	0.0	0.0	0.0	22.1	9.2	19.6	17.7	4,000
Comparison between countries[b]	**$F_{13,v}=7.9$* $P<0.001$**		**$F_{13,v}=4.0$* $P<0.001$**		**$F_{13,v}=3.5$* $P<0.001$**		**$F_{13,v}=0.9$, $P=0.506$**		**$F_{13,v}=0.8$, $P=0.701$**		
Comparison between low-, middle-, and high-income country groups[b]	**$F_{2,v}=18.2$* $P<0.001$**		**$F_{2,v}=4.2$* $P=0.015$**		**$F_{2,v}=3.0$* $P=0.049$**		**$F_{2,v}=2.8$, $P=0.059$**		**$F_{2,v}=0.7$ $P=0.509$**		
Comparison between WHO regions[b]	**$F_{3,v}=24.9$* $P<0.001$**		**$F_{3,v}=16.5$* $P<0.001$**		**$F_{3,v}=14.6$* $P<0.001$**		**$F_{3,v}=1.3$, $P=0.264$**		**$F_{3,v}=0.8$, $P=0.487$**		

*Significant at the 0.05 level, two-sided test.
[a]**Region of the Americas** (Colombia, Mexico, Brazil, Peru, United States); **Western Pacific region** (New Zealand); **Western European region** (Belgium, France, Germany, Netherlands, Spain, Northern Ireland, Portugal); **Eastern European region** (Poland).
[b]Wald design-corrected F-tests were used to determine if there is variation in prevalence estimates across countries. The denominator degree of freedom, v, is 658.

respondents with 12-month BED (Table 18.5) and 31.7% of those with 12-month BN (Table 18.6). Prevalence of these severe role impairments is relatively similar in the four role domains assessed by the SDS: home (11.1% for BED vs. 16.2% for BN); work (9.8% vs. 11.7%); relationships (10.2% vs. 15.1%); and social life (13.3% vs. 17.5%). None of these aggregate differences between BED and BD is statistically significant.

Socio-demographic Correlates

Thirty-day prevalences of BED (Table 18.7) and BN (Table 18.8) are significantly less common among respondents ages 60+ than younger respondents and higher among those 18–44 than those aged 45–59. However, BED is somewhat more common among respondents ages 30–44 than those 18–29, while BN

Table 18.3 Age at selected percentiles on the standardized age-of-onset distributions of DSM-IV binge-eating disorder (BED) with projected lifetime risk at age 75

Country	Ages at selected percentiles								Lifetime prevalence of BED		Projected risk at age 75	
	5	10	25	50	75	90	95	99	%	SE	%	SE
Low/lower-middle-income countries	10	16	21	36	53	56	56	56	0.8	0.2	1.5	0.4
Colombia[a]	13	16	20	36	41	53	53	53	0.9	0.2	1.5	0.4
Peru[a]	10	16	21	37	56	56	56	56	0.8	0.3	1.6	0.7
Upper-middle-income countries	14	17	20	27	41	52	58	67	3.8	0.3	5.6	0.4
Brazil	14	17	20	26	41	52	58	61	4.7	0.3	6.8	0.5
Mexico[a]	15	17	25	29	37	43	49	49	1.6	0.4	2.4	0.6
High-income countries	11	14	18	23	36	51	56	62	1.5	0.1	2.1	0.1
Belgium	15	21	22	26	41	41	43	43	1.2	0.4	1.7	0.7
France	5	5	5	26	57	57	59	59	1.7	0.8	2.6	1.1
Germany	18	18	20	21	43	51	51	51	0.5	0.2	0.7	0.3
New Zealand	11	14	17	21	31	46	51	64	1.9	0.2	2.4	0.2
Northern Ireland	10	10	16	17	29	33	37	55	1.5	0.3	1.8	0.4
Poland[b]	20	20	21	31	51	56	56	56	0.6	0.1	0.9	0.2
Portugal	11	13	17	25	33	40	54	54	2.4	0.6	2.9	0.8
Spain	17	18	20	33	33	33	36	38	0.8	0.3	1.0	0.5
Netherlands	12	12	12	21	25	28	28	28	0.9	0.5	0.9	0.5
United States	11	15	20	28	41	54	60	60	2.6	0.3	3.8	0.6
All countries combined	12	15	19	24	38	51	56	62	1.8	0.1	2.5	0.1
WHO regions												
Region of the Americas	13	16	20	28	41	54	58	61	2.7	0.2	4.1	0.3
Western Pacific region	11	14	17	21	31	46	51	64	1.9	0.2	2.4	0.2
Western European region	5	12	16	25	33	41	55	57	1.2	0.2	1.6	0.2
Eastern European region	20	20	21	31	51	56	56	56	0.6	0.1	0.9	0.2

[a]The projected risk for these countries is at age 65 because the age range of these surveys is between 18 and 65.
[b]The projected risk for this country is at age 64 because the age range of this survey is between 18 and 64.

is somewhat less common among respondents 30–44 than 18–29. These age differences are due to inverse association of age-at-interview with increased lifetime prevalence rather than to associations of either AOO or time-since-onset with persistence (12-month/lifetime). This pattern is consistent with either an increase in eating disorders over time in more recent cohorts, differential recall error for prior lifetime cases, and/or differential mortality. Thirty-day prevalence is also significantly higher among women than men (BED OR 2.2; BN OR 3.8) and, as with age, this is due to significantly elevated odds of lifetime prevalence among women compared to men rather than to gender differences in disorder or episode persistence. Employment status (χ^2_4=3.5–4.7, P = 0.47–0.32) and marital status (χ^2_2 = 0.1–3.0, P = 0.96–0.22), in comparison, are unrelated to 30-day prevalence of BED and BN. The associations of education level and household income with 30-day prevalence, finally, differ across the two disorders, with these associations significant but non-monotonic in predicting 30-day BED but nonsignificant in predicting 30-day BN.

Comorbidity

The vast majority of respondents with lifetime BED (79.6%) and BN (87.8%) meet lifetime criteria for other DSM-IV disorders (Tables 18.9 and 18.10). More detailed analyses presented in an earlier WMH report show that ORs of BN and BED with each of the other disorders are positive and significant (BN Median = 4.3, IQR = 3.5–4.6; BED Median = 2.8, IQR = 2.7–3.3)

Table 18.4 Age at selected percentiles on the standardized age-of-onset distributions of DSM-IV bulimia nervosa (BN) with projected lifetime risk at age 75

Country	Ages at selected percentiles								Lifetime prevalence of BN		Projected risk at age 75	
	5	10	25	50	75	90	95	99	%	SE	%	SE
Low/lower-middle-income countries	14	15	16	21	30	40	40	40	0.4	0.1	0.5	0.1
Colombia[a]	14	14	15	17	24	36	36	36	0.4	0.1	0.4	0.2
Peru[a]	21	21	21	21	30	40	40	40	0.4	0.2	0.5	0.2
Upper-middle-income countries	12	15	19	25	36	43	48	66	1.6	0.2	2.3	0.2
Brazil	12	15	19	24	36	41	45	66	2.0	0.2	2.7	0.3
Mexico[a]	13	18	19	26	43	48	48	48	0.8	0.2	1.3	0.4
High-income countries	11	14	16	20	26	39	43	51	0.9	0.1	1.0	0.1
Belgium	15	19	21	23	23	33	34	34	1.1	0.5	1.2	0.5
France	11	18	18	21	21	23	33	33	0.7	0.4	0.8	0.4
Germany	15	15	18	43	43	43	43	43	0.4	0.1	0.6	0.2
New Zealand	12	14	16	19	24	39	47	57	1.3	0.1	1.6	0.1
Northern Ireland	15	16	20	22	41	51	51	51	0.5	0.1	0.6	0.2
Poland[b]	17	17	20	21	21	26	51	51	0.2	0.1	0.3	0.1
Portugal	18	18	30	36	36	43	43	43	0.8	0.3	1.1	0.5
Spain	16	17	18	19	36	36	45	45	0.7	0.4	0.9	0.4
Netherlands	11	11	11	18	22	27	37	37	0.9	0.5	1.0	0.5
United States	9	14	16	19	24	36	39	40	1.0	0.2	1.2	0.2
All countries combined	11	14	17	21	30	41	43	57	1.0	0.1	1.2	0.1
WHO regions												
Region of the Americas	11	14	18	21	33	41	43	66	1.2	0.1	1.5	0.1
Western Pacific region	12	14	16	19	24	39	47	57	1.3	0.1	1.6	0.1
Western European region	11	16	18	21	33	43	43	51	0.7	0.1	0.8	0.1
Eastern European region	17	17	20	21	21	26	51	51	0.2	0.1	0.3	0.1

[a]The projected risk for these countries is at age 65 because the age range of these surveys is between 18 and 65.
[b]The projected risk for this country is at age 64 because the age range of this survey is between 18 and 64.

(Kessler *et al.* 2013). Highest rates of BED and BN comorbidity are with anxiety (54.6–63.3%) and mood (45.2–57.1%) disorders. Rates of comorbidity are lower with disruptive behaviour/impulse-control disorders (23.7–32.3%) and substance-use disorders (23.9–26.8%). Rates of comorbidity between lifetime BED-BN and *12-month* comorbid disorders are generally similar to those of lifetime BED-BN with *lifetime* comorbid disorders. Rates of comorbidity between 12-month BED-BN and 12-month comorbid disorders, in comparison, are lower (e.g., 61.0–73.4% overall vs 82.6–84.9% for lifetime BED-BN).

Comparison of AOO reports suggests that BED and BN typically have first onsets at later ages than the other DSM-IV disorders with which they are comorbid. More detailed analyses presented in an earlier WMH report used retrospective AOO reports to estimate reciprocal survival models of (i) temporally primary eating disorders predicting subsequent first onset of other mental disorders and (ii) temporally primary other mental disorders predicting subsequent first onset of eating disorders (Kessler *et al.* 2013). The time-lagged ORs were mostly elevated and significant in both directions, but generally higher for other disorders predicting eating disorders than the reverse. Median (IQR) ORs of BN predicting other disorders were generally higher than those of BED predicting the same disorders (BN 3.3 [2.8–4.4]) vs. BED (2.3 [2.0–2.7]). ORs in reciprocal models showed that other disorders predicted subsequent first onset of BN somewhat more powerfully than first onset of BED (BN 5.1 [3.8–6.0] vs. BED 3.4 [3.3–3.9]).

Treatment

Somewhat more than one-third (37.3%) of respondents with 12-month BED and 44.4% with 12-month

Table 18.5 Severity of role impairment (Sheehan Disability Scale) associated with 12-month binge-eating disorder, by country

Country	Proportion with severe role impairment (SDS score: 7–10)										Number of 12-month cases
	Home		Work		Relationship		Social		Any[a]		
	%	SE	%	SE	%	SE	%	SE	%	SE	
Low/lower-middle-income countries	**19.7**	**17.0**	**19.7**	**17.0**	**19.7**	**17.0**	**19.7**	**17.0**	**19.7**	**17.0**	**13**
Colombia	36.5	27.1	36.5	27.1	36.5	27.1	36.5	27.1	36.5	27.1	7
Peru	–	–	–	–	–	–	–	–	–	–	6
Upper-middle-income countries	**16.0**	**4.0**	**16.0**	**4.4**	**19.0**	**7.3**	**22.9**	**8.3**	**29.3**	**7.2**	**102**
Brazil	17.9	4.4	18.1	5.0	20.6	8.2	25.0	9.3	32.0	7.8	89
Mexico	–	–	–	–	5.9	6.2	5.9	6.2	6.2	6.6	13
High-income countries	**8.7**	**2.3**	**6.9**	**2.3**	**6.3**	**1.8**	**9.0**	**2.1**	**18.1**	**3.3**	**242**
Belgium	–	–	–	–	–	–	–	–	–	–	5
France	–	–	–	–	–	–	–	–	–	–	4
Germany	–	–	–	–	–	–	–	–	–	–	2
New Zealand	7.4	2.9	9.7	3.8	5.0	2.6	5.0	1.6	17.4	4.6	134
Northern Ireland	28.0	17.0	23.7	17.2	11.3	6.7	20.5	13.3	42.9	18.3	14
Poland	5.9	5.9	5.6	5.6	9.6	7.0	4.0	4.1	10.0	7.3	15
Portugal	–	–	–	–	–	–	–	–	–	–	9
Spain	–	–	–	–	11.3	10.2	7.2	8.1	11.3	10.2	7
Netherlands	–	–	–	–	–	–	–	–	–	–	1
United States	10.7	4.7	–	–	6.3	4.0	17.7	6.6	20.9	7.0	51
All countries combined	**11.1**	**2.0**	**9.8**	**2.0**	**10.2**	**2.4**	**13.3**	**2.9**	**21.3**	**3.1**	**357**
WHO regions											
Region of the Americas	14.4	3.0	10.4	2.7	14.6	4.6	20.9	5.5	25.8	5.0	166
Western Pacific region	7.4	2.9	9.7	3.8	5.0	2.6	5.0	1.6	17.4	4.6	134
Western European region	10.8	6.4	9.0	6.2	8.4	3.5	10.4	5.2	19.3	7.8	42
Eastern European region	5.9	5.9	5.6	5.6	9.6	7.0	4.0	4.1	10.0	7.3	15
Comparison between countries[b]	**$F_{13,v} = 1.4$, P = 0.133**		**$F_{13,v} = 1.7$, P = 0.051**		**$F_{13,v} = 0.9$, P = 0.580**		**$F_{13,v} = 1.1$, P = 0.385**		**$F_{13,v} = 1.3$, P = 0.196**		
Comparison between low-, middle-, and high-income countries[b]	**$F_{2,v} = 1.4$, P = 0.241**		**$F_{2,v} = 2.0$, P = 0.143**		**$F_{2,v} = 1.7$, P = 0.180**		**$F_{2,v} = 1.4$, P = 0.238**		**$F_{2,v} = 1.0$, P = 0.372**		
Comparison between WHO regions[b]	**$F_{3,v} = 1.1$, P = 0.365**		**$F_{3,v} = 0.2$, P = 0.909**		**$F_{3,v} = 1.1$, P = 0.342**		**$F_{3,v} = 2.6$, P = 0.051**		**$F_{3,v} = 0.9$, P = 0.423**		

A dash indicates low cell count (<5 cases).
[a]Highest severity category across four SDS role domains.
[b]Wald design-corrected F-tests were used to determine if there is variation in impairment severity across countries. The denominator degree of freedom, v, is 658.

Table 18.6 Severity of role impairment (Sheehan Disability Scale) associated with 12-month bulimia nervosa, by country

Country	Proportion with severe role impairment (SDS score: 7–10)										Number of 12-month cases
	Home		Work		Relationship		Social		Any[a]		
	%	SE	%	SE	%	SE	%	SE	%	SE	
Low/lower-middle-income countries	–	–	–	–	–	–	–	–	–	–	**6**
Colombia	–	–	–	–	–	–	–	–	–	–	3
Peru	–	–	–	–	–	–	–	–	–	–	3
Upper-middle-income countries	**7.8**	**4.7**	**5.9**	**2.7**	**20.0**	**5.7**	**16.4**	**5.8**	**27.0**	**7.7**	**45**
Brazil	7.7	5.0	5.6	2.9	21.0	6.1	17.0	6.3	28.7	8.2	38
Mexico	9.4	9.9	9.4	9.9	9.4	9.9	9.4	9.9	9.4	9.9	7
High-income countries	**21.0**	**5.6**	**14.2**	**4.5**	**13.2**	**4.5**	**18.8**	**4.9**	**34.2**	**6.1**	**115**
Belgium	–	–	–	–	–	–	–	–	–	–	1
France	–	–	–	–	–	–	–	–	–	–	2
Germany	–	–	–	–	–	–	–	–	–	–	3
New Zealand	15.6	6.0	12.5	4.9	14.7	6.2	19.0	6.5	26.6	7.0	73
Northern Ireland	15.1	14.6	15.1	14.6	38.5	26.5	–	–	53.6	24.0	5
Poland	–	–	–	–	–	–	14.1	13.6	14.1	13.6	5
Portugal	40.2	30.6	–	–	40.2	30.6	40.2	30.6	40.2	30.6	5
Spain	–	–	–	–	–	–	–	–	–	–	3
Netherlands	–	–	–	–	–	–	–	–	–	–	2
United States	26.7	15.9	27.9	16.5	7.1	5.2	32.7	13.9	45.3	16.7	16
All countries combined	**16.2**	**4.1**	**11.7**	**3.2**	**15.1**	**3.5**	**17.5**	**3.7**	**31.7**	**4.8**	**166**
WHO regions											
Region of the Americas	12.0	5.5	12.0	5.0	15.9	4.5	19.1	5.4	31.4	7.1	67
Western Pacific region	15.6	6.0	12.5	4.9	14.7	6.2	19.0	6.5	26.6	7.0	73
Western European region	39.8	15.8	9.0	6.4	16.8	11.4	5.1	4.5	55.5	14.3	21
Eastern European region	–	–	–	–	–	–	14.1	13.6	14.1	13.6	5
Comparison between countries[b]	**$F_{13,v}=0.7$, $P=0.782$**		**$F_{13,v}=0.7$, $P=0.769$**		**$F_{13,v}=0.8$, $P=0.612$**		**$F_{13,v}=0.8$, $P=0.633$**		**$F_{13,v}=0.8$, $P=0.707$**		
Comparison between low-, middle-, and high-income countries[b]	**$F_{2,v}=1.9$, $P=0.144$**		**$F_{2,v}=1.2$, $P=0.290$**		**$F_{2,v}=1.6$, $P=0.195$**		**$F_{2,v}=1.3$, $P=0.287$**		**$F_{2,v}=0.3$ $P=0.753$**		
Comparison between WHO regions[b]	**$F_{3,v}=1.7$, $P=0.171$**		**$F_{3,v}=0.9$, $P=0.467$**		**$F_{3,v}=1.4$, $P=0.252$**		**$F_{3,v}=1.1$, $P=0.340$**		**$F_{3,v}=1.0$, $P=0.379$**		

A dash indicates low cell count (<5 cases).
[a]Highest severity category across four SDS role domains.
[b]Wald design-corrected F-tests were used to determine if there is variation in impairment severity across countries. The denominator degree of freedom, v, is 658.

Table 18.7 Bivariate associations between socio-demographic correlates and DSM-IV binge-eating disorder (BED), all countries combined

Correlates	30-day BED[a]		Lifetime BED[b]		12-month BED among lifetime cases[c]		30-day BED among 12-month cases[c]	
	OR	(95% CI)	OR	(95% CI)	OR	(95% CI)	OR	(95% CI)
Age-cohort								
18–29	**3.5***	(1.4–8.7)	**26.7***	(14.7–48.7)				
30–44	**4.6***	(1.8–11.6)	**13.5***	(7.9–23.0)				
45–59	**2.8***	(1.1–7.0)	**4.5***	(2.8–7.2)				
60+	**1.0**		**1.0**					
Age-cohort difference[d]	$\chi^2_3 = 11.5^*, P < 0.001$		$\chi^2_3 = 154.3^*, P < 0.001$					
Age-of-onset								
Early					**0.5***	(0.3–1.0)	**1.2**	(0.5–3.2)
Early-average					**0.7**	(0.4–1.1)	**0.9**	(0.4–2.1)
Late-average					**0.9**	(0.5–1.5)	**0.9**	(0.4–2.3)
Late					**1.0**		**1.0**	
Age-of-onset difference[d]					$\chi^2_3 = 5.8, P = 0.123$		$\chi^2_3 = 0.5, P = 0.918$	
Time since onset (continuous)					**1.00**	(0.99–1.02)	**1.02**	(0.99–1.05)
Gender								
Female	**2.2***	(1.4–3.6)	**2.3***	(1.8–2.9)	**1.1**	(0.7–1.9)	**0.8**	(0.4–1.6)
Male	**1.0**		**1.0**		**1.0**		**1.0**	
Gender difference[d]	$\chi^2_1 = 11.3^*, P = 0.001$		$\chi^2_1 = 40.3^*, P < 0.001$		$\chi^2_1 = 0.3, P = 0.591$		$\chi^2_1 = 0.4, P = 0.526$	
Employment status								
Student	**1.5**	(0.7–3.4)	**1.3**	(0.7–2.2)	**1.5**	(0.6–4.1)	**2.2**	(0.6–8.1)
Homemaker	**1.2**	(0.7–2.0)	**0.9**	(0.6–1.2)	**1.4**	(0.8–2.3)	**1.2**	(0.4–3.5)
Retired	**0.5**	(0.2–1.5)	**1.2**	(0.6–2.3)	**1.5**	(0.5–4.4)	**0.1***	(0.0–0.4)
Other	**0.9**	(0.5–1.6)	**1.4***	(1.0–2.0)	**0.9**	(0.5–1.5)	**0.7**	(0.2–1.9)
Employed	**1.0**		**1.0**		**1.0**		**1.0**	
Employment status difference[d]	$\chi^2_4 = 3.5, P = 0.471$		$\chi^2_4 = 6.9, P = 0.141$		$\chi^2_4 = 3.8, P = 0.439$		$\chi^2_4 = 10.9^*, P = 0.028$	

(cont.)

Table 18.7 *(cont.)*

Correlates	30-day BED[a]		Lifetime BED[b]		12-month BED among lifetime cases[c]		30-day BED among 12-month cases[c]	
	OR	(95% CI)	OR	(95% CI)	OR	(95% CI)	OR	(95% CI)
Marital status								
Never married	**1.0**	(0.6–1.6)	**1.6***	(1.2–2.0)	**0.6***	(0.4–0.9)	**1.8**	(0.8–4.0)
Divorced/separated/widowed	**1.1**	(0.6–1.9)	**1.4***	(1.0–1.8)	**1.1**	(0.6–2.0)	**0.5**	(0.3–1.2)
Currently married	**1.0**		**1.0**		**1.0**		**1.0**	
Marital status difference[d]	$\chi^2_2 = 0.1$, P = 0.957		$\chi^2_2 = 14.6$*, P = 0.001		$\chi^2_2 = 6.2$*, P = 0.045		$\chi^2_2 = 5.4$, P = 0.066	
Education level								
No education and some primary	**1.1**	(0.5–2.5)	**1.2**	(0.7–1.9)	**1.4**	(0.6–3.8)	**0.4**	(0.1–1.4)
Finished primary	**0.9**	(0.4–2.4)	**1.1**	(0.6–1.9)	**1.1**	(0.4–2.9)	**0.4**	(0.1–1.6)
Some secondary	**0.9**	(0.5–1.8)	**1.5***	(1.0–2.1)	**0.9**	(0.4–1.7)	**0.7**	(0.2–2.2)
Finished secondary	**1.2**	(0.6–2.2)	**1.2**	(0.8–1.6)	**1.2**	(0.6–2.5)	**0.8**	(0.3–2.2)
Some college	**0.7**	(0.3–1.4)	**1.2**	(0.8–1.7)	**1.0**	(0.5–2.0)	**0.3***	(0.1–1.0)
Finished college	**1.0**		**1.0**		**1.0**		**1.0**	
Education level difference[d]	$\chi^2_5 = 2.3$, P = 0.803		$\chi^2_5 = 5.7$, P = 0.337		$\chi^2_5 = 2.3$, P = 0.806		$\chi^2_5 = 7.6$, P = 0.179	
Household income								
Low	**1.1**	(0.6–1.8)	**1.4***	(1.0–1.8)	0.7	(0.3–1.2)	**1.2**	(0.5–3.0)
Low-average	**0.6**	(0.3–1.2)	**1.1**	(0.8–1.5)	0.5	(0.3–1.0)	**1.0**	(0.4–2.4)
High-average	**0.4***	(0.2–0.8)	**1.2**	(0.8–1.7)	0.4*	(0.2–0.7)	**0.4**	(0.2–1.2)
High	**1.0**		**1.0**		1.0		**1.0**	
Household income difference[d]	$\chi^2_4 = 12.9$*, P = 0.005		$\chi^2_4 = 4.6$, P = 0.204		$\chi^2_4 = 13.5$*, P = 0.004		$\chi^2_4 = 5.2$, P = 0.157	
N[e]	**25,764**		**1,091,645**		**753**		**357**	

*Significant at the 0.05 level, two-sided test.
[a]These estimates are based on logistic regression models adjusted for age, gender, and country.
[b]These estimates are based on survival models adjusted for age-cohorts, gender, person-years, and country.
[c]These estimates are based on logistic regression models adjusted for time since BED onset, age of BED onset, gender, and country.
[d]Chi-square test of significant differences between blocks of socio-demographic variables.
[e]Denominator N: 25,764 = total sample; 1,091,645 = number of person-years in the survival models; 753 = number of lifetime BED cases; 357 = number of 12-month BED cases.

Table 18.8 Bivariate associations between socio-demographic correlates and DSM-IV bulimia nervosa (BN), all countries combined

Correlates	30-day BN[a]		Lifetime BN[b]		12-month BN among lifetime cases[c]		30-day BN among 12-month cases[c]	
	OR	(95% CI)	OR	(95% CI)	OR	(95% CI)	OR	(95% CI)
Age-cohort								
18–29	**7.8***	(2.7–22.5)	**41.4***	(22.2–77.4)				
30–44	**5.5***	(1.9–16.0)	**20.4***	(11.9–35.0)				
45–59	**5.9***	(1.9–17.8)	**10.7***	(6.1–18.7)				
60+	**1.0**		**1.0**					
Age-cohort difference[d]	$\chi^2_3 = 14.8^*$, P = 0.002		$\chi^2_3 = 142.3^*$, P < 0.001					
Age-of-onset								
Early					**1.1**	(0.6–2.2)	**2.3**	(0.9–5.8)
Early-average					**0.5***	(0.3–1.0)	**0.6**	(0.2–1.8)
Late-average					**1.1**	(0.5–2.3)	**0.7**	(0.2–2.4)
Late					**1.0**		**1.0**	
Age-of-onset difference[d]					$\chi^2_3 = 6.7$, P = 0.083		$\chi^2_3 = 6.8$, P = 0.078	
Time since onset (continuous)					**0.98**	(0.96–1.00)	**1.01**	(0.96–1.05)
Gender								
Female	**3.8***	(2.0–7.2)	**3.5***	(2.6–4.7)	**0.8**	(0.4–1.6)	**1.7**	(0.6–4.8)
Male	**1.0**		**1.0**		**1.0**		**1.0**	
Gender difference[d]	$\chi^2_1 = 16.7^*$, P < 0.001		$\chi^2_1 = 70.3^*$, P < 0.001		$\chi^2_1 = 0.3$, P = 0.603		$\chi^2_1 = 1.1$, P = 0.290	
Employment status								
Student	**1.7**	(0.6–5.2)	**1.3**	(0.7–2.3)	**1.2**	(0.3–4.6)	**4.0**	(0.6–24.6–
Homemaker	**1.1**	(0.5–2.4)	**1.0**	(0.7–1.5)	**1.2**	(0.6–2.4)	**0.8**	(0.2–2.7)
Retired	**1.5**	(0.3–7.7)	**1.6**	(0.4–5.7)	**2.5**	(0.4–13.9)	–	–
Other	**2.0**	(1.0–4.3)	**1.9***	(1.3–2.7)	**1.3**	(0.7–2.5)	**1.1**	(0.4–3.2)
Employed	**1.0**		**1.0**		**1.0**		**1.0**	
Employment status difference[d]	$\chi^2_4 = 4.7$, P = 0.318		$\chi^2_4 = 11.8^*$, P = 0.019		$\chi^2_4 = 1.8$, P = 0.771		$\chi^2_4 = 3.1$, P = 0.540	
Marital status								
Never married	**0.7**	(0.3–1.7)	**0.9**	(0.6–1.3)	**1.0**	(0.5–1.8)	**1.3**	(0.4–3.9)
Divorced/separated/widowed	**1.8**	(0.9–3.7)	**1.3**	(0.9–1.8)	**1.3**	(0.7–2.3)	**1.7**	(0.5–5.2)
Currently married	**1.0**		**1.0**		**1.0**		**1.0**	

(cont.)

Table 18.8 (*cont.*)

Correlates	30-day BN[a]		Lifetime BN[b]		12-month BN among lifetime cases[c]		30-day BN among 12-month cases[c]	
	OR	(95% CI)	OR	(95% CI)	OR	(95% CI)	OR	(95% CI)
Marital status difference[d]	$\chi^2_2 = 3.0, P = 0.223$		$\chi^2_2 = 2.7, P = 0.255$		$\chi^2_2 = 0.6, P = 0.751$		$\chi^2_2 = 0.9, P = 0.643$	
Education level								
No education	–	–	–	–	–	–	–	–
Some primary	**1.2**	(0.3–4.5)	**1.1**	(0.7–1.7)	**2.0**	(0.6–7.1)	**0.3**	(0.0–2.0)
Finished primary	–	–	**0.8**	(0.4–1.4)	**4.2***	(1.0–17.8)	–	–
Some secondary	**1.9**	(0.8–4.5)	**1.3**	(0.8–1.9)	**2.5***	(1.0–6.2)	**0.7**	(0.1–3.3)
Finished secondary	**1.5**	(0.6–3.5)	**1.1**	(0.8–1.6)	**2.2**	(0.9–5.2)	**0.5**	(0.1–2.5)
Some college	**2.5**	(1.0–6.6)	**1.3**	(0.9–2.0)	**3.3***	(1.3–8.4)	**0.5**	(0.1–3.3)
Finished college	**1.0**		**1.0**		**1.0**		**1.0**	
Education level difference[d]	$\chi^2_6 = 7.3, P = 0.298$		$\chi^2_6 = 6.6, P = 0.360$		$\chi^2_6 = 9.3, P = 0.157$		$\chi^2_6 = 88.2^*, P < 0.001$	
Household income								
Low	**1.6**	(0.6–3.8)	**1.1**	(0.8–1.6)	**2.3***	(1.1–5.1)	**0.5**	(0.1–2.0)
Low-average	**0.9**	(0.4–2.3)	**0.8**	(0.6–1.3)	**1.0**	(0.5–2.1)	**1.5**	(0.3–6.5)
High-average	**1.7**	(0.7–4.0)	**0.8**	(0.6–1.2)	**1.8**	(0.8–3.8)	**2.0**	(0.4–8.7)
High	**1.0**		**1.0**		**1.0**		**1.0**	
Household income difference[d]	$\chi^2_4 = 4.2, P = 0.241$		$\chi^2_4 = 4.4, P = 0.223$		$\chi^2_4 = 8.1^*, P = 0.043$		$\chi^2_4 = 5.2, P = 0.161$	
N[e]	**25,764**		**1,094,214**		**484**		**166**	

*Significant at the 0.05 level, two-sided test.

[a]These estimates are based on logistic regression models adjusted for age, gender, and country.

[b]These estimates are based on survival models adjusted for age-cohorts, gender, person-years, and country.

[c]These estimates are based on logistic regression models adjusted for time since BN onset, age of BN onset, gender, and country.

[d]Chi-square test of significant differences between blocks of socio-demographic variables.

[e]Denominator N: 25,764 = total sample; 1,094,214 = number of person-years in the survival models; 484 = number of lifetime BN cases; 166 = number of 12-month BN cases.

Table 18.9 Comorbidity of binge-eating disorder with other DSM-IV disorders

	Binge-eating disorder cases with comorbid disorders									
	Mood disorder[a]		Anxiety disorder[b]		Disruptive behaviour/ impulse-control disorder[c]		Substance-use disorder[d]		Any mental disorder[e]	
	%	SE	%	SE	%	SE	%	SE	%	SE
Lifetime comorbidity[f]										
Lifetime	**45.2**	2.2	**54.6**	2.4	**23.7**	2.2	**23.9**	2.1	**79.6**	2.5
12-month	**53.6**	3.8	**58.0**	3.6	**30.1**	3.1	**25.0**	3.3	**82.6**	3.3
12-month comorbidity[g]										
12-month	**36.1**	3.4	**44.3**	3.5	**10.4**	1.9	**8.7**	1.7	**61.0**	3.5
Temporal priority of binge-eating disorder[h]										
Lifetime	**35.9**	3.1	**12.6**	2.0	**5.6**	2.7	**35.1**	4.8	**16.2**	1.9
12-month	**35.0**	4.6	**9.5**	2.4	–	–	**31.1**	5.8	**13.9**	2.8

A dash indicates low cell count (<5 cases).
[a]Respondents with major depressive episode or bipolar spectrum disorder.
[b]Respondents with panic disorder, generalized anxiety disorder, social phobia, specific phobia, agoraphobia, posttraumatic stress disorder, or separation anxiety disorder.
[c]Respondents with intermittent explosive disorder, attention deficit disorder, conduct disorder, oppositional defiant disorder, or bulimia nervosa.
[d]Respondents with alcohol abuse with or without dependence or drug abuse with or without dependence.
[e]Respondents with any disorder listed above.
[f]Percentage of respondents with either lifetime or 12-month BED who also meet lifetime criteria for at least one of the other DSM-IV disorders.
[g]Percentage of respondents with 12-month BED who also meet 12-month criteria for at least one of the other disorders.
[h]Percentage of respondents with either lifetime or 12-month BED and at least one of the other disorders, whose AOO of BED is reported to be younger than the AOO of all comorbid disorders under consideration.

BN report receiving some type of treatment in the 12 months before interview for problems with their emotions, nerves, mental health, or substance use. Treatment is somewhat more likely in the general medical sector than the specialty mental health sector (24.8% vs 18.4% for BED; 30.6% vs 25.2% for BN), with much lower treatment rates in the human services (5.3–7.0%) and CAM (7.0–5.2%) sectors. Treatment rates appear to be higher in high-income than upper-middle-income countries, but the numbers of 12-month cases are too small to make reliable statements. The numbers of 12-month cases in low/lower-middle-income countries are too small to estimate treatment rates. No consistent association of severity, as indicated by SDS scores, can be seen with treatment rates for either BED or BN (Tables 18.11 and 18.12).

An earlier WMH report also examined lifetime treatment of eating disorders (Kessler *et al.* 2013). We found there that the majority of respondents with lifetime BN (67.3%) and BED (57.7%) received lifetime treatment for emotional problems and that the most common treatment sector was the mental health specialty sector (43.3–57.7%) followed by the general medical sector (34.3–43.2%), with lower proportions in the human services (10.3–14.3%) and CAM (15.0–18.8%) sectors. However, smaller proportions of lifetime cases (BN 47.4%, BED 38.3%) ever received treatment specifically for eating disorders, representing roughly two-thirds of those who received lifetime treatment for emotional problems. Roughly half of those with 12-month BN and one-fourth of those with BED who received 12-month treatment for any emotional problems reported receiving treatment specifically for eating disorders. These results suggest that in the majority of cases of BED and in roughly half of those of BN, eating disorders were not the focus of complaint when seeking treatment for emotional problems. The WMH

Table 18.10 Comorbidity of bulimia nervosa with other DSM-IV disorders

	Bulimia nervosa cases with comorbid disorders									
	Mood disorder[a]		Anxiety disorder[b]		Disruptive behaviour/ impulse-control disorder[c]		Substance-use disorder[d]		Any mental disorder[e]	
	%	SE	%	SE	%	SE	%	SE	%	SE
Lifetime comorbidity[f]										
Lifetime	**57.1**	2.9	**63.3**	2.9	**32.3**	2.8	**26.8**	2.7	**87.8**	2.0
12-month	**62.9**	4.6	**67.9**	5.0	**26.3**	4.6	**31.2**	4.4	**84.9**	3.7
12-month comorbidity[g]										
12-month	**46.4**	5.1	**53.9**	5.2	**19.5**	4.0	**12.8**	3.1	**73.4**	4.5
Temporal priority of bulimia nervosa[h]										
Lifetime	**50.6**	3.9	**17.6**	3.0	**44.6**	6.0	**43.4**	5.8	**25.7**	3.1
12-month	**41.2**	6.0	**9.7**	2.8	–	–	**38.1**	7.1	**15.8**	4.4

A dash indicates low cell count (<5 cases).
[a]Respondents with major depressive episode or bipolar spectrum disorder.
[b]Respondents with panic disorder, generalized anxiety disorder, social phobia, specific phobia, agoraphobia, posttraumatic stress disorder, or separation anxiety disorder.
[c]Respondents with intermittent explosive disorder, attention deficit disorder, conduct disorder, oppositional defiant disorder, or BED.
[d]Respondents with alcohol abuse with or without dependence or drug abuse with or without dependence.
[e]Respondents with any disorder listed above.
[f]Percentage of respondents with either lifetime or 12-month bulimia nervosa who also meet lifetime criteria for at least one of the other DSM-IV disorders.
[g]Percentage of respondents with 12-month bulimia nervosa who also meet 12-month criteria for at least one of the other disorders.
[h]Percentage of respondents with either lifetime or 12-month bulimia nervosa and at least one of the other disorders, whose AOO of bulimia nervosa is reported to be younger than the AOO of all comorbid disorders under consideration.

data do not tell, though, how often clinicians treating these patients for emotional problems are aware of their patients' eating disorders.

Discussion

The results reported here must be interpreted in the context of several WMH limitations: that response rates varied considerably across surveys; sample sizes were too small to produce country-specific results other than for a few estimates; and that lifetime disorders were assessed retrospectively using fully structured rather than semi-structured interviews, probably leading to underestimation of lifetime prevalence and overestimation of AOO and of the effects of age-at-interview and comorbidity. Although an earlier version of CIDI under-diagnosed eating disorders (Thornton *et al.* 1998), the more recent version of CIDI used here modified probes to address this problem (Kessler & Üstün 2004). Nonetheless, the absence of CIDI validation studies is a limitation. Because of this limitation, prevalence estimates should be considered lower bounds.

Notwithstanding these limitations, the data reported here provide the most complete population-based estimates of the prevalence and correlates of BED in comparison to BN ever presented among adults across a diverse set of countries. The number of correlates considered was necessarily limited by virtue of the constraints on interview length and the fact that epidemiological surveys are not able to assess all types of correlates, resulting in the literatures on some correlates of eating disorders not being addressed (e.g., Sansone & Sansone 2011; Culbert *et al.* 2015). But the results nonetheless extend findings from previous epidemiological research, which has largely concentrated on females (e.g., Cachelin *et al.* 1999; Kinzl *et al.* 1999; Fairburn *et al.* 2000; Favaro *et al.* 2003; Striegel-Moore *et al.* 2003, 2005; Wade *et al.* 2006; Keski-Rahkonen *et al.* 2009; Field *et al.* 2012), adolescents (see Striegel-Moore & Franko 2003, 2008; Wade *et al.* 2011, for reviews), and particular races or ethnic groups (e.g.,

Table 18.11 Among those with 12-month binge-eating disorder, percent reporting treatment in the past 12 months by Sheehan impairment severity

Sector of treatment	Sheehan Disability Scale category[a]											
	Mild impairment (score: 1–3)			Moderate impairment (score: 4–6)			Severe impairment (score: 7–10)			Any impairment		
	%	SE	Comparison between country income groups[b]	%	SE	Comparison between country income groups[b]	%	SE	Comparison between country income groups[b]	%	SE	Comparison between country income groups[b]
Specialty mental health[c]												
Low/lower-middle-income countries	–	–		–	–		–	–		–	–	$F_{2,v} = 0.6$,
Upper-middle-income countries	–	–	–	–	–	–	–	–	–	**14.3**	5.2	$P = 0.58$
High-income countries	**30.8**	12.4		**19.4**	7.8		**24.7**	7.2		**19.8**	3.1	
All countries combined	**29.6**	12.0		**19.6**	6.7		**17.7**	4.7		**18.4**	2.6	
General medical[d]												
Low/lower-middle-income countries	–	–		–	–		–	–		–	–	$F_{2,v} = 5.8$*,
Upper-middle-income countries	–	–	–	–	–	–	–	–	–	**16.5**	5.0	$P < 0.001$
High-income countries	**24.3**	9.9		**24.0**	8.4		**34.5**	8.7		**29.3**	4.1	
All countries combined	**23.4**	9.6		**23.6**	7.2		**21.8**	5.8		**24.8**	3.2	
Any health care[e]												
Low/lower-middle-income countries	–	–	–	–	–	$F_{2,v} = 0.4$,	–	–	$F_{2,v} = 4.9$*,	–	–	$F_{2,v} = 1.5$,
Upper-middle-income countries	–	–		**42.8**	18.6	$P = 0.68$	**9.4**	3.1	$P = 0.01$	**26.2**	5.2	$P = 0.22$
High-income countries	**43.6**	12.2		**28.5**	8.7		**46.0**	9.0		**37.6**	4.1	
All countries combined	**41.9**	11.8		**31.0**	7.6		**30.6**	6.3		**34.0**	3.3	
Human services[f]												
Low/lower-middle-income countries	–	–	–	–	–	–	–	–	–	–	–	$F_{2,v} = 3.0$,
Upper-middle-income countries	–	–		–	–		–	–		**4.7**	2.4	$P = 0.05$
High-income countries	–	–		**5.0**	2.6		**5.9**	3.9		**5.7**	1.7	
All countries combined	–	–		**4.1**	2.1		**8.9**	3.7		**5.3**	1.4	
CAM[g]												
Low/lower-middle-income countries	–	–	–	–	–	–	–	–	–	–	–	–
Upper-middle-income countries	–	–		–	–		–	–		–	–	
High-income countries	**13.3**	6.1		**11.3**	6.9		**16.5**	7.2		**9.2**	2.5	
All countries combined	**13.2**	5.8		**10.6**	5.8		**10.1**	4.5		**6.7**	1.8	

(cont.)

Table 18.11 (*cont.*)

Sector of treatment	Sheehan Disability Scale category[a]											
	Mild impairment (score: 1–3)			Moderate impairment (score: 4–6)			Severe impairment (score: 7–10)			Any impairment		
	%	SE	Comparison between country income groups[b]	%	SE	Comparison between country income groups[b]	%	SE	Comparison between country income groups[b]	%	SE	Comparison between country income groups[b]
Any non-health care[h]												
Low/lower-middle-income countries	–	–	–	–	–	–	–	–	–	–	–	$F_{2,v} = 1.8$, $P = 0.17$
Upper-middle-income countries	–	–		–	–		–	–		**4.7**	2.4	
High-income countries	**13.3**	6.1		**13.5**	6.9		**17.3**	7.2		**11.7**	2.6	
All countries combined	**13.2**	5.8		**12.4**	5.8		**15.6**	5.1		**9.6**	1.9	
Any treatment[i]												
Low/lower-middle-income countries	–	–	–	–	–	$F_{2,v} = 0.2$, $P = 0.80$	–	–	$F_{2,v} = 4.6^*$, $P = 0.01$	–	–	$F_{2,v} = 2.0$, $P = 0.13$
Upper-middle-income countries	–	–		**42.8**	18.6		**17.5**	6.8		**28.5**	5.1	
High-income countries	**48.2**	12.2		**31.8**	8.9		**54.8**	9.0		**41.5**	4.2	
All countries combined	**46.8**	11.8		**33.7**	7.7		**39.0**	6.6		**37.3**	3.3	

*Significant at the 0.05 level, two-sided test.
A dash indicates low cell count (<5 cases).
[a]Highest severity category across four SDS role domains.
[b]Wald design-corrected F-tests were used to determine if there is variation in treatment estimates across country income groups. The denominator degree of freedom, v, is 658. Wald tests only generated where there is more than one stable cell (≥5 cases) for each combination of treatment sector and Sheehan impairment.
[c]The mental health specialist sector, which includes psychiatrist and non-psychiatrist mental health specialists (psychiatrist, psychologist, or other non-psychiatrist mental health professional; social worker or counsellor in a mental health specialty setting; use of a mental health helpline; or overnight admissions for a mental health or drug or alcohol problems, with a presumption of daily contact with a psychiatrist).
[d]The general medical sector (general practitioner, other medical doctor, nurse, occupational therapist, or any healthcare professional).
[e]The mental health specialist sector or the general medical sector.
[f]The human services sector (religious or spiritual advisor or social worker or counsellor in any setting other than a specialty mental health setting).
[g]The CAM (complementary and alternative medicine) sector (any other type of healer such as herbalist or homeopath, participation in an internet support group, or participation in a self-help group).
[h]The human services sector or CAM.
[i]Any treatment listed above.

Table 18.12 Among those with 12-month bulimia nervosa, percent reporting treatment in the past 12 months by Sheehan impairment severity

Sector of treatment	Sheehan Disability Scale category[a]											
	Mild impairment (score: 1–3)			Moderate impairment (score: 4–6)			Severe impairment (score: 7–10)			Any impairment		
	%	SE	Comparison between country income groups[b]	%	SE	Comparison between country income groups[b]	%	SE	Comparison between country income groups[b]	%	SE	Comparison between country income groups[b]
Specialty mental health[c]												
Low/lower-middle-income countries	–	–	–	–	–	–	–	–	$F_{2,v} = 0.7$, $P = 0.51$	–	–	$F_{2,v} = 2.5$, $P = 0.09$
Upper-middle-income countries	–	–		–	–		**50.8**	18.4		**27.0**	7.4	
High-income countries	–	–		–	–		**36.5**	11.0		**26.6**	5.1	
All countries combined	**24.6**	11.8		**25.4**	10.5		**40.0**	9.5		**25.2**	4.1	
General medical[d]												
Low/lower-middle-income countries	–	–	–	–	–	–	–	–	–	–	–	$F_{2,v} = 8.1^*$, $P < 0.001$
Upper-middle-income countries	–	–		–	–		–	–		**10.0**	4.2	
High-income countries	–	–		**31.2**	12.1		**55.6**	11.1		**44.3**	6.4	
All countries combined	–	–		**24.9**	9.9		**47.2**	9.7		**30.6**	4.7	
Any health care[e]												
Low/lower-middle-income countries	–	–	–	–	–	–	–	–	$F_{2,v} = 0.6$, $P = 0.58$	–	–	$F_{2,v} = 3.0$, $P = 0.05$
Upper-middle-income countries	–	–		–	–		**50.8**	18.4		**31.5**	7.8	
High-income countries	–	–		**31.2**	12.1		**58.1**	10.9		**48.9**	6.4	
All countries combined	**31.2**	12.5		**33.1**	11.4		**56.7**	9.3		**40.7**	4.9	
Human services[f]												
Low/lower-middle-income countries	–	–	–	–	–	–	–	–	–	–	–	–
Upper-middle-income countries	–	–		–	–		–	–		–	–	
High-income countries	–	–		–	–		–	–		**4.8**	2.3	
All countries combined	–	–		–	–		–	–		**7.0**	2.9	

(cont.)

Table 18.12 *(cont.)*

Sector of treatment	Sheehan Disability Scale category[a]											
	Mild impairment (score: 1–3)			Moderate impairment (score: 4–6)			Severe impairment (score: 7–10)			Any impairment		
	%	SE	Comparison between country income groups[b]	%	SE	Comparison between country income groups[b]	%	SE	Comparison between country income groups[b]	%	SE	Comparison between country income groups[b]
CAM[g]												
Low/lower-middle-income countries	–	–	–	–	–	–	–	–	–	–	–	$F_{2,v}=1.8$
Upper-middle-income countries	–	–		–	–		–	–		**7.6**	4.1	P = 0.17
High-income countries	–	–		–	–		–	–		**4.4**	1.7	
All countries combined	–	–		–	–		–	–		**5.2**	1.7	
Any non-health care[h]												
Low/lower-middle-income countries	–	–	–	–	–	–	–	–	–	–	–	$F_{2,v}=1.9$
Upper-middle-income countries	–	–		–	–		–	–		**14.6**	7.4	P = 0.16
High-income countries	–	–		–	–		**9.9**	5.8		**8.6**	2.8	
All countries combined	–	–			–	–	**8.9**	4.4		**10.1**	3.1	
Any treatment[i]												
Low/lower-middle-income countries	–	–	–	–	–	–	–	–	$F_{2,v}=0.6$,	–	–	$F_{2,v}=2.4$,
Upper-middle-income countries	–	–		–	–		**50.8**	18.4	P = 0.54	**39.1**	8.6	P = 0.10
High-income countries	–	–		**31.2**	12.1		**61.7**	10.9		**50.9**	6.3	
All countries combined	**49.7**	14.9		**33.1**	11.4		**59.2**	9.3		**44.4**	5.0	

[*]Significant at the 0.05 level, two-sided test.
A dash indicates low cell count (<5 cases).
[a]Highest severity category across four SDS role domains.
[b]Wald design-corrected F-tests were used to determine if there is variation in treatment estimates across country income groups. The denominator degree of freedom, v, is 658. Wald tests only generated where there is more than one stable cell (≥5 cases) for each combination of treatment sector and Sheehan impairment.
[c]The mental health specialist sector, which includes psychiatrist and non-psychiatrist mental health specialists (psychiatrist, psychologist, or other non-psychiatrist mental health professional; social worker or counsellor in a mental health specialty setting; use of a mental health helpline; or overnight admissions for a mental health or drug or alcohol problems, with a presumption of daily contact with a psychiatrist).
[d]The general medical sector (general practitioner, other medical doctor, nurse, occupational therapist, or any healthcare professional).
[e]The mental health specialist sector or the general medical sector.
[f]The human services sector (religious or spiritual advisor or social worker or counsellor in any setting other than a specialty mental health setting).
[g]The CAM (complementary and alternative medicine) sector (any other type of healer such as herbalist or homeopath, participation in an internet support group, or participation in a self-help group).
[h]The human services sector or CAM.
[i]Any treatment listed above.

Striegel-Moore *et al.* 2003, 2005; Alegria *et al.* 2007; Taylor *et al.* 2007; Marques *et al.* 2011; Swanson *et al.* 2012). Indeed, apart from the DSM field trial, which established a population prevalence of 2.0% for BED (Spitzer *et al.* 1992) and some seminal but now dated Western studies (Bushnell *et al.* 1994; Garfinkel *et al.* 1995; Gotestam & Agras 1995; Hay 1998), few epidemiological studies describe eating disorders in broadly representative samples of men and women. Although one regional Italian study examined adult mixed-gender rates (Faravelli *et al.* 2006), the overly restrictive screener in that study undermined the representativeness of the tiny resultant sample of 32 cases. To our knowledge, other contemporary mixed-gender surveys are limited to WMH subsamples in Europe and the United States, with estimates between 0.5% to 1.0% for BN and 1.1% to 2.6% for BED (Hudson *et al.* 2007; Preti *et al.* 2009), consistent with the WMH pooled estimates reported here of 1.0% for BN and 1.9% for BED.

Data on eating disorder AOO are also not well established, given methodological heterogeneity of studies, although the WMH finding of relatively early AOO is broadly consistent with previous research (Striegel-Moore & Franko 2008; Wade *et al.* 2011; Javaras & Hudson 2017). Our finding of somewhat earlier AOO for BN than BED is also consistent with previous studies of DSM-defined eating *disorders* (Wade *et al.* 2011; Javaras & Hudson 2017), but differs from more general studies of eating *behaviours*, which tend to show binge-eating behaviours peaking before compensatory behaviours (Raymond *et al.* 1995; Fairburn *et al.* 2000; Stice *et al.* 2009). The wider AOO range found here for BED than BN possibly reflects diagnostic heterogeneity of BED (Grilo *et al.* 2001; Mond *et al.* 2006; Pope *et al.* 2006; Wade *et al.* 2006; Mond *et al.* 2007b; Goldschmidt *et al.* 2011).

The WMH finding of relatively low persistence of BED and BN is consistent with most research (Keel & Brown 2010), but clinical samples show higher persistence, presumably due to the fact that the cases in clinical samples are more severe than those that do not come to clinical attention. With regard to our somewhat lower persistence of BED than BN, it is noteworthy that lower persistence of BED than BN was also found in several longitudinal clinical studies that found lower remission for BN than BED (Agras *et al.* 2009; Castellini *et al.* 2011), higher relapse for BN than BED (Stice *et al.* 2009), and higher diagnostic crossover from BED to BN than the reverse (Fichter *et al.* 1998; Castellini *et al.* 2011; Keel *et al.* 2012).

The finding that age-at-interview is inversely related to lifetime risk is consistent with previous evidence suggesting that BN (Kendler *et al.* 1991; Hoek & van Hoeken 2003; Hay *et al.* 2008) and BED (Hudson *et al.* 2007; Hay *et al.* 2008; Mitchison *et al.* 2012) have increased in prevalence over time. However, it should be noted that studies of the incidence of eating disorders over time – which are not subject to potential recall bias from retrospective assessments, but which unfortunately have other methodologic limitations – have not yielded consistent or reliable data (Wade *et al.* 2011).

The finding that BN and BED are more prevalent among females than males is consistent with much previous research (Striegel-Moore & Franko 2003; Wade *et al.* 2011; Smink *et al.* 2012; Javaras & Hudson 2017). The WMH gender differences are smaller, though, than in treatment studies (Fairburn & Beglin 1990; Hoek & van Hoeken 2003), presumably reflecting the lower help-seeking rates of men than women (Striegel *et al.* 2012). The higher proportion of males found here in BED than BN is consistent with previous findings (Wade *et al.* 2011), further supporting the clinical differentiation of BED from BN.

Our finding that BN and BED are associated with an equivalently high prevalence of current overweight and obesity is consistent with some (Dansky *et al.* 1998, Darby *et al.* 2007, Zachrisson *et al.* 2008), but not all (Hay 1998; Fairburn *et al.* 2000; Striegel-Moore *et al.* 2001; Field *et al.* 2012) previous community-based surveys. All of these other studies found a high prevalence of obesity in BED, but only some also found a high prevalence of obesity in BN. The exception is a pair of national trend surveys in Norway, where equivalently, an elevated prevalence of obesity was found for BN and BED in the first survey (1991), but only for BN (that is, not for BED) in the second survey (2004) (Zachrisson *et al.* 2008). In light of these diverse results, it is striking that the WMH finding of equivalently high BMI in BN and BED was found consistently in surveys in the United States, Latin America, Western Europe, and New Zealand. It is noteworthy, in view of this consistency, that none of the previous community surveys other than the two in Norway was based on a nationally representative mixed-gender sample, raising the possibility that the inconsistent association of BN with obesity in these studies might reflect genuine variation in this association across segments of the population that were differentially sampled in these surveys. Future studies should include systematic investigations of such possible specifications.

A complicating factor in such future studies is the possibility of time trends. As noted above, the Norwegian trend studies showed that BN versus BED differences in obesity changed in that country in the years between those two surveys. In addition, while clinical studies have traditionally found high obesity rates among patients with BED but not BN (Ramacciotti *et al.* 2005; Peterson *et al.* 2010), recent studies have begun to find a rising prevalence of obesity also among patients with BN (Bulik *et al.* 2012; Villarejo *et al.* 2012). This development might reflect changing patterns of differential selection into treatment on the basis of BMI among community cases with BN versus BED. Another possibility is that age patterns of BN prevalence and/or help-seeking are changing, as the association of BN with obesity is stronger among older cases (Gendall *et al.* 1999). Future studies of these possibilities, while well beyond the scope of the WMH data, are clearly warranted in light of inconsistences across community and clinical studies in the associations of BED and BN with obesity.

The high comorbidities of BED and BN with other DSM-IV disorders are broadly consistent with previous studies of both BED and BN (Wade *et al.* 2011). However, only a few of these previous studies examined associations between early-onset mental disorders and subsequent eating disorders (Johnson *et al.* 2002b; Biederman *et al.* 2007; Sihvola *et al.* 2009) or between early-onset eating disorders and other subsequent mental disorders (Johnson *et al.* 2002a). The WMH results are consistent with those few studies in finding significant reciprocal bivariate time-lagged associations, although our multivariate analysis did not find the dominance of major depression as the primary predictor of eating disorders suggested in one previous study (Johnson *et al.* 2002b).

Although we know of no previous study of the relative sizes of cross-lagged ORs between eating disorders and other mental disorders, one cross-lagged evaluation of eating behaviours and substance-use problems revealed no concurrent or temporal associations between binge-eating symptoms and alcohol or illicit substance use (Dunn *et al.* 2009). In addition, two separate papers from one prospective study (Johnson *et al.* 2002a,b) found other mental disorders predicting eating disorders somewhat more strongly than vice versa. To the extent that this asymmetry reflects causal influences of other mental disorders on subsequent eating disorders, a question can be raised whether successful early intervention to treat other disorders would help prevent subsequent eating disorders. This question is of considerable public health importance and deserves empirical investigation (Kessler & Price 1993).

As shown in Chapter 22, the proportions of WMH respondents reporting severe impairment range between 18.7% (specific phobia) and 57% (major depressive disorder). The rates of severe role impairment associated with 12-month BED (21.3%) and BN (31.7%) are at the lower end of that range. This might reflect the well-known lack of insight and tendency of people with eating disorders to minimize their symptom severity (Johnson-Sabine *et al.* 1988; Beglin & Fairburn 1992).

The finding that low proportions of people with eating disorders receive treatment is broadly consistent with previous reports from component WMH surveys in the United States (Hudson *et al.* 2007) and Western Europe (Fairburn *et al.* 2000; Preti *et al.* 2009). These are lower treatment rates than for many other mental disorders found in the WMH surveys (Wang *et al.* 2007). Consistent with previous research on health-service utilization in eating disorders (Mond *et al.* 2007a), a substantial proportion of WMH eating disorder cases who received treatment were treated for comorbid emotional problems rather than for their eating disorders. This finding, coupled with the observation that physicians seldom assess and often fail to recognize eating disorders (Johnson *et al.* 2001; Crow *et al.* 2004), highlights the importance of clinicians questioning about eating problems even when patients do not include them among presenting complaints.

Acknowledgement

The earlier analyses of the WMH eating disorders data summarized in this chapter were supported in part by Shire Pharmaceuticals.

References

Agras, W. S., Crow, S., Mitchell, J. E., Halmi, K. A., & Bryson, S. (2009). A 4-year prospective study of eating disorder NOS compared with full eating disorder syndromes. *International Journal of Eating Disorders* 42, 565–70.

Alegria, M., Woo, M., Cao, Z., *et al.* (2007). Prevalence and correlates of eating disorders in Latinos in the United States. *International Journal of Eating Disorders* 40(Suppl S3), S15–21.

American Psychiatric Association (2013). *Diagnostic and Statistical Manual of Mental Disorders: Fifth Edition (DSM-5)*. Washington, DC: American Psychiatric Publishing.

Beglin, S. J., & Fairburn, C. G. (1992). Women who choose not to participate in surveys on eating disorders. *International Journal of Eating Disorders* 12, 113–6.

Biederman, J., Ball, S. W., Monuteaux, M. C., *et al.* (2007). Are girls with ADHD at risk for eating disorders? Results from a controlled, five-year prospective study. *Journal of Developmental and Behavioral Pediatrics* 28, 302–7.

Bulik, C. M., Marcus, M. D., Zerwas, S., Levine, M. D., & La Via, M. (2012). The changing "weightscape" of bulimia nervosa. *American Journal of Psychiatry* 169, 1031–6.

Bushnell, J. A., Wells, J. E., McKenzie, J. M., *et al.* (1994). Bulimia comorbidity in the general population and in the clinic. *Psychological Medicine* 24, 605–11.

Cachelin, F. M., Striegel-Moore, R. H., Elder, K. A., *et al.* (1999). Natural course of a community sample of women with binge eating disorder. *International Journal of Eating Disorders* 25, 45–54.

Castellini, G., Lo Sauro, C., Mannucci, E., *et al.* (2011). Diagnostic crossover and outcome predictors in eating disorders according to DSM-IV and DSM-V proposed criteria: a 6-year follow-up study. *Psychosomatic Medicine* 73, 270–9.

Crow, S. J., Peterson, C. B., Levine, A. S., Thuras, P., & Mitchell, J. E. (2004). A survey of binge eating and obesity treatment practices among primary care providers. *International Journal of Eating Disorders* 35, 348–53.

Culbert, K. M., Racine, S. E., & Klump, K. L. (2015). Research review: what we have learned about the causes of eating disorders – a synthesis of sociocultural, psychological, and biological research. *Journal of Child Psychology and Psychiatry and Allied Disciplines* 56, 1141–64.

Dansky, B. S., Brewerton, T. D., Kilpatrick, D. G., *et al.* (1998). The nature and prevalence of binge eating disorder in a national sample of women. In T. A. Widiger, A. J. Frances, H. A. Pincus, *et al.*, eds., *DSM-IV Sourcebook, Volume 4*. Washington, DC: American Psychiatric Association, pp. 515–31.

Darby, A., Hay, P., Mond, J., Rodgers, B., & Owen, C. (2007). Disordered eating behaviours and cognitions in young women with obesity: relationship with psychological status. *International Journal of Obesity* 31, 876–82.

Dunn, E. C., Neighbors, C., Fossos, N., & Larimer, M. E. (2009). A cross-lagged evaluation of eating disorder symptomatology and substance-use problems. *Journal of Studies on Alcohol and Drugs* 70, 106–16.

Fairburn, C. G., & Beglin, S. J. (1990). Studies of the epidemiology of bulimia nervosa. *American Journal of Psychiatry* 147, 401–8.

Fairburn, C. G., Cooper, Z., Doll, H. A., Norman, P., & O'Connor, M. (2000). The natural course of bulimia nervosa and binge eating disorder in young women. *Archives of General Psychiatry* 57, 659–65.

Faravelli, C., Ravaldi, C., Truglia, E., *et al.* (2006). Clinical epidemiology of eating disorders: results from the Sesto Fiorentino study. *Psychotherapy and Psychosomatics* 75, 376–83.

Favaro, A., Ferrara, S., & Santonastaso, P. (2003). The spectrum of eating disorders in young women: a prevalence study in a general population sample. *Psychosomatic Medicine* 65, 701–8.

Fichter, M. M., Quadflieg, N., & Gnutzmann, A. (1998). Binge eating disorder: treatment outcome over a 6-year course. *Journal of Psychosomatic Research* 44, 385–405.

Field, A. E., Sonneville, K. R., Micali, N., *et al.* (2012). Prospective association of common eating disorders and adverse outcomes. *Pediatrics* 130, e289–95.

Garfinkel, P. E., Lin, E., Goering, P., *et al.* (1995). Bulimia nervosa in a Canadian community sample: prevalence and comparison of subgroups. *American Journal of Psychiatry* 152, 1052–8.

Gendall, K. A., Bulik, C. M., Sullivan, P. F., *et al.* (1999). Body weight in bulimia nervosa. *Eating and Weight Disorders* 4, 157–64.

Goldschmidt, A. B., Le Grange, D., Powers, P., *et al.* (2011). Eating disorder symptomatology in normal-weight vs. obese individuals with binge eating disorder. *Obesity* 19, 1515–8.

Gotestam, K. G., & Agras, W. S. (1995). General population-based epidemiological study of eating disorders in Norway. *International Journal of Eating Disorders* 18, 119–26.

Grilo, C. M., Masheb, R. M., & Wilson, G. T. (2001). Subtyping binge eating disorder. *Journal of Consulting and Clinical Psychology* 69, 1066–72.

Hay, P. (1998). The epidemiology of eating disorder behaviors: an Australian community-based survey. *International Journal of Eating Disorders* 23, 371–82.

Hay, P. J., Mond, J., Buttner, P., & Darby, A. (2008). Eating disorder behaviors are increasing: findings from two sequential community surveys in South Australia. *PLoS ONE* 3, e1541.

Hoek, H. W., & van Hoeken, D. (2003). Review of the prevalence and incidence of eating disorders. *International Journal of Eating Disorders* 34, 383–96.

Hudson, J. I., Hiripi, E., Pope, H. G., Jr., & Kessler, R. C. (2007). The prevalence and correlates of eating disorders in the National Comorbidity Survey Replication. *Biological Psychiatry* 61, 348–58.

Javaras, K., & Hudson, J. (2017). Epidemiology of eating disorders. In T. Wade, eds., *Encyclopedia of Feeding and Eating Disorders*. Singapore: Springer.

Johnson-Sabine, E., Wood, K., Patton, G., Mann, A., & Wakeling, A. (1988). Abnormal eating attitudes in London schoolgirls – a prospective epidemiological study: factors associated with abnormal response on screening questionnaires. *Psychological Medicine* 18, 615–22.

Johnson, J. G., Cohen, P., Kasen, S., & Brook, J. S. (2002a). Eating disorders during adolescence and the risk for physical and mental disorders during early adulthood. *Archives of General Psychiatry* 59, 545–52.

Johnson, J. G., Cohen, P., Kotler, L., Kasen, S., & Brook, J. S. (2002b). Psychiatric disorders associated with risk for the development of eating disorders during adolescence and early adulthood. *Journal of Consulting and Clinical Psychology* 70, 1119–28.

Johnson, J. G., Spitzer, R. L., & Williams, J. B. (2001). Health problems, impairment and illnesses associated with bulimia nervosa and binge eating disorder among primary care and obstetric gynaecology patients. *Psychological Medicine* 31, 1455–66.

Keel, P. K., & Brown, T. A. (2010). Update on course and outcome in eating disorders. *International Journal of Eating Disorders* 43, 195–204.

Keel, P. K., Brown, T. A., Holland, L. A., & Bodell, L. P. (2012). Empirical classification of eating disorders. *Annual Review of Clinical Psychology* 8, 381–404.

Kendler, K. S., MacLean, C., Neale, M., *et al.* (1991). The genetic epidemiology of bulimia nervosa. *American Journal of Psychiatry* 148, 1627–37.

Keski-Rahkonen, A., Hoek, H. W., Linna, M. S., *et al.* (2009). Incidence and outcomes of bulimia nervosa: a nationwide population-based study. *Psychological Medicine* 39, 823–31.

Kessler, R. C., Berglund, P. A., Chiu, W. T., *et al.* (2013). The prevalence and correlates of binge eating disorder in the World Health Organization World Mental Health Surveys. *Biological Psychiatry* 73, 904–14.

Kessler, R. C., & Price, R. H. (1993). Primary prevention of secondary disorders: a proposal and agenda. *American Journal of Community Psychology* 21, 607–33.

Kessler, R. C., Shahly, V., Hudson, J. I., *et al.* (2014). A comparative analysis of role attainment and impairment in binge-eating disorder and bulimia nervosa: results from the WHO World Mental Health Surveys. *Epidemiology and Psychiatric Sciences* 23, 27–41.

Kessler, R. C., & Üstün, T. B. (2004). The World Mental Health (WMH) Survey Initiative Version of the World Health Organization (WHO) Composite International Diagnostic Interview (CIDI). *International Journal of Methods in Psychiatric Research* 13, 93–121.

Kinzl, J. F., Traweger, C., Trefalt, E., Mangweth, B., & Biebl, W. (1999). Binge eating disorder in females: a population-based investigation. *International Journal of Eating Disorders* 25, 287–92.

Marques, L., Alegria, M., Becker, A. E., *et al.* (2011). Comparative prevalence, correlates of impairment, and service utilization for eating disorders across US ethnic groups: implications for reducing ethnic disparities in health care access for eating disorders. *International Journal of Eating Disorders* 44, 412–20.

Mitchison, D., Hay, P., Slewa-Younan, S., & Mond, J. (2012). Time trends in population prevalence of eating disorder behaviors and their relationship to quality of life. *PLoS ONE* 7, e48450.

Mond, J., Hay, P., Rodgers, B., *et al.* (2006). Use of extreme weight control behaviors with and without binge eating in a community sample: implications for the classification of bulimic-type eating disorders. *International Journal of Eating Disorders* 39, 294–302.

Mond, J. M., Hay, P. J., Rodgers, B., & Owen, C. (2007a). Health service utilization for eating disorders: findings from a community-based study. *International Journal of Eating Disorders* 40, 399–408.

(2007b). Recurrent binge eating with and without the "undue influence of weight or shape on self-evaluation": implications for the diagnosis of binge eating disorder. *Behaviour Research and Therapy* 45, 929–38.

Peterson, C. B., Thuras, P., Ackard, D. M., *et al.* (2010). Personality dimensions in bulimia nervosa, binge eating disorder, and obesity. *Comprehensive Psychiatry* 51, 31–6.

Pope, H. G., Jr., Lalonde, J. K., Pindyck, L. J., *et al.* (2006). Binge eating disorder: a stable syndrome. *American Journal of Psychiatry* 163, 2181–3.

Preti, A., Girolamo, G., Vilagut, G., *et al.* (2009). The epidemiology of eating disorders in six European countries: results of the ESEMeD-WMH project. *Journal of Psychiatric Research* 43, 1125–32.

Ramacciotti, C. E., Coli, E., Paoli, R., *et al.* (2005). The relationship between binge eating disorder and non-purging bulimia nervosa. *Eating and Weight Disorders* 10, 8–12.

Raymond, N. C., Mussell, M. P., Mitchell, J. E., de Zwaan, M., & Crosby, R. D. (1995). An age-matched comparison of subjects with binge eating disorder and bulimia nervosa. *International Journal of Eating Disorders* 18, 135–43.

Sansone, R. A., & Sansone, L. A. (2011). Personality pathology and its influence on eating disorders. *Innovations in Clinical Neuroscience* 8, 14–8.

Sihvola, E., Keski-Rahkonen, A., Dick, D. M., *et al.* (2009). Prospective associations of early-onset Axis I disorders with developing eating disorders. *Comprehensive Psychiatry* 50, 20–5.

Smink, F. R., van Hoeken, D., & Hoek, H. W. (2012). Epidemiology of eating disorders: incidence, prevalence and mortality rates. *Current Psychiatry Reports* 14, 406–14.

Spitzer, R. L., Devlin, M., Walsh, B. T., *et al.* (1992). Binge eating disorder: a multisite field trial of the diagnostic criteria. *International Journal of Eating Disorders* 11, 191–203.

Stice, E., Marti, C. N., Shaw, H., & Jaconis, M. (2009). An 8-year longitudinal study of the natural history of threshold, subthreshold, and partial eating disorders from a community sample of adolescents. *Journal of Abnormal Psychology* 118, 587–97.

Striegel-Moore, R. H., Cachelin, F. M., Dohm, F. A., *et al.* (2001). Comparison of binge eating disorder and bulimia nervosa in a community sample. *International Journal of Eating Disorders* 29, 157–65.

Striegel-Moore, R. H., Dohm, F. A., Kraemer, H. C., *et al.* (2003). Eating disorders in white and black women. *American Journal of Psychiatry* 160, 1326–31.

Striegel-Moore, R. H., Fairburn, C. G., Wilfley, D. E., *et al.* (2005). Toward an understanding of risk factors for binge-eating disorder in black and white women: a community-based case-control study. *Psychological Medicine* 35, 907–17.

Striegel-Moore, R. H., & Franko, D. L. (2003). Epidemiology of binge eating disorder. *International Journal of Eating Disorders* 34 (Suppl S1), S19–29.

(2008). Should binge eating disorder be included in the DSM-V? A critical review of the state of the evidence. *Annual Review of Clinical Psychology* 4, 305–24.

Striegel, R. H., Bedrosian, R., Wang, C., & Schwartz, S. (2012). Why men should be included in research on binge eating: results from a comparison of psychosocial impairment in men and women. *International Journal of Eating Disorders* 45, 233–40.

Swanson, S. A., Saito, N., Borges, G., *et al.* (2012). Change in binge eating and binge eating disorder associated with migration from Mexico to the U.S. *Journal of Psychiatric Research* 46, 31–7.

Taylor, J. Y., Caldwell, C. H., Baser, R. E., Faison, N., & Jackson, J. S. (2007). Prevalence of eating disorders among Blacks in the National Survey of American Life. *International Journal of Eating Disorders* 40 (Suppl S1), S10–4.

Thornton, C., Russell, J., & Hudson, J. (1998). Does the Composite International Diagnostic Interview underdiagnose the eating disorders? *International Journal of Eating Disorders* 23, 341–5.

Villarejo, C., Fernandez-Aranda, F., Jimenez-Murcia, S., *et al.* (2012). Lifetime obesity in patients with eating disorders: increasing prevalence, clinical and personality correlates. *European Eating Disorders Review* 20, 250–4.

Wade, T. D., Bergin, J. L., Tiggemann, M., Bulik, C. M., & Fairburn, C. G. (2006). Prevalence and long-term course of lifetime eating disorders in an adult Australian twin cohort. *Australian and New Zealand Journal of Psychiatry* 40, 121–8.

Wade, T. D., Keski-Rahkonen, A., & Hudson, J. I. (2011). Epidemiology of eating disorders. In M. T. Tsuang, M. Tohen, & P. Jones, eds., *Textbook of Psychiatric Epidemiology*, 3rd Edition. New York, NY: John Wiley & Sons, pp. 343–60.

Wang, P. S., Aguilar-Gaxiola, S., Alonso, J., *et al.* (2007). Use of mental health services for anxiety, mood, and substance disorders in 17 countries in the WHO world mental health surveys. *Lancet* 370, 841–50.

Wonderlich, S. A., Gordon, K. H., Mitchell, J. E., Crosby, R. D., & Engel, S. G. (2009). The validity and clinical utility of binge eating disorder. *International Journal of Eating Disorders* 42, 687–705.

Zachrisson, H. D., Vedul-Kjelsas, E., Gotestam, K. G., & Mykletun, A. (2008). Time trends in obesity and eating disorders. *International Journal of Eating Disorders* 41, 673–80.

Chapter

19 Psychotic Experiences

John J. McGrath, Sukanta Saha, Carmen C. W. Lim, Oye Gureje, Silvia Florescu

Introduction

Community-based surveys have identified that a substantial proportion of individuals who do not have a confirmed psychotic disorder endorse items related to the presence of hallucinations and delusions (psychotic experiences, PEs). For example, a meta-analysis (based on 61 studies) reported a median lifetime prevalence of PEs of 7.2% (Linscott & van Os 2013). These estimates were substantially higher than the lifetime prevalence of psychotic disorders such as schizophrenia (median estimate 0.4%) (Saha *et al.* 2005), and the field of psychiatric epidemiology has reappraised how these experiences 'fit' into the epidemiologic landscape of psychotic disorders. The terminology to describe these experiences has also been revised in recent years. Sometimes referred to as psychotic-like experiences or psychosis-like symptoms, we will use the general term psychotic experiences (PEs), and the specific terms hallucinatory experiences (HEs) and delusional experiences (DEs) in this chapter.

Understandably, early work on the epidemiology of PEs was focused on the utility of these experiences as risk indicators for later conversion to full psychosis (Hanssen *et al.* 2005; Werbeloff *et al.* 2012). There was an appealing logic to this research, as many of the risk factors associated with PEs are also associated with schizophrenia/psychosis (e.g. cannabis, trauma, physical health) (Scott *et al.* 2007; Kelleher & Cannon 2010; Saha *et al.* 2011a). More recently, the evidence has indicated that PEs are also associated with a wide array of common mental disorders including anxiety, mood, and substance-use disorders (Johns *et al.* 2004; Freeman & Fowler 2009; Saha *et al.* 2011a; Varghese *et al.* 2011b; Yung *et al.* 2011; Saha *et al.* 2012). A prospective population-based study from Israel confirmed that those with PEs at baseline had an increased risk of being hospitalized for both psychotic disorders and non-psychotic (mental) disorders over the following 24 years (Kaymaz *et al.* 2012). There is also evidence that individuals who report PEs have a significantly increased risk of suicidal ideation, intent, and attempts (Nishida *et al.* 2010; Saha *et al.* 2011a–2011e; Kelleher and Cannon 2010; Kelleher *et al.* 2014). As the empirical data have accumulated, there has been debate about whether PEs represent a continuum of psychopathology (analogous with mild vs. severe depression), and/or a '*form fruste*' or attenuated expression of psychosis that may persist and worsen over time (David 2010; Kaymaz & van Os 2010; Lawrie *et al.* 2010; Sommer 2010).

The first wave of studies on PEs had several major limitations. First, the studies contributing to the systematic reviews have assessed PEs using a wide array of scales and diagnostic instruments – 20 different instruments were identified in the most recent systematic review (Linscott & van Os 2013). In order to allow synthesis of these data, PE data are usually dichotomized (lifetime prevalence present/absent). There is a need for studies that can efficiently measure different types of PEs and retain more fine-grain data related to PEs. Second, much of the previous research has examined associations between lifetime PEs and lifetime mental disorders regardless of temporal priority. There is a lack of empirical data on whether temporally primary common mental disorders are associated with an increased risk of subsequent first onset of PEs, and conversely, which mental disorders are predicted by pre-existing PEs. The World Mental Health (WMH) surveys provide a suitable cross-national platform to explore the epidemiology of PEs. For example, WMH analyses provide more textured information about comorbidity between PEs and other mental disorders, and can take into account the temporal order of these events based on retrospective reports of ages of onset. The surveys also allow us to provide much more detailed information than previous studies about risk factors, with a special focus on parental psychopathology, childhood adversities, and exposure to traumatic experiences that precede the onset of the PEs. The aim of this chapter is to present the lifetime and 12-month prevalence of PEs, DEs and HEs and explore key socio-demographic correlates of PEs based on the WMH surveys data.

Methods

Eighteen WMH surveys completed the Composite International Diagnostic Interview (CIDI) Psychosis Module (Kessler & Üstün 2008). In keeping with previous studies of PEs (Scott *et al.* 2007; Saha *et al.* 2011a–e, 2012, 2013; Varghese *et al.* 2011a), we made the *a priori* decision to exclude individuals who had PEs but who also screened positive for possible schizophrenia/psychosis, and manic-depression/mania. Thus, we excluded respondents who (a) reported (1) *schizophrenia/psychosis* or (2) *manic-depression/mania* in response to the question '*What did the doctor say was causing (this/these) experiences?*' or (b) reported lifetime use of an antipsychotic medication for these symptoms. This resulted in the exclusion of 140 respondents (0.4% of all respondents), leaving 31,261 respondents for this study. Analyses in this chapter were based on the weighted Part II subsample of respondents administered the CIDI Psychosis Module.

The CIDI Psychosis Module included questions about six PE types – two related to HEs (visual hallucinations, auditory hallucinations) and four related to DEs (two 'bizarre' delusional items – thought insertion/withdrawal, mind control/passivity; two 'paranoid' delusional items – ideas of reference, plot to harm/follow). For example, respondents were asked if they ever experienced PEs (e.g. '*Have you ever heard any voices that other people said did not exist?*') (Table 19.1). This was followed by a probe question to determine if the reported PEs ever occurred when the person was '*not dreaming, not half-asleep, or not under the influence of alcohol or drugs*'. Only responses of the latter type are considered here.

Respondents who reported PEs were then asked about: (a) presence of the PEs in the past 12 months and (b) frequency/occurrences of the PEs in their lifetime. We present prevalence estimates for any PEs, any HEs (with or without associated DEs), any DEs (with or without associated HEs), 'pure' HEs (without DEs), and 'pure' DEs (without HEs). In addition, we present key PE-related metrics: (a) count of types of PEs (henceforth referred to as *PEs type metric*) and (b) cumulative or annual frequency of occurrence of PEs episodes. Respondents who reported PEs were also asked probe questions about the age-of-onset (AOO) of PEs (i.e. *How old were you the very first time (this/either of these things/any of these things)* happened to you?).

Generic statistical methods are detailed in Chapter 3. This chapter includes an additional analysis that investigated bi-directionality in comorbidity with mental disorders. For this, discrete-time survival analyses (Singer & Willett 1993) with person-year as the unit of analysis and time-varying measures for prior onset of other mental disorders were used to examine the predictive associations of temporally prior disorders with the subsequent onset of each mental disorder considered in the analysis. We estimated survival models that examined bivariate associations between PEs and only one common mental disorder at a time (with adjustment for age-cohorts, gender, person-year, education, marital and employment status, and country) as well as multivariate models that included information on all temporally primary common mental disorders to predict the outcome disorder. The latter models included measures of number of prior mental disorders.

Table 19.1 Six CIDI psychotic experiences items

Saw a vision: Did you ever see something that wasn't really there that other people could not see?
Heard voices: Did you ever hearing things that other people said did not exist, like strange voices coming from inside your head talking to you or about you, or voices coming out of the air when there was no one around?
Thought insertion: Did you ever believe that some mysterious force was inserting many different strange thoughts – that were definitely not your own thoughts – directly into your head by means of x-rays or laser beams or other methods?
Mind control/passivity: Did you ever feel that your mind had been taken over by strange forces with laser beams or other methods that were making you do things you did not choose to do?
Ideas of reference: Did you ever believe that some strange force was trying to communicate directly with you by sending special signs or signals that you could understand but that no one else could understand. Sometimes this happens by special signs coming through the radio or television?
Plot to harm/follow: Did you ever believe that there was an unjust plot going on to harm you or to have people follow you that your family and friends did not believe existed?

Results

Prevalence

Table 19.2 presents country-specific lifetime PEs prevalence estimates. In all countries combined, lifetime prevalence of any PE is 5.8%, of any HE it is 5.2%, and of any DE it is 1.3%. Twelve-month prevalence of any PEs is 2.0%. From additional analyses reported in a prior publication, prevalence of lifetime PEs is

Table 19.2 Prevalence of psychotic experiences in the World Mental Health surveys

Country	Lifetime prevalence										12-month prevalence		12-month prevalence of PEs among lifetime cases		Sample size used
	Psychotic experiences		Hallucinatory experiences		Delusional experiences		Pure hallucinatory experiences		Pure delusional experiences		Psychotic experiences				
	%	SE	%	SE	%	SE	%	SE	%	SE	%	SE	%	SE	
Low/lower-middle-income countries	**3.2**	**0.3**	**2.6**	**0.2**	**0.9**	**0.1**	**2.3**	**0.2**	**0.6**	**0.1**	**1.2**	**0.2**	**36.3**	**3.8**	**9,466**
Colombia	7.5	1.2	7.1	1.2	0.9	0.3	6.7	1.2	0.4	0.2	2.1	0.5	27.5	6.5	722
Iraq	1.2	0.2	1.1	0.2	0.4	0.2	0.8	0.2	0.1	0.1	0.7	0.2	54.9	10.7	4,329
Nigeria	2.2	0.5	1.7	0.4	1.0	0.4	1.2	0.4	0.4	0.3	1.0	0.4	46.7	12.7	1,417
Peru	6.4	1.4	6.1	1.4	1.1	0.4	5.3	1.2	0.3	0.2	3.3	0.9	52.3	9.3	530
PRC (Shenzhen)	5.3	0.8	3.8	0.6	1.8	0.4	3.4	0.6	1.5	0.4	1.4	0.3	25.7	5.0	2,468
Upper-middle-income countries	**7.2**	**0.4**	**6.4**	**0.4**	**1.7**	**0.1**	**5.5**	**0.4**	**0.8**	**0.1**	**2.7**	**0.2**	**37.2**	**3.0**	**7,023**
Brazil	14.9	0.9	13.3	0.9	3.6	0.3	11.3	0.8	1.6	0.3	5.6	0.4	37.4	3.4	2,922
Lebanon	1.9	0.4	1.6	0.4	0.6	0.3	1.3	0.4	0.3	0.1	0.9	0.4	50.3	12.5	1,029
Mexico	4.1	1.0	3.6	0.9	0.8	0.4	3.3	0.9	0.5	0.3	1.4	0.4	33.2	10.3	715
Romania	1.0	0.4	0.9	0.4	0.1	0.1	0.8	0.4	0.1	0.0	0.3	0.1	27.3	8.6	2,357
High-income countries	**6.8**	**0.3**	**6.2**	**0.3**	**1.4**	**0.1**	**5.4**	**0.3**	**0.7**	**0.1**	**2.2**	**0.2**	**32.0**	**2.0**	**14,772**
Belgium	8.3	2.5	5.0	1.6	5.7	2.3	2.6	1.2	3.2	1.9	4.1	2.4	49.3	18.6	319
France	5.7	1.4	4.9	1.3	1.6	0.6	4.2	1.4	0.8	0.3	1.3	0.7	22.6	10.5	301
Germany	2.8	0.5	1.8	0.4	1.3	0.3	1.5	0.3	0.9	0.3	1.0	0.2	37.0	7.1	408
Italy	4.5	0.8	3.5	1.0	1.9	0.6	2.6	0.9	0.9	0.4	1.3	0.5	29.2	11.5	617
New Zealand	6.9	0.4	6.5	0.4	0.9	0.1	6.0	0.4	0.4	0.1	2.4	0.2	34.0	2.7	7,263
Portugal	5.2	0.7	3.9	0.5	2.6	0.5	2.6	0.5	1.3	0.4	1.7	0.3	32.1	6.2	2,053
Spain	6.7	1.5	5.8	1.5	1.4	0.4	5.3	1.5	0.9	0.3	0.9	0.2	13.4	4.4	1,159
Netherlands	10.8	2.5	10.1	2.5	1.6	0.5	9.2	2.4	0.7	0.4	3.0	1.2	27.9	10.3	348
United States	8.6	0.9	8.2	0.9	1.3	0.2	7.3	0.9	0.4	0.1	2.8	0.4	32.4	4.2	2,304
All countries combined	**5.8**	**0.2**	**5.2**	**0.2**	**1.3**	**0.1**	**4.5**	**0.2**	**0.7**	**0.1**	**2.0**	**0.1**	**34.2**	**1.5**	**31,261**
WHO regions[a]															
Region of the Americas	10.4	0.5	9.5	0.5	2.1	0.2	8.3	0.5	0.9	0.1	3.7	0.2	35.8	2.4	7,193
African region	2.2	0.5	1.7	0.4	1.0	0.4	1.2	0.4	0.4	0.3	1.0	0.4	46.7	12.7	1,417
Western Pacific region	6.5	0.3	5.8	0.3	1.1	0.1	5.4	0.3	0.7	0.1	2.1	0.2	32.3	2.4	9,731
Eastern Mediterranean region	1.4	0.2	1.2	0.2	0.5	0.1	0.9	0.2	0.2	0.1	0.7	0.2	53.7	8.5	5,358
Western European region	5.8	0.5	4.6	0.4	2.2	0.3	3.6	0.4	1.2	0.2	1.7	0.2	28.4	3.9	5,205
Eastern European region	1.0	0.4	0.9	0.4	0.1	0.1	0.8	0.4	0.1	0.0	0.3	0.1	27.3	8.6	2,357
Comparison between countries[b]	**$F_{17,v}$ = 24.7*, P < 0.001**		**$F_{17,v}$ = 23.4*, P < 0.001**		**$F_{17,v}$ = 13.6*, P < 0.001**		**$F_{17,v}$ = 21.7*, P < 0.001**		**$F_{17,v}$ = 4.8*, P < 0.001**		**$F_{17,v}$ = 13.6*, P < 0.001**		**$F_{17,v}$ = 1.3, P = 0.185**		
Comparison between low-, middle-, and high-income country groups[b]	**$F_{2,v}$ = 49.5*, P < 0.001**		**$F_{2,v}$ = 58.3*, P < 0.001**		**$F_{2,v}$ = 7.1*, P = 0.001**		**$F_{2,v}$ = 52.0*, P < 0.001**		**$F_{2,v}$ = 0.8, P = 0.446**		**$F_{2,v}$ = 21.3*, P < 0.001**		**$F_{2,v}$ = 1.3, P = 0.284**		
Comparison between WHO regions[b]	**$F_{5,v}$ = 75.8*, P < 0.001**		**$F_{5,v}$ = 70.6*, P < 0.001**		**$F_{5,v}$ = 42.5*, P < 0.001**		**$F_{5,v}$ = 67.3*, P < 0.001**		**$F_{5,v}$ = 14.4*, P < 0.001**		**$F_{5,v}$ = 38.3*, P < 0.001**		**$F_{5,v}$ = 1.7, P = 0.128**		

*Significant at the 0.05 level, two-sided test.

[a] **Region of the Americas** (Colombia, Mexico, Brazil, Peru, United States); **African region** (Nigeria); **Western Pacific region** (PRC Shen Zhen, New Zealand); **Eastern Mediterranean region** (Iraq, Lebanon); **Western European region** (Belgium, France, Germany, Italy, Netherlands, Spain, Portugal); **Eastern European region** (Romania).

[b] Wald design-corrected F-tests were used to determine if there is variation in prevalence estimates across countries. The denominator degree of freedom, v, is 841.

PRC: People's Republic of China

significantly higher among women than men (6.6% vs. 5.0%) (McGrath *et al.* 2015). Similar gender differences are found for prevalence of HEs but not DEs. The significant gender difference is also found for respondents with 'pure' HEs, but not 'pure' DEs. Significant differences are evident across the three country income groups in lifetime prevalence of any different PEs (Table 19.2). In each comparison the prevalence estimates are lower among respondents in low/lower-middle-income countries than in upper-middle- and high-income countries. Significant differences are also found between WHO regions. For example, regions of the Americas, Western Pacific, and Western European have higher prevalence compared to other regions that represent low-income countries.

More detailed analyses reported in our prior publication found the most common PE type overall to be visual hallucinations (3.8%) followed by auditory hallucinations (2.5%) (McGrath *et al.* 2015). Prevalence estimates of individual DEs types were low (0.3–0.7%). Among those with any lifetime PEs, 72.0% (representing 4.2% of the total sample) reported only one PE type, 21.1% (representing 1.2% of the total sample) exactly two types, and 6.8% (representing 0.4% of the total sample) three or more types. We also found that PEs are typically infrequent, with 32.2% of the respondents with lifetime PEs reporting only one solitary episode. An additional 31.8% of respondents with lifetime PEs experienced only 2–5 PEs episodes. Thus, for nearly two-thirds of respondents (64.0%) with lifetime PEs, these experiences occurred only 1–5 times in their lives. This lack of persistence of PEs across the lifetime is also indicated in Table 19.2 by the proportion of lifetime cases of PE with 12-month prevalence being relatively low (34.2% in all countries combined). This 12-month/lifetime ratio is an indicator of the course of symptoms (persistence or recurrence) and it is notable that at 34%, this proportion is substantially lower than the corresponding proportions observed for most of the mental disorders featured in this volume (see Chapter 22).

Socio-demographic Correlates

Table 19.3 shows the association of socio-demographic variables with lifetime onset of PEs, HEs, and DEs, and course of any PE, in bivariate models. Several socio-demographic variables are associated with increased lifetime risk of PEs, HEs, and DEs: (a) being younger (compared to those over 60 years); (b) being classified as 'other' employment (looking for work, disabled, etc.) (vs. employed); (c) being separated/widowed/divorced (vs. married); and (d) lower household income (vs. high income). In addition to these findings, several socio-demographic variables are associated with only one type of PE. Female gender is associated with HE and through this with any PE, but not with DE (as also noted in the section above on prevalence). Being never married is associated with DE, but not PE or HE. Lower education is associated with any PE and HE, but less consistently with DE. In general, associations between socio-demographic variables and the pure subtypes of HE and DE are similar to those for PEs in general.

In contrast to these associations between a wide range of socio-demographic variables and lifetime onset of PEs, it is notable that few socio-demographic factors are associated with course/persistence of PEs (12 months/lifetime). Employment status and educational outcomes warrant closer attention in future studies.

Age-of-Onset

Most people experience PEs early in their lives; 5% of all cases will have experienced a PE by age eight years, 25% by age 17, 50% by age 26, 75% by age 41, and 99% by age 62 (Table 19.4). The age-of-onset (AOO) distributions for PEs, DEs, and HEs do not differ by gender. The projected AOO distribution is marginally earlier for low/low-middle- (median AOO = 23, IQR = 15–41) and high-income countries (median AOO = 24, IQR = 16–40) when compared to upper-middle-income countries (median AOO = 28, IQR = 18–42) ($\chi^2_2 = 18.3$, $P < 0.001$).

The projected lifetime risk for all countries combined at age 75 is 7.8%. This is higher than the lifetime prevalence estimate (5.8%). The gap between lifetime prevalence estimates and the projected lifetime risk is 2.0%. This suggests that a small proportion of respondents who had not experienced PEs prior to survey interview can be expected to experience PEs before 75 years. Across the three country income groups, the projected lifetime risk is 53%, 38%, and 21% higher among high-, upper-middle-, and low/lower-middle-income countries respectively, compared to lifetime prevalence estimates. When classified by WHO regions, the highest projected lifetime risk for PEs is found in the Americas (14.2%) followed by Western Pacific regions (8.2%), and Western European regions (7.4%).

Table 19.3 Bivariate associations between socio-demographic correlates and psychotic experiences, all countries combined

Correlates	Lifetime PE[a,b]		Lifetime HE[a,b]		Lifetime DE[a,b]		Lifetime pure HE[a,b]		Lifetime pure DE[a,b]		12-month PE among lifetime cases[c]	
	OR	(95% CI)	OR	(95% CI)	OR	(95% CI)	OR	(95% CI)	OR	(95% CI)	OR	(95% CI)
Age-cohort												
18–29	**5.4***	(4.2–7.1)	**4.6***	(3.5–5.9)	**14.0***	(7.4–26.4)	**4.2***	(3.2–5.6)	**36.6***	(12.3–109.14)		
30–44	**2.6***	(2.0–3.2)	**2.3***	(1.8–2.9)	**4.9***	(2.8–8.4)	**2.2***	(1.7–2.8)	**9.8***	(3.8–25.3)		
45–59	**1.7***	(1.3–2.0)	**1.5***	(1.2–1.8)	**2.9***	(1.7–4.8)	**1.4***	(1.1–1.8)	**5.6***	(2.5–12.6)		
60+	**1.0**		**1.0**		**1.0**		**1.0**		**1.0**			
Age-cohort difference[d]	$\chi^2_3 = 210.3^*$, P < 0.001		$\chi^2_3 = 170.3^*$, P < 0.001		$\chi^2_3 = 92.8^*$, P < 0.001		$\chi^2_3 = 122.7^*$, P < 0.001		$\chi^2_3 = 55.5^*$, P < 0.001			
Gender												
Female	**1.3***	(1.1–1.5)	**1.4***	(1.2–1.6)	**1.1**	(0.8–1.3)	**1.4***	(1.2–1.6)	**1.0**	(0.7–1.3)	**1.0**	(0.8–1.3)
Male	**1.0**		**1.0**		**1.0**		**1.0**		**1.0**		**1.0**	
Gender difference[d]	$\chi^2_1 = 12.6^*$, P < 0.001		$\chi^2_1 = 15.3^*$, P < 0.001		$\chi^2_1 = 0.2$, P = 0.627		$\chi^2_1 = 15.2^*$, P < 0.001		$\chi^2_1 = 0.1$, P = 0.818		$\chi^2_1 = 0.0$, P = 0.878	
Employment status												
Student	**1.3**	(0.9–1.9)	**1.3**	(0.9–2.0)	**0.9**	(0.5–1.7)	**1.4**	(0.9–2.2)	**1.1**	(0.4–2.7)	**1.3**	(0.7–2.3)
Homemaker	**1.2**	(1.0–1.4)	**1.2***	(1.0–1.5)	**1.0**	(0.7–1.5)	**1.2**	(1.0–1.5)	**0.6**	(0.3–1.1)	**1.2**	(0.9–1.8)
Retired	**0.7***	(0.5–1.0)	**0.7***	(0.5–0.9)	**1.1**	(0.5–2.2)	**0.7***	(0.5–0.9)	**1.8**	(0.7–4.4)	**0.9**	(0.5–1.6)
Other	**1.5***	(1.2–1.8)	**1.5***	(1.2–1.8)	**2.2***	(1.6–3.0)	**1.2**	(1.0–1.6)	**1.4**	(0.9–2.3)	**1.5***	(1.0–2.1)
Employed	**1.0**		**1.0**		**1.0**		**1.0**		**1.0**		**1.0**	
Employment status difference[d]	$\chi^2_4 = 25.8^*$, P < 0.001		$\chi^2_4 = 25.6^*$, P < 0.001		$\chi^2_4 = 26.6^*$, P < 0.001		$\chi^2_4 = 14.3^*$, P = 0.006		$\chi^2_4 = 11.4^*$, P = 0.023		$\chi^2_4 = 6.4$, P = 0.174	
Marital status												
Never married	**1.2**	(1.0–1.4)	**1.1**	(0.9–1.3)	**1.9***	(1.4–2.6)	**1.0**	(0.8–1.2)	**2.1***	(1.3–3.3)	**1.2**	(0.9–1.7)
Divorced/separated/widowed	**1.6***	(1.3–1.9)	**1.5***	(1.2–1.8)	**1.8***	(1.3–2.6)	**1.5***	(1.2–1.9)	**2.3***	(1.4–3.8)	**1.0**	(0.7–1.4)
Currently married	**1.0**		**1.0**		**1.0**		**1.0**		**1.0**		**1.0**	
Marital status difference[d]	$\chi^2_2 = 20.0^*$, P < 0.001		$\chi^2_2 = 14.1^*$, P = 0.001		$\chi^2_2 = 25.7^*$, P < 0.001		$\chi^2_2 = 13.5^*$, P = 0.001		$\chi^2_2 = 17.5^*$, P < 0.001		$\chi^2_2 = 1.6$, P = 0.453	
Education level												
No education	**1.9***	(1.0–3.6)	**1.9**	(1.0–3.7)	**3.4***	(1.0–11.0)	**1.5**	(0.7–3.2)	–		**2.8***	(1.1–7.0)
Some primary	**1.6**	(0.9–2.8)	**1.8***	(1.0–3.2)	**1.7**	(0.6–5.1)	**1.6**	(0.9–2.9)	**0.4**	(0.2–1.2)	**1.3**	(0.7–2.2)
Finished primary	**0.9**	(0.6–1.4)	**0.9**	(0.6–1.4)	**0.9**	(0.3–2.6)	**0.9**	(0.5–1.5)	**0.8**	(0.2–3.6)	**1.9**	(1.0–3.8)
Some secondary	**1.3**	(1.0–1.8)	**1.3**	(1.0–1.8)	**1.4**	(0.8–2.7)	**1.3**	(0.9–1.8)	**1.0**	(0.4–2.6)	**1.0**	(0.6–1.6)
Finished secondary	**1.4***	(1.0–1.8)	**1.4***	(1.0–1.9)	**1.4**	(0.7–2.7)	**1.3**	(1.0–1.8)	**1.0**	(0.4–2.7)	**0.9**	(0.5–1.5)
Some college	**1.6***	(1.2–2.1)	**1.6***	(1.2–2.2)	**1.3**	(0.6–2.6)	**1.6***	(1.2–2.2)	**1.2**	(0.4–3.4)	**1.0**	(0.6–1.6)
Finished college	**1.0**		**1.0**		**1.0**		**1.0**		**1.0**		**1.0**	

Table 19.3 (*cont.*)

Correlates	Lifetime PE[a,b]		Lifetime HE[a,b]		Lifetime DE[a,b]		Lifetime pure HE[a,b]		Lifetime pure DE[a,b]		12-month PE among lifetime cases[c]	
	OR	(95% CI)	OR	(95% CI)	OR	(95% CI)	OR	(95% CI)	OR	(95% CI)	OR	(95% CI)
Education level difference[d]	$\chi^2_6 = 17.7^*$, $P = 0.007$		$\chi^2_6 = 19.0^*$, $P = 0.004$		$\chi^2_6 = 5.7$, $P = 0.457$		$\chi^2_6 = 14.6^*$, $P = 0.024$		$\chi^2_6 = 7.9$, $P = 0.247$		$\chi^2_6 = 10.7$, $P = 0.097$	
Household income												
Low	**1.6***	(1.4–1.9)	**1.7***	(1.4–2.0)	**1.7***	(1.3–2.3)	**1.6***	(1.3–1.9)	**1.3**	(0.8–2.0)	**1.4**	(1.0–2.0)
Low-average	**1.2**	(1.0–1.4)	**1.2**	(1.0–1.5)	**1.0**	(0.7–1.3)	**1.2**	(1.0–1.5)	**0.8**	(0.5–1.2)	**1.3**	(0.9–2.0)
High-average	**1.1**	(0.9–1.3)	**1.1**	(0.9–1.3)	**1.0**	(0.7–1.4)	**1.1**	(0.9–1.4)	**0.9**	(0.6–1.4)	**1.1**	(0.7–1.6)
High	**1.0**		**1.0**		**1.0**		**1.0**		**1.0**		**1.0**	
Household income difference[d]	$\chi^2_3 = 38.6^*$, $P < 0.001$		$\chi^2_3 = 32.4^*$, $P < 0.001$		$\chi^2_3 = 22.0^*$, $P < 0.001$		$\chi^2_3 = 20.1^*$, $P < 0.001$		$\chi^2_3 = 5.6$, $P = 0.133$		$\chi^2_3 = 4.6$, $P = 0.203$	
Age-of-onset												
Early											**1.5***	(1.0–2.3)
Early-average											**1.0**	(0.7–1.4)
Late-average											**1.1**	(0.7–1.6)
Late											**1.0**	
Age-of-onset difference[d]											$\chi^2_3 = 6.4$, $P = 0.096$	
Time since onset (continuous)											**0.98***	(0.97–0.99)
N[e]	**1,278,613**		**12,282,275**		**1,308,724**		**1,288,506**		**1,314,955**		**2,385**	

*Significant at the 0.05 level, two-sided test.
[a]PE, Psychotic Experiences; HE, Hallucinatory Experiences; DE, Delusional Experiences.
[b]These estimates are based on survival models adjusted for age-cohorts, gender, person-years, and country.
[c]These estimates are based on logistic regression models adjusted for time since PE onset, age of PE onset, gender, and country.
[d]Chi-square test of significant differences between blocks of socio-demographic variables.
[e]Denominator N: 2,385 = number of lifetime PE cases. The denominator in other models are referring to the number of person-years in the survival models.

Table 19.4 Standardized age-of-onset distributions of psychotic experiences (PE) with projected lifetime risk at age 75

Country	Ages at selected percentiles								Lifetime prevalence of PE		Projected risk at age 75	
	5	10	25	50	75	90	95	99	%	SE	%	SE
Low/lower-middle-income countries	**7**	**10**	**16**	**23**	**41**	**54**	**56**	**56**	**3.2**	**0.3**	**4.9**	**0.5**
Colombia[a]	13	13	24	41	56	56	56	56	7.5	1.2	13.8	3.8
Iraq	17	17	22	26	45	46	49	49	1.2	0.2	1.9	0.4
Nigeria	6	6	14	21	41	41	41	41	2.2	0.5	3.3	0.8
Peru[a]	13	13	21	25	39	50	50	50	6.4	1.4	8.8	2.5
PRC (Shenzhen)	6	8	16	27	54	54	54	54	5.3	0.8	8.3	1.8
Upper-middle-income countries	**8**	**12**	**18**	**28**	**42**	**49**	**50**	**61**	**7.2**	**0.4**	**9.9**	**0.7**
Brazil	8	14	18	27	42	49	49	61	14.9	0.9	20.8	1.8
Lebanon	29	32	50	50	50	50	50	50	1.9	0.4	3.8	1.2
Mexico[a]	8	8	8	18	36	38	38	38	4.1	1.0	6.9	1.4
Romania	6	8	19	20	29	29	29	29	1.0	0.4	1.0	0.4
High-income countries	**7**	**9**	**16**	**24**	**40**	**54**	**54**	**65**	**6.8**	**0.3**	**8.2**	**0.4**
Belgium	19	19	45	48	52	52	52	52	8.3	2.5	14.6	4.7
France	9	9	9	15	19	36	36	36	5.7	1.4	5.9	1.4
Germany	8	8	8	11	23	23	23	23	2.8	0.5	3.3	0.7
Italy	6	6	16	26	36	44	44	44	4.5	0.8	5.0	1.0
New Zealand	8	9	15	22	36	46	54	54	6.9	0.4	8.1	0.5
Portugal	5	10	16	36	40	54	54	54	5.2	0.7	6.1	1.1
Spain	13	13	14	19	48	62	62	62	6.7	1.5	8.8	2.1
Netherlands	5	5	17	21	54	65	65	65	10.8	2.5	15.3	4.3
United States	7	11	19	26	40	54	61	62	8.6	0.9	10.1	1.5
All countries combined	**8**	**10**	**17**	**26**	**41**	**52**	**54**	**62**	**5.8**	**0.2**	**7.8**	**0.3**
WHO regions												
Region of the Americas	8	12	18	26	41	49	58	62	10.4	0.5	14.2	0.9
African region	6	6	14	21	41	41	41	41	2.2	0.5	3.3	0.8
Western Pacific region	6	8	15	20	35	48	54	54	6.5	0.3	8.2	0.5
Eastern Mediterranean region	17	19	23	31	49	50	50	50	1.4	0.2	2.3	0.4
Western European region	6	10	15	26	48	54	62	65	5.8	0.5	7.4	0.8
Eastern European region	6	8	19	20	29	29	29	29	1.0	0.4	1.0	0.4

[a]The projected risk for these countries is at age 65 because the age range of these surveys is between 18 and 65.
PRC: People's Republic of China.

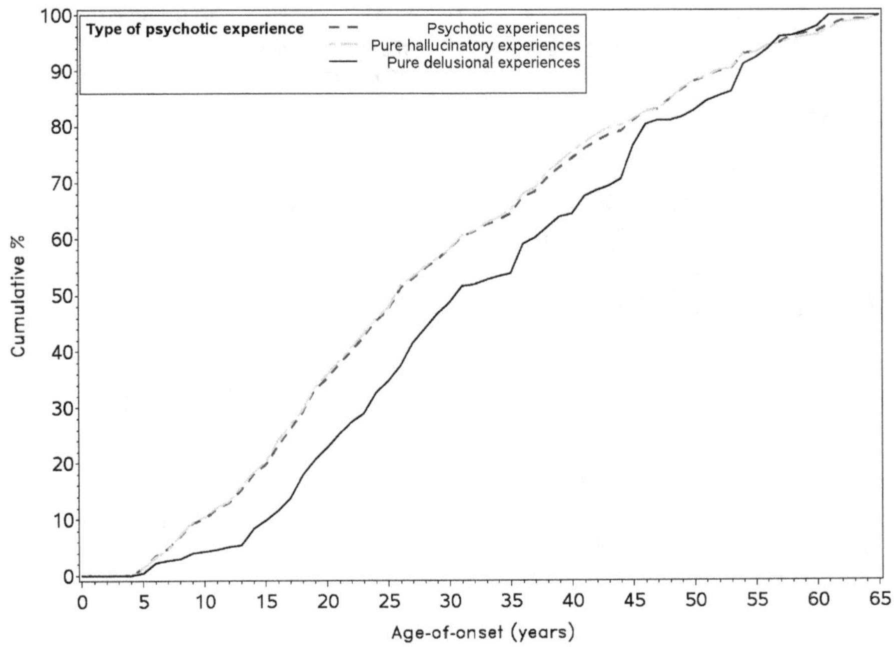

Figure 19.1 Cumulative age-of-onset distribution of psychotic experiences, all countries combined.

Figure 19.1 shows the cumulative AOO distributions of PEs and related subtypes based on projected data for the various PEs subgroups, including those with PEs, pure HEs, and pure DEs. A key feature that emerges from these distributions relates to the delayed AOO for those with pure DEs. Those with pure DEs have a later AOO distribution. The AOO for pure HEs is significantly earlier than that for pure DEs ($X^2_1 = 590.5, P < 0.001$).

The Bi-directional Associations between PEs and Mental Disorders

When we examined the prevalence of mental disorders among respondents with and without PEs (without considering temporal sequence), compared to those with no PEs those with PEs had significantly higher odds of having 20 of the 21 mental disorders examined (McGrath *et al.* 2016b). In this chapter we present summary results of these associations from multivariate models in Figure 19.2. We first examined temporally prior PEs and found in these models that those with PEs are significantly more likely to subsequently experience 8 of 21 disorders (major depressive disorder, bipolar disorder, generalized anxiety disorder, social phobia, posttraumatic stress disorder, adult separation anxiety disorder, bulimia nervosa, alcohol abuse). When we examined the associations between preceding mental disorders and the subsequent onset of PEs in multivariate models, we found that 18 of the 21 mental disorders are significantly associated with the later onset of PEs.

Discussion

Based on these 18 WMH samples, we found that 5.8% of respondents reported having one or more psychotic experiences at least once in their lifetime and 2.0% in the previous year. These overall estimates are broadly consistent with the previous literature (Linscott & van Os 2013). Our data have contributed important new information regarding the count of psychotic experiences types and frequency of psychotic experiences that go beyond the issues considered in previous community-based studies of psychotic experiences. Perhaps the most striking finding is that psychotic experiences were not persistent for most of the individuals who experience them, with 32.2% reporting only one psychotic experience episode in their life; 64.0% reporting no more than five lifetime occurrences and only around a third of lifetime cases reporting PEs in the past year. This suggests that in the general population,

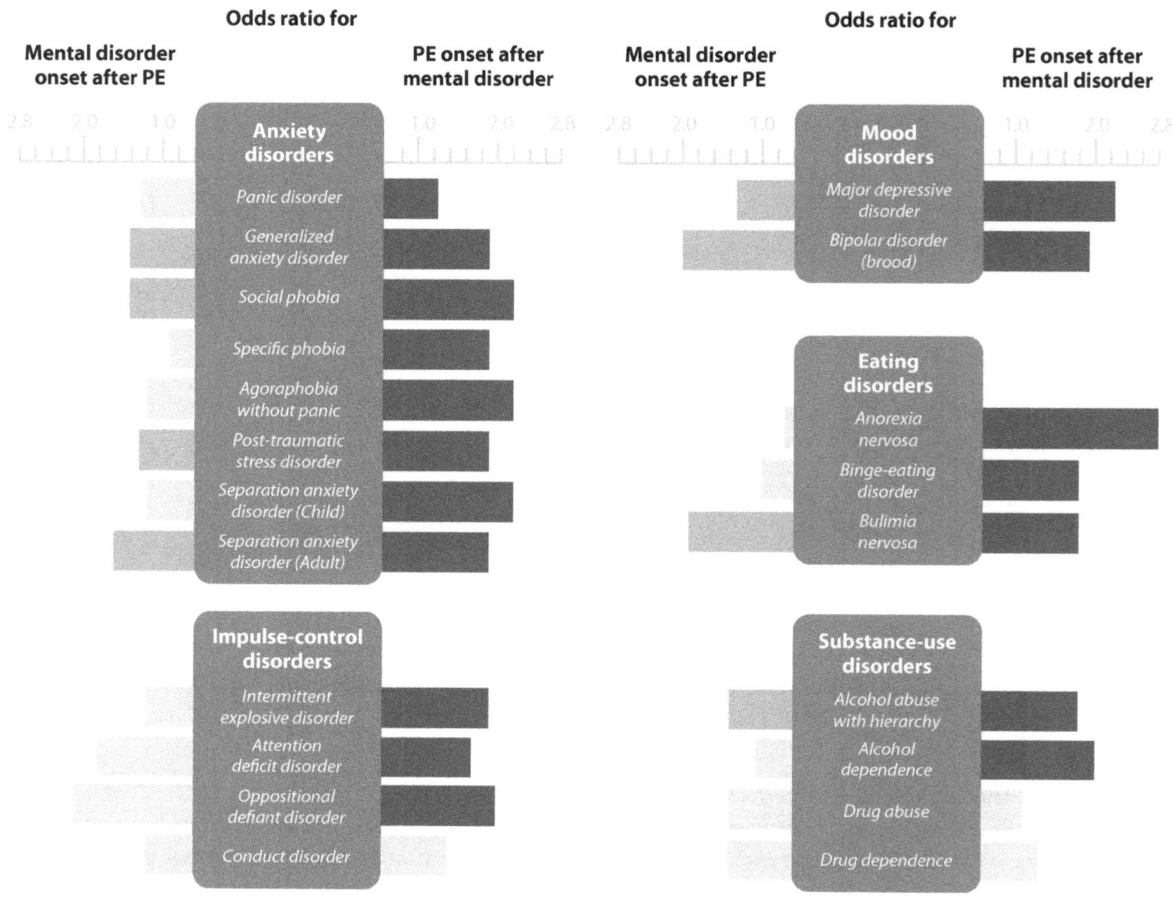

Figure 19.2 Summary of bi-directional associations between psychotic experiences (PEs) and mental disorders (odds ratios for insignificant associations are shown in the lightest grey bars).

only a small subgroup of individuals has multiple types of psychotic experiences and experiences these types of psychotic experiences more frequently. The CIDI only explores a subset of PEs (e.g. there are many types of DEs), and this needs to be taken into account when comparing prevalence estimates between studies that use difference scales to assess PEs.

The WMH data found that hallucinatory experiences are more common than delusional experiences (5.2% vs. 1.3%) and this general pattern was consistent across the three country income groups. Lifetime prevalence of psychotic experiences was lower in the low/lower-middle-income countries compared with the upper-middle- and high-income countries, reflecting a similar pattern observed in the prevalence of schizophrenia (Saha *et al.* 2005).

Based on projected AOO values, the median AOO for PEs was 26 years. Strikingly, approximately a quarter of individuals who will experience PEs during their life will have their first experience after age 40 years (McGrath *et al.* 2016a). In contrast to the AOO of schizophrenia (Thorup *et al.* 2007), we found no gender difference in the AOO of PEs (nor in HEs and DEs). The projected AOO for pure DEs was significantly right-shifted (encompassing older AOOs) compared to that for pure HEs while the AOO of PEs that contain any HEs show closely overlapping distributions. It will be of interest to explore if the risk factors associated with PEs in general differ according to AOO. For example, are respondents who have the onset of PEs later in life more likely to have a preceding mental disorder? The WMH surveys have provided us with many new research questions to guide future research.

The time-lagged associations between PEs and mental disorders provide new insights into the bi-directional relationship between psychotic experiences and mental disorders. The analysis demonstrates that individuals with PEs are at increased risk of experiencing a wide range of mental disorders at some stage in their life compared with other people in the population. On the other hand, we found a very consistent increased odds of psychotic experience onset after nearly all of the mental disorders we examined. That is, most mental disorders were associated with an increased likelihood of subsequent psychotic experiences, even in multivariate models. Of the 21 disorders examined in this study, only three externalizing disorders did not significantly predict subsequent psychotic experiences in the multivariate model (conduct disorder, drug abuse, and drug dependence). These findings call into the question the specificity of the association between psychotic experiences and psychotic disorders (Kelleher & Cannon 2010).

Our research has provided new insights into the fine-grained epidemiology of PEs, and also provided new insights into the bi-directional relationship between psychotic experiences and mental disorders. Epidemiologists have increasingly recognised the importance of considering psychotic experiences in the causal pathways of psychotic disorders. These new findings provide a heuristic framework for the generation of new hypotheses related to psychotic experiences.

Acknowledgements

Figure 19.2 appeared previously in: McGrath, J.J., Saha, S., Al-Hamzawi, A., Andrade, L., Benjet, C., Bromet, E.J., Browne, M.O., Caldas de Almeida, J.M., Chiu, W.T., Demyttenaere, K., Fayyad, J., Florescu, S., de Girolamo, G., Gureje, O., Haro, J.M., ten Have, M., Hu, C., Kovess-Masfety, V., Lim, C.C., Navarro-Mateu, F., Sampson, N., Posada-Villa, J., Kendler, K.S., Kessler, R.C. (2016). The bi-directional associations between psychotic experiences and DSM-IV mental disorders. *The American Journal of Psychiatry*, 173 (10), 997–1006, used with permission from The American Psychiatric Association (Journals).

References

David, A. S. (2010). Why we need more debate on whether psychotic symptoms lie on a continuum with normality. *Psychological Medicine*, 40, 1–8.

Freeman, D. & Fowler, D. (2009). Routes to psychotic symptoms: trauma, anxiety and psychosis-like experiences. *Psychiatry Research*, 169, 107–12.

Hanssen, M., Bak, M., Bijl, R., *et al.* (2005). The incidence and outcome of subclinical psychotic experiences in the general population. *British Journal of Clinical Psychology*, 44, 181–91.

Johns, L. C., Cannon, M., Singleton, N., *et al.* (2004). Prevalence and correlates of self-reported psychotic symptoms in the British population. *British Journal of Psychiatry*, 185, 298–305.

Kaymaz, N., Drukker, M., Lieb, R., *et al.* (2012). Do subthreshold psychotic experiences predict clinical outcomes in unselected non-help-seeking population-based samples? A systematic review and meta-analysis, enriched with new results. *Psychological Medicine*, 42, 2239–53.

Kaymaz, N. & van Os, J. (2010). Extended psychosis phenotype – yes: single continuum – unlikely. *Psychological Medicine*, 40, 1963–6.

Kelleher, I. and Cannon, M. (2010). Psychotic-like experiences in the general population: characterizing a high-risk group for psychosis. *Psychological Medicine*, 41, 1–6.

(2014). Whither the psychosis-neurosis borderline. *Schizophrenia Bulletin*, 40, 266–8.

Kelleher, I., Devlin, N., Wigman, J. T., *et al.* (2014). Psychotic experiences in a mental health clinic sample: implications for suicidality, multimorbidity and functioning. *Psychological Medicine*, 44, 1615–24.

Kessler, R. C. & Üstün, T. B. (2008). The World Health Organization Composite International Diagnostic Interview. *The WHO World Mental Health Surveys: Global Perspectives on the Epidemiology of Mental Disorders*. R. C. Kessler and T. B. Üstün, eds. New York: Cambridge University Press, 58–90.

Lawrie, S. M., Hall, J., McIntosh, A. M., *et al.* (2010). The 'continuum of psychosis': scientifically unproven and clinically impractical. *British Journal of Psychiatry*, 197, 423–5.

Linscott, R. J. & van Os, J. (2013). An updated and conservative systematic review and meta-analysis of epidemiological evidence on psychotic experiences in children and adults: on the pathway from proneness to persistence to dimensional expression across mental disorders. *Psychological Medicine*, 43, 1133–49.

McGrath, J. J., Saha, S., Al-Hamzawi, A., *et al.* (2015). Psychotic experiences in the general population: a cross-national analysis based on 31261 respondents from 18 countries. *JAMA Psychiatry*, 72, 697–705.

McGrath, J. J., Saha, S., Al-Hamzawi, A. O., *et al.* (2016a). Age of onset and lifetime projected risk of psychotic experiences: cross-national data from the World Mental Health Survey. *Schizophrenia Bulletin*, 42, 933–41.

McGrath, J. J., Saha, S., Al-Hamzawi, A., *et al.* (2016b). The bidirectional associations between psychotic experiences and DSM-IV mental disorders. *The American Journal of Psychiatry*, 173(10), 997–1006.

Nishida, A., Sasaki, T., Nishimura, Y., *et al.* (2010). Psychotic-like experiences are associated with suicidal feelings and deliberate self-harm behaviors in adolescents aged 12–15 years. *Acta Psychiatrica Scandinavica*, 121, 301–7.

Saha, S., Chant, D., Welham, J., *et al.* (2005). A systematic review of the prevalence of schizophrenia. *PLoS Medicine*, 2, e141.

Saha, S., Scott, J., Varghese, D., *et al.* (2011a). The association between physical health and delusional-like experiences: a general population study. *PLoS ONE*, 6, e18566.

Saha, S., Scott, J., Varghese, D., *et al.* (2012). Anxiety and depressive disorders are associated with delusional-like experiences: a replication study based on a National Survey of Mental Health and Wellbeing. *BMJ Open*, 2, e001001.

Saha, S., Scott, J. G., Johnston, A. K., *et al.* (2011b). The association between delusional-like experiences and suicidal thoughts and behaviour. *Schizophrenia Research*, 132, 197–202.

Saha, S., Scott, J. G., Varghese, D., *et al.* (2011c). The association between delusional-like experiences, and tobacco, alcohol or cannabis use: a nationwide population-based survey. *BMC Psychiatry*, 11, 202–10.

Saha, S., Scott, J. G., Varghese, D., *et al.* (2011d). The association between general psychological distress and delusional-like experiences: a large population-based study. *Schizophrenia Research*, 127, 246–51.

Saha, S., Scott, J. G., Varghese, D., *et al.* (2013). Socio-economic disadvantage and delusional-like experiences: A nationwide population-based study. *European Psychiatry*, 28, 59–63.

Saha, S., Varghese, D., Slade, T., *et al.* (2011e). The association between trauma and delusional-like experiences. *Psychiatry Research*, 189, 259–64.

Scott, J., Chant, D., Andrews, G., *et al.* (2007). Association between trauma exposure and delusional experiences in a large community-based sample. *British Journal of Psychiatry*, 190, 339–43.

Singer, J. D. & Willett, J. B. (1993). It's about time: using discrete-time survival analysis to study duration and the timing of events. *Journal of Educational Statistics*, 18, 155–95.

Sommer, I. E. (2010). The continuum hypothesis of psychosis: David's criticisms are timely. *Psychological Medicine*, 40, 1959–61.

Thorup, A., Waltoft, B. L., Pedersen, C. B., *et al.* (2007). Young males have a higher risk of developing schizophrenia: a Danish register study. *Psychological Medicine*, 37, 479–84.

Varghese, D., Saha, S., Scott, J. D., *et al.* (2011a). The association between family history of mental disorder and delusional-like experiences: a general population study. *American Journal of Medical Genetics Part B-Neuropsychiatric Genetics*, 156B, 478–83.

Varghese, D., Scott, J., Welham, J., *et al.* (2011b). Psychotic-like experiences in major depression and anxiety disorders: a population-based survey in young adults. *Schizophrenia Bulletin*, 37, 389–93.

Werbeloff, N., Drukker, M., Dohrenwend, B. P., *et al.* (2012). Self-reported attenuated psychotic symptoms as forerunners of severe mental disorders later in life. *Archives of General Psychiatry*, 69, 467–75.

Yung, A. R., Phillips, L. J., Nelson, B., *et al.* (2011). Randomized controlled trial of interventions for young people at ultra high risk for psychosis: 6-month analysis. *Journal of Clinical Psychiatry*, 72, 430–40.

Chapter 20

Comorbidity: The Cross-national Structure of Mental Disorders

Klaas J. Wardenaar, Yueqin Huang, Bogdan Wojtyniak, Peter de Jonge

Introduction

The previous chapters have described the cross-national epidemiology of each of the mental disorders separately. However, comorbidity is the rule rather than the exception among mental disorders. Many surveys (e.g., Kessler *et al.* 1994; Bijl *et al.* 1998; Teesson *et al.* 2009; Hasin & Kilcoyne 2012) have shown high rates of current and lifetime comorbidity between mental disorders, which is important both from a scientific and a clinical perspective. Associations (lifetime comorbidity) between the mental disorders included in this volume are shown in Table 20.1.

The high comorbidity rates among mental disorders indicate that these disorders are not strictly discrete entities and that the disorder diagnostic classifications do not reflect the natural way in which mental disorders occur (Sher & Trull 1996; Mineka *et al.* 1998; Widiger & Clark 2000). The observed patterns of comorbidity are considered to reflect the actual underlying structure of psychopathology and investigating this latent structure is important to gain knowledge that can be used for the development of evidence-based classifications of mental disorders (Carragher *et al.* 2015). Over the past decades, much scientific work has been dedicated to gaining a better understanding of comorbidity. Many studies have been focused on understanding comorbidity between particular pairs of disorders, such as bipolar disorder and borderline personality disorder (Frías *et al.* 2016) or attention deficit hyperactivity disorder (ADHD) and conduct disorder (CD; Knecht *et al.* 2015). Another line of research has focused on understanding the more general 'meta structure' of mental disorders (reviews: Mineka *et al.* 1998; Krueger & Markon 2006; Carragher *et al.* 2015; Eaton *et al.* 2015). The current chapter focuses on this latter, general line of research. The point of departure for this work has been the observation that some patterns of comorbidity are observed more often than others, suggesting that some sets of disorders have more in common than others and that perhaps higher-order factors may be present that can explain the high levels of comorbidity between specific mental disorders. Indeed, factor-analytical research has consistently shown that patterns of comorbidity between common mental disorders can be explained by at least two general underlying factors that have been labelled the 'internalizing' and 'externalizing' domains (Krueger *et al.* 1998; Krueger 1999; Krueger & Markon 2006) in line with earlier two-factor conceptualizations of child psychopathology (Achenbach & Edelbroek 1978, 1984). In this model, depressive and anxiety disorders have been shown to load most strongly on an internalizing dimension, whereas substance-abuse disorders, CD, and antisocial problems have been shown to load most strongly on an externalizing dimension.

Although the existence of internalizing and externalizing domains has been confirmed repeatedly, it has been suggested that the structure is more complex than that, with the existence of multiple underlying subdomains. Most consistently, it has been shown that the internalizing domain has two lower-order subdomains that explain clustering of, respectively, 'distress' disorders (major depressive episode [MDE], dysthymia, generalized anxiety disorder [GAD], and posttraumatic stress disorder [PTSD]) and 'fear' disorders (social anxiety disorder [SAD], specific phobia, agoraphobia, panic disorder and obsessive compulsive disorder [OCD]); e.g., Krueger *et al.* 1998; Krueger 1999; Vollebergh *et al.* 2001; Watson 2005; Krueger & Markon 2006; Slade & Watson 2006; Miller *et al.* 2008; Eaton *et al.* 2013a.

Studies investigating the structure of associations among the externalizing disorders have also found some evidence for subfactors that distinguish 'oppositional behaviour' disorders (ADHD, oppositional defiant disorder [ODD]) from 'norm-violations' disorders (CD and substance-use disorders; Farmer *et al.* 2009). One other study (Verona *et al.* 2011) found that substance-use disorders load on a separate factor alongside an externalizing and internalizing factor. It has also been

Table 20.1 Bivariate associations (odds ratios) of lifetime mental disorders without hierarchy

	Major depressive episode	Panic disorder	PTSD	Social anxiety disorder	Specific phobia	AGO	GAD	ADHD	ODD	Conduct disorder	Substance disorder	Bipolar disorder	Eating disorder	IED
Panic disorder	**5.3*** (4.3–6.4)													
PTSD	**7.4*** (5.9–9.4)	**5.3*** (4.0–7.1)												
Social anxiety disorder	**5.1*** (4.4–5.9)	**5.4*** (4.3–6.7)	**4.6*** (3.6–5.9)											
Specific phobia	**3.7*** (3.2–4.2)	**5.5*** (4.4–7.0)	**4.0*** (3.2–4.9)	**6.2*** (5.3–7.2)										
AGO	**6.3*** (4.9–8.2)	**13.7*** (10.5–18.0)	**5.5*** (3.8–7.8)	**19.6*** (14.8–26.0)	**12.2*** (9.5–15.6)									
GAD	**10.9*** (9.1–13.0)	**6.4*** (5.0–8.1)	**6.5*** (5.2–8.1)	**6.0*** (4.8–7.4)	**3.9*** (3.2–4.9)	**7.0*** (5.0–9.9)								
ADHD	**3.5*** (2.7–4.6)	**3.5*** (2.7–4.6)	**4.2*** (3.0–5.9)	**4.4*** (3.5–5.6)	**2.8*** (2.3–3.5)	**4.4*** (3.0–6.5)	**3.3*** (2.5–4.3)							
ODD	**3.2*** (2.7–3.9)	**3.1*** (2.2–4.4)	**4.3*** (3.4–5.4)	**4.1*** (3.3–5.1)	**2.8*** (2.2–3.5)	**3.4*** (2.5–4.6)	**3.4*** (2.5–4.5)	**12.6*** (9.8–16.2)						
Conduct disorder	**2.7*** (2.2–3.3)	**3.5*** (2.5–4.9)	**3.8*** (2.8–5.1)	**3.0*** (2.4–3.7)	**2.4*** (2.0–2.9)	**2.7*** (1.9–3.7)	**2.7*** (2.1–3.6)	**7.6*** (5.9–9.8)	**17.7*** (13.9–22.4)					
Substance disorder	**2.3*** (2.0–2.6)	**2.9*** (2.2–3.8)	**2.8*** (2.3–3.5)	**2.5*** (2.2–2.9)	**1.8*** (1.5–2.1)	**2.4*** (1.8–3.1)	**2.6*** (2.1–3.1)	**3.9*** (3.1–5.0)	**5.8*** (4.9–6.9)	**8.3*** (6.7–10.4)				
Bipolar disorder	**7.3*** (6.0–8.9)	**5.7*** (4.3–7.7)	**4.4*** (3.3–5.9)	**5.0*** (4.1–6.2)	**4.2*** (3.5–5.2)	**8.9*** (6.4–12.2)	**5.9*** (4.6–7.5)	**6.1*** (4.7–7.9)	**5.9*** (4.7–7.4)	**5.0*** (3.9–6.5)	**5.0*** (4.1–6.1)			
Eating disorder	**3.0*** (2.4–3.7)	**2.8*** (1.9–4.2)	**3.4*** (2.4–4.9)	**3.6*** (2.9–4.6)	**2.9*** (2.2–4.0)	**5.1*** (3.4–7.6)	**3.2*** (2.2–4.5)	**4.9*** (3.1–7.9)	**3.4*** (2.4–4.8)	**2.2*** (1.5–3.3)	**2.9*** (2.3–3.6)	**5.0*** (3.5–7.1)		
IED	**3.3*** (2.8–3.9)	**3.6*** (2.6–5.0)	**2.7*** (2.1–3.5)	**3.3*** (2.7–4.1)	**2.6*** (2.1–3.2)	**3.7*** (2.6–5.4)	**3.8*** (2.9–5.1)	**4.1*** (3.0–5.4)	**4.5*** (3.5–5.6)	**4.8*** (3.8–6.1)	**3.2*** (2.7–3.8)	**5.2*** (4.1–6.6)	**3.1*** (2.3–4.1)	
Psychotic Experiences	**2.8*** (2.2–3.6)	**3.6*** (2.5–5.1)	**4.0*** (2.7–5.9)	**2.5*** (1.9–3.3)	**2.8*** (2.2–3.5)	**3.2*** (2.0–5.1)	**2.8*** (2.0–4.0)	**2.4*** (1.5–3.8)	**2.9*** (1.9–4.3)	**2.1*** (1.4–3.2)	**1.8*** (1.3–2.3)	**3.7*** (2.5–5.6)	**2.8*** (1.9–4.2)	**2.3*** (1.8–3.0)

PTSD, Posttraumatic stress disorder; AGO, Agoraphobia; GAD, Generalized anxiety disorder; ADHD, Attention deficit hyperactivity disorder; ODD, Oppositional defiant disorder; IED, Intermittent explosive disorder.

Data are shown as odds ratios (OR) (95% CI).

*Significant at the 0.05 level, two-sided test.

All estimates were based on 10 WMH surveys: Colombia, Peru, Romania, Brazil, Northern Ireland, Poland, Murcia, Medellin, Mexico, and the United States with the exception of IED estimates which utilized data from seven WMH surveys: Colombia, Peru, Romania, Brazil, Northern Ireland, Poland, and the United States and psychotic experiences estimates which utilized data from six WMH surveys: Colombia, Peru, Romania, Brazil, Mexico, and the United States. All logistic regression models controlled for dummy variables representing country.

suggested that externalizing disorders have a hierarchical structure, with a general externalizing factor and two subordinate subfactors for aggression-related and substance-related problems (Krueger *et al.* 2007). However, empirical evidence for these various externalizing disorder subtyping distinctions is less consistent than the evidence for fear and distress disorders among the internalizing disorders, with many studies failing to find evidence for externalizing disorder subfactors beyond the single continuous externalizing dimension (e.g., Krueger *et al.*, 2005; Markon & Krueger 2005; Vrieze *et al.* 2012). A complicating factor here appears to be that the number of externalizing disorders assessed in epidemiological studies is less than the number of internalizing disorders, with the results of structural studies of externalizing disorders seeming to vary depending on the number and type of analysed externalizing disorders.

Although some questions about the lower-order structure remain, the higher-order distinction between internalizing and externalizing psychopathology domains has been shown to be very robust and, as such, has been argued to reflect a natural classification of common mental illness (Krueger 1999; Watson 2005; Krueger & Markon 2006; Kotov *et al.* 2011b; Carragher *et al.* 2015). This notion has been supported by studies showing that the domains reflect variations on separate genetic risk factors (Kendler *et al.* 2011). Also, using data from the WMH surveys, it has been shown that the internalizing and externalizing domains account for a considerable part of time-lagged lifetime comorbidity patterns: time-lagged associations between disorders were shown to be stronger within each domain than between domains, although residual associations between specific sets of disorders exist as well (Kessler *et al.* 2011a–c). Importantly, it has been shown that associations of specific disorders with important outcomes (e.g., suicide) can often be largely explained by domain-specific rather than disorder-specific variance (e.g., Eaton *et al.* 2012). In addition, the internalizing and/or externalizing domains have been shown to be structurally invariant across gender (Hicks *et al.* 2007; Kramer *et al.* 2008; Eaton *et al.* 2012) and ethnic groups in the United States (Eaton *et al.* 2013b); and to be stable over time within persons (e.g., Vollebergh *et al.* 2001; Eaton *et al.* 2011).

There is also some evidence for the stability of the internalizing-externalizing distinction across cultures and countries. First, the structure has been replicated with survey data from different countries around the world (e.g., Australia: Slade & Watson 2006; the Netherlands: Vollebergh *et al.* 2001; Norway: Røysamb *et al.* 2012), although much of this work has been done in Western, high-income countries. Second, Krueger *et al.* (2003) conducted a cross-national study using data from the WHO Collaborative Study of Psychological Problems in General Health Care, which were collected in 15 countries (Brazil, Chile, the People's Republic of China, France, Germany, Greece, India, Italy, Japan, the Netherlands, New Zealand, Nigeria, Turkey, the United Kingdom, and the United States). The authors showed that a two-factor structure (internalizing vs. alcohol problems) fit best in the complete cross-national data and in most of the individual country datasets. Formal evaluations of measurement invariance (MI; Meredith 1993) showed *configural invariance* and invariant factor loadings across countries, which means that the configuration of the factor structure was invariant but that factor means and residual variances varied across countries. However, a limitation of this cross-national study was that only one externalizing disorder ('hazardous use of alcohol') was included, making it impossible to gain any deeper insight into the structural stability of the externalizing disorders in a broader sense. The WMH surveys provide a much richer assessment of externalizing disorders, as they assess ADHD, CD, IED, and ODD in addition to alcohol and drug abuse and dependence.

The latent model of mental disorders remains a work in progress and some of the most important open research questions regard the placement of new and less common mental disorders in the model. The two-factor model was originally developed to describe the latent structure of common anxiety, mood, and substance disorders, a choice that was dictated by the availability of data. Older mental-health studies usually did not assess uncommon disorders because of their low prevalence and if uncommon disorders were assessed, they could not be incorporated in analyses due to low endorsement rates. However, in recent years much larger epidemiological datasets have become available, making it possible to investigate the underlying structure of both common and uncommon mental disorders. Studies using this data have shown that the two-factor model could be extended to include a broader range of disorders. For instance, it has been found that psychotic symptoms or experiences load on a separate 'thought disorders' or 'psychosis' factor (Kotov *et al.* 2011a,b; Markon 2010; Keyes *et al.* 2013; Wright *et al.* 2013), that autism-related problems load on a separate 'autism' factor (Noordhof *et al.* 2015) and that bipolar disorders load on a 'bipolar/mania' subfactor of the internalizing factor (Forbush & Watson 2013; Kotov *et al.* 2015). However, others have found that mania loads on the 'thought disorders' factor, together with psychotic disorders (Kotov *et al.* 2011b) and in another study, it was shown that bipolar disorders can be fit into the existing two-factor structure (Eaton *et al.* 2013a). Much of the variations in the results so far could be related to variations across studies in the symptoms or disorders that were assessed and used for modelling.

Although the internalizing and externalizing factors are regarded as separate domains, they are in fact substantially correlated. Recently, researchers have started to focus on explaining this interrelatedness by using *bifactor* models. In these models, all disorders load on a 'general' factor that accounts for the shared variance between all disorders, and on a specific 'group'-factor ('internalizing', 'externalizing', or 'thought disorder') that accounts for the variance shared with disorders in the same domain. In empirical studies, these bifactor models have been shown to fit well to disorder data and often better than regular two- or three-factor models (e.g., Lahey *et al.* 2012; Caspi *et al.* 2014; Brodbeck *et al.* 2014).

This chapter aims to provide a cross-national overview of the latent structure of mental disorders using the data of the WMH surveys. There are various areas where the WMH data can be used to clarify open questions in the literature. First, apart from the study by Krueger *et al.* (2003) that included only one externalizing disorder ('hazardous use of alcohol'), research of the underlying dimensional structure of mental disorders in multiple countries with a larger range of both internalizing and externalizing disorders has been limited so far. Second, the placement of less common disorders in the latent model remains a subject of continued debate. The WMH surveys provide a unique opportunity to contribute to this work because several less common mental problems (i.e. bipolar disorder, eating disorders [i.e. bulimia and binge-eating disorder] and psychotic experiences [delusions and hallucinations]) were assessed in subsets of the surveys. Third, the large scale and cross-national nature of the WMH surveys enables evaluation of the stability the latent structure of mental disorders across country income groups.

Analyses

Mental Disorders

For this chapter, analyses were conducted with lifetime Composite International Diagnostic Interview (CIDI) DSM-IV diagnoses (present/absent), without hierarchy rules. The following core set of mental disorders were included: MDE, dysthymia, GAD, SAD, specific phobia, panic disorder, agoraphobia, PTSD, alcohol abuse, drug abuse, IED, ADHD, ODD, and CD. Because alcohol and drug abuse are very strongly correlated, these were combined into a single variable for substance-abuse disorders (with or without dependence). In addition, less common disorders were included. Bipolar I, bipolar II, and subthreshold bipolar disorders were combined into a single bipolar disorder variable. Bulimia and binge-eating disorder were combined into a eating-disorder variable. Finally, psychotic experiences (PEs) were used to determine the presence of hallucinations (visual and auditory) and/or delusions (thought insertion/withdrawal, mind control/passivity, ideas of reference [e.g., telepathy], plot to harm/follow). These psychotic symptoms were used as six individual input variables instead of merging them into an overall 'hallucinations' variable and an overall 'delusions' variable (as done in Chapter 19) because the latter would limit modelling possibilities in confirmatory factor analyses (CFAs). In Chapter 19, those with a psychotic disorder were excluded from the analyses. No such restriction was applied in the current analyses because the aim was to model a continuous latent variable that represents the full severity spectrum of psychotic symptomatology, running from absent PEs through single and/or minimal PEs to multiple PEs (in and outside the context of a full-blown psychotic disorder). Here, restricting variance in PE symptomatology by excluding PE cases would impose a limit on the range of the modelled spectrum.

Datasets

Analyses were run in the Part II sample with the age-range limited to 18–44 because several common externalizing disorders (ADHD, CD, and ODD) were assessed only among subjects within this range to limit recall bias. In addition, as bipolar disorder, eating disorders and psychosis were not assessed in all countries, we used separate subsamples for models with these disorders including subsets of countries and/or surveys in which they were assessed.

The structure of all common mental disorders and the subsequent investigation of the optimal placement of bipolar disorder in the larger model was investigated in one large cross-national subsample, consisting of the Part II country samples for those countries that assessed all the disorders required for the model

(Colombia, Peru, Romania, Brazil, Northern Ireland, Poland, Spain (Murcia), Colombia (Medellin), Mexico, and the United States). The weighted sample size for this subsample was n = 15,499.

The placement of IED into this model was investigated in a subsample of countries that assessed IED in addition to the common mental disorders. This sample consisted of the Part II country samples for Colombia, Peru, Romania, Brazil, Northern Ireland, Poland, and the United States. The weighted sample size for this subsample was n = 12,162.

The placement of eating disorders was investigated in a subsample of the sample in which all common disorders were assessed. In most of the countries, eating disorders were assessed in a randomly selected subsample and only those who had received the eating disorders assessment were included in this sample (n = 10,585)

The placement of psychotic symptoms in the larger model was investigated in a smaller subsample consisting of the Part II samples in countries in which psychosis was assessed in addition to the common mental disorders and bipolar disorders (Brazil, Colombia, the United States, Peru, Romania, and Mexico). Psychotic experiences were assessed in a random subsample in each country and only those who had completed the psychosis section were included. This subsample had a sample size of n = 5,478.

Separation anxiety disorder was left out of these current analyses because it was only assessed in part of each sample.

Analyses

A series of analyses were conducted, starting with exploratory factor analyses (EFA) to gain insight into the number of factors and the loading-patterns of different disorders. After this, CFA were used to fit and compare hypothesized structural models from the literature to the WMH surveys data. In addition, multigroup-CFA (MG-CFA) was used to investigate the invariance of the model across country income groups.

All analyses were conducted with Mplus (version 7; Muthén & Muthén 1998–2012). Model estimation was done with mean and variance adjusted Weighted Least Squares estimation for categorical data (WLSMV). All analyses were weighted and run including WMH surveys design variables (clusters and strata) to account for effects of the complex design (Asparouhov 2005). In the EFAs, the Eigenvalues were inspected to determine the optimal number of factors to extract (select factors with Eigenvalues > 1). After an oblique (Promax) rotation, factor loadings were inspected, paying particular attention to the presence of salient factor loadings (≥0.30), the highest loading of each included disorder and the presence of cross-loadings (strong loadings on two or more factors).

In the CFAs, several previously presented structural models were fit to the data as structural equation models. The fit of each model was assessed with the Comparative Fit Index (CFI) and the Root Mean Square Error of Approximation (RMSEA), with a CFI ≥ 0.95 and an RMSEA ≤ 0.06 indicating good fit to the data (Hu & Bentler 1999).

After identification of the best-fitting model, the extent of invariance of this model across country income groups was investigated with MG-CFA. In these analyses, models were fit with different levels of invariance across groups. In the model with *configural invariance* the patterns of factor loadings and item-thresholds were set to be the same across groups but their values were freely estimated for each group. In the model with *scalar invariance*, factor loadings and item-thresholds were constrained to be similar across groups, implying strong MI. To evaluate the level of MI across the grouping of interest, the scalar invariance model was compared to the configural invariance model. The Mplus DIFFTEST procedure (Asparouhov & Muthén 2006) was used to compare fit across the models, with a significant difference between the scalar and configural invariance model implying that there is only configural invariance and scalar non-invariance across groups.

Results

Common Mental Disorders

EFAs show that the latent structure of common mental disorders (Table 20.2) in the WMH surveys is described well by a two-factor structure, as indicated by Eigenvalues of 5.70, 1.55, and 0.98, respectively, for the first three factors. In this model, MDE, Dysthymia, GAD, SAD, specific phobia, agoraphobia, and panic disorder load highest on the first factor and ADHD, ODD, CD, and substance abuse load highest on the second factor. A correlation of 0.58 indicates considerable interrelatedness between the two identified latent domains.

In the next step of the analyses, several competing models from the literature are fit to the common mental disorder data (Figure 20.1): (a) a simple two-factor

Table 20.2 Rotated factor loadings from exploratory factor analyses of mental disorders in the WMH surveys

Disorders	Common mental disorders (n = 15,499)		Common mental disorders and bipolar disorder (n = 15,499)		Common mental disorders and eating disorders (n = 10,585)		Common mental disorders and IED (n = 12,162)	
Disorders	2-Factor[a]		2-Factor[a]		2-Factor[a]		2-Factor[a]	
	F1	F2	F1	F2	F1	F2	F1	F2
MDE	**0.86**	−0.06	**0.87**	−0.07	**0.90**	−0.11	**0.85**	−0.04
Dysthymia	**0.91**	−0.10	**0.92**	−0.12	**0.91**	−0.11	**0.90**	−0.10
Panic disorder	**0.56**	0.15	**0.56**	0.15	**0.58**	0.15	**0.57**	0.14
PTSD	**0.51**	0.21	**0.51**	0.20	**0.53**	0.19	**0.49**	0.23
SAD	**0.61**	0.16	**0.61**	0.15	**0.59**	0.20	**0.62**	0.15
Specific phobia	**0.57**	0.05	**0.57**	0.04	**0.56**	0.09	**0.58**	0.04
Agoraphobia	**0.80**	−0.08	**0.80**	−0.08	**0.78**	−0.03	**0.83**	−0.12
GAD	**0.72**	0.02	**0.73**	0.01	**0.75**	0.00	**0.71**	0.05
ADHD	0.13	**0.64**	0.12	**0.65**	0.16	**0.62**	0.13	**0.65**
ODD	−0.04	**0.87**	−0.06	**0.88**	−0.02	**0.84**	−0.07	**0.88**
Conduct disorder	−0.09	**0.90**	−0.12	**0.91**	−0.13	**0.94**	−0.11	**0.91**
Substance abuse[b]	−0.00	**0.60**	−0.01	**0.62**	−0.00	**0.60**	−0.01	**0.62**
Bipolar disorder	–	–	**0.40**	**0.34**	–	–	–	–
Eating disorder	–	–	–	–	**0.36**	0.15	–	–
IED	–	–	–	–	–	–	0.23	**0.43**
Factor-correlation	0.58		0.60		0.63		0.61	

All factor loadings ≥0.3 printed in bold font.
[a]Promax-rotated factor loadings.
[b]Including abuse and dependence.
[c]Including bipolar I, bipolar II, and subthreshold bipolar disorder.

model, (b) a higher-order model with distress and fear subfactors, and (c) a hierarchical ('bifactor') model with a general factor and two group-factors, defined along the lines of the internalizing and externalizing domains. Of these models, the bifactor model shows the best fit to the data (CFI = 0.992; RMSEA = 0.013). In this model, most disorders show considerable loadings on the general factor, with the highest loading for the internalizing disorders. In addition, most disorders also load on their respective group-factors. Interestingly, all 'distress'-disorders (i.e. MDE, dysthymia, GAD, PTSD) show positive loadings on the first group-factor, whereas all 'fear'-disorders show negative loadings, indicating that variations on the first group-domain may reflect the clustering of distress versus fear disorders. The very low loading of PTSD on the first group-factor could indicate that it is related to both clusters. ODD and CD are the disorders with the highest loadings on the second group-factor.

The invariance of the bifactor model across country income groups (low/lower-middle-income: Colombia and Peru [n = 3,018]; upper-middle-income: Romania, Brazil, Medellin and Mexico [n = 5,470]; high-income: the United States, Murcia, Poland, and Northern Ireland [n = 7,011]) is tested with MG-CFA. The analyses show that the bifactor model with configural invariance across the country income groups fits well to the data (CFI = 0.992; RMSEA = 0.012). However, constraining factor loadings and item-thresholds to be the same across country income groups in the scalar-invariance model leads to estimation difficulties and a significantly lower model fit (CFI = 0.989; RMSEA = 0.013; DIFFTEST, $\Delta\chi^2 = 90.9$; degrees of freedom [d.f.] = 36; $P < 0.001$). These results indicate that the model

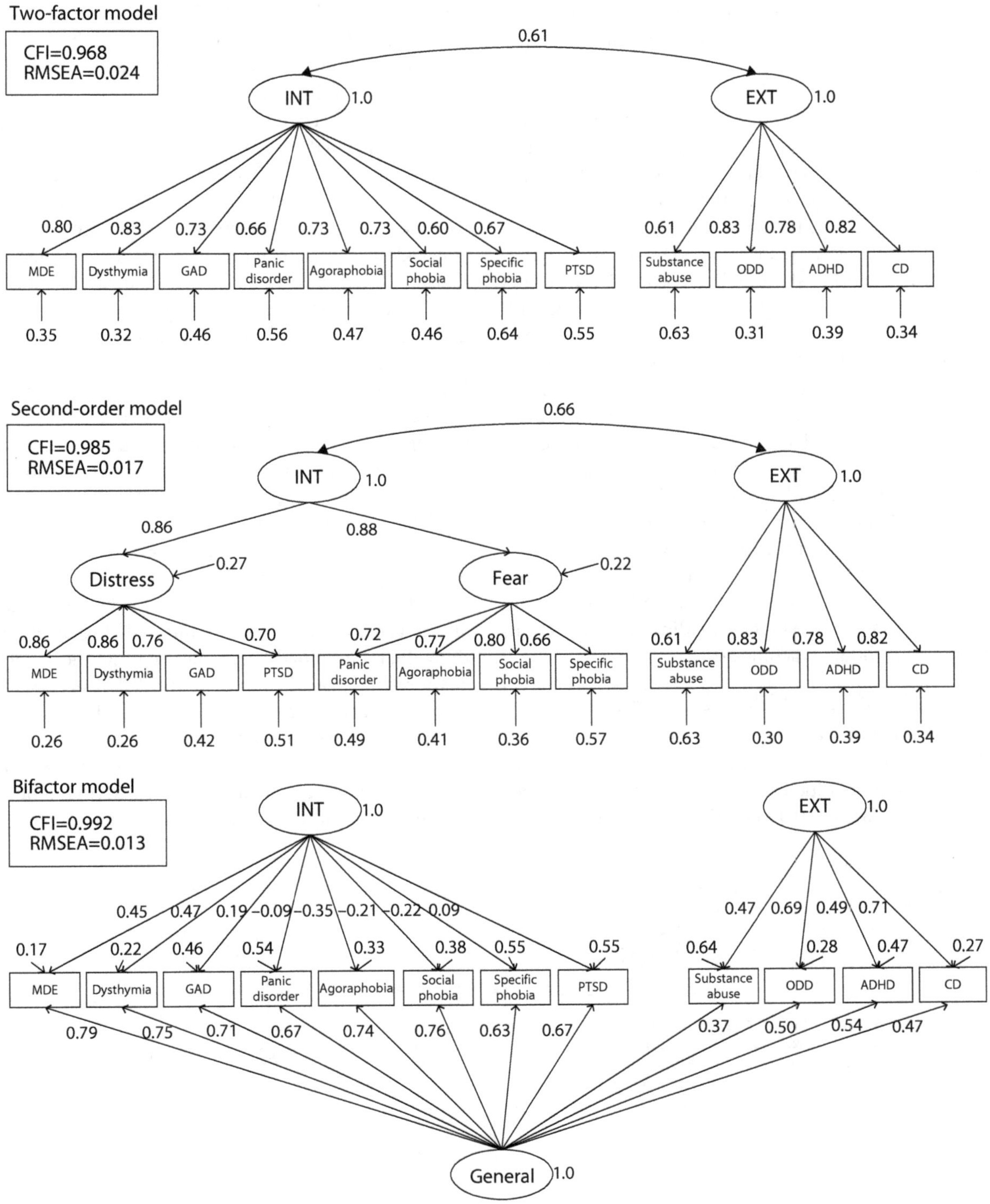

Figure 20.1 Configuration, parameters, and fit of the confirmatory factor models fit to the common mental disorders in the WMH surveys (n = 15,499)

has configural invariance but no measurement non-invariance across country income groups. Indeed, inspection of the model parameters in the model with configural MI showed that the values of the factor loadings varied somewhat across the country income groups. However, several consistencies across groups could also be seen in the directions (positive vs. negative) of the loadings and in the ordering/patterns of loadings per factor. First, specific phobia, SAD, agoraphobia and panic disorder loaded negatively and GAD, MDE, and dysthymia loaded positively on the first group-factor in all groups. Second, the loadings on the second group-factor of CD (0.68–0.79 across groups) and ODD (0.61–0.74) were highest in all country income groups and lower for ADHD (0.45–0.58) and substance-use disorders (0.39–0.52). Third, externalizing disorders showed the lowest loadings on the general factor in all country income groups (substance-use disorders: 0.24–0.39 across groups; CD: 0.34–0.48; ODD: 0.45–0.49; ADHD: 0.47–0.54). In contrast, the internalizing disorders GAD (0.55–0.72), MDE (0.77–0.80), dysthymia (0.66–0.81), SAD (0.68–0.78), and agoraphobia (0.70–0.82) were among the disorders with the highest loadings on the general factor in all country income groups.

The Placement of Bipolar Disorders

EFAs show that the structure of the common mental disorders and bipolar disorder (bipolar I, bipolar II, or subthreshold bipolar disorder) is best described with a two-factor structure (Table 20.2; first three Eigenvalues: 6.15, 1.55, and 0.98). The common disorders load on the same respective factors as in the previous EFA. Bipolar disorders cross-load on both the internalizing and externalizing factor.

CFAs to determine which model configuration of common mental disorders and bipolar disorder fits best to the data show that higher-order models provide better fit than regular two-factor models. A higher-order model with bipolar disorder as a separate internalizing domain alongside the distress and fear subfactors (Forbush & Watson 2013; Kotov *et al.* 2015; CFI = 0.982; RMSEA = 0.017) shows better fit than a configuration with bipolar disorder cross-loading on the fear and distress subfactors (Eaton *et al.* 2013a; CFI = 0.980; RMSEA = 0.018). However, of all models, a bifactor configuration shows the best fit. Of the tested bifactor models, a model with bipolar disorder loading on the general factor and on the second, 'externalizing' group-factor fits best to the data (see Figure 20.2; CFI = 0.992; RMSEA = 0.012). Modelling bipolar disorder as a separate domain (following e.g., Kotov *et al.* 2015) leads to a worse fitting model (CFI = 0.986; RMSEA = 0.016).

In the final model, all disorders load considerably on the general factor, but the internalizing disorders show the highest loadings, indicating that the general factor reflects shared variance among all disorders, but among internalizing disorders in particular. The first group-factor explains additional clustering among distress disorders versus fear disorders and the second group-factor explains additional clustering among externalizing disorders and bipolar disorder.

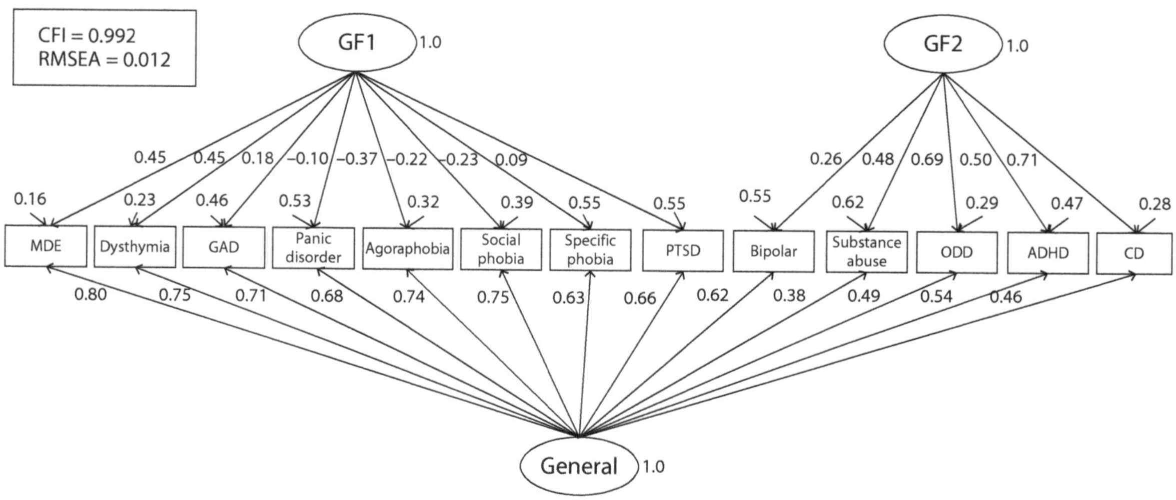

Figure 20.2 The best-fitting confirmatory factor model of the common mental disorders and bipolar disorder (n = 15,499).
GF1 = Group-factor 1; GF2 = Group-factor 2

The Placement of Eating Disorders

EFAs in the subsample in which all common mental disorders and eating disorders were assessed (n = 10,585; Table 20.2) show that eating disorders load most strongly on the internalizing factor, although the factor loading (0.36) is lower than those of the other internalizing disorders (0.53–0.91). In CFAs with the regular two-factor model, grouping the eating disorders with the internalizing disorders (CFI = 0.973; RMSEA = 0.020) leads to better fit than grouping them with the externalizing disorders (CFI = 0.968; RMSEA = 0.022). Higher-order models showed better fit but the placement of eating disorders in the higher-order structure remains unclear as different configurations (eating disorders loading on [1] the distress subfactor, [2] the fear subfactor, and [3] both subfactors) show comparable fit (CFI = 0.984/0.986; RMSEA = 0.015). As before, a bifactor model shows the best fit of all model variants. Comparisons of different configurations reveal that a model with eating disorders only loading on the general factor (Figure 20.3) shows good fit (CFI = 0.993; RMSEA = 0.011) and that model fit is not significantly improved when eating disorders are set to load freely on the first group-factor (DIFFTEST: $\Delta\chi^2 = 0.06$, d.f. = 1, P = 0.81) and does improve only somewhat (but significantly) when set to load on the second group-factor (DIFFTEST: $\Delta\chi^2 = 5.38$, d.f. = 1, P = 0.02). In this model, however, eating disorders showed a very low loading (0.09) on the second group factor. The more parsimonious model with eating disorders only loading on the general factor is shown in Figure 20.3. The patterns of the other disorders' factor loadings in the bifactor model were very similar to those in the previously estimated bifactor models.

The Placement of IED

EFAs in the subsample with IED (n = 12,162; Table 20.2) show that the structure of common mental disorders and IED is best described by two factors (first three Eigenvalues: 6.12, 1.55, and 0.94). In this model, IED shows the highest loading on the second factor, together with the externalizing disorders, although its loading (0.43) is lower than those of the other externalizing disorders (0.62–0.91). Further CFAs show that a two-factor model with IED loading on the externalizing factor fits the data well (CFI = 0.971; RMSEA = 0.022) and a higher-order model, with IED loading on the externalizing factor fits the data even better (CFI = 0.983; RMSEA = 0.017). However, the best fit is observed for a bifactor structure (Figure 20.4; CFI = 0.993; RMSEA = 0.012) with all disorders loading on a general factor, internalizing disorders loading on the first group-factor and externalizing disorders and IED loading on the second group-factor. The factor-loading patterns of the bifactor model looked very similar to the previously estimated bifactor models.

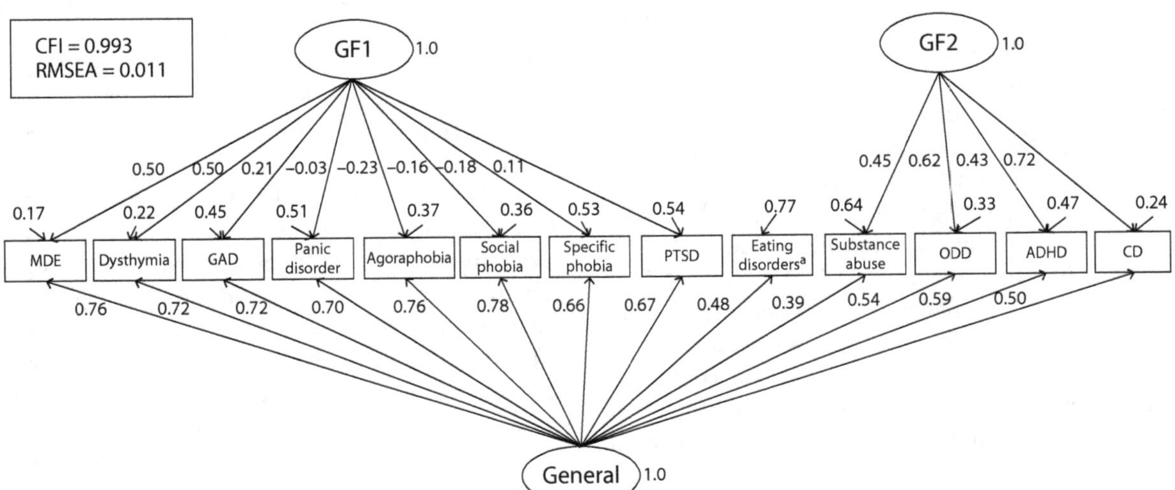

Figure 20.3 The best-fitting confirmatory factor model of the common mental disorders and eating disorders (n = 10,585).

GF1 = Group-factor 1; GF2 = Group-factor 2

[a]Bulimia nervosa and/or binge-eating disorder.

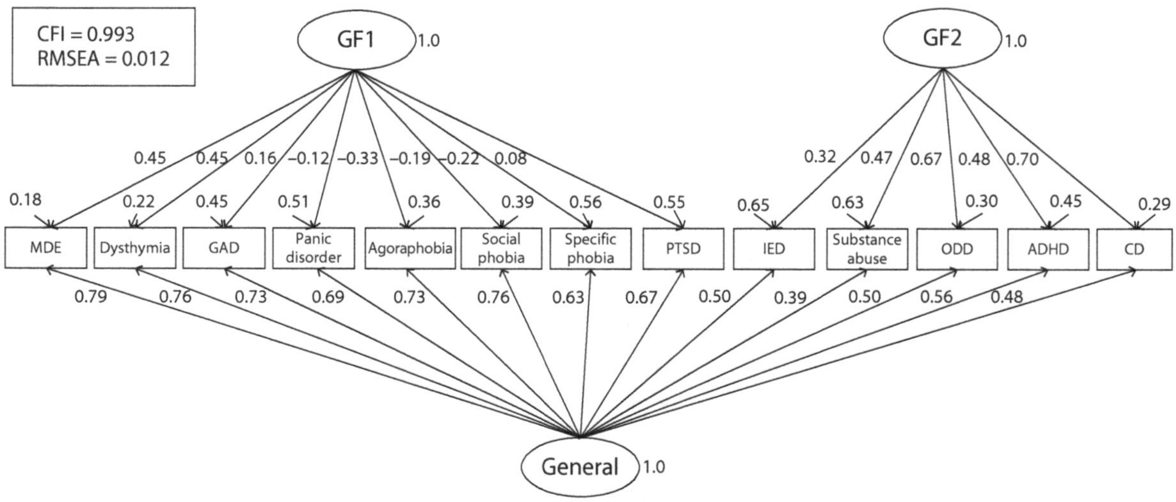

Figure 20.4 The best-fitting confirmatory factor model of the common mental disorders and IED (n = 12,162)
GF1 = Group-factor 1; GF2 = Group-factor 2

The Placement of Psychotic Experiences

EFAs with PEs and common mental disorders in the selected subsample (n = 5,478) indicate that the latent structure could be described with up to four factors (Table 20.3; first five Eigen values: 7.58, 2.65, 1.62, 1.08, 0.82). In the two-factor model, PEs load highest on the first factor and all other disorders load highest on the second factor; in this model MDE and dysthymia cross-load on both factors. In the three-factor model, the internalizing disorders, externalizing disorders, and PEs all load most strongly on their own respective factors. In the four-factor model the internalizing factor is split up into fear and distress subfactors. Together, these results suggest that PEs can be seen to reflect a separate mental health domain, in line with previous reports (e.g., Markon 2010; Wright *et al.* 2013).

In line with the EFA results and previous literature, a CFA model with three factors (internalizing, externalizing, and PEs) fits the data well (CFI = 0.972; RMSEA = 0.015). However, a higher-order model with distress and fear subfactors fits the data even better (CFI = 0.984; RMSEA = 0.011). Again, a bifactor configuration (Figure 20.5) fits the data best of all (CFI = 0.993; RMSEA = 0.008). In this model, all disorders load on the general factor, with the highest loadings for the internalizing disorders. In addition, the group-factors explain additional clustering among distress versus fear disorders (group-factor 1), PEs (group-factor 2) and behavioural externalizing problems (group-factor 3).

Complete Model with Common Disorders, PEs and Bipolar Disorder

A model with all common disorders, bipolar disorder, and PEs is estimated next in the sample with assessed psychosis (n = 5,478). IED and eating disorders were not included because they were only assessed in smaller subsamples.

EFAs of all common mental disorders, bipolar disorder, and PEs (Table 20.4) show that the latent structure of these disorders can be explained by up to four factors (the first five Eigenvalues: 8.01, 2.72, 1.62, 1.08, 0.82). In the two-factor model, the PEs load highest on the first factor and the other disorders load on the second factor. MDE and dysthymia cross-load on both factors.

In the three-factor model, PEs, internalizing disorders, and externalizing disorders all group with their own respective factors. Bipolar disorders load roughly equally on the internalizing and externalizing factors. Factor-loading patterns in the four-factor model show a fear, distress, externalizing, and PE factor. Here, bipolar disorder does not show a very distinct loading on either one factor, but does show its strongest loading (0.37) on the externalizing factor. PTSD shows equal loadings on the fear and distress factors.

Given the superior fit of the bifactor models in all above-described CFAs, only a bifactor model with all disorders was estimated. A model with one general

Table 20.3 Rotated factor solutions for one- to four-factor exploratory factor models of mental disorders, including psychotic symptoms, in a subsample of the WMH surveys (n = 5,478)

Disorders		1-factor model[a]	2-factor model[a]		3-factor model[a]			4-factor model[a]			
		F1	F1	F2	F1	F2	F3	F1	F2	F3	F4
MDE		0.76	**0.43**	**0.50**	0.15	**0.76**	−0.03	0.03	**0.90**	−0.04	0.06
Dysthymia		0.81	**0.47**	**0.49**	0.17	**0.78**	−0.06	0.05	**0.88**	0.01	−0.05
Panic disorder		0.66	0.21	**0.55**	0.03	**0.60**	0.12	0.07	0.06	0.12	**0.57**
PTSD		0.62	0.27	**0.47**	0.12	**0.52**	0.11	0.10	**0.30**	0.11	**0.30**
SAD		0.65	0.04	**0.68**	−0.16	**0.65**	0.22	−0.13	0.06	0.24	**0.62**
Specific phobia		0.59	0.16	**0.52**	−0.07	**0.66**	0.03	−0.02	−0.01	0.02	**0.72**
Agoraphobia		0.65	0.18	**0.56**	−0.16	**0.90**	−0.12	−0.07	−0.07	−0.14	**0.99**
GAD		0.67	0.27	**0.53**	0.07	**0.65**	0.06	0.03	**0.47**	0.07	0.27
ADHD		0.64	−0.12	**0.78**	−0.01	0.13	**0.69**	−0.01	0.04	**0.71**	0.08
ODD		0.64	−0.22	**0.84**	0.01	0.00	**0.81**	0.01	−0.06	**0.83**	0.02
Conduct disorder		0.68	−0.31	**0.92**	−0.05	−0.01	**0.91**	−0.05	−0.04	**0.92**	−0.02
Substance abuse[b]		0.46	−0.11	**0.57**	0.06	−0.04	**0.62**	0.05	0.06	**0.64**	−0.13
Visual hallucination		0.57	**0.78**	−0.08	**0.79**	−0.03	0.03	**0.85**	−0.18	0.04	0.08
Auditory hallucination		0.61	**0.78**	−0.06	**0.78**	0.03	−0.03	**0.79**	−0.05	−0.02	0.08
Thought insertion/withdrawal		0.86	**0.87**	0.03	**0.79**	0.20	−0.03	**0.79**	0.07	−0.04	0.15
Mind control/passivity		0.81	**1.01**	−0.21	**0.94**	0.06	−0.16	**0.93**	0.18	−0.17	−0.10
Ideas of reference		0.74	**0.89**	−0.09	**0.93**	−0.19	0.16	**0.93**	0.04	0.17	−0.27
Plot to harm/follow		0.68	**0.61**	0.20	**0.54**	0.29	0.05	**0.56**	−0.04	0.05	0.33
Factor-correlations	F1	–	1.00	–	1.00	–	–	1.00	–	–	–
	F2	–	0.46	1.00	0.46	1.00	–	0.46	1.00	–	–
	F3	–	–	–	0.31	0.54	1.00	0.33	0.51	1.00	–
	F4	–	–	–	–	–	–	0.43	0.60	0.51	1.00

All factor loadings ≥0.3 printed in bold font.
Note that factor loadings are standardized regression coefficients and, hence can be larger than one (Deegan 1978).

[a]Promax-rotated factor loadings.
[b]Including abuse and dependence.

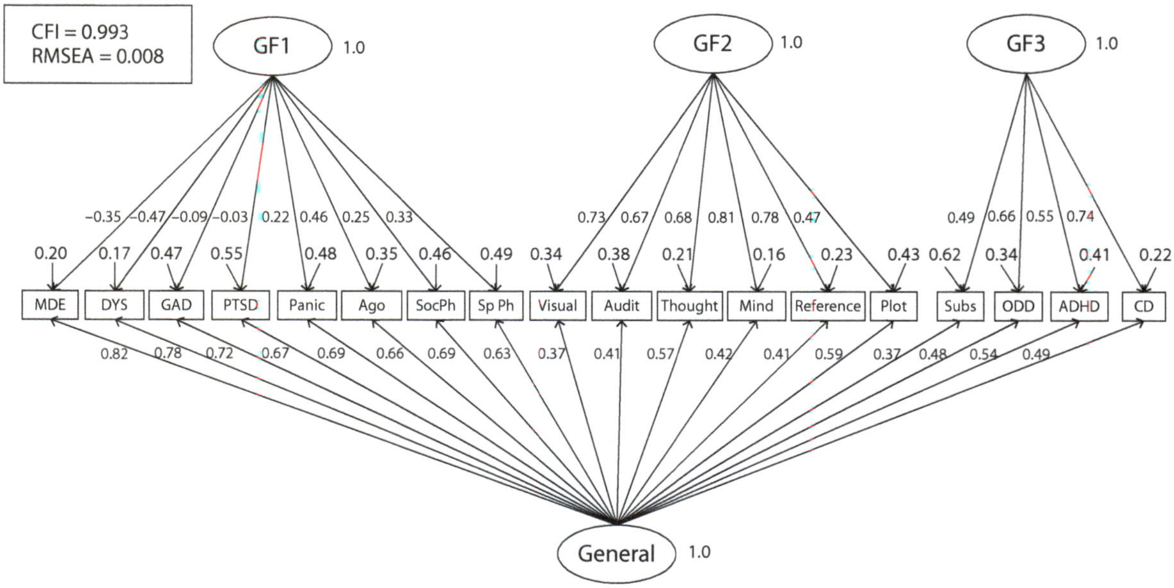

Figure 20.5 The best-fitting confirmatory factor model of the common mental disorders and psychotic experiences (n = 5,478).

GF1 = Group-factor 1; GF2 = Group-factor 2; GF3 = Group-factor 3; Visual = visual hallucination; Audit = Auditory hallucination; Thought = ideas of thought insertion/extraction; Mind = feeling that mind was taken over; Reference = feeling that strange force tries to communicate with you; Plot = believing that there is an unjust plot going on to harm you

factor and three group-factors fits well to the data (Figure 20.6; CFI = 0.994; RMSEA = 0.007). In line with the above-described findings, bipolar disorders were set to load on the same group-factor as the externalizing disorders in this model. Grouping bipolar disorders either with the PE group-factor (following e.g., Keyes *et al.* 2013) or with the internalizing disorder group-factor (following e.g., Eaton *et al.* 2013a; Forbush & Watson 2013) led to lower model fit (both: CFI = 0.989; RMSEA = 0.009).

Discussion

The underlying structure of disorders in the WMH surveys are best described by a bifactor structure, with a general factor reflecting the overall common variance shared among disorders, especially the internalizing disorders, as indicated by their comparatively high factor loadings. In addition, several group-factors explain clustering among disorders up and above the variance explained by the general factor.

In all estimated bifactor models the patterns of factor loadings of internalizing disorders on the first group-factor consistently suggests that this factor reflects the variance explained by clustering of, respectively, distress disorders and fear disorders, in line with many previous findings on the importance of this distinction (e.g., Krueger *et al.* 1998; Krueger 1999; Vollebergh *et al.* 2001; Watson 2005; Krueger & Markon 2006; Slade & Watson 2006; Miller *et al.* 2008; Eaton *et al.* 2015). These previous studies have mostly used higher-order models that impose the distinction between distress and fear subfactors in a top-down fashion. Although the structure was not imposed in the current bifactor CFAs, the distinction between distress and fear did manifest itself in the group-factor loadings. This provides additional empirical support for the existence and robustness of the distress versus fear-disorder distinction.

The high factor loadings of the PEs on the second group-factor suggest that these experiences cluster into a separate domain relatively strongly. Still, although loadings of PEs on the general factor are comparatively smaller, they indicate that part of the variance in PEs is shared with other disorders. The observation that variations in PEs are partly domain-specific and partly related to a broader spectrum of psychopathology is in line with previous work showing their role as cross-diagnostic predictors of adverse psychopathology outcomes (Rössler *et al.* 2011; Fusar-Poli *et al.* 2012; Werbeloff *et al.* 2012).

Table 20.4 Rotated factor solutions for one- to four-factor exploratory factor models of mental disorders, including bipolar disorders and psychotic experiences in a subsample of the WMH surveys (n = 5,478)

Disorders		1-factor model[a]	2-factor model[a]		3-factor model[a]			4-factor model[a]			
		F1	F1	F2	F1	F2	F3	F1	F2	F3	F4
MDE		0.77	**0.42**	**0.51**	0.15	**0.77**	−0.04	0.03	**0.92**	0.05	−0.05
Dysthymia		0.80	**0.47**	**0.49**	0.17	**0.79**	−0.08	0.05	**0.89**	−0.06	0.00
Bipolar disorder		0.67	0.09	**0.64**	0.03	**0.41**	**0.36**	0.02	0.22	0.23	**0.37**
Panic disorder		0.67	0.20	**0.56**	0.02	**0.60**	0.12	0.07	0.05	**0.58**	0.12
PTSD		0.62	0.27	**0.46**	0.12	**0.52**	0.10	0.10	**0.29**	**0.30**	0.10
SAD		0.64	0.05	**0.67**	−0.15	**0.64**	0.20	−0.12	0.04	**0.62**	0.22
Specific phobia		0.59	0.15	**0.52**	−0.07	**0.66**	0.02	−0.02	−0.02	**0.73**	0.01
Agoraphobia		0.65	0.18	**0.57**	−0.17	**0.91**	−0.13	−0.08	−0.08	**1.01**	−0.15
GAD		0.67	0.26	**0.54**	0.06	**0.66**	0.06	0.02	**0.47**	0.27	0.07
ADHD		0.65	−0.13	**0.79**	−0.01	0.12	**0.70**	−0.02	0.03	0.06	**0.72**
ODD		0.65	−0.23	**0.84**	0.00	−0.02	**0.82**	0.01	−0.08	0.01	**0.85**
Conduct disorder		0.68	−0.32	**0.93**	−0.05	−0.03	**0.91**	−0.05	−0.06	−0.03	**0.94**
Substance abuse[b]		0.47	−0.13	**0.59**	0.06	−0.05	**0.64**	0.04	0.04	−0.14	**0.67**
Visual hallucination		0.55	**0.78**	−0.08	**0.80**	−0.04	0.03	**0.85**	−0.18	0.08	0.04
Auditory hallucination		0.59	**0.78**	−0.05	**0.78**	0.04	−0.03	**0.79**	−0.04	0.06	−0.02
Thought insertion/withdrawal		0.86	**0.87**	0.03	**0.79**	0.20	−0.03	**0.79**	0.06	0.17	−0.05
Mind control/passivity		0.80	**1.01**	−0.20	**0.94**	0.06	−0.16	**0.94**	0.19	−0.10	−0.17
Ideas of reference		0.73	**0.88**	−0.08	**0.93**	−0.19	0.16	**0.93**	0.04	−0.28	0.17
Plot to harm/follow		0.68	**0.61**	0.21	**0.54**	0.29	0.05	**0.56**	−0.04	0.34	0.04
Factor-correlations	F1	–	1.00	–	1.00	–	–	1.00	–	–	–
	F2	–	0.47	1.00	0.46	1.00	–	0.47	1.00	–	–
	F3	–	–	–	0.32	0.56	1.00	0.43	0.63	1.00	–
	F4	–	–	–	–	–	–	0.34	0.54	0.54	1.00

All factor loadings ≥0.3 printed in bold font.
Note that factor loadings are standardized regression coefficients and, hence can be larger than one (Deegan 1978).
[a]Promax-rotated factor loadings.
[b]Including abuse and dependence.

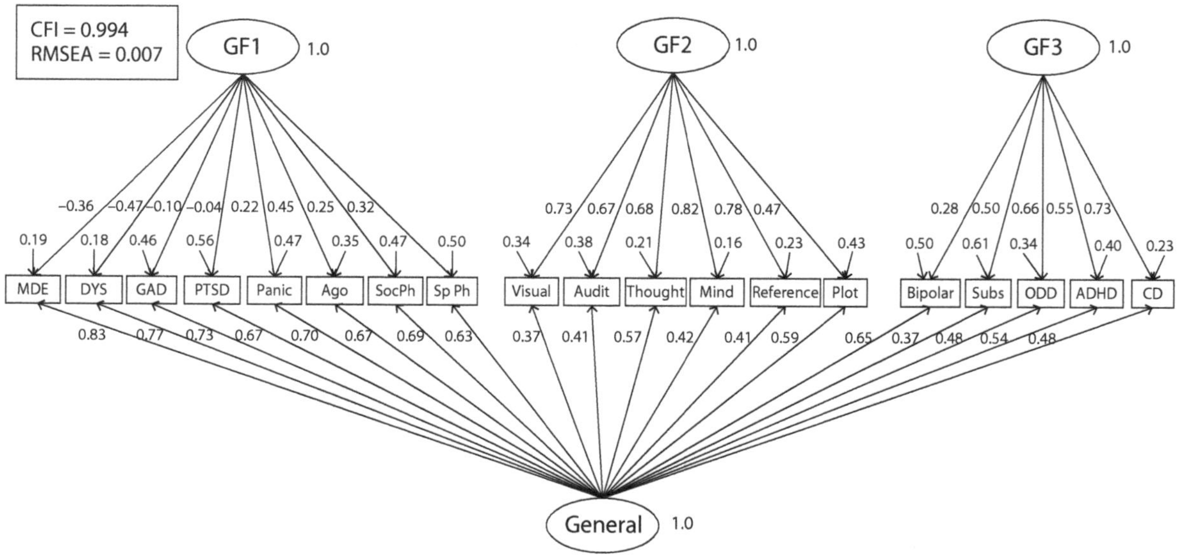

Figure 20.6 The best-fitting confirmatory factor model of the common mental disorders, bipolar disorder and psychotic experiences (n = 5,478).

GF1 = Group-factor 1; GF2 = Group-factor 2; GF3 = Group-factor 3; Visual = visual hallucination; Audit = Auditory hallucination; Thought = ideas of thought insertion/extraction; Mind = feeling that mind was taken over; Reference = feeling that strange force tries to communicate with you; Plot = believing that there is an unjust plot going on to harm you

The third group-factor reflects clustering among externalizing disorders and bipolar disorders. This clustering could lie in the disorders' shared aspects of norm-breaking, oppositional and/or aggressive behaviour. Indeed, disorders in which these behaviours play a central role (ODD and CD) load highest on the group-factor, whereas bipolar disorders, where these behaviours can occur in the context of mania/hypomania, but play a less central role, show a lower factor loading on the externalizing group-factor and a higher loading on the internalizing factor, in line with previous observations of bipolar disorder/mania being related to the internalizing disorders (Eaton *et al.* 2013a; Forbush & Watson 2013; Kotov *et al.* 2015). Unlike these previous studies, the current bifactor model does not directly group bipolar disorders in a single domain with all other internalizing disorders. Rather, their interrelatedness is modelled via their common loadings on the general factor. Here, the group-factor with all internalizing disorders mainly reflects the clustering of distress versus fear disorders, which may be less relevant in explaining the presence of bipolar disorders.

These results show that the occurrence of mental disorders is substantially related to the occurrence of other disorders, as reflected by the disorders' loadings on the general and group-factors. However, there are considerable residual variances for many of the disorders, suggesting that their presence is also partly unrelated to other disorders but related to disorder-specific factors and/or random noise. For research, this could mean that part of the etiology and clinical characteristics/outcomes of a disorder is shared with all other disorders, part is shared with a cluster of related disorders and part is disorder-specific. General and group-factor scores from the bifactor model could be used as covariates when analysing associations between specific disorders and correlates of interest (e.g., psychosocial functioning, experienced disability, service use) to gain insight into the extent to which associations are disorder-specific or explained by their membership of a cluster of disorders. For instance, one could investigate how much of GAD's association with functional limitations is GAD-specific, how much of the association is specific to the cluster of distress disorders, and how much of the association is related to the overall presence of psychopathology.

Previously, Kessler *et al.* (2011a–c) used a novel analytical method in the WMH surveys data to investigate the role of the internalizing and externalizing domains in explaining the development of comorbidity over time. These analyses showed that an important part of time-lagged patterns of comorbidity is explained by clustering within either the internalizing or externalizing domain. In line with this, the currently presented EFA and CFA results showed that the two-factor model provided an adequate description of the latent structure of mental disorders. However, the current analyses also aimed to expand on the previous WMH surveys results and to gain more detailed insight into the fine-grained structure of mental disorders by evaluating the fit of higher-order and bifactor models. These results could be used to further fine-tune research seeking to explain the clustering of disorders and to distinguish between common, domain-specific and disorder-specific vulnerability factors and, in particular, to expand the cross-sectional lifetime focus used here to consider more dynamic analyses that take into consideration the temporal unfolding of these disorders over the life course. This is a line of investigation we are currently pursuing.

Although these results provide interesting and comprehensive insights into the latent structure underlying observed patterns of co-occurring mental disorders, there are some limitations that should be kept in mind. First, the analyses were limited to those WMH surveys with data on all disorders and to subjects in the age-range of 18 to 45 years, which may limit the generalizability of the findings to other populations. Second, the number of fitted CFA models was limited and included only models that built on hypotheses from previous literature. Although the final models were statistically and conceptually sound, it cannot be completely ruled out that an unknown, better-fitting alternative model does exist. Third, the models were fitted on cross-national datasets but prevalence rates could differ across surveys. Investigations of measurement invariance indicated only configural invariance across country income groups, which suggests that factor scores should be compared across countries with care. Tests of measurement invariance were not presented for individual countries, but for country income groups because individual survey samples were comparatively small and some disorder combinations were not present in some of the countries. However, given the presented results for invariance across country income groups, it is unlikely that the bifactor model has full measurement invariance across countries. Further research could investigate the presence of partial measurement invariance or could focus on measurement invariance of a less complex model configuration or of a part of the model (e.g., only internalizing disorders). Fourth, PEs, rather than psychotic disorders and schizophrenia were assessed and included in the analyses. On the one hand, this could seem somewhat inconsistent, as all other modelled mental problems were included as formal disorders. On the other hand, PEs are more common than full-blown psychotic disorders, which provides more possibilities to model the full PE spectrum, irrespective of diagnosis. However, it is possible that some of the observed clustering of PEs in the analyses can be explained by the fact that they were assessed differently from the other diagnoses.

In conclusion, the results presented here suggest that patterns of lifetime comorbidity between common and uncommon mental disorders can be explained with general, cluster-specific and disorder-specific factors.

Acknowledgement

A modified version of this chapter appears in: de Jonge, P., Wardenaar, K.J., Lim, C.C.W., Aguilar-Gaxiola, S., Alonso, J., Andrade, L.H., Bunting, B., Chatterji, S., Ciutan, M., Gureje, O., Karam, E.G., Lee, S., Medina-Mora, M.E., Moskalewicz, J., Navarro-Mateu, F., Pennell, B., Piazza, M., Posada-Villa, J., Torres, Y., Kessler, R.C., & Scott, K.M. (In press). The cross-national structure of mental disorders: results from the World Mental Health Surveys. *Psychological Medicine*; used with permission from Cambridge University Press.

References

Achenbach, T. M., Edelbroek, C. S. (1978). The classification of child psychopathology: a review and analysis of empirical efforts. *Psychological Bulletin*, 85, 1275–301.
(1984). Psychopathology of childhood. *Annual Review of Psychology*, 35, 227–56.

Asparouhov, T. (2005). Sampling weights in latent variable modeling. *Structural Equation Modeling*, 12(3), 411–34.

Asparouhov, T., Muthén, B. (2006). Robust chi square difference testing with mean and variance adjusted test statistics. *Mplus Web Notes*, 10, 1–6.

Bijl, R. V., Ravelli, A., van Zessen G. (1998). Prevalence of psychiatric disorder in the general population: results of The Netherlands Mental Health Survey and Incidence Study (NEMESIS). *Social Psychiatry and Psychiatric Epidemiology*, 33(12), 587–95.

Brodbeck, J., Stulz, N., Itten, S., *et al.* (2014). The structure of psychopathological symptoms and the associations with DSM-diagnoses in treatment seeking individuals. *Comprehensive Psychiatry*, 55(3), 714–26.

Carragher, N., Krueger, R. F., Eaton, N. R., Slade, T. (2015). Disorders without borders: current and future directions in the meta-structure of mental disorders. *Social Psychiatry and Psychiatric Epidemiology*, 50(3), 339–50.

Caspi, A., Houts, R. M., Belsky, D. W., *et al.* (2014). The p factor: one general psychopathology factor in the structure of psychiatric disorders? *Clinical Psychological Science*, 2(2), 119–37.

Deegan, J. R. (1978). On the occurrence of standardized regression coefficients greater than 1. *Educational and Psychological Measurement*, 38, 873–88.

Eaton, N. R., Keyes, K. M., Krueger, R. F., *et al.* (2012). An invariant dimensional liability model of gender differences in mental disorder prevalence: evidence from a national sample. *Journal of Abnormal Psychology*, 121(1), 282–8.

Eaton, N. R., Keyes, K. M., Krueger, R. F., *et al.* (2013b). Ethnicity and psychiatric comorbidity in a national sample: evidence for latent comorbidity factor invariance and connections with disorder prevalence. *Social Psychiatry and Psychiatric Epidemiology*, 48(5), 701–10.

Eaton, N. R., Krueger, R. F., Markon, K. E., *et al.* (2013a). The structure and predictive validity of the internalizing disorders. *Journal of Abnormal Psychology*, 122(1), 86–92.

Eaton, N. R., Krueger, R. F., Oltmanns, T. F. (2011). Aging and the structure and long-term stability of the internalizing spectrum of personality and psychopathology. *Psychology and Aging*, 26(4), 987–93.

Eaton, N. R., Rodriguez-Seijas, C., Carragher, N., *et al.* (2015). Transdiagnostic factors of psychopathology and substance use disorders: a review. *Social Psychiatry and Psychiatric Epidemiology*, 50(2), 171–82.

Farmer, R. F., Seeley, J. R., Kosty, D. B., *et al.* (2009) Refinements in the hierarchical structure of externalizing psychiatric disorders: patterns of lifetime liability from mid-adolescence through early adulthood. *Journal of Abnormal Psychology*, 118(4), 699–710.

Forbush, K. T., Watson, D. (2013). The structure of common and uncommon mental disorders. *Psychological Medicine*, 43(1), 97–108.

Frías, Á., Baltasar, I., Birmaher, B. (2016). Comorbidity between bipolar disorder and borderline personality disorder: prevalence, explanatory theories, and clinical impact. *Journal of Affective Disorders*, 202, 210–9.

Fusar-Poli, P., Bonoldi, I., Yung, A. R., *et al.* (2012). Predicting psychosis: meta-analysis of transition outcomes in individuals at high clinical risk. *Archives of General Psychiatry*, 69(3), 220.

Hasin, D., Kilcoyne, B. (2012). Comorbidity of psychiatric and substance use disorders in the United States: current issues and findings from the NESARC. *Current Opinion-in Psychiatry*, 25(3), 165–71.

Hicks, B. M., Blonigen, D. M., Kramer, M. D., *et al.* (2007). Gender differences and developmental change in externalizing disorders from late adolescence to early adulthood: a longitudinal twin study. *Journal of Abnormal Psychology*, 116(3), 433–47.

Hu, L., Bentler, P. M. (1999). Cutoff criteria for fit indexes in covariance structure analysis: conventional criteria versus new alternatives. *Structural Equation Modeling*, 6, 1–55.

Kelleher, I., Cannon, M. (2011). Psychotic-like experiences in the general population: characterizing a high-risk group for psychosis. *Psychological Medicine*, 41(1), 1–6.

Kendler, K. S., Aggen, S. H., Knudsen, G. P., *et al.* (2011). The structure of genetic and environmental risk factors for syndromal and subsyndromal common DSM-IV axis I and all axis II disorders. *American Journal of Psychiatry*, 168(1), 29–39.

Kessler, R. C., Cox, B. J., Green, J. G., *et al.* (2011c) The effects of latent variables in the development of comorbidity among common mental disorders. *Depression and Anxiety*, 28(1), 29–39.

Kessler, R. C., McGonagle, K. A., Zhao S., *et al.* (1994). Lifetime and 12-month prevalence of DSM-III-R psychiatric disorders in the United States. Results from the National Comorbidity Survey. *Archives of General Psychiatry*, 51(1), 8–19.

Kessler, R. C., Ormel, J., Petukhova, M., *et al.* (2011a). Development of lifetime comorbidity I the World Health Organization world mental health surveys. *Archives of General Psychiatry*, 68(1), 90–100.

Kessler, R. C., Petukhova, M., Zaslavsky, A. M. (2011b). The role of latent internalizing and externalizing predispositions in accounting for the development of comorbidity among common mental disorders. *Current Opinion in Psychiatry*, 24(4), 307–12.

Keyes, K. M., Eaton, N. R., Krueger, R. F., *et al.* (2013). Thought disorder in the meta-structure of psychopathology. *Psychological Medicine*, 43(8), 1673–83.

Knecht, C., de Alvaro, R., Martinez-Raga, J., Balanza-Martinez, V. (2015). Attention-deficit hyperactivity disorder (ADHD), substance use disorders, and criminality: a difficult problem with complex solutions. *International Journal of Adolescent Medicine and Health*, 27(2), 163–75.

Kotov, R., Chang, S. W., Fochtmann, L. J., *et al.* (2011a) Schizophrenia in the internalizing-externalizing framework: a third dimension? *Schizophrenia Bulletin*, 37(6), 1168–78.

Kotov, R., Perlman, G., Gámez, W., *et al.* (2015). The structure and short-term stability of the emotional disorders: a dimensional approach. *Psychological Medicine*, 45(8), 1687–98.

Kotov, R., Ruggero, C. J., Krueger, R. F., *et al.* (2011b). New dimensions in the quantitative classification of mental illness. *Archives of General Psychiatry*, 68(10), 1003–11.

Kramer, M. D., Krueger, R. F., Hicks, B. M. (2008). The role of internalizing and externalizing liability factors in accounting for gender differences in the prevalence of common psychopathological syndromes. *Psychological Medicine*, 38(1), 51–61.

Krueger, R. F. (1999). The structure of common mental disorders. *Archives of General Psychiatry*, 56(10), 921–6.

Krueger, R. F., Caspi, A., Moffitt, T. E., *et al.* (1998). The structure and stability of common mental disorders (DSM-III-R): a longitudinal-epidemiological study. *Journal of Abnormal Psychology*, 107(2), 216–27.

Krueger, R. F., Chentsova-Dutton, Y. E., Markon, K. E., *et al.* (2003). A cross-cultural study of the structure of comorbidity among common psychopathological syndromes in the general health care setting. *Journal of Abnormal Psychology*, 112(3), 437–47.

Krueger, R. F., Markon, K. E. (2006). Reinterpreting comorbidity: a model-based approach to understanding and classifying psychopathology. *Annual Review of Clinical Psychology*, 2, 111–33.

Krueger, R. F., Markon, K. E., Patrick, C. J., *et al.* (2005). Externalizing psychopathology in adulthood: a dimensional-spectrum conceptualization and its implications for DSM-V. *Journal of Abnormal Psychology*, 114(4), 537–50.

Krueger, R. F., Markon, K. E., Patrick, C. J., *et al.* (2007). Linking antisocial behavior, substance use, and personality: an integrative quantitative model of the adult externalizing spectrum. *Journal of Abnormal Psychology*, 116(4), 645–66.

Lahey, B. B., Applegate, B., Hakes, J. K., *et al.* (2012). Is there a general factor of prevalent psychopathology during adulthood? *Journal of Abnormal Psychology*, 121(4), 971–7.

Markon, K. E. (2010). Modeling psychopathology structure: a symptom-level analysis of Axis I and II disorders. *Psychological Medicine*, 40(2), 273–88.

Markon, K. E., Krueger, R. F. (2005). Categorical and continuous models of liability to externalizing disorders: a direct comparison in NESARC. *Archives of General Psychiatry*, 62(12), 1352–9.

Meredith, W. (1993). Measurement invariance, factor analysis and factorial invariance. *Psychometrika*, 58, 525–43.

Miller, M. W., Fogler, J. M., Wolf, E. J., *et al.* (2008). The internalizing and externalizing structure of psychiatric comorbidity in combat veterans. *Journal of Traumatic Stress*, 21(1), 58–65.

Mineka, S., Watson, D., Clark, L. A. (1998). Comorbidity of anxiety and unipolar mood disorders. *Annual Review of Psychology*, 49, 377–412.

Muthén, L. K., Muthén, B. O. (1998-2012). *Mplus User's Guide.* Seventh Edition. Los Angeles, CA: Muthén & Muthén.

Noordhof, A., Krueger, R. F., Ormel, J., *et al.* (2015). Integrating autism-related symptoms into the dimensional internalizing and externalizing model of psychopathology. The TRAILS Study. *Journal of Abnormal Child Psychology*, 43(3), 577–87.

Rössler, W., Hengartner, M. P., Ajdacic-Gross, V., *et al.* (2011). Sub-clinical psychosis symptoms in young adults are risk factors for subsequent common mental disorders. *Schizophrenia Research*, 131(1), 18–23.

Røysamb, E., Kendler, K. S., Tambs, K. *et al.* (2010). The joint structure of DSM-IV Axis I and Axis II disorders. *Journal of Abnormal Psychology*, 120(1), 198–209.

Sher, K. J., Trull, T. J. (1996). Methodological issues in psychopathology research. *Annual Review of Psychology*, 47, 371–400.

Slade, T., Watson, D. (2006). The structure of common DSM-IV and ICD-10 mental disorders in the Australian general population. *Psychological Medicine*, 36(11), 1593–600.

Teesson, M., Slade, T., Mills, K. (2009). Comorbidity in Australia: findings of the 2007 National Survey of Mental Health and Wellbeing. *Australian and New Zealand Journal of Psychiatry*, 43(7), 606–14.

Verona, E., Javdani, S., Sprague, J. (2011). Comparing factor structures of adolescent psychopathology. *Psychological Assessment*, 23(2), 545–51.

Vollebergh, W. A., Iedema, J., Bijl, R. V., *et al.* (2001). The structure and stability of common mental disorders: the NEMESIS study. *Archives of General Psychiatry*, 58(6), 597–603.

Vrieze, S. I., Perlman, G., Krueger, R. F., *et al.* (2012) Is the continuity of externalizing psychopathology the same in adolescents and middle-aged adults? A test of the externalizing spectrum's developmental coherence. *Journal of Abnormal Child Psychology*, 40(3), 459–70.

Watson, D. (2005). Rethinking the mood and anxiety disorders: a quantitative hierarchical model for DSM-V. *Journal of Abnormal Psychology*, 114(4), 522–36.

Werbeloff, N., Drukker, M., Dohrenwend, B. P., *et al.* (2012). Self-reported attenuated psychotic symptoms as forerunners of severe mental disorders later in life. *Archives of General Psychiatry*, 69(5), 467–75.

Widiger, T. A., Clark, L. A. (2000). Toward DSM-V and the classification of psychopathology. *Psychological Bulletin*, 126(6), 946–63.

Widiger, T. A., Samuel, D. B. (2005). Diagnostic categories or dimensions? A question for the *Diagnostic And Statistical Manual Of Mental Disorders* – fifth edition. *Journal of Abnormal Psychology*, 114(4), 494–504.

Wright, A. G., Krueger, R. F., Hobbs, M. J., *et al.* (2013). The structure of psychopathology: toward an expanded quantitative empirical model. *Journal of Abnormal Psychology*, 122(1), 281–94.

Chapter 21

Service Use

Sara Evans-Lacko, Hisateru Tachimori, Viviane Kovess-Masféty, Somnath Chatterji, Graham Thornicroft

Introduction

The large difference between the number of people who need treatment for mental disorders and the number who receive this treatment, known as the mental health treatment gap, represents one of the main public mental health challenges in the world. This is clearly shown by the fact that even though mental disorders represent a leading cause of disability worldwide (Murray *et al.* 2012; World Health Organization 2012; Whiteford *et al.* 2015; Vigo *et al.* 2016), only a minority of individuals with mental disorders receive any treatment (Wang *et al.* 2007). Some research suggests that the treatment gap is even greater for individuals from low socio-economic groups and for those living in low-income countries (Steele *et al.* 2007; Ormel *et al.* 2008) which may rely more on informal providers (Kovess-Masfety *et al.* 2017). One of the most pressing health policy issues in addressing this gap is the achievement of horizontal equity in health services, whereby access to high-quality health care depends on treatment need, rather than socio-economic factors. It has been suggested that mental health care is particularly vulnerable to horizontal inequities in access (Gureje & Thornicroft 2015; Tsai & Tomlinson 2015).

Most studies suggest that at the individual level, illness severity is one of the strongest and most consistent predictors of service use. Certain clinical and socio-demographic characteristics may also be associated with greater predisposition for mental illness, help-seeking and service use (Mojtabai 2010; Andrade *et al.* 2014). For instance, systematic reviews have shown that individuals with low education and low income are at higher risk of mental disorders (Muntaner *et al.* 2004; Fryers *et al.* 2005). Moreover, previous research has noted that these marked socio-economic inequalities in mental disorder risk and prevalence increase with severity of mental disorder (Mangalore *et al.* 2007). Area level studies further support this relationship in relation to service use in that individuals from deprived neighbourhoods tend to use more mental health care than those from affluent neighbourhoods, likely due to greater levels of need among lower socio-economic groups (Thornicroft 1991; Tello *et al.* 2005).

Certain subgroups may also be more or less likely to use certain sectors of care. For example, because specialist mental health care resources are more limited compared with general medical care, access is often restricted through a gatekeeper system that requires referral so that scarce resources are allocated to those individuals with the most severe and/or complex problems (Thornicroft & Tansella 2013). Given their lower supply, we might expect greater barriers to accessing specialist mental health care and hence greater impact of socio-demographic characteristics when accessing specialist versus general medical, or non-health care.

The World Mental Health (WMH) Surveys Initiative provides an opportunity to investigate clinical and socio-demographic variations in the mental health treatment gap. This chapter describes the prevalence of treatment received among people experiencing mental disorders in the past year across mental health specialist, general medical, and non-health care sectors. Next, we present findings on the extent to which the treatment gap varies depending on socio-demographic and clinical characteristics of individuals with mental disorders. We do this first by examining these variables as predictors of receiving any treatment and then, among individuals receiving treatment, by examining whether the same variables are associated with the type of care received. We look in particular at characteristics associated with whether care is received from the specialist mental health sector, which is likely to provide better care quality but might be more limited and protected through a gatekeeper model, rather than from some other sector.

Methods

Service use was assessed in 28 of the 29 surveys included in this volume (Australia was excluded because not all the requisite data were available) (see Table 21.1).

Because we were interested in describing service use among those with 12-month mental disorders, we included data from 71,239 respondents assessed in the Part II sample. Respondents with these disorders were classified as being either severe, moderate, or mild (ten Have *et al.* 2013). Respondents were classified as severe if at least one of their 12-month DSM-IV disorders included either bipolar I disorder, substance dependence with a physiological dependence syndrome, a disorder associated with making a 12-month suicide attempt, or any disorder associated with severe impairment in any domain of the expanded version of the Sheehan Disability Scales (SDS). Respondents not classified severe were classified moderate if at least one of their 12-month disorders included substance dependence without a physiological dependence syndrome or at least one disorder with moderate interference in any SDS domain. All other disorders were classified as mild. To assess 12-month mental health service use, we used categories described in Chapter 3 and elsewhere (Wang *et al.* 2007). As noted in Chapter 3, respondents were asked if they ever obtained professional treatment for "problems with emotions, nerves, mental health or use of alcohol or drugs", and if so, whether they had received such treatment at any time in the 12 months before interview. So this question about treatment was not disorder-specific, but the responses to it were analysed among people meeting criteria for specific mental disorders in this and the other chapters in this volume.

Results

Type of Service Use

Service use by setting is displayed for each country/region in Table 21.1. Among people with any mental disorders in the prior 12 months, service use in the health care sectors is significantly different across high-income (33.8%), compared with upper-middle-income (18.9%) and low/lower-middle-income (10.8%) countries ($F = 249.3$ $P < 0.001$). There is a similar gradient by country income group for non-health care use of complementary and alternative medical services (CAM) and/or human services. Overall, looking at any treatment for mental disorder, service use is highest in Murcia in Spain (49.6%) and lowest in Shenzhen in the People's Republic of China (6.7%). In general, the majority of respondents who received treatment reported receiving care from general medical providers.

Likelihood of Receiving Treatment across Service Sectors by Clinical Characteristics

Table 21.2 shows the relative odds of receiving treatment in the mental health specialist, general medical, human services, or CAM sectors, by clinical characteristics. There is a clear gradient in relation to severity in that individuals with more severe conditions have higher odds (OR 2.5) of using services across all health and non-health care sectors compared to those with mild conditions (reference group). Among those using services, those with the most severe conditions are more likely to receive care from the specialist mental health and CAM sectors relative to those with mild conditions.

In relation to diagnostic groups, individuals with anxiety disorders, in particular panic disorder, are most likely to receive treatment overall (OR 3.3) relative to the reference group of individuals without that specific disorder (i.e., in the case of panic disorder the reference group is those with other 12-month disorders). Individuals with generalized anxiety disorder and posttraumatic stress disorder (PTSD) have higher service use across all sectors, while those with panic disorder or agoraphobia without panic disorder have higher utilization in the health care sectors specifically. Individuals with specific phobia have lower likelihood of any treatment (OR 0.8). Individuals with major depressive disorder (MDD) have a similarly elevated likelihood of receiving treatment in the specialist mental health sector (OR 2.4) as those with panic disorder (OR 2.4). People with MDD also have a higher likelihood of receiving treatment in the general medical or CAM sectors. Those with bipolar spectrum disorder have higher use of specialist mental health care (OR 2.0).

After restricting the analysis to individuals who have received some treatment (second half of Table 21.2), we find that people with MDD (OR 1.5) and bipolar spectrum disorder (OR 1.6) are still more likely than those without these disorders to receive treatment from the specialist mental health sector (OR 1.6). Similarly, among those who received some treatment, individuals with alcohol- (OR 1.7) or drug- (OR 1.5) use disorders are more likely to receive specialist care, possibly because individuals who seek treatment are more severe.

Likelihood of Receiving Treatment across Service Sectors by Socio-demographic Characteristics

Table 21.3 presents the socio-demographic characteristics associated with receiving treatment across sectors, first among individuals with any mental disorder and then more specifically among those with mental

Table 21.1 Among people with any mental disorder in the past 12 months, percent with service use for mental health problems, by service sectors and by country

Country	Specialist mental health care	General medical care	Any health care	Human services	CAM	Any treatment	Unweighted N with mental disorder
	% (SE)	% (SE)	% (SE)	% (SE)	% (SE)	% (SE)	
Low/lower-middle-income countries	**5.1 (0.6)**	**6.5 (0.7)**	**10.8 (0.8)**	**2.6 (0.5)**	**1.4 (0.3)**	**13.7 (0.9)**	3,043
Colombia	7.4 (1.2)	5.8 (1.0)	12.7 (1.5)	1.1 (0.6)	0.5 (0.3)	13.5 (1.6)	785
Iraq	3.6 (1.6)	4.1 (1.4)	6.7 (1.9)	4.6 (1.5)	0.5 (0.4)	11.7 (2.3)	467
Nigeria	1.5 (0.8)	10.3 (2.5)	10.7 (2.4)	1.3 (0.7)	0.0 (0.0)	11.7 (2.5)	204
PRC (Beijing/Shanghai)	3.7 (1.5)	8.5 (4.4)	11.4 (4.5)	0.3 (0.3)	4.8 (4.0)	12.1 (4.5)	205
PRC (Shenzhen)	2.4 (1.0)	2.6 (0.9)	3.8 (1.1)	1.1 (0.7)	2.4 (0.804)	6.7 (1.6)	404
Peru	10.2 (1.4)	5.4 (1.4)	15.4 (2.1)	2.7 (0.8)	2.9 (0.9)	19.0 (2.6)	358
Ukraine	4.0 (1.0)	11.4 (1.0)	14.5 (2.1)	3.9 (1.0)	1.6 (0.5)	18.6 (2.4)	620
Upper-middle-income countries	**10.1 (0.6)**	**11.3 (0.7)**	**18.9 (0.8)**	**3.2 (0.5)**	**3.1 (0.3)**	**22.0 (0.9)**	3,911
Brazil	15.5 (1.1)	8.8 (0.8)	21.4 (1.2)	3.5 (0.7)	3.4 (0.6)	24.1 (1.0)	1,174
Bulgaria	6.5 (1.2)	16.6 (2.5)	19.5 (2.4)	1.0 (0.9)	0.05 (0.05)	20.5 (2.7)	390
Colombia (Medellin)	11.7 (1.5)	6.9 (1.4)	17.5 (1.9)	1.5 (0.6)	1.6 (0.6)	18.7 (2.1)	513
Lebanon	3.4 (1.1)	7.2 (1.4)	9.9 (1.7)	1.2 (0.6)	0.0 (0.0)	11.1 (1.8)	307
Mexico	10.3 (1.5)	6.1 (1.0)	15.6 (1.7)	0.6 (0.3)	3.1 (1.0)	18.1 (1.8)	653
Romania	11.2 (2.3)	13.6 (2.7)	22.6 (2.9)	0.8 (0.5)	0.0 (0.0)	23.4 (3.0)	174
South Africa	5.8 (1.3)	16.9 (1.9)	19.3 (2.0)	6.4 (1.4)	5.8 (1.0)	25.7 (2.5)	700
High-income countries	**17.8 (0.5)**	**24.2 (0.5)**	**33.8 (0.6)**	**4.3 (0.3)**	**4.7 (0.3)**	**36.8 (0.6)**	9,659
Belgium	20.7 (2.9)	30.0 (4.7)	37.0 (4.2)	0.9 (0.7)	1.2 (0.7)	37.8 (4.2)	220
France	12.0 (1.6)	23.6 (2.8)	28.8 (2.7)	1.6 (0.8)	1.1 (0.6)	30.9 (3.1)	382
Germany	13.5 (2.5)	16.9 (2.8)	24.01 (3.3)	1.8 (0.7)	1.2 (0.5)	25.4 (3.4)	260
Israel	17.4 (1.9)	17.4 (1.8)	29.7 (2.2)	5.7 (1.1)	3.1 (0.8)	34.9 (2.3)	482
Italy	8.7 (2.3)	23.4 (2.8)	26.4 (3.0)	1.3 (0.6)	0.6 (0.4)	27.4 (2.9)	266
Japan	15.3 (2.5)	11.2 (2.1)	20.5 (3.0)	1.3 (0.7)	5.6 (2.2)	23.0 (3.3)	235
Netherlands	16.3 (2.9)	24.4 (4.2)	29.4 (4.4)	1.7 (0.7)	2.3 (0.8)	30.6 (4.5)	271
New Zealand	16.1 (1.0)	28.4 (1.0)	35.3 (1.1)	4.9 (0.5)	6.5 (0.7)	38.4 (1.2)	2,727
Northern Ireland	14.9 (1.8)	38.0 (2.8)	40.3 (3.2)	2.7 (0.7)	6.2 (1.4)	42.4 (3.0)	528
Poland	13.7 (1.4)	9.9 (1.1)	19.7 (1.9)	2.6 (0.8)	3.7 (0.9)	21.3 (1.9)	620
Portugal	17.5 (1.7)	24.0 (1.7)	34.8 (2.0)	2.1 (0.6)	1.7 (0.4)	36.2 (2.0)	723
Spain	20.6 (2.3)	23.1 (2.4)	34.3 (3.2)	1.0 (0.5)	1.7 (0.6)	34.5 (3.2)	386
Spain (Murcia)	28.0 (4.2)	26.9 (2.6)	48.9 (3.3)	0.0 (0.0)	1.0 (0.6)	49.6 (3.4)	361
United States	22.1 (0.9)	23.0 (0.8)	36.4 (1.0)	8.1 (0.8)	6.9 (0.6)	41.5 (0.9)	2,198
All countries	**13.6 (0.3)**	**17.8 (0.4)**	**26.0 (0.4)**	**3.7 (0.2)**	**3.7 (0.2)**	**29.0 (0.5)**	16,613
Wald design-corrected F-test for country income group differences	**$F_{2,5366} = 132.7$ $P < 0.001$**	**$F_{2,5366} = 231.4$ $P < 0.001$**	**$F_{2,5366} = 249.3$ $P < 0.001$**	**$F_{2,5366} = 6.0$ $P < 0.001$**	**$F_{2,5366} = 33.2$ $P < 0.001$**	**$F_{2,5366} = 221.1$ $P < 0.001$**	

PRC: People's Republic of China.

Table 21.2 Multivariable associations (odds ratios) of mental disorders with type of service sector contact among those with any 12-month mental disorder, and among those with any 12-month disorder who made service contact[a]

	Respondents with 12-month mental disorder					Respondents with 12-month mental disorder using services			
	Any treatment	Specialist mental health care	General medical	Human services	CAM	Specialist mental health care	General medical	Human services	CAM
	OR (95% CI)	OR (95% CI)	OR (95% CI)	OR (95% CI)	OR (95% CI,	OR (95% CI)	OR (95% CI)	OR (95% CI)	OR (95% CI)
Type of mental disorder[b]									
Generalized anxiety disorder	1.8* (1.5, 2.1)	1.6* (1.3, 1.9)	1.7* (1.4, 2.0)	1.5* (1.1, 2.0)	1.4* (1.0, 1.9)	1.2 (0.9, 1.5)	1.2 (1.0, 1.5)	1.1 (0.8, 1.5)	1.0 (0.8, 1.4)
Panic disorder	3.3* (2.7, 4.0)	2.4* (1.9, 2.9)	3.2* (2.6, 4.0)	1.4 (0.9, 2.0)	1.3 (0.9, 2.0)	1.2 (0.9, 1.5)	1.7* (1.2, 2.2)	0.8 (0.5, 1.1)	0.8 (0.6, 1.2)
Agoraphobia without panic disorder	1.7* (1.4, 2.2)	1.6* (1.1, 2.1)	1.9* (1.5, 2.5)	0.8 (0.5, 1.4)	1.0 (0.6, 1.6)	1.0 (0.7, 1.5)	1.4 (1.0, 2.0)	0.6 (0.4, 1.1)	0.8 (0.5, 1.2)
Social anxiety disorder	1.1 (1.0, 1.3)	1.2* (1.0, 1.5)	1.2 (1.0, 1.4)	1.1 (0.8, 1.6)	1.1 (0.9, 1.5)	1.2 (0.9, 1.5)	1.2 (0.9, 1.5)	1.0 (0.7, 1.5)	1.1 (0.8, 1.5)
Specific phobia	0.8* (0.7, 1.0)	0.9 (0.7, 1.0)	0.9 (0.8, 1.1)	0.8 (0.6, 1.1)	1.0 (0.8, 1.4)	0.9 (0.7, 1.2)	1.2 (1.0, 1.6)	0.9 (0.7, 1.3)	1.1 (0.8, 1.5)
Adult separation anxiety disorder	1.1 (0.8, 1.4)	1.2 (0.9, 1.6)	1.0 (0.7, 1.3)	1.2 (0.7, 2.0)	1.1 (0.7, 1.7)	1.1 (0.8, 1.6)	0.9 (0.6, 1.3)	1.1 (0.6, 2.0)	1.0 (0.6, 1.6)
Posttraumatic stress disorder	2.0* (1.7, 2.3)	1.7* (1.4, 2.2)	1.8* (1.5, 2.1)	1.4* (1.0, 2.0)	1.7* (1.2, 2.3)	1.1 (0.9, 1.5)	1.1 (0.8, 1.4)	1.0 (0.7, 1.5)	1.1 (0.8, 1.6)
Major depressive disorder	2.2* (1.9, 2.5)	2.4* (2.0, 2.8)	2.0* (1.7, 2.3)	1.3 (0.9, 1.8)	1.5* (1.1, 2.1)	1.5* (1.1, 1.8)	1.1 (0.9, 1.4)	0.9 (0.6, 1.2)	1.0 (0.7, 1.4)
Bipolar spectrum disorder	1.6 (1.3, 1.9)	2.0* (1.6, 2.5)	1.6* (1.2, 2.0)	1.4 (1.0, 1.2)	1.1 (0.8, 1.7)	1.6* (1.2, 2.2)	1.3 (0.9, 1.7)	1.0 (0.7, 1.5)	0.8 (0.6, 1.2)
Alcohol abuse or dependence	0.7* (0.6, 0.9)	1.0 (0.8, 1.3)	0.6* (0.5, 0.8)	0.7* (0.4, 1.0)	0.9 (0.6, 1.4)	1.7* (1.2, 2.3)	0.7* (0.5, 1.0)	0.8 (0.5, 1.3)	1.2 (0.8, 1.8)
Drug abuse or dependence	1.6* (1.2, 2.1)	1.6* (1.2, 2.1)	1.4 (0.9, 2.1)	1.0 (0.6, 1.8)	1.8* (1.1, 3.0)	1.5* (1.0, 2.2)	0.9 (0.6, 1.5)	0.7 (0.4, 1.2)	1.5 (0.9, 2.5)
Level of disorder severity									
Severity: severe	2.5* (2.2, 2.8)	3.0* (2.5, 3.5)	2.2* (1.9, 2.6)	2.0* (1.5, 2.7)	2.4* (1.8, 3.2)	1.8* (1.5, 2.3)	1.0 (0.8, 1.3)	1.1 (0.8, 1.5)	1.4* (1.0, 1.9)
Severity: moderate	1.3* (1.2, 1.5)	1.3* (1.1, 1.6)	1.4* (1.2, 1.6)	1.3 (1.0, 1.8)	1.5* (1.1, 2.0)	1.1 (0.9, 1.3)	1.1 (0.9, 1.4)	1.0 (0.7, 1.4)	1.2 (0.8, 1.6)
Mild	1.0	1.0	1.0	1.0	1.0	1.0	1.0	1.0	1.0
Number of disorders									
Four+ disorders	0.8 (0.6, 1.2)	0.6 (0.4, 1.0)	0.7 (0.4, 1.1)	1.2 (0.6, 2.3)	1.1 (0.5, 2.4)	0.8 (0.5, 1.2)	0.6 (0.4, 1.1)	1.4 (0.7, 2.8)	1.4 (0.6, 2.9)
Three disorders	1.0 (0.8, 1.3)	0.9 (0.6, 1.2)	0.9 (0.7, 1.1)	1.1 (0.7, 1.7)	1.1 (0.7, 1.7)	0.8 (0.5, 1.2)	0.7 (0.5, 1.0)	1.0 (0.6, 1.6)	1.0 (0.6, 1.6)
Two disorders	1.0	1.0	1.0	1.0	1.0	1.0	1.0	1.0	1.0

*Significant at the 0.05 level, two-sided test.

[a]Analyses adjusted for number of 12-month mood, anxiety, substance and disruptive behaviour disorders, and country.

[b]The reference group for type of mental disorders is individuals with all other 12-month disorders , e.g., in the first row the reference group for people with generalized anxiety disorder is everyone who did not meet criteria for generalized anxiety disorder.

Table 21.3 Multivariable associations (odds ratios) of socio-demographic characteristics with type of service sector contact among those with any 12-month mental disorder, and among those with any 12-month disorder who made service contact[a]

Socio-demographic characteristics	Respondents with 12-month mental disorder					Respondents with 12-month mental disorder using services			
	Specialist mental health care	General medical	Human services	CAM	Any treatment	Special-ist mental health care	General medical	Human services	CAM
	OR (95% CI)	OR (95% CI)	OR (95% CI)	OR (95% CI)	OR (95% CI)	OR (95% CI)	OR (95% CI)	OR (95% CI)	OR (95% CI)
Gender									
Male	1.0 (0.8, 1.1)	0.7* (0.6, 0.8)	0.7* (0.6, 0.9)	0.7* (0.5, 0.9)	0.8* (0.7, 0.8)	1.3* (1.1, 1.6)	0.8* (0.7, 1.0)	0.8 (0.7, 1.1)	0.8 (0.6, 1.1)
Female	1.0	1.0	1.0	1.0	1.0	1.0	1.0	1.0	1.0
Age									
18–34	1.3 (1.0, 1.8)	0.5* (0.4, 0.7)	1.5 (0.9, 2.5)	2.0* (1.2, 3.4)	0.8 (0.7, 1.0)	2.0* (1.4, 2.9)	0.3* (0.2, 0.5)	1.6* (1.0, 2.7)	2.4* (1.4, 4.1)
35–49	1.8* (1.4, 2.3)	0.8* (0.7, 1.0)	1.5* (1.0, 2.3)	2.8* (1.8, 4.3)	1.2* (1.0, 1.4)	1.9* (1.4, 2.7)	0.4* (0.3, 0.6)	1.3 (0.9, 2.1)	2.6* (1.6, 4.1)
50–64	1.7* (1.3, 2.2)	1.0 (0.8, 1.2)	1.2 (0.8, 1.9)	2.5* (1.6, 4.0)	1.3* (1.1, 1.6)	1.7* (1.2, 2.3)	0.5* (0.4, 0.7)	1.1 (0.7, 1.7)	2.2* (1.4, 3.6)
65+	1.0	1.0	1.0	1.0	1.0	1.0	1.0	1.0	1.0
Household income									
Low	0.8* (0.7, 1.0)	1.0 (0.8, 1.2)	1.5* (1.0, 2.1)	1.2 (0.9, 1.6)	0.9 (0.8, 1.1)	0.9 (0.7, 1.1)	1.0 (0.8, 1.3)	1.7* (1.2, 2.5)	1.3 (0.9, 1.8)
Low-average	0.8* (0.7, 1.0)	1.0 (0.8, 1.1)	1.7* (1.2, 2.4)	1.1 (0.8, 1.5)	0.9 (0.8, 1.0)	0.8 (0.7, 1.0)	1.0 (0.8, 1.3)	2.0* (1.4, 2.8)	1.1 (0.8, 1.6)
High-average	0.8* (0.7, 1.0)	0.9 (0.8, 1.1)	1.3 (0.9, 1.8)	1.1 (0.8, 1.6)	0.9 (0.8, 1.0)	0.9 (0.7, 1.1)	1.0 (0.8, 1.2)	1.5* (1.0, 2.2)	1.3 (0.9, 1.8)
High	1.0	1.0	1.0	1.0	1.0	1.0	1.0	1.0	1.0
Marital status									
Never married	1.3* (1.1, 1.6)	0.7* (0.6, 0.9)	0.7* (0.6, 1.0)	1.2 (0.9, 1.5)	0.9 (0.8, 1.1)	1.7* (1.4, 2.1)	0.6* (0.5, 0.8)	0.8 (0.6, 1.1)	1.2 (0.9, 1.6)
Separated/widowed/ divorced	1.4* (1.2, 1.6)	1.0 (0.8, 1.1)	1.1 (0.8, 1.4)	1.4* (1.0, 1.8)	1.2* (1.1,1.4)	1.3* (1.1, 1.5)	0.7* (0.6, 0.8)	1.0 (0.8, 1.3)	1.2 (0.9, 1.6)
Married/cohabitating	1.0	1.0	1.0	1.0	1.0	1.0	1.0	1.0	1.0
Education									
Low	0.6* (0.5, 0.8)	1.0 (0.8, 1.2)	0.6* (0.4, 0.8)	0.4* (0.3, 0.7)	0.8* (0.7, 0.9)	0.7* (0.5, 0.9)	1.5* (1.1, 1.9)	0.7* (0.5, 1.0)	0.5* (0.3, 0.7)
Low-average	0.6* (0.5, 0.8)	0.9 (0.8, 1.1)	0.8 (0.6, 1.1)	0.7* (0.5, 0.9)	0.8* (0.7, 0.9)	0.6* (0.5, 0.8)	1.4* (1.1, 1.7)	0.8 (0.6, 1.2)	0.8 (0.6, 1.1)
High-average	0.7* (0.6, 0.9)	1.0 (0.8, 1.2)	0.8 (0.6, 1.1)	0.7* (0.5, 0.9)	0.8* (0.7, 0.9)	0.7* (0.6, 0.9)	1.3* (1.0, 1.6)	0.9 (0.7, 1.3)	0.7* (0.6, 1.0)
High	1.0	1.0	1.0	1.0	1.0	1.0	1.0	1.0	1.0

France is excluded from these analyses, as education was missing for all participants. *Significant at the 0.05 level, two-sided test.
[a]Analyses adjusted for number of 12-month mood, anxiety, substance, and disruptive behaviour disorders, number of disorders, severity, and country.

disorders who are service users. In general, men with mental disorders are less likely than women with mental disorders to use general medical, human services or CAM care. Among service users, however, males with mental disorders are more likely to receive care from the specialist mental health sector (OR 1.3) and less likely to receive care from the general medical sector (OR 0.8) compared to women. Age and marital status are also associated with different types of service use. Those who are younger are more likely to use specialist mental health, human services, and CAM care relative to individuals over 65 years of age. The same pattern applies for those in treatment. In relation to marital status, individuals who never married and those who are separated, widowed, or divorced have higher utilization of specialist mental health care. Those who never married have lower rates of general medical care and human services (OR 0.7) and those who are separated, widowed, or divorced have higher rates of specialist mental health care and CAM services (OR 1.4). Among service users, having never married or being separated, widowed, or divorced is associated with higher use of specialist and lower use of general medical care compared to individuals who are married.

Individuals with low, low-average or high-average incomes are all less likely to receive specialist mental health care compared with individuals with high incomes, though individuals with lower incomes have a higher likelihood of receiving care from the human services sector. There is a clear gradient in relation to service use and education, in that individuals with the lowest levels of education have the lowest relative odds of service use in specialist mental health, human services, and CAM care. However, there are no differences by level of education associated with general medical care use. Among service users, individuals with lower education levels are also less likely than those with high levels of education to receive specialist mental health care, human services, and CAM services and more likely to receive services in the general medical sector.

Interaction between Disorder Severity and Socio-demographic Characteristics

Although services in general are clearly targeted to those with more severe needs, there are disparities in service use by socio-demographic characteristics even among those with the same level of severity. In order to evaluate this, we estimated models with interactions for severity of disorder with socio-demographic characteristics (detailed results not shown). These findings provide a more nuanced picture than the results presented in Table 21.3, where associations are simply averaged across levels of severity. The interaction results indicate that the comparatively low odds of receiving treatment associated with low socio-economic status are especially pronounced for specialist treatment. For example, in relation to use of specialist mental health care, there were significant interactions for mental disorder severity by income ($\chi^2_9 = 23.7$, $P = 0.005$), and education ($\chi^2_9 = 44.6$, $P < 0.001$), such that the socio-economic disparities in accessing specialist care were most pronounced among those with greatest clinical severity. Individuals with low levels of education and higher clinical severity appear to be at the greatest disadvantage. Among those with the most severe disorder, those with low levels of education are less likely than those with high education to receive general medical care (low education OR 0.5, 95% CI: 0.3, 0.7), specialist mental health care (low education OR 0.6, 95% CI: 0.4, 0.7) or CAM care (low education: OR 0.4, 95% CI: 0.2, 0.8).

Discussion

These results should be interpreted taking into account the following limitations. Earlier studies suggest self-reports of service use may overestimate administrative records, especially among respondents with more distressing disorders. Commitment probes were used to minimize such inaccuracies (i.e., questions measuring a subject's commitment to the survey) and respondents who failed to endorse that they would think carefully and answer honestly were excluded. Nevertheless, potentially biased recall of service use remains possible and may have led to overestimation of service use. Finally, some analyses involved small numbers of respondents and may have rendered our conclusions less certain, especially in countries with lower prevalence of mental disorders and service use. In addition, we did not incorporate or control for differences in health care organization or financing, which varies across countries.

Despite these limitations the findings presented in this chapter add to the literature demonstrating low levels of access to mental health treatment across the world (Wang *et al.* 2007; Ormel *et al.* 2008; Thornicroft *et al.* 2017). We identified a significant treatment gap with only a small minority of people across high, middle, and low-income countries receiving any treatment for their mental disorder during the past 12 months. We also identified particular groups who experienced greater disadvantage in accessing care and thus, an even wider treatment gap. For example, being from a low/lower-middle-income and upper-middle-income country, being male, separated, widowed, or divorced, or having low education further decreased an individual's likelihood of receiving any treatment. Moreover, some disadvantaged groups with the greatest needs faced additional difficulties in accessing the specialist care they need. These findings suggest there is a pyramid of disadvantage whereby levels of need are inversely related to levels of mental health care access. For example, we found that socio-economic barriers to service use were more pronounced among individuals with the most severe disorders: in this group the disparity of access as a function of level of education and income was even greater than among those with less severe disorders.

There were specific clinical characteristics associated with greater odds of receiving treatment. As has been found previously (Roy-Byrne *et al.* 1999), panic disorder was the mental disorder most likely to result in treatment, followed by major depressive disorder. In contrast, individuals with alcohol abuse or dependence tended to have the lowest likelihood of treatment receipt. This suggests some disorders are more important in driving treatment. They may be perceived as more serious or as more of a medical problem. Others, in particular substance-use disorders, may be associated with greater stigma and be perceived more as a social problem not warranting medical treatment and thus individuals with these disorders may have greater barriers to treatment (Evans-Lacko & Thornicroft 2010; Schomerus *et al.* 2011). Of greater impact than type of disorder, however, our findings suggest disorder severity was one of the most significant factors associated with greater use of health and non-health care (Bebbington *et al.* 2000; Wang *et al.* 2007; Brown *et al.* 2014). Moreover, among service users, those with greater disorder severity were more likely to receive specialist mental health care and CAM services than those with less severe disorders. It is plausible that the higher rate of CAM service use could be based on 'perceived access', resulting from the individual's experience and beliefs about their own state, while higher rates of specialist mental health care are more likely due to 'evaluated access', resulting from professional evaluation of a patient's condition (Andersen 1995, 2008). By contrast, among service users general medical care and human services were not associated with greater severity, perhaps because they are often more available and play a gatekeeping role so have fewer access barriers.

Overall, these findings show that after adjustment for mental disorder severity and comorbidity, the treatment gap was greater for males, younger age groups, and those with low levels of education. Moreover, there was a threefold higher prevalence of service use among those with disorders in high-income countries relative to those with disorders in low/lower-middle-income countries. When we examined service use among those with a 12-month disorder by sector, certain sectors were especially poor at reaching disadvantaged groups. Individuals with low levels of education seemed to be most disadvantaged in accessing care. They had the lowest specialist mental health, human services, and CAM service use; however, there were no differences associated with general medical care use. Individuals with low-average incomes were also less likely to receive specialist mental health care relative to individuals with high incomes, though they had higher utilization of human services, potentially due to fewer financial barriers to access. In contrast to education and income, although men were less likely to receive care overall, it is interesting to note that men in treatment were more likely to receive specialist care while women were more likely to receive general medical care for their mental disorder. It may be that general practitioners are more likely to refer men than women to specialist care, or that men delay treatment until the problem is severe but then are more likely to demand access. Other studies have noted that females are more likely to access services compared to males, possibly due to greater stigma among men or greater difficulty in recognizing feelings of distress and seeking help (Wang *et al.* 2007; Mojtabai 2010; Kovess-Mafesty *et al.* 2014; Evans-Lacko *et al.* 2014; Boyd *et al.* 2015). Structural barriers may be greater for certain sectors of care; however, distinct barriers related to individual values or social and economic resources may also drive the type of services sought and/or influence accessibility.

The low utilization rates of specialist mental health care among those with low education and low income deserve further attention. There is little research examining the relationship between socio-economic status and access to specialist mental health care. This has important implications for distribution of mental health care resources, particularly given what we know about the relationship between mental disorders and low socio-economic status (Mangalore *et al.* 2007; Lund *et al.* 2010). A small study from Brazil found that individuals with high relative to low education and income levels were more likely to see a specialist physician for minor psychiatric disorder (De Lima *et al.* 1999). Another study from Belgium found that individuals from low socio-economic groups were less likely to receive antidepressants and psychotherapy, but more likely to receive care in a non-teaching or psychiatric hospital, to have an unexpectedly long average length of stay, or to have an involuntary psychiatric admission (Lorant *et al.* 2003); some of these effects may be due to these individuals experiencing greater barriers to accessing timely care (Amaddeo & Jones 2007; Young & Rabiner 2015). To our knowledge, however, this is the first study to provide evidence of greater socio-economic disparities in access to specialist mental health care compared with general medical care across a range of high-income and low- to middle-income countries.

Even for individuals who were able to access care, socio-economic disparities persisted. Among those who received care, individuals with low education and low incomes were less likely to receive specialist mental health care. Given that all individuals in this group had sought treatment and no socio-economic disparities were identified for use of general medical care, these disparities are unlikely to be explained purely by awareness of mental illness or treatments and/or individual help-seeking behaviour. Thus, it is likely that individuals from low socio-economic groups face structural barriers in accessing care. Individuals with low education had the greatest disadvantage, after adjustment for income. In addition to lower access to specialist mental health care, individuals with low education were also less likely than those with high levels of education to receive human services and CAM services. Importantly, this suggests that the barriers were not only related to financial constraints. A study among 15 OECD countries also identified disparities for general health visits among individuals with low income and low education, which were greater for specialist compared to primary care (Devaux & de Looper 2012). Their findings also suggested that structural factors such as broader health insurance coverage were associated with better access, while higher out-of-pocket payments and more care delivered by the private sector were associated with lower access. Other studies have shown how health system structures can influence whether access is based on need or ability to pay (Kessler *et al.* 1997). Given the importance of education, the treatment gap cannot be resolved with financial solutions only and thus additional structural interventions that focus on individuals with low levels of education should be explored.

In conclusion, the findings in this chapter point to clear variations in the treatment gap, which are driven by socio-economic characteristics, in particular education, and that the gap is greater for specialist mental health care. The gaps we identified seem to indicate inequality in the way that health systems, particularly mental health specialist care, identify, refer and respond to mental health needs. Reducing this treatment gap requires commitment from governments to parity for mental health care. Universal access to mental health care and reduced out-of-pocket payments for low-income individuals would be an important step to reducing some socio-economic inequalities (Saxena *et al.* 2007; Gureje & Thornicroft 2015). Currently, however, more than a third of low-income countries rely on out-of-pocket payments as a primary source of finance for mental health care (Saxena *et al.* 2007). Moreover, low education seemed to represent an even greater barrier to mental health care in comparison with income and additional initiatives are needed to facilitate access to care for individuals with low levels of education. Policies will continue to be shaped by the resources and values of the country context (Evans-Lacko *et al.* 2016) and these results suggest that national and international mental health policies should specifically focus upon reducing disparities in access to treatment and care for the most socio-economically disadvantaged and hence rebalance this pyramid of disadvantage.

References

Amaddeo, F. & Jones, J. (2007) What is the impact of socioeconomic inequalities on the use of mental health services? *Epidemiologia e Psichiatria Sociale*, 16, 16–9.

Andersen, R. M. (1995). Revisiting the behavioral model and access to medical care: does it matter? *Journal of Health and Social Behavior*, 36, 1–10.

(2008). National health surveys and the behavioral model of health services use. *Medical Care*, 46, 647–53.

Andrade, L. H., Alonso, J., Mneimneh, Z. *et al.* (2014). Barriers to mental health treatment: results from the WHO World Mental Health surveys. *Psychological Medicine*, 44, 1303–17.

Bebbington, P. E., Meltzer, H., Brugha, T. S., *et al.* (2000). Unequal access and unmet need: neurotic disorders and the use of primary care services. *Psychological Medicine*, 30, 1359–67.

Boyd, A., Van de Velde, S., Pivette, M., *et al.* (2015). Gender differences in psychotropic use across Europe: Results from a large cross-sectional, population-based study. *European Psychiatry*, 30, 778–88.

Brown, J., Evans-Lacko, S., Aschan, L., *et al.* (2014). Seeking informal and formal help for mental health problems in the community: a secondary analysis from a psychiatric morbidity survey in South London. *BMC Psychiatry*, 14, 275.

De Lima, M. S., Hotopf, M., Mari, J. J., *et al.* (1999). Psychiatric disorder and the use of benzodiazepines: an example of the inverse care law from Brazil. *Social Psychiatry and Psychiatric Epidemiology*, 34, 316–22.

Devaux, M. & de Looper, M. (2012). *Income-Related Inequalities in Health Service Utilisation in 19 OECD Countries, 2008–2009*, Paris. Available at: www.oecd-ilibrary.org/ (Accessed 1 October 2016).

Evans-Lacko, S., Corker, E., Williams, P., *et al.* (2014). Trends in mental illness related public stigma among the English population in 2003–2013: influence of the Time to Change anti-stigma campaign. *Lancet Psychiatry*, 1, 121–8.

Evans-Lacko, S., Ribeiro, W., Brietzke, E., *et al.* (2016). Lean economies and innovation in mental health systems. *The Lancet*, 387, 1356–8.

Evans-Lacko, S. & Thornicroft, G. (2010). Stigma among people with dual diagnosis and implications for health services. *Advances in Dual Diagnosis*, 3, 4–7.

Fryers, T., Melzer, D., Jenkins, R., *et al.* (2005). The distribution of the common mental disorders: social inequalities in Europe. *Clinical Practice and Epidemiology in Mental Health: CP & EMH*, 1, 14.

Gureje, O. & Thornicroft, G. (2015). Health equity and mental health in post-2015 sustainable development goals. *The Lancet Psychiatry*, 2, 12–4.

Kessler, R. C., Frank, R. G., Edlund, M., *et al.* (1997). Differences in the use of psychiatric outpatient services between the United States and Ontario. *The New England Journal of Medicine*, 336, 551–7.

Kovess-Masfety V., Boyd, A., van de Velde, S., *et al.* (2014). Are there gender differences in service use for mental disorders across countries in the European Union? Results from the EU-World Mental Health survey. *Journal of Epidemiology and Community Health*, 68, 649–56.

Kovess-Mafesty, V., Evans-Lacko, S., Williams, D., *et al.* (2017). The role of religious advisors in mental health care in the World Mental Health surveys. *Social Psychiatry and Psychiatric Epidemiology*, 52, 353–67.

Lorant, V., Kampfl, D., Seghers, A., *et al.* (2003). Socioeconomic differences in psychiatric in-patient care. *Acta Psychiatrica Scandinavica*, 107, 170–7.

Lund, C., Breen, A., Flisher, A. J., *et al.* (2010). Poverty and common mental disorders in low and middle income countries: A systematic review. *Social Science & Medicine*, 71, 517–28.

Mangalore, R., Knapp, M. & Jenkins, R. (2007). Income-related inequality in mental health in Britain: the concentration index approach. *Psychological Medicine*, 37, 1037–45.

Mojtabai, R. (2010). Mental illness stigma and willingness to seek mental health care in the European Union. *Social Psychiatry and Psychiatric Epidemiology*, 45, 705–12.

Muntaner, C., Eaton, W. W., Miech, R., *et al.* (2004). Socioeconomic position and major mental disorders. *Epidemiologic Reviews*, 26, 53–62.

Murray, C. J., Vos, T., Lozano, R., *et al.* (2012). Disability-adjusted life years (DALYs) for 291 diseases and injuries in 21 regions, 1990–2010: a systematic analysis for the Global Burden of Disease Study 2010. *Lancet*, 380, 2197–223.

Ormel, J., Petukhova, M., Chatterji, S., *et al.* (2008). Disability and treatment of specific mental and physical disorders across the world. *The British Journal of Psychiatry*, 192, 368–75.

Roy-Byrne, P. P., Stein, M. B., Russo, J., *et al.* (1999). Panic disorder in the primary care setting: Comorbidity, disability, service utilization, and treatment. *The Journal of Clinical Psychiatry*, 60, 492–9.

Saxena, S., Thornicroft, G., Knapp, M., *et al.* (2007). Resources for mental health: scarcity, inequity, and inefficiency. *Lancet*, 370, 878–89.

Schomerus, G., Lucht, M., Holzinger, A., *et al.* (2011). The stigma of alcohol dependence compared with other mental disorders: a review of population studies. *Alcohol and Alcoholism*, 47, 105–12.

Steele, L., Dewa, C. & Lee, K. (2007). Socioeconomic status and self-reported barriers to mental health service use. *Canadian Journal of Psychiatry*, 52, 201–6.

Tello, J. E., Mazzi, M., Tansella, M., *et al.* (2005). Does socioeconomic status affect the use of community-based psychiatric services? A South Verona case register study. *Acta Psychiatrica Scandinavica*, 112, 215–23.

ten Have, M., Nuyen, J., Beekman, A., *et al.* (2013). Common mental disorder severity and its association with treatment contact and treatment intensity for mental health problems. *Psychological Medicine*, 43, 2203–13.

Thornicroft, G. (1991). Social deprivation and rates of treated mental disorder. Developing statistical models to predict psychiatric service utilisation. *The British Journal of Psychiatry*, 158, 475–84.

Thornicroft, G., Chatterji, S., Evans-Lacko, S., *et al.* (2017). Under-treatment of people with major depressive disorder in 21 countries. *British Journal of Psychiatry*, 210, 119–24.

Thornicroft, G. & Tansella, M. (2013). The balanced care model for global mental health. *Psychological Medicine*, 43, 849–63.

Tsai, A. C. & Tomlinson, M., (2015). Inequitable and ineffective: Exclusion of mental health from the post-2015 development agenda. *PLoS Medicine*, 12, e1001846.

Vigo, D., Thornicroft, G. & Atun, R. (2016). Estimating the true global burden of mental illness. *The Lancet Psychiatry*, 3, 171–8.

Wang, P. S., Aguilar-Gaxiola, S., Alonso, J., *et al.* (2007). Use of mental health services for anxiety, mood, and substance disorders in 17 countries in the WHO world mental health surveys. *Lancet*, 370, 841–50.

Whiteford, H. A., Ferrari, A. J., Degenhardt, L., *et al.* (2015). The global burden of mental, neurological and substance use disorders: an analysis from the Global Burden of Disease Study 2010. *PLoS One*, 10, e0116820.

World Health Organization (2012). *Global Burden of Mental Disorders and the Need for Comprehensive, Coordinated Response from Health and Social Sectors at the Country Level. Document EB130.R8*, Geneva: World Health Organization.

Young, A. S. & Rabiner, D., (2015). Racial/ethnic differences in parent-reported barriers to accessing children's health services. *Psychological Services*, 12, 267–73.

Chapter 22

Discussion

Kate M. Scott, Dan J. Stein, Peter de Jonge, Ronald C. Kessler

Introduction

Most of the prior chapters in this volume have focused on individual mental disorders, reviewing their descriptive epidemiology and presenting the World Mental Health (WMH) findings on each disorder. This chapter discusses and integrates these findings, taking (i) a *cross-disorder* perspective that highlights key differences as well as commonalities among disorders on epidemiological parameters, and (ii) a *cross-national* perspective, discussing the possible methodological and substantive factors that could be contributing to cross-national variation in findings. The first part of the chapter is structured as a response to a series of key questions about the epidemiology of mental disorders concerning their *prevalence*, *persistence*, *age-of-onset*, *associated impairment*, and *comorbidity*. A section on *study limitations* then follows, and the chapter finishes with a discussion of *policy implications* and *future directions for research*.

How Prevalent are Mental Disorders?

Variation across Disorders

Unsurprisingly, prevalence estimates vary greatly by disorder. Considering lifetime prevalence, and averaging estimates across all surveys, we find major depressive disorder (MDD) to be the most prevalent single disorder among those considered in this volume (10.6%) and intermittent explosive disorder (IED) to be the least prevalent disorder (0.8%) (Table 22.1). Other disorders not included in the WMH surveys (e.g., schizophrenia), or not included in this volume (e.g., anorexia) would also be expected to have low prevalence. Among the anxiety disorders included here the most prevalent are the two that usually have early onset (social anxiety disorder and specific phobia at 4.0 and 7.4%, respectively), while agoraphobia is less prevalent (1.2%). Adult separation anxiety disorder (SEPAD) emerges with a prevalence of 3.1% that falls between the estimate for generalized anxiety disorder (GAD) of 2.7% and for posttraumatic disorder (PTSD) of 3.9%. This supports the argument for increasing recognition of adult SEPAD put forward in Chapter 12. Although MDD is the single most prevalent disorder considered here, anxiety disorders are the most prevalent class of disorders. Alcohol-use disorders collectively rank second to MDD in prevalence (AUD: 8.6%) while the disruptive behaviour disorders and the eating disorders are for the most part clustered at the lower end of the prevalence spectrum (from 1.0% for bulimia nervosa to 2.7% for oppositional defiant disorder).

In all countries, these lifetime prevalence estimates are undoubtedly conservative due to recall failure, conscious nondisclosure, and survival bias. The estimates of lifetime risk from survival models presented in the disorder-specific chapters adjust for another issue: that the lifetime prevalence estimates reported here represent estimates of prevalence-to-date rather than lifetime risk. The latter is higher than prevalence-to-date due to the fact that not all respondents have passed through the age-of-risk of onset of the disorders. However, the projections of lifetime risk do not adjust for the under-counting due to recall bias, conscious nondisclosure, or survival bias. A study that illustrates how conservative our prevalence estimates may be compared prospectively assessed lifetime prevalence (the cumulative prevalence obtained from repeated past-year measures of the common mental disorders from age 18 to 32) in a New Zealand birth cohort with the retrospectively assessed lifetime prevalence estimates in the same age group in the New Zealand and American WMH surveys (Moffitt *et al.* 2010). That study found that the prospective lifetime estimates were approximately double the retrospective lifetime estimates for all the major classes of mental disorders. An even greater discrepancy between lifetime prevalence estimates obtained from retrospective versus

Table 22.1 Key epidemiological parameters of mental disorders in the World Mental Health surveys

Type of mental disorder	Lifetime prevalence		12-month prevalence among lifetime cases		Median age-of-onset	Proportion of 12-month cases with severe role impairment		Lifetime comorbidity		Proportion of 12-month cases seeking treatment from the health care sector[a]	
	%	SE	%	SE		%	SE	%	SE	%	SE
Major depressive disorder	**10.6**	0.1	**42.1**	0.5	**38**	**57.0**	0.9	**57.9**	0.5	**38.9**	0.7
Bipolar spectrum disorder	**1.9**	0.1	**60.3**	1.2	**25**	**54.1**	1.8	**77.3**	1.2	**39.4**	1.2
Generalized anxiety disorder	**2.7**	0.1	**44.8**	0.9	**38**	**45.7**	1.5	**75.6**	0.9	**40.0**	1.4
Panic disorder	**1.7**	0.0	**57.1**	1.3	**32**	**45.7**	1.7	**80.4**	1.1	**56.0**	1.6
Agoraphobia	**1.2**	0.0	**62.9**	1.4	**21**	**41.9**	2.0	**88.3**	1.4	**46.9**	1.9
Social anxiety disorder	**4.0**	0.1	**60.2**	0.8	**14**	**37.6**	1.0	**78.8**	0.8	**34.9**	0.9
Specific phobia	**7.4**	0.1	**74.2**	0.6	**8**	**18.7**	0.6	**60.5**	0.9	**21.0**	0.6
Posttraumatic stress disorder	**3.9**	0.1	**50.5**	1.0	**35**	**49.8**	2.1	**78.1**	1.1	**42.9**	1.6
Separation anxiety disorder (adult)	**3.1**	0.1	**30.8**	1.5	**27**	**38.3**	2.7	**78.5**	1.6	**27.7**	2.4
Intermittent explosive disorder	**0.8**	0.0	**53.6**	2.5	**17**	**38.9**	2.9	**81.7**	2.2	**25.0**	2.6
Conduct disorder	**2.3**	0.1	**14.5**	1.6	**13**	–	–	**87.3**	1.8	**23.5**	5.3
Oppositional defiant disorder	**2.7**	0.1	**17.4**	1.7	**12**	**41.2**	5.3	**87.5**	1.7	**39.7**	5.1
Alcohol-use disorder	**8.6**	0.1	**25.4**	0.6	**23**	**30.8**	2.9	**51.7**	0.8	**18.0**	1.0
Drug-use disorder	**3.5**	0.1	**21.4**	0.9	**20**	**45.8**	6.8	**81.8**	1.0	**33.4**	2.3
Binge-eating disorder	**1.8**	0.1	**44.4**	2.8	**24**	**21.3**	3.1	**79.6**	2.5	**34.0**	3.3
Bulimia nervosa	**1.0**	0.1	**36.7**	3.0	**21**	**31.7**	4.8	**87.8**	2.0	**40.7**	4.9
Psychotic experiences	**5.8**	0.2	**34.2**	1.5	**26**	–	–	**57.7**	1.9	**18.0**	1.5

[a]The specialty mental health sector or the general medical sector.

prospective methods was observed in long term follow up of the Baltimore Epidemiological Catchment Area Study (Takayanagi *et al.* 2014). Retrospective methods particularly undercount individuals with single, mild episodes (Wells & Horwood 2004; Moffitt *et al.* 2010) so the WMH lifetime prevalence estimates are likely to be somewhat more representative of the more persistent and severe disorders.

Variation across Countries

The results reported in this volume show clearly that there is a great deal of variation in disorder prevalence across countries as well as within each of the three country income groups. It is quite striking to note, though, that when we examine the cross-national *patterns* in lifetime prevalence – that is, the average prevalence for any given disorder in each of the three country income groups (see Table 22.2) – there is a consistent pattern in 17/18 disorders (SEPAD being the exception) of prevalence being lower in the low/lower-middle-income countries than in the high-income countries. In 15/18 disorders prevalence is lowest in the low/lower-middle-income countries and in 10/18 disorders there is a significant positive gradient of increasing prevalence across the three country income groups. This positive association between prevalence of mental disorders and income level of country is consistent with recent systematic reviews from the Global Burden of Disease (GBD) studies (Baxter *et al.* 2013; Ferrari *et al.* 2013a; Steel *et al.* 2014). This gradient is intriguing given that it is opposite in direction to what might be expected based on individual-level inverse associations between socio-economic status and mental disorder prevalence within countries. However, the cross-national variation we find in the WMH surveys is difficult to interpret because of the unknown role of methodological influences on the differences in prevalence estimates across countries.

As Chapter 3 details, enormous effort went into making the WMH surveys as methodologically consistent as possible, but inevitable differences occurred across surveys in sampling frame, fieldwork quality control, disorders surveyed, length of the interview, oversampling of population subgroups, use of the two-part interview, degree of clustering and stratification, and obtained response rate. Methodological variation may also arise due to the formidable set of challenges involved in the successful application of the CIDI in cross-cultural research, with a long period of development required to ensure the cultural relevance and cross-cultural equivalence of the constructs and concepts being measured (Prince 2008; Harkness *et al.* 2010; Ghimire *et al.* 2013). Although all WMH surveys adhered in general terms to the WHO translation guidelines for cross-cultural research, it is likely that not all the several steps in this process were followed with equal rigour in every country (Ghimire *et al.* 2013). A further potential source of variation in prevalence across countries may come from cross-national variation in the degree to which mental disorders are stigmatized (Gureje *et al.* 2005; Lasalvia *et al.* 2013), with flow-on effects on willingness to disclose symptoms (Reavley & Jorm 2014). There is some evidence that stigmatizing attitudes associated with mental disorders are greater in less developed countries (Alonso *et al.* 2009), although other studies do not find clear cut patterns in this regard (Pescosolido *et al.* 2013). Besides stigma, other factors may affect response patterns. Low-income countries have less of a tradition of health surveys and this may also inhibit willingness to disclose symptoms to lay interviewers (Gureje *et al.* 2008).

Our finding of lower prevalence in the lower-income countries could also reflect variation in substantive factors. For example, while mental disorders are generally correlated with social disadvantage and stressful exposures within all countries, there may be factors that promote mental health or buffer the effects of these exposures that are more concentrated in lower-income countries or non-Westernized cultures. Such factors might include greater social capital and opportunities for community engagement (De Silva *et al.* 2005; Diener *et al.* 2010; Axinn *et al.* 2015) as well as a greater degree of support from extended family (Daatland *et al.* 2011; Yeh *et al.* 2013). Value orientations could also be relevant. In an earlier WMH study we found that associations between subjective social status and mental disorders were significantly less strong in the low/lower-middle-income countries than in the higher-income countries (Scott *et al.* 2014). One interpretation of this finding is that non-Westernized cultures that place less emphasis on individual achievement and status might render their citizens less vulnerable to invidious social comparisons that undermine mental health. In a related vein, some researchers have suggested that the easy access to material things and sense of entitlement that characterizes affluent cultures undermines motivation and wellbeing, thereby creating the conditions for a mismatch

Table 22.2 Mean lifetime prevalence of mental disorders in the World Mental Health surveys in the country income groups, and in all countries combined

Type of mental disorder	Low/lower-middle-income countries		Upper-middle-income countries		High-income countries		All countries combined			
	%	SE	%	SE	%	SE	%	SE	F	[P]
Major depressive disorder	7.1	0.2	9.2	0.3	12.6	0.2	10.6	0.1	259.6*	<0.001
Bipolar spectrum disorder	1.0	0.1	1.6	0.1	2.5	0.1	1.9	0.0	88.6*	<0.001
Generalized anxiety disorder	1.1	0.1	2.1	0.1	3.7	0.1	2.7	0.1	253.3*	<0.001
Panic disorder	0.8	0.1	1.1	0.1	2.2	0.1	1.7	0.0	129.9*	<0.001
Agoraphobia	0.7	0.1	1.5	0.1	1.4	0.1	1.2	0.0	32.3*	<0.001
Social anxiety disorder	1.6	0.1	2.9	0.1	5.5	0.1	4.0	0.1	387.5	<0.001
Specific phobia	5.7	0.2	8.0	0.2	8.1	0.1	7.4	0.1	51.1*	<0.001
Posttraumatic stress disorder	2.1	0.2	2.3	0.1	5.0	0.1	3.9	0.1	135.8*	<0.001
Separation anxiety disorder (adult)	3.4	0.3	3.2	0.2	2.9	0.2	3.1	0.1	2.1	0.120
Intermittent explosive disorder	0.6	0.1	0.7	0.1	1.1	0.1	0.8	0.0	19.1*	<0.001
Conduct disorder	1.5	0.2	1.5	0.1	3.2	0.2	2.3	0.1	21.7*	<0.001
Oppositional defiant disorder	2.6	0.3	2.1	0.2	3.0	0.2	2.7	0.1	5.3*	0.005
Alcohol-use disorder	5.9	0.2	7.2	0.2	10.4	0.2	8.6	0.1	163.2*	<0.001
Drug-use disorder	0.9	0.1	2.5	0.1	4.8	0.1	3.5	0.1	300.8*	<0.001
Binge-eating disorder	0.8	0.2	3.8	0.3	1.5	0.1	1.8	0.1	38.6*	<0.001
Bulimia nervosa	0.4	0.1	1.6	0.2	0.9	0.1	1.0	0.1	18.2*	<0.001
Psychotic experiences	3.2	0.3	7.2	0.4	6.8	0.3	5.8	0.2	49.5*	<0.001

*Significant difference in prevalence across the three country income groups.

between expectations and outcomes that could lead to mental illness (Koplewicz *et al.* 2009; Luthar *et al.* 2013).

It is also interesting to note the remarkable consistency between the cross-national patterning of mental disorders found in the WMH (and GBD) data and the cross-national patterning of chronic medical conditions such as cardiovascular disease (Lozano *et al.* 2013). This consistency may be due in part to the well-established bi-directional associations of mental disorders with chronic physical conditions (Prince *et al.* 2007; Scott *et al.* 2016), but it may also reflect shared underlying dietary and lifestyle factors that are more prevalent in wealthy countries (Logan & Jacka 2014; Prescott *et al.* 2016).

To conclude this section, the WMH data are interesting in that they show inverse associations between socio-economic status and disorder prevalence within countries, yet positive associations between country income level and disorder prevalence across countries. However, interpretation of this cross-national pattern is complicated by the possible contribution of between-survey methodological variation. As mentioned in Chapter 3, the WMH surveys were optimized to discern consistent within-country patterns rather than to examine reasons for cross-national differences.

How Persistent are Mental Disorders?

If we compare the indirect indicator of disorder persistence (the ratio of 12-month to lifetime prevalence) across the adult disorders (Table 22.1), we see that approximately one-quarter to two-thirds of respondents with a given lifetime disorder experience persistence of that disorder in the 12 months prior to interview. This is an upper-bound estimate to the extent that lifetime prevalence is underestimated (see below). The lower persistence of MDD (42.1%) relative to bipolar spectrum disorder (60.3%) is illustrative of the episodic nature of MDD. The substance-use disorders have even lower rates of persistence (21.4–25.4%) that also denote the waxing and waning of symptoms with these disorders. The relatively low rate of persistence for bulimia nervosa (36.7%) may seem surprising, but because these persistence rates are averaged across all ages this lower rate for bulimia may obscure an age-related pattern of bulimia symptoms being more severe and persistent when sufferers are younger. Several of the anxiety disorders, by contrast, are marked by quite high persistence, especially the phobias. Specific phobia for example, a disorder that many people would consider among the least severe of the disorders considered here (a characterization supported by it having the lowest rate of impairment in Table 22.1), is nonetheless the most persistent disorder with a 12-month/lifetime ratio of 74.2%; this indicates the capacity of this disorder to have an enduring influence on those who develop it.

One important limitation to note is that these persistence estimates based on the 12-month/lifetime ratio are likely to be overestimates due to the fact that lifetime prevalence is underestimated and recall failure is higher among those with non-persistent disorders, as noted in the earlier section on prevalence. The likelihood that persistence is overestimated by the 12-month/lifetime ratio is supported by prospective epidemiological studies finding that disorder persistence across multiple study waves is rare (Paksarian *et al.* 2016). It is noteworthy that we observe a cross-national pattern of disorder persistence being, for most disorders, higher in the lower-income countries than in the higher-income countries. This could be a methodological artefact if lifetime prevalence is underestimated to a greater degree in the lower-income countries. On the other hand, the higher persistence of disorders in lower-income countries could also be a substantive finding related to the more limited treatment availability in poor countries. More research will be required to adjudicate between these explanations.

When in the Life Course do Mental Disorders First Occur?

The median estimated ages-of-onset (AOOs) are shown for each disorder in the third column of Table 22.1. Although they vary considerably across disorders, these estimates indicate that for many of the mental disorders under consideration, half of the people who will ever experience the disorder will have first developed it by adolescence or in the first decade of adulthood. There are some notable exceptions to this, with MDD, GAD, and PTSD having median AOOs in the mid to late thirties. It is also important to note that the dementias and other neurocognitive disorders of ageing (not included in the WMH surveys) have much later median AOOs. Nonetheless, these data suggest that most mental disorders typically onset within the first decades of life, emphasizing the need for early diagnosis and intervention (Birchwood & Singh 2013). And in fact, these AOO estimates may be biased upwards if older respondents forget disorder episodes occurring earlier in life or if the sample is biased by earlier mortality associated with mental disorders, especially if this is more true for early-onset than later-onset disorders (Walker *et al.* 2015). As explained in Chapter 3, a series of approaches to minimize recall bias in AOO reports was adopted and there is some evidence of their success in the absence of the pattern found in previous surveys of AOOs being over-represented in the five years before interview. Nonetheless, it is likely that some recall bias remains in the WMH AOO estimates.

The median AOOs shown in Table 22.1 are averaged across all WMH countries and it is worth pointing out that they are somewhat higher than those reported in our earlier publications based on high-income WMH countries like the United States (Kessler *et al.* 2005). They are also somewhat higher than earlier cross-national reports based on WMH surveys (Kessler *et al.* 2007). This is because the AOO distributions tend to be higher (i.e., with an older median AOO) in lower-income countries and a greater number of low-income countries are included in this volume compared with earlier WMH publications. But in addition to the general problem of basing AOO estimates on retrospective data there are additional methodological factors that may have compromised our ability to estimate AOO comparably across countries and so may have contributed to this cross-national variation in AOO estimates. These factors include the possibility of differential early mortality associated with mental disorders across countries, differences in age structure across countries, and cross-national variation in the cognitive representation of time and temporal sequencing (Fuhrman & Boroditsky 2010; Ghimire *et al.* 2013).

What Impact do Mental Disorders have on Functioning?

Variation across Disorders

As can be seen from the Sheehan Disability Scale estimates shown in column 4 of Table 22.1, most active mental disorders are associated with severe impairment in at least one domain of role functioning in around one-third to one-half of cases. Among the disorders considered here, mood disorders appear to be more impairing than other disorders, with 57% of 12-month MDD cases associated with severe impairment in the worst month of the year. Some caveats are important to note here. The Sheehan estimate for bipolar disorder is for the bipolar spectrum category and so underestimates the degree of impairment associated with bipolar I or II. Additionally, this relative ranking of impairment is limited by omissions of disorders that are known to be highly impairing such as schizophrenia, dementia, and obsessive compulsive disorder. Nonetheless, our finding that MDD is associated with high impairment is consistent with the recent GBD study that found depression to be the second leading contributor to years lived with disability worldwide (Ferrari *et al.* 2013b). In both the GBD study and the WMH surveys, the degree of impairment associated with mental disorders is based on self-report. Some researchers have suggested that the high degree of self-reported impairment associated with MDD is because depressed individuals 'over-report' disability as a function of the pessimistic outlook that is intrinsic to depression (Morgado *et al.* 1991). A counterpoint to that criticism comes from the ample research showing that depression and other mental disorders can impact motivation, cognition, emotional regulation, and behaviour in ways that can be more disabling than the activity limitations associated with physical disabilities (Ormel *et al.* 2008; Alonso *et al.* 2013). These functional limitations, as well as the potentially profound long-term impacts associated with mental disorders, are extensively detailed in our earlier volume (Alonso *et al.* 2013).

Based on the Sheehan data, some mental disorders are less impairing than others. Specific phobia is the least impairing of those considered here (although, as noted above, it is also the most persistent), probably because many individuals with the disorder are able to organize their lives so as to avoid encountering the feared object or situation. Substance-use disorders are also associated with lower reported functional impairment, but this might be because minimization or lack of recognition of the deleterious impact of substance use on self or others is a frequent concomitant of these disorders. Reluctance to admit to, or lack of understanding of, the impact of disorder symptoms may also contribute to the relatively low level of reported impairment associated with IED.

Variation across Countries

An interesting cross-national pattern in the impairment data emerges whereby for 10/12 disorders (the two exceptions being binge-eating disorder and PTSD) the percent with severe impairment is higher in the high-income countries than in the low/lower-middle-income countries. Furthermore, for 6 of the 12 disorders with comparable data there is a significant positive gradient across the three country income groups of increasing impairment with increasing county income level. As noted earlier in this chapter, there is also a positive gradient of increasing disorder *prevalence* with increasing country income level. The conjunction of these two trends implies that there is a positive association between prevalence and severe impairment across countries. As noted in an earlier WMH report on depression (Bromet *et al.* 2011), this positive country-level association between prevalence and impairment contrasts with an earlier cross-national WHO study of major depression in primary-care patients that found countries with the highest prevalence estimates to report the lowest levels of impairment associated with depression (Simon *et al.* 2002).

Our finding that impairment associated with mental disorders is generally greater in the high-income countries than in the lower-income countries is surprising given the more limited treatment resources (Saxena *et al.* 2007) and lower treatment uptake for mental disorders (Chapter 21) in poorer countries. It is possible that this cross-national pattern is a methodological artefact attributable to the same factors that may have led to lower disorder prevalence in low-income countries. Inconsistent with that suggestion, however, is the fact that the pattern we observe of both lower impairment *and* lower prevalence in the low/lower-middle-income countries is the opposite of what we would expect to see if prevalence estimates were biased downwards in low-income countries, or if the CIDI diagnosis thresholds were inappropriately high in low-income countries. This is because a more conservative (higher) diagnostic threshold would normally capture the more severe cases and miss more of the mild cases, resulting in those meeting diagnostic criteria reporting higher rather than lower impairment in the countries where prevalence was underestimated. Yet we find the opposite pattern in the WMH data.

Based on this observation, although we cannot rule out a methodological explanation for this cross-national variation in impairment, it is worth considering a substantive interpretation: that there is genuinely less impairment associated with mental disorders in lower- than in higher-income countries. This could be because mental disorder symptoms interfere less with role demands in lower-income countries, either because of cross-national differences in role or performance expectations, or because greater family or community support may help meet role demands among the mentally ill in lower-income countries. There is some indirect evidence in support of this latter suggestion from other WMH data showing that the burden among family caregivers of those with mental health problems is 2–3-fold higher in the lower-income countries than in the higher-income countries (Shahly *et al.* 2013). Moreover, our finding of lower impairment in the lower-income countries is consistent with the findings of earlier cross-national studies that found the course and outcomes associated with schizophrenia to be more benign in developing countries than in developed countries (Jablensky *et al.* 1992; Harrison *et al.* 2001). The conclusions drawn from those earlier studies have been disputed (Cohen *et al.* 2008; Jääskeläinen *et al.* 2013) and the WMH surveys do not shed any further light on the issue as it relates to schizophrenia. But in relation to other mental disorders, the rather consistent cross-national patterning of impairment we observe in the WMH data does suggest that there may be potent cultural modifiers of the disability burden associated with mental disorders. This is an important area for further research as policy initiatives may more easily reduce the impairment associated with disorders than the prevalence of disorders.

What Can We Learn from Comorbidity between Disorders?

In most chapters, high levels of comorbidity are reported between focal disorders and the other DSM-IV disorders assessed in the WMH surveys. Indeed, the average proportion of people with a lifetime comorbid disorder exceeds 50% among those with each of the lifetime disorders considered here (Table 22.1). Importantly, though, there is considerable variation between disorders in this regard. For instance, 51.7% of people with a lifetime alcohol-use disorder met criteria for another lifetime disorder, while for lifetime agoraphobia this figure was 88.3%. Also, specific patterns of comorbidity emerged for the different mental disorders, with some specific comorbid disorder combinations more common than others. There are important lessons to be learnt from these comorbidity patterns as they may inform us about the latent structure of psychopathology, as explored in Chapter 20. In the WMH surveys data, support was found for both a general psychopathology factor and for a distinction between internalizing and externalizing disorders.

These findings are in line with previous findings on both cross-sectional and longitudinal data regarding the role of the internalizing and externalizing domains in explaining the development of comorbidity over time (Kessler *et al.* 2011). Taken together, these results may be used to distinguish between common, domain-specific, and disorder-specific vulnerability factors, and formulate or fine-tune treatments aimed at those factors. Several recent reports have extended the work on the structure of psychopathology to work on the structure of personality and of etiological factors. For example, Lahey *et al.* (2017) recently proposed a taxonomy of psychopathology distinguishing between genetic and environmental influences that are either common to multiple dimensions of psychopathology or unique to each dimension. In this taxonomy a central role is dedicated to the distinction between the higher-order domains of internalizing and externalizing psychopathology and their associated genetic and environmental risk factors. Future research dedicated to the development of comorbidity over time may reveal early warning signals and specific trajectories of poor mental health with associated risk factors and treatment options, thus informing future psychiatric classification systems.

Study Limitations

As emphasized throughout this volume, the WMH surveys have several important limitations. They rely on fully structured diagnostic assessments rather than on semi-structured diagnostic assessments made by trained clinicians. They rely on retrospective recall of respondents' past experience of disorders, which, together with the possibility of sample survival bias, means that the lifetime prevalence estimates are conservative. The estimates of AOO are similarly based on respondent recall and thus are likely to be biased to some degree and possibly to vary in magnitude across countries. Our indirect indicators of persistence are likely to be overestimates due to lifetime prevalence being underestimated and recall failure being higher among those with non-persistent disorders. The cross-sectional design of the surveys means that we rely on respondent recall for the temporal ordering of life events and disorders. Finally, we are limited in the ability to interpret cross-national differences due to the unknown degree of between-surveys methodological variation that may have contributed to the lower estimates of prevalence and impairment in the low-income countries.

Policy Implications

Even with the caveats resulting from the limitations noted above, the WMH surveys provide the most comprehensive cross-national data on the epidemiology of mental disorders ever assembled. Given the complexity of mounting coordinated cross-national surveys, this will probably remain true for some time to come. The use of probability sampling methods together with a standardized, validated, face-to-face diagnostic interview; the central oversight of data collection and analysis; and the achievement of good response rates in most surveys means that these data are able to provide a firm foundation for policy and planning.

As discussed earlier in this chapter, there is considerable variation in WMH estimates of prevalence and other epidemiological parameters across disorders and across countries. But from a policy point of view what is most important is the consistent pattern that emerges from the WMH surveys as a whole: that mental disorders are common; that they occur world wide; that most disorders begin relatively early in the lifespan; that they are most prevalent among the young and the socially disadvantaged; that they are often highly impairing, persistent, and comorbid with other disorders; and that they are greatly under-treated. These central features of the epidemiology of mental disorders underscore the call for health policy and services to place much greater emphasis on the needs of adolescents and young adults with mental disorders given that it is in this age group that most mental disorders first emerge and are most prevalent (Patton *et al.* 2016). Intervention early in the course of the disorder offers significant potential for long-term social, health, and economic benefits to individuals and societies. This can occur through the reduction of disorder persistence and secondary comorbidity (Kessler & Price 1993; Kessler *et al.* 2011), reduced likelihood of lost educational and employment opportunities (Alonso *et al.* 2013), and delayed development of chronic physical diseases (Scott *et al.* 2016). That said, our present understanding of the public health implications of early intervention is still at an early stage because of the lack of focus on this issue in clinical studies.

The WMH data offer the most detailed information about treatment seeking among people with mental disorders in general populations worldwide. These data make clear that the majority of people with mental disorders are not getting treatment at all and that even fewer are being treated in a timely fashion or in accordance with current evidence of best practices for effective intervention (Thornicroft *et al.* 2017). This huge treatment gap is especially pronounced among individuals with low socio-economic status within all countries, and in low/lower-middle-income countries. These findings indicate that for the reduction in prevalence of disorders and prevention of secondary comorbidity there is much more that could be achieved through better planning and funding of mental health services that are well integrated with primary care (WHO 2015b) and able to target those most in need (Thornicroft *et al.* 2010; Patel *et al.* 2016). These results also underscore how much more is required in terms of the scaling up and provision of mental disorder treatment services in low- and middle-income countries (Saxena *et al.* 2007; Patel *et al.* 2009). The latter is the focus of the World Health Organization (WHO) Mental Health Gap Action Programme (WHO 2016). Addressing this formidable problem will require a much greater investment in mental health service research and delivery than is currently being made by any country in the world, an investment that would help redress the lack of parity in service provision between mental and physical disorders (Wykes *et al.* 2015). Improved mental health service provision and integration should happen in the context of moving towards universal health coverage (WHO 2015a). This is a target of the WHO for people in countries at all levels of development to ensure that they receive the quality, essential health services they need without suffering financial hardship. Universal health coverage is a specific component of one of the United Nation's new Sustainable Development Goals (UN 2015).

Reducing the prevalence and incidence of mental disorders requires a response that extends beyond the responsibilities of the health sector. As evident in the findings presented for each mental disorder in this volume, the onset likelihood and current prevalence of mental disorders are highest among the most socially vulnerable: those with less education and low incomes; those who are divorced, separated, or widowed; those who are unemployed or disabled. These WMH findings replicate much prior research in high- (Fryers *et al.* 2003; Wells *et al.* 2006) and low- (Patel and Kleinman 2003; Lund *et al.* 2010) income countries. The direction of causality in the associations between mental disorders and disadvantaged social status is unclear, although evidence exists for both social causation (disadvantaged social status leading to mental disorders) and social selection (mental disorders leading to disadvantaged social status) pathways (Johnson *et al.* 1999; Miech *et al.* 1999; Stansfeld *et al.* 2011; Olesen *et al.* 2013). Of all the social correlates we studied, the one that was the most systematically associated with lifetime prevalence of mental disorders was being out of the labour force through unemployment or disability (the 'other' category of labour force status). In this regard it is relevant to note that most of the surveys included in this volume were conducted prior to the Global Financial Crisis and that the latter has been associated with substantially increased rates of unemployment (especially among those with existing mental disorders), economic hardship, and associated mental health problems in many affected countries (Evans-Lacko *et al.* 2013; Karanikolos *et al.* 2013). The associations of social disadvantage with mental disorders have important policy implications, suggesting that mental disorders and/or their effects on functioning may be amenable to amelioration through a range of social, employment, and welfare policy measures that aim to protect jobs and improve access to financial and housing support (Karanikolos *et al.* 2013; Barr *et al.* 2015). This will require a multi-sectoral strategy where health is embedded in all policies and the health system stewards the other sectors to ensure the mental health and wellbeing of the population.

Future Directions

Discussions of the future of psychiatric epidemiology research tend to emphasize the need to move beyond the kind of descriptive epidemiology of mental disorders from cross-sectional surveys featured in this volume to prospective studies that can better illuminate the causes and course of mental disorders (Susser *et al.* 2006; Tsuang *et al.* 2011; Toyokawa *et al.* 2012). But priorities for psychiatric epidemiological research vary by country and country income level. The WMH Surveys Initiative was mounted because for many low- and middle-income countries (and indeed for a number of high-income countries) basic descriptive epidemiological data on the prevalence and burden of mental disorders was lacking. And despite the achievements of the WMH surveys, their global coverage is limited. This means that notwithstanding the limitations of cross-sectional surveys, there remains a pressing need for more surveys of this kind, especially in the many low-income countries and global regions not currently represented in the WMH surveys (Sharan *et al.* 2009). In addition, there is a need for ongoing trend surveys to monitor changes in prevalence and correlates over time associated with changes in policy initiatives.

Realistically too, study of the cross-national epidemiology of mental disorders is likely to continue to rely on cross-sectional surveys because these can be more readily standardized across countries in terms of methodology. In this respect, to advance the study of cross-national variation in mental disorders the most urgent research need is for further careful methodological research that can better delineate and thereby help reduce the contribution of methodological variation to cross-national variation in estimates. There is already an active research programme devoted to the methodology of comparative cross-national survey design (Harkness *et al.* 2010; Johnson *et al.* 2018) and the WMH surveys have built on some of the accrued insights from this past research. But the challenges in interpretation of our cross-national findings discussed in this chapter highlight the need for extensive further methodological research in certain specific areas. For example, further studies that investigate individual social and cultural factors that affect willingness to disclose mental health symptoms (Mneimneh 2012) would be useful, although future surveys are likely to utilize audio computer-assisted self-interviews that can reduce the social effects that may occur with face-to-face interviews. More in-depth studies of the kind conducted in Nepal that seek to optimize the validation of the translation protocol for diagnostic interviews (Ghimire *et al.* 2013) are needed; these studies can uncover cultural differences in understanding of key concepts that may have a bearing on prevalence estimates. More clinical validation studies in a wider range of countries will be important to test the validity of lay-administered, fully structured interviews. To further examine the cultural validity of the DSM/ICD classifications themselves, it may be informative to conduct studies within some countries that include both DSM/ICD-based measurement of disorders alongside measures of culture-specific concepts of distress (Kohrt *et al.* 2014). Although cross-national comparative research is likely to rely on current diagnostic systems for the foreseeable future, ongoing research into alternative, biologically based ways of conceptualizing and classifying mental disorders is important, as highlighted in Chapter 2.

Future research could also explore some of the possible substantive reasons put forward above in the discussion of cross-national variation in disorder prevalence and impairment. Such studies could include expanded measurement of attitudes and values as well as individual and community-level indicators of social support and social capital. We need a better understanding of variation in the lived experience of those with mental illness in different countries and cultural settings; of what factors help buffer the impact of the disorder on the individual sufferers; and of how individuals and families cope in settings where the treatment gap is most pronounced. As suggested by the WMH findings (and prior research), culture appears to influence the outcomes and impairment associated with mental disorders, but exactly how and through what mechanisms requires further study. Future studies of mental disorder epidemiology that include measures of diet and lifestyle would be very valuable to test hypotheses about common causal pathways underpinning mental and physical disorders and their co-variation. Mounting multiple-country studies on the scale of the WMH surveys is hugely resource-demanding, but cross-national studies of more limited scope can be conducted in a smaller number of countries known to vary on factors of interest, laying the ground work for subsequent larger studies.

Conclusion

As the data presented in this volume attest, the WMH Surveys Initiative has generated a wealth of epidemiological information on prevalence and sociodemographic patterning of a wide range of DSM-IV disorders in the general populations of a broad range of countries. For most WMH countries these surveys provide the first such descriptive information on the burden of mental disorders in their citizens, and as such they provide an invaluable foundation for health service policy and planning. The findings featured in this volume document many consistent patterns of association across countries: in all countries surveyed mental disorders begin relatively early in the lifespan; they are most prevalent among the young and the socially disadvantaged; they are often highly impairing and frequently comorbid with other disorders; and they are greatly under-treated. These findings have important policy implications indicating the need to prioritize the detection and treatment of mental disorders in young people, to upscale treatment services in low- and middle-income countries in particular, and to coordinate the health policy response with other relevant agencies to reduce the incidence and improve the outcomes of mental disorders among the socially vulnerable. Substantial cross-national variation is also evident with both prevalence and impairment being lower in low-income countries than in high-income countries. These cross-national patterns are provocative but difficult to interpret given the inability to tease apart the respective contributions of methodological and substantive factors to the cross-national variation observed. The WMH surveys demonstrate the enormous challenges but rich rewards of cross-national comparative studies of mental disorders in providing an essential foundation for future policy and research.

References

Alonso J., Buron A., Bruffaerts R., *et al.* (2009). Association of perceived stigma and mood and anxiety disorders: results from the World Mental Health Surveys. *Acta Psychiatrica Scandinavica.*

Alonso J., Chatterji S., He Y. (2013). *The Burdens of Mental Disorders: Global Perspectives from the WHO World Mental Health Surveys.* New York: Cambridge University Press.

Axinn W. G., Ghimire D. J., Williams N. E., *et al.* (2015). Associations between the social organization of communities and psychiatric disorders in rural Asia. *Social Psychiatry and Psychiatric Epidemiology*, 50, 1537–45.

Barr B., Kinderman P., Whitehead M. (2015). Trends in mental health inequalities in England during a period of recession, austerity and welfare reform 2004 to 2013. *Social Science & Medicine*, 147, 324–31.

Baxter A. J., Scott K. M., Vos T., *et al.* (2013). Global prevalence of anxiety disorders: a systematic review and meta-regression. *Psychological Medicine*, 43, 897–910.

Birchwood M., Singh S. P. (2013). Mental health services for young people: matching the service to the need. *The British Journal of Psychiatry*, 202, s1–s2.

Bromet E., Andrade L., Hwang I., *et al.* (2011). Cross-national epidemiology of DSM-IV major depressive episode. *BMC Medicine*, 9, 90.

Cohen A., Patel V., Thara R., *et al.* (2008). Questioning an axiom: better prognosis for schizophrenia in the developing world? *Schizophrenia Bulletin*, 34, 229–44.

Daatland S. O., Herlofson K., Lima I. A. (2011). Balancing generations: on the strength and character of family norms in the West and East of Europe. *Ageing and Society*, 31, 1159–79.

De Silva M. J., McKenzie K., Harpham T., *et al.* (2005). Social capital and mental illness: a systematic review. *Journal of Epidemiology and Community Health*, 59, 619–27.

Diener E., Ng W., Harter J., *et al.* (2010). Wealth and happiness across the world: material prosperity predicts life evaluation, whereas psychosocial prosperity predicts positive feeling. *Journal of Personality and Social Psychology*, 99, 52.

Evans-Lacko S., Knapp M., McCrone P., *et al.* (2013). The mental health consequences of the recession: economic hardship and employment of people with mental health problems in 27 European countries. *PLoS ONE*, 8, e69792.

Ferrari A., Somerville A., Baxter A., *et al.* (2013a). Global variation in the prevalence and incidence of major depressive disorder: a systematic review of the epidemiological literature. *Psychological Medicine*, 43, 471–81.

Ferrari A. J., Charlson F. J., Norman R. E., *et al.* (2013b). Burden of depressive disorders by country, sex, age, and year: findings from the global burden of disease study 2010. *PLoS Medicine*, 10, e1001547.

Fryers T., Melzer D., Jenkins R. (2003). Social inequalities and the common mental disorders. *Social Psychiatry and Psychiatric Epidemiology*, 38, 229–37.

Fuhrman O., Boroditsky L. (2010). Cross-cultural differences in mental representations of time: evidence from an implicit nonlinguistic task. *Cognitive Science*, 34, 1430–51.

Ghimire D. J., Chardoul S., Kessler R. C., *et al.* (2013). Modifying and validating the Composite International Diagnostic Interview (CIDI) for use in Nepal. *International Journal of Methods in Psychiatric Research*, 22, 71–81.

Gureje O., Adeyemi O., Enyidah N., *et al.* (2008). Mental disorders among adult Nigerians: risks, prevalence and treatment. In *The WHO World Mental Health Surveys: Global Perspectives on the Epidemiology of Mental Disorders* (eds R. C. Kessler and T. B. Ustun). New York: Cambridge University Press.

Gureje O., Lasebikan V. O., Ephraim-Oluwanuga O., *et al.* (2005). Community study of knowledge of and attitude to mental illness in Nigeria. *The British Journal of Psychiatry*, 186, 436–41.

Harkness J. A., Braun M., Edwards B., *et al.* (2010). *Survey Methods in Multinational, Multiregional, and Multicultural Contexts.* Hoboken, NJ: Wiley.

Harrison G., Hopper K., Craig T., *et al.* (2001). Recovery from psychotic illness: a 15-and 25-year international follow-up study. *The British Journal of Psychiatry*, 178, 506–17.

Jääskeläinen E., Juola P., Hirvonen N., *et al.* (2013). A systematic review and meta-analysis of recovery in schizophrenia. *Schizophrenia Bulletin*, 39, 1296–306.

Jablensky A., Sartorius N., Ernberg G., *et al.* (1992). Schizophrenia: manifestations, incidence and course in different cultures. A World Health Organization Ten-Country Study. *Psychological Medicine. Monograph Supplement*, 20, 1–97.

Johnson J. G., Cohen P., Dohrenwend B. P., *et al.* (1999). A longitudinal investigation of social causation and social selection processes involved in the association between socioeconomic status and psychiatric disorders. *Journal of Abnormal Psychology*, 108, 490–99.

Johnson T., Pennell B.-E., Stoop I., *et al.* (eds) (2018). *Advances in Comparative Survey Methods:*

Multinational, Multiregional and Multicultural Contexts (3MC). New York: John Wiley & Sons.

Karanikolos M., Mladovsky P., Cylus J., *et al.* (2013). Financial crisis, austerity, and health in Europe. *The Lancet*, 381, 1323–31.

Kessler R. C., Angermeyer M., Anthony J. C., *et al.* (2007). Lifetime prevalence and age-of-onset distributions of mental disorders in the World Health Organization's World Mental Health Surveys. *World Psychiatry*, 6, 168–76.

Kessler R. C., Berglund P., Demler O., *et al.* (2005). Lifetime prevalence and age-of-onset distributions of DSM-IV disorders in the National Comorbidity Survey Replication. *Archives of General Psychiatry*, 62, 593–602.

Kessler R. C., Ormel J., Petukhova M., *et al.* (2011). Development of lifetime comorbidity in the World Health Organization World Mental Health Surveys. *Archives of General Psychiatry*, 68, 90.

Kessler R. C., Price R. H. (1993). Primary prevention of secondary disorders: a proposal and agenda. *American Journal of Community Psychology*, 21, 607–33.

Kohrt B. A., Rasmussen A., Kaiser B. N., *et al.* (2014). Cultural concepts of distress and psychiatric disorders: literature review and research recommendations for global mental health epidemiology. *International Journal of Epidemiology*, 43, 365–406.

Koplewicz H. S., Gurian A., Williams K. (2009). The era of affluence and its discontents. *Journal of the American Academy of Child & Adolescent Psychiatry*, 48, 1053–5.

Lahey B. B., Krueger R. F., Rathouz P. J., *et al.* (2017). A hierarchical causal taxonomy of psychopathology across the life span. *Psychological Bulletin*, 143, 142–86.

Lasalvia A., Zoppei S., Van Bortel T., *et al.* (2013). Global pattern of experienced and anticipated discrimination reported by people with major depressive disorder: a cross-sectional survey. *The Lancet*, 381, 55–62.

Logan A. C., Jacka F. N. (2014). Nutritional psychiatry research: an emerging discipline and its intersection with global urbanization, environmental challenges and the evolutionary mismatch. *Journal of Physiological Anthropology*, 33, 22.

Lozano R., Naghavi M., Foreman K., *et al.* (2013). Global and regional mortality from 235 causes of death for 20 age groups in 1990 and 2010: a systematic analysis for the Global Burden of Disease Study 2010. *The Lancet*, 380, 2095–128.

Lund C., Breen A., Flisher A. J., *et al.* (2010). Poverty and common mental disorders in low and middle income countries: a systematic review. *Social Science & Medicine*, 71, 517–28.

Luthar S. S., Barkin S. H., Crossman E. J. (2013). "I can, therefore I must": Fragility in the upper-middle classes. *Development and Psychopathology*, 25, 1529–49.

Miech R. A., Caspi A., Moffitt T. E., *et al.* (1999). Low socioeconomic status and mental disorders: a longitudinal study of selection and causation during young adulthood 1. *American Journal of Sociology*, 104, 1096–131.

Mneimneh Z. N. (2012). *Interview Privacy and Social Conformity Effects on Socially Desirable Reporting Behavior: Importance of Cultural, Individual, Question, Design and Implementation Factors*. Ph.D. dissertation. The University of Michigan.

Moffitt T., Caspi A., Taylor A., *et al.* (2010). How common are common mental disorders? Evidence that lifetime prevalence rates are doubled by prospective versus retrospective ascertainment. *Psychological Medicine*, 40, 899.

Morgado A., Raoux N., Jourdain G., *et al.* (1991). Over-reporting of maladjustment by depressed subjects. Findings from retesting after recovery. *Social Psychiatry & Psychiatric Epidemiology*, 26, 68–74.

Olesen S. C., Butterworth P., Leach L. S., *et al.* (2013). Mental health affects future employment as job loss affects mental health: findings from a longitudinal population study. *BMC Psychiatry*, 13, 1.

Ormel J., Petukhova M., Chatterji S., *et al.* (2008). Disability and treatment of specific mental and physical disorders across the world: results from the WHO World Mental Health Surveys. *British Journal of Psychiatry*, 192, 368–75.

Paksarian D., Cui L., Angst J., *et al.* (2016). Latent trajectories of common mental health disorder risk across 3 decades of adulthood in a population-based cohort. *JAMA Psychiatry*, 73, 1023–31.

Patel V., Chisholm D., Parikh R., *et al.* (2016). Addressing the burden of mental, neurological, and substance use disorders: key messages from *Disease Control Priorities*, 3rd edition. *The Lancet*, 387, 1672–85.

Patel V., Goel D. S., Desai R. (2009). Scaling up services for mental and neurological disorders in low-resource settings. *International Health*, 1, 37–44.

Patel V., Kleinman A. (2003). Poverty and common mental disorders in developing countries. *Bulletin of the World Health Organization*, 81, 609–15.

Patton G. C., Sawyer S. M., Santelli J. S., *et al.* (2016). Our future: a Lancet commission on adolescent health and wellbeing. *The Lancet*, 10036, 2423–78.

Pescosolido B. A., Medina T. R., Martin J. K., *et al.* (2013). The "backbone" of stigma: identifying the global core of public prejudice associated with mental illness. *American Journal of Public Health*, 103, 853–60.

Prescott S. L., Millstein R. A., Katzman M. A., *et al.* (2016). Biodiversity, the human microbiome and mental health: moving toward a new clinical ecology for the 21st century? *International Journal of Biodiversity*. Article ID 2718275, doi: 10.1155/2016/2718275.

Prince M. (2008). Measurement validity in cross-cultural comparative research. *Epidemiology and Psychiatric Sciences*, 17, 211–20.

Prince M., Patel V., Saxena S., *et al.* (2007). Global Mental Health 1: No health without mental health. *The Lancet*, 370, 859–77.

Reavley N. J., Jorm A. F. (2014). Willingness to disclose a mental disorder and knowledge of disorders in others:

changes in Australia over 16 years. *Australian and New Zealand Journal of Psychiatry*, 48, 162–8.

Saxena S., Thornicroft G., Knapp M., *et al.* (2007). Resources for mental health: scarcity, inequity, and inefficiency. *The Lancet*, 370, 878–89.

Scott K., Al-Hamzawi A., Andrade L., *et al.* (2014). Associations between subjective social status and DSM-IV mental disorders: results from the World Mental Health Surveys. *JAMA Psychiatry*, 71, 1400–8.

Scott K. M., Lim C., Al-Hamzawi A., *et al.* (2016). Association of mental disorders with subsequent chronic physical conditions: world mental health surveys from 17 countries. *JAMA Psychiatry*, 73, 150–8.

Shahly V., Chatterji S., Gruber M., *et al.* (2013). Cross-national differences in the prevalence and correlates of burden among older family caregivers in the World Health Organization World Mental Health (WMH) Surveys. *Psychological Medicine*, 43, 865–79.

Sharan P., Gallo C., Gureje O., *et al.* (2009). Mental health research priorities in low- and middle-income countries of Africa, Asia, Latin America and the Caribbean. *The British Journal of Psychiatry*, 195, 354–63.

Simon G., Goldberg D., Von Korff M., *et al.* (2002). Understanding cross-national differences in depression prevalence. *Psychological Medicine*, 32, 585–94.

Stansfeld S. A., Clark C., Rodgers B., *et al.* (2011). Repeated exposure to socioeconomic disadvantage and health selection as life course pathways to mid-life depressive and anxiety disorders. *Social Psychiatry and Psychiatric Epidemiology*, 46, 549–58.

Steel Z., Marnane C., Iranpour C., *et al.* (2014). The global prevalence of common mental disorders: a systematic review and meta-analysis 1980–2013. *International Journal of Epidemiology*, 43, 476–93.

Susser E., Schwartz S., Morabia A., *et al.* (2006). *Psychiatric Epidemiology: Searching for the Causes of Mental Disorders*. New York: Oxford University Press.

Takayanagi Y., Spira A. P., Roth K. B., *et al.* (2014). Accuracy of reports of lifetime mental and physical disorders: results from the Baltimore Epidemiological Catchment Area Study. *JAMA Psychiatry*, 71, 273–80.

Thornicroft G., Alem A., Santos R. A., *et al.* (2010). WPA guidance on steps, obstacles and mistakes to avoid in the implementation of community mental health care. *World Psychiatry*, 9, 67–77.

Thornicroft G., Chatterji S., Evans-Lacko S., *et al.* (2017). Undertreatment of people with major depressive disorder in 21 countries. *The British Journal of Psychiatry*, 210, 119–24.

Toyokawa S., Uddin M., Koenen K. C., *et al.* (2012). How does the social environment 'get into the mind'? Epigenetics at the intersection of social and psychiatric epidemiology. *Social Science & Medicine*, 74, 67–74.

Tsuang M. T., Tohen M., Jones P. (2011) (eds.). *Textbook of Psychiatric Epidemiology*. Chichester: John Wiley & Sons.

UN (2015). Sustainable Development Goals. www.un.org/sustainabledevelopment/health/

Walker E. R., McGee R. E., Druss B. G. (2015). Mortality in mental disorders and global disease burden implications: a systematic review and meta-analysis. *JAMA Psychiatry*, 72, 334–41.

Wells J. E., Horwood L. J. (2004). How accurate is recall of key symptoms of depression?: a comparison of recall and longitudinal reports. *Psychological Medicine*, 34, 1001–11.

Wells J. E., Oakley Browne M. A., Scott K. M., *et al.* (2006). Te Rau Hinengaro: the New Zealand Mental Health Survey (NZMHS): overview of methods and findings. *Australian and New Zealand Journal of Psychiatry*, 40, 835–44.

WHO (2015a). Tracking Universal Health Coverage: First Global Monitoring Report. www.who.int.

(2015b). People-centred and integrated health services: an overview of the evidence. www.who.int.

(2016). MhGAP Intervention Guide for mental, neurological and substance use disorders in non-specialized health settings: Version 2. www.who.int.

Wykes T., Haro J. M., Belli S. R., *et al.* (2015). Mental health research priorities for Europe. *The Lancet Psychiatry*, 2, 1036–42.

Yeh K. H., Yi C. C., Tsao W. C., *et al.* (2013). Filial piety in contemporary Chinese societies: a comparative study of Taiwan, Hong Kong, and China. *International Sociology*, 28, 277–96.

Appendices

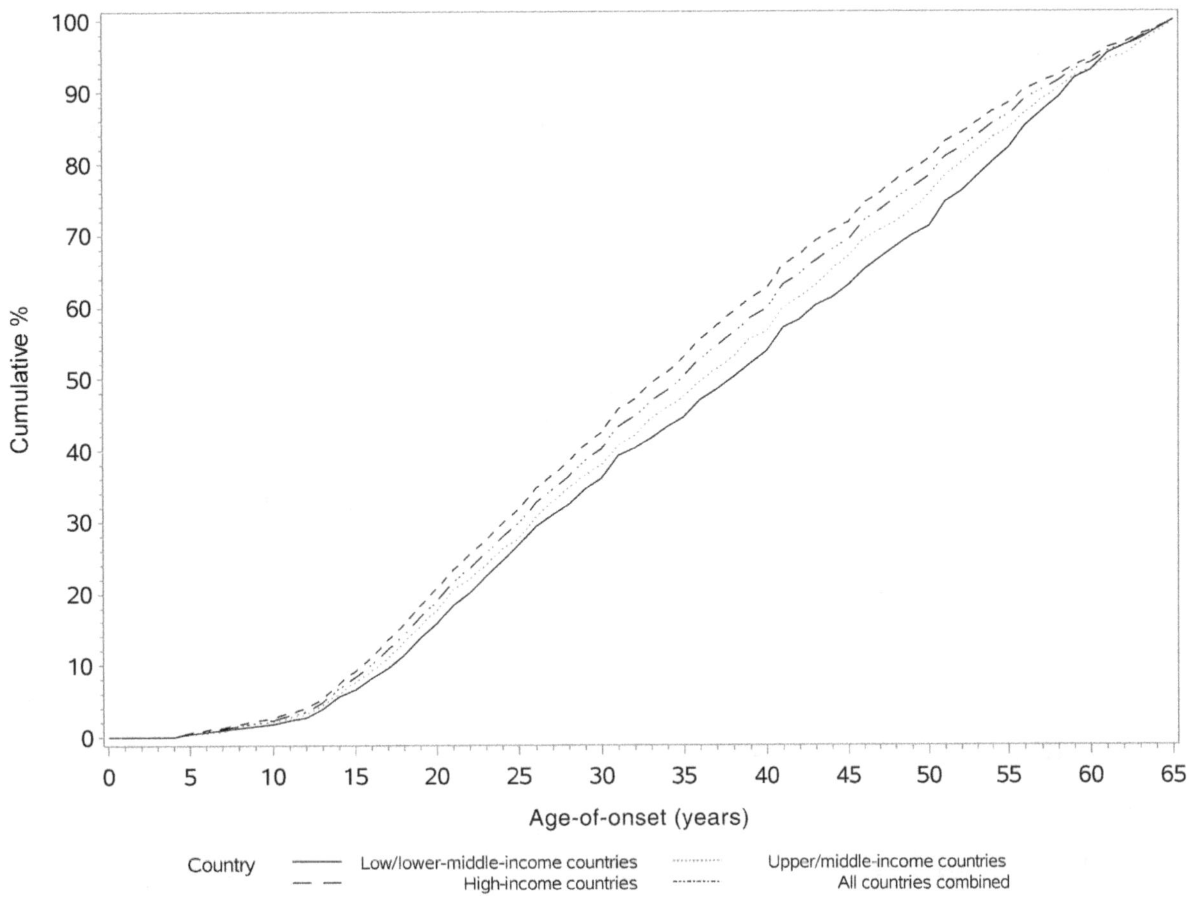

Figure 4A.1 Cumulative age-of-onset distribution for major depressive disorder by country income groups and in all countries combined.

Table 4A.1 Prevalence of DSM-IV major depressive disorder (MDD) in the World Mental Health surveys (males only)

Country	Lifetime prevalence		12-month prevalence		30-day prevalence		12-month prevalence of MDD among lifetime cases		30-day prevalence of MDD among 12-month cases		Sample size used
	%	SE	%	SE	%	SE	%	SE	%	SE	
Low/lower-middle-income countries	**5.4**	**0.2**	**2.7**	**0.2**	**0.9**	**0.1**	**50.6**	**2.1**	**33.2**	**2.8**	**16,805**
Colombia	8.4	0.8	3.6	0.5	0.8	0.2	42.9	5.3	21.3	6.2	1,700
Iraq	5.1	0.5	2.8	0.5	0.9	0.3	55.5	6.3	32.9	7.6	2,091
Nigeria	2.8	0.3	1.1	0.2	0.3	0.1	39.3	6.8	24.5	8.6	3,315
Peru	5.2	0.6	2.2	0.3	0.6	0.2	43.3	5.7	25.9	7.3	1,759
PRC (Beijing/Shanghai)	3.8	0.5	2.0	0.4	0.5	0.2	53.4	7.9	26.3	9.1	2,533
PRC (Shenzhen)	5.7	0.6	3.2	0.4	1.0	0.2	56.4	4.3	30.9	6.6	3,614
Ukraine	8.6	0.7	4.9	0.5	2.6	0.3	56.5	3.8	53.7	5.2	1,793
Upper-middle-income countries	**5.9**	**0.3**	**2.7**	**0.2**	**1.0**	**0.1**	**45.4**	**2.5**	**38.2**	**3.5**	**12,129**
Brazil	10.0	0.7	5.3	0.6	1.9	0.4	52.8	5.5	36.4	6.1	2,187
Bulgaria	3.2	0.5	1.3	0.3	0.7	0.2	40.6	6.6	55.4	10.9	2,430
Colombia (Medellin)	6.1	1.1	1.5	0.4	0.8	0.4	25.1	5.6	53.0	14.1	1,120
Lebanon	7.0	1.0	3.2	0.7	0.9	0.3	45.7	5.9	26.6	8.7	1,297
Mexico	4.6	0.6	2.3	0.4	1.0	0.2	49.9	6.0	45.0	7.8	2,285
Romania	2.5	0.5	1.4	0.5	0.3	0.2	54.6	11.2	24.1	9.8	1,092
South Africa	7.1	0.8	3.1	0.5	1.0	0.3	43.0	5.9	32.1	8.8	1,718
High-income countries	**9.0**	**0.2**	**3.3**	**0.1**	**1.1**	**0.1**	**36.3**	**1.1**	**34.0**	**1.7**	**37,326**
Australia	10.5	0.7	3.9	0.5	1.8	0.3	37.1	4.0	47.1	5.3	3,843
Belgium	10.3	1.2	3.9	0.8	1.7	0.5	37.5	5.6	43.2	10.6	1,190
France	14.8	1.2	4.4	0.7	1.7	0.6	29.6	4.4	38.3	11.0	1,329
Germany	7.3	0.8	2.2	0.4	0.5	0.2	30.2	4.3	24.2	6.4	1,660
Israel	7.4	0.6	4.4	0.4	1.1	0.2	58.6	3.8	26.0	4.6	2,380
Italy	6.4	0.4	1.7	0.3	0.8	0.2	26.9	4.4	46.0	7.7	2,321
Japan	3.6	0.5	1.1	0.3	0.2	0.1	31.3	6.3	18.8	9.9	1,868
New Zealand	11.6	0.6	4.3	0.5	1.3	0.2	36.6	3.0	31.5	4.0	5,537
Northern Ireland	11.4	0.8	4.9	0.6	1.3	0.2	43.2	4.2	25.7	4.3	1,899
Poland	1.9	0.2	0.8	0.1	0.1	0.0	41.2	5.1	9.9	5.1	4,883
Portugal	10.7	0.8	3.6	0.5	1.2	0.3	33.6	3.9	33.4	5.9	1,632
Spain	6.4	0.5	2.2	0.3	0.9	0.2	33.7	3.9	41.3	9.4	2,421
Spain (Murcia)	9.4	0.8	3.3	0.5	1.5	0.4	35.4	6.0	44.1	9.8	1,192
Netherlands	13.0	1.5	3.0	0.5	0.6	0.2	23.2	3.8	18.9	8.6	1,032
United States	13.2	0.8	4.9	0.4	1.7	0.2	36.9	2.5	35.6	3.3	4,139

Table 4A.1 *(cont.)*

Country	Lifetime prevalence		12-month prevalence		30-day prevalence		12-month prevalence of MDD among lifetime cases		30-day prevalence of MDD among 12-month cases		Sample size used
	%	SE	%	SE	%	SE	%	SE	%	SE	
All countries combined	**7.5**	**0.1**	**3.0**	**0.1**	**1.0**	**0.0**	**40.3**	**0.9**	**34.5**	**1.3**	**66,260**
WHO regions[a]											
Region of the Americas	8.7	0.3	3.6	0.2	1.3	0.1	41.4	1.9	35.0	2.5	13,190
African region	4.4	0.4	1.8	0.2	0.5	0.1	41.5	4.5	29.3	6.5	5,033
Western Pacific region	8.2	0.3	3.3	0.2	1.1	0.1	40.2	2.0	34.6	2.8	17,395
Eastern Mediterranean region	6.5	0.4	3.5	0.3	1.0	0.1	54.4	2.9	28.2	3.7	5,768
Western European region	9.5	0.3	3.1	0.2	1.1	0.1	33.1	1.5	34.4	2.9	14,676
Eastern European region	3.6	0.2	1.8	0.1	0.8	0.1	49.3	2.8	42.5	4.0	1,0198
Comparison between countries[b]	**$F_{28,v} = 35.6^*$, $P < 0.001$**		**$F_{28,v} = 15.7^*$, $P < 0.001$**		**$F_{28,v} = 10.6^*$, $P < 0.001$**		**$F_{28,v} = 4.2^*$, $P < 0.001$**		**$F_{28,v} = 2.2^*$, $P < 0.001$**		
Comparison between low-, middle-, and high-income country groups[b]	**$F_{2,v} = 88.3^*$, $P < 0.001$**		**$F_{2,v} = 5.5^*$, $P = 0.004$**		**$F_{2,v} = 1.8$, $P = 0.160$**		**$F_{2,v} = 19.8^*$, $P < 0.001$**		**$F_{2,v} = 0.7$, $P = 0.489$**		
Comparison between WHO regions[b]	**$F_{5,v} = 83.8^*$, $P < 0.001$**		**$F_{2,v} = 21.3^*$, $P < 0.001$**		**$F_{5,v} = 5.1^*$, $P < 0.001$**		**$F_{5,v} = 10.6^*$, $P < 0.001$**		**$F_{5,v} = 1.5$, $P = 0.190$**		

*Significant at the 0.05 level, two-sided test.

[a]**Region of the Americas** (Colombia, Mexico, Brazil, Peru, United States, Colombia (Medellin)); **African region** (South Africa, Nigeria); **Western Pacific region** (PRC (Shenzhen), PRC (Beijing and Shanghai), Japan, Australia, New Zealand); **Eastern Mediterranean region** (Israel, Iraq, Lebanon); **Western European region** (Belgium, France, Germany, Italy, Netherlands, Spain, Northern Ireland, Portugal, Spain (Murcia)); **Eastern European region** (Romania, Poland, Bulgaria, Ukraine).

[b]Wald design-corrected F-tests were used to determine if there is variation in prevalence estimates across countries. The denominator degree of freedom, v, is 5429.

PRC: People's Republic of China.

Table 4A.2 Prevalence of DSM-IV major depressive disorder (MDD) in the World Mental Health surveys (females only)

Country	Lifetime prevalence		12-month prevalence		30-day prevalence		12-month prevalence of MDD among lifetime cases		30-day prevalence of MDD among 12-month cases		Sample size used
	%	SE	%	SE	%	SE	%	SE	%	SE	
Low/lower-middle-income countries	**8.8**	**0.3**	**4.5**	**0.2**	**2.0**	**0.1**	**50.7**	**1.5**	**44.8**	**2.2**	**19,693**
Colombia	15.0	0.9	6.8	0.6	2.3	0.3	45.5	3.1	34.1	4.8	2,726
Iraq	9.3	0.9	4.9	0.8	2.0	0.4	53.2	6.6	41.1	7.2	2,241
Nigeria	3.5	0.4	1.1	0.2	0.1	0.1	30.5	4.8	12.7	5.4	3,437
Peru	7.5	0.4	3.1	0.3	0.8	0.2	41.2	3.6	25.9	5.6	2,171
PRC (Beijing/Shanghai)	3.2	0.5	1.6	0.3	0.6	0.2	49.0	6.0	40.7	8.3	2,668
PRC (Shenzhen)	6.4	0.5	3.7	0.4	1.9	0.3	57.3	3.7	50.2	5.7	3,518
Ukraine	19.5	0.9	11.3	0.8	6.6	0.7	58.2	2.2	58.2	3.5	2,932
Upper-middle-income countries	**12.2**	**0.4**	**6.3**	**0.3**	**2.8**	**0.1**	**51.3**	**1.3**	**44.8**	**1.6**	**16,798**
Brazil	23.0	1.3	13.2	1.0	6.3	0.5	57.2	2.1	47.8	2.2	2,850
Bulgaria	7.9	0.6	3.6	0.4	2.2	0.3	46.2	3.9	61.2	5.4	2,888
Colombia (Medellin)	13.3	1.1	5.7	0.6	1.9	0.4	43.0	3.4	33.2	5.0	2,141
Lebanon	12.8	1.1	6.4	0.9	3.1	0.5	50.0	4.0	48.3	5.3	1,560
Mexico	9.7	0.6	4.7	0.4	2.1	0.2	48.9	2.9	44.9	4.4	3,497
Romania	3.3	0.6	1.5	0.3	0.5	0.2	46.5	5.8	33.4	11.2	1,265
South Africa	12.1	1.0	6.5	0.7	2.2	0.4	53.6	3.8	33.8	5.0	2,597
High-income countries	**16.0**	**0.2**	**6.2**	**0.1**	**2.2**	**0.1**	**38.9**	**0.7**	**36.1**	**1.0**	**44,513**
Australia	16.4	0.8	6.0	0.5	2.2	0.3	36.7	2.2	36.9	3.7	4,620
Belgium	17.7	1.5	6.0	0.8	2.2	0.4	34.0	4.2	36.4	7.6	1,229
France	26.6	1.4	7.2	0.9	1.4	0.4	27.1	2.8	19.4	4.4	1,565
Germany	12.4	0.9	3.7	0.5	1.5	0.3	30.1	3.1	39.9	6.3	1,895
Israel	12.0	0.7	7.2	0.5	2.2	0.3	60.4	2.9	30.4	3.6	2,479
Italy	13.2	0.8	4.2	0.4	1.9	0.3	31.7	2.5	45.1	6.2	2,391
Japan	8.4	0.6	3.1	0.4	0.4	0.1	36.7	3.9	13.6	4.0	2,261
New Zealand	20.7	0.6	7.1	0.4	2.0	0.2	34.5	1.6	27.7	2.3	7,253
Northern Ireland	20.8	1.2	10.6	0.7	5.0	0.5	50.7	2.5	47.4	3.7	2,441
Poland	4.0	0.3	1.7	0.2	0.7	0.1	42.2	3.2	43.8	5.2	5,198
Portugal	22.3	1.2	9.7	0.8	4.2	0.5	43.6	2.5	43.7	3.3	2,217
Spain	14.5	0.8	5.7	0.5	2.5	0.3	39.0	2.3	43.5	4.2	3,052

Table 4A.2 (*cont.*)

Country	Lifetime prevalence		12-month prevalence		30-day prevalence		12-month prevalence of MDD among lifetime cases		30-day prevalence of MDD among 12-month cases		Sample size used
	%	SE	%	SE	%	SE	%	SE	%	SE	
Spain (Murcia)	18.2	1.1	8.7	0.8	3.8	0.6	47.7	2.8	43.4	5.4	1,429
Netherlands	22.6	1.5	6.7	0.8	2.2	0.7	29.6	3.3	32.9	8.2	1,340
United States	20.2	0.5	8.6	0.4	3.2	0.2	42.7	1.6	37.0	2.4	5,143
All countries combined	**13.5**	**0.2**	**5.8**	**0.1**	**2.3**	**0.1**	**43.0**	**0.6**	**39.7**	**0.8**	**81,004**
WHO regions[a]											
Region of the Americas	15.7	0.4	7.4	0.3	2.9	0.1	47.1	1.0	39.7	1.4	18,528
African region	6.9	0.5	3.2	0.3	1.0	0.2	46.7	3.0	29.6	4.3	6,034
Western Pacific region	13.4	0.3	5.1	0.2	1.7	0.1	37.8	1.2	32.8	1.8	20,320
Eastern Mediterranean region	11.2	0.5	6.2	0.4	2.3	0.2	55.5	2.6	37.7	2.9	6,280
Western European region	18.1	0.4	6.9	0.2	2.8	0.1	37.9	1.0	40.8	1.7	17,559
Eastern European region	8.3	0.3	4.3	0.2	2.4	0.2	51.6	1.7	55.4	2.5	12,283
Comparison between countries[b]	**$F_{28,v} = 79.4^*$, $P < 0.001$**		**$F_{28,v} = 37.0^*$, $P < 0.001$**		**$F_{28,v} = 25.8^*$, $P < 0.001$**		**$F_{28,v} = 9.6^*$, $P < 0.001$**		**$F_{28,v} = 5.7^*$, $P < 0.001$**		
Comparison between low-, middle-, and high-income country groups[b]	**$F_{2,v} = 226.8^*$, $P < 0.001$**		**$F_{2,v} = 29.2^*$, $P < 0.001$**		**$F_{2,v} = 8.8^*$, $P < 0.001$**		**$F_{2,v} = 50.0^*$, $P < 0.001$**		**$F_{2,v} = 13.4^*$, $P < 0.001$**		
Comparison between WHO regions[b]	**$F_{5,v} = 130.5^*$, $P < 0.001$**		**$F_{5,v} = 37.2^*$, $P < 0.001$**		**$F_{5,v} = 24.0^*$, $P < 0.001$**		**$F_{5,v} = 22.0^*$, $P < 0.001$**		**$F_{2,v} = 10.4^*$, $P < 0.001$**		

*Significant at the 0.05 level, two-sided test.

[a]**Region of the Americas** (Colombia, Mexico, Brazil, Peru, United States, Colombia (Medellin)); **African region** (South Africa, Nigeria); **Western Pacific region** (PRC (Shenzhen), PRC (Beijing and Shanghai), Japan, Australia, New Zealand); **Eastern Mediterranean region** (Israel, Iraq, Lebanon); **Western European region** (Belgium, France, Germany, Italy, Netherlands, Spain, Northern Ireland, Portugal, Spain (Murcia)); **Eastern European region** (Romania, Poland, Bulgaria, Ukraine).

[b]Wald design-corrected F-tests were used to determine if there is variation in prevalence estimates across countries. The denominator degree of freedom, v, is 5429.

PRC: People's Republic of China.

Table 7A.1 12-month prevalence of panic attack (PA) and panic disorder (PD) in the World Mental Health surveys

Country	Among the total population										Part 1 sample sizes	Sample size used[a]
	12-month PA with or without lifetime PD		12-month PA without lifetime PD cases		12-month PD		12-month PA among lifetime PA cases without lifetime PD		12-month PD among lifetime PD			
	%	SE	%	SE	%	SE	%	SE	%	SE		
Low/lower-middle-income countries	**2.9**	**0.1**	**2.4**	**0.1**	**0.5**	**0.1**	**38.4**	**1.3**	**64.4**	**3.6**	**36,498**	**36,395**
Colombia	6.1	0.4	5.4	0.4	0.7	0.1	31.2	2.2	53.7	9.0	4,426	4,422
Iraq	3.7	0.5	2.7	0.4	1.0	0.3	43.5	4.6	71.5	6.5	4,332	4,295
Nigeria	1.3	0.2	1.1	0.2	0.1	0.1	46.7	5.3	76.2	16.1	6,752	6,713
Peru	3.0	0.2	2.7	0.2	0.3	0.1	40.3	2.1	70.5	6.4	3,930	3,929
PRC (Beijing/Shanghai)	1.0	0.2	0.8	0.2	0.2	0.1	47.6	8.4	50.1	13.0	5,201	5,197
PRC (Shenzhen)	0.9	0.1	0.7	0.1	0.2	0.1	33.4	4.1	78.9	7.7	7,132	7,129
Ukraine	6.2	0.4	4.8	0.3	1.4	0.3	42.6	2.4	64.4	6.2	4,725	4,710
Upper-middle-income countries	**4.3**	**0.2**	**3.7**	**0.2**	**0.7**	**0.1**	**36.4**	**1.2**	**62.1**	**3.5**	**28,927**	**24,565**
Brazil	5.1	0.3	4.0	0.3	1.0	0.2	40.2	2.2	61.8	8.2	5,037	5,023
Bulgaria	2.7	0.3	2.2	0.3	0.6	0.1	43.7	4.4	53.5	5.4	5,318	5,301
Colombia (Medellin)	7.1	0.7	6.1	0.6	0.9	0.2	32.6	2.4	73.8	7.2	3,261	3,260
Lebanon	4.8	0.5	4.6	0.5	0.3	0.1	34.1	2.7	49.2	10.3	2,857	2,851
Mexico	3.3	0.4	2.6	0.3	0.7	0.1	38.6	3.1	65.3	7.1	5,782	5,781
Romania	4.7	0.4	4.2	0.4	0.4	0.1	32.0	3.3	63.3	12.1	2,357	2,349
High-income countries	**6.0**	**0.1**	**4.8**	**0.1**	**1.2**	**0.1**	**33.3**	**0.5**	**55.2**	**1.4**	**81,839**	**81,754**
Australia	7.3	0.4	5.5	0.4	1.8	0.2	30.8	1.7	50.0	3.9	8,463	8,461
Belgium	3.5	0.7	2.7	0.5	0.9	0.3	31.4	4.0	54.6	11.4	2,419	2,417
France	3.2	0.4	2.3	0.2	1.0	0.3	25.2	2.3	46.0	9.7	2,894	2,894
Germany	3.2	0.4	2.5	0.4	0.7	0.2	28.9	3.3	46.9	7.2	3,555	3,555
Israel	5.0	0.3	4.4	0.3	0.6	0.1	48.7	2.5	62.6	7.5	4,859	4,853
Italy	2.7	0.3	2.1	0.3	0.7	0.1	32.1	3.4	42.5	5.8	4,712	4,708
Japan	2.0	0.3	1.7	0.2	0.3	0.1	28.8	3.1	45.0	10.6	4,129	4,126
New Zealand	9.2	0.3	7.5	0.3	1.7	0.1	30.5	1.1	60.3	3.2	12,790	12,781
Northern Ireland	9.5	0.5	7.2	0.5	2.3	0.2	34.1	1.8	70.7	3.6	4,340	4,335
Poland	2.5	0.1	2.3	0.1	0.2	0.1	41.4	2.1	62.8	8.5	10,081	10,049
Portugal	6.9	0.4	6.0	0.4	0.9	0.2	33.3	1.9	52.9	6.9	3,849	3,841
Spain	3.7	0.3	3.1	0.3	0.6	0.1	36.9	2.7	49.2	6.8	5,473	5,472
Spain (Murcia)	6.0	0.5	5.3	0.6	0.7	0.1	36.3	2.7	45.7	6.5	2,621	2,617
Netherlands	4.5	0.4	3.2	0.4	1.3	0.3	29.1	3.1	41.5	6.2	2,372	2,370
United States	10.7	0.4	8.0	0.4	2.7	0.2	35.2	1.2	57.9	3.0	9,282	9,275

Table 7A.1 *(cont.)*

Country	Among the total population										Part 1 sample sizes	Sample size used[a]
	12-month PA with or without lifetime PD		12-month PA without lifetime PD cases		12-month PD		12-month PA among lifetime PA cases without lifetime PD		12-month PD among lifetime PD			
	%	SE	%	SE	%	SE	%	SE	%	SE		
All countries combined	**4.9**	**0.1**	**4.0**	**0.1**	**1.0**	**0.0**	**34.5**	**0.5**	**57.1**	**1.3**	**147,264**	**142,714**
WHO regions[b]												
Region of the Americas	6.5	0.2	5.2	0.2	1.3	0.1	35.3	0.8	60.0	2.4	31,718	31,690
African region	1.3	0.2	1.1	0.2	0.1	0.1	46.7	5.3	76.2	16.1	11,067	6,713
Western Pacific region	5.3	0.2	4.2	0.1	1.1	0.1	30.9	0.9	55.4	2.4	37,715	37,694
Eastern Mediterranean region	4.5	0.3	3.8	0.2	0.6	0.1	42.3	1.8	65.3	4.9	12,048	11,999
Western European region	4.9	0.1	3.9	0.1	1.0	0.1	32.8	0.9	52.5	2.2	32,235	32,209
Eastern European region	3.6	0.1	3.0	0.1	0.6	0.1	40.4	1.4	61.1	3.8	22,481	22,409
Comparison between countries[c]	**$F_{27,v} = 55.3^*$, $P < 0.001$**		**$F_{27,v} = 43.8^*$, $P < 0.001$**		**$F_{27,v} = 15.9^*$, $P < 0.001$**		**$F_{27,v} = 4.7^*$, $P < 0.001$**		**$F_{27,v} = 2.1^*$, $P = 0.001$**			
Comparison between low-, middle-, and high-income country groups[c]	**$F_{2,v} = 183.1^*$, $P < 0.001$**		**$F_{2,v} = 147.3^*$, $P < 0.001$**		**$F_{2,v} = 50.8^*$, $P < 0.001$**		**$F_{2,v} = 8.4^*$, $P < 0.001$**		**$F_{2,v} = 3.8^*$, $P = 0.024$**			
Comparison between WHO regions[c]	**$F_{5,v} = 71.7^*$, $P < 0.001$**		**$F_{5,v} = 52.8^*$, $P < 0.001$**		**$F_{5,v} = 35.7^*$, $P < 0.001$**		**$F_{5,v} = 12.4^*$, $P < 0.001$**		**$F_{5,v} = 2.1$, $P = 0.063$**			

*Significant at the 0.05 level, two-sided test.

[a] Sample size used after excluding lifetime panic attack cases with missing age-of-onset.

[b] **Region of the Americas** (Colombia, Mexico, Brazil, Peru, United States, Colombia (Medellin)); **African region** (Nigeria); **Western Pacific region** (PRC (Shenzhen), PRC Beijing and Shanghai, Japan, Australia, New Zealand); **Eastern Mediterranean region** (Israel, Iraq, Lebanon); **Western European region** (Belgium, France, Germany, Italy, Netherlands, Spain, Northern Ireland, Portugal, Spain (Murcia)); **Eastern European region** (Romania, Bulgaria, Poland, Ukraine).

[c] Wald design-corrected F-tests were used to determine if there is variation in prevalence estimates across countries. The denominator degree of freedom, v, is 5367.

PRC: People's Republic of China.

Table 7A.2 30-day prevalence of panic attack (PA) and panic disorder (PD) in the World Mental Health surveys

Country	Among the total population										Part 1 sample sizes	Sample size used[a]
	30-day PA		30-day PA without lifetime PD cases		30-day PD		30-day PA among 12-month PA cases without lifetime PD		30-day PD among 12-month PD			
	%	SE	%	SE	%	SE	%	SE	%	SE		
Low/lower-middle-income countries	**1.0**	**0.1**	**0.8**	**0.1**	**0.3**	**0.0**	**32.4**	**1.9**	**50.4**	**4.7**	**36,498**	**36,395**
Colombia	1.6	0.2	1.3	0.2	0.3	0.1	24.9	3.2	44.8	10.6	4,426	4,422
Iraq	1.9	0.3	1.2	0.3	0.7	0.3	45.1	7.0	71.4	10.3	4,332	4,295
Nigeria	0.3	0.1	0.3	0.1	0.0	0.0	24.6	7.2	17.2	14.0	6,752	6,713
Peru	0.9	0.1	0.8	0.1	0.1	0.0	30.8	4.8	35.6	13.1	3,930	3,929
PRC (Beijing/Shanghai)	0.3	0.1	0.3	0.1	0.1	0.1	30.4	7.6	36.3	22.4	5,201	5,197
PRC (Shenzhen)	0.3	0.1	0.3	0.1	0.1	0.0	34.6	9.3	36.1	14.6	7,132	7,129
Ukraine	2.5	0.3	1.8	0.2	0.7	0.2	37.1	2.9	52.4	6.3	4,725	4,710
Upper-middle-income countries	**1.4**	**0.1**	**1.2**	**0.1**	**0.3**	**0.0**	**31.7**	**1.9**	**38.9**	**4.8**	**28,927**	**24,565**
Brazil	1.7	0.2	1.3	0.2	0.4	0.1	32.9	3.6	37.0	8.8	5,037	5,023
Bulgaria	1.2	0.2	0.9	0.2	0.3	0.1	41.0	5.6	49.4	11.4	5,318	5,301
Colombia (Medellin)	1.7	0.3	1.4	0.2	0.3	0.1	22.9	3.6	34.1	11.1	3,261	3,260
Lebanon	1.5	0.3	1.4	0.3	0.1	0.1	31.0	5.0	33.0	16.4	2,857	2,851
Mexico	1.0	0.2	0.7	0.1	0.2	0.1	28.5	4.4	30.9	8.9	5,782	5,781
Romania	2.1	0.3	1.8	0.3	0.3	0.1	42.2	5.9	67.6	21.2	2,357	2,349
High-income countries	**1.8**	**0.1**	**1.3**	**0.1**	**0.5**	**0.0**	**27.9**	**0.8**	**39.1**	**2.0**	**81,839**	**81,754**
Australia	1.9	0.2	1.3	0.2	0.6	0.1	24.3	2.6	33.0	4.9	8,463	8,461
Belgium	1.2	0.5	0.8	0.3	0.5	0.3	28.9	8.3	50.8	15.8	2,419	2,417
France	0.8	0.2	0.5	0.1	0.2	0.1	24.3	5.2	22.6	10.3	2,894	2,894
Germany	1.0	0.2	0.6	0.1	0.4	0.2	23.3	4.5	53.1	12.0	3,555	3,555
Israel	1.4	0.2	1.3	0.2	0.2	0.1	28.3	3.2	32.8	8.8	4,859	4,853
Italy	1.0	0.2	0.7	0.2	0.3	0.1	31.8	5.9	46.5	9.8	4,712	4,708
Japan	0.5	0.1	0.3	0.1	0.2	0.1	20.3	5.7	46.2	14.1	4,129	4,126
New Zealand	2.9	0.2	2.2	0.2	0.7	0.1	29.3	1.7	41.3	3.8	12,790	12,781
Northern Ireland	3.3	0.3	2.2	0.2	1.1	0.2	30.9	3.0	45.8	4.8	4,340	4,335
Poland	0.7	0.1	0.6	0.1	0.0	0.0	26.7	3.0	19.4	9.4	10,081	10,049
Portugal	2.0	0.2	1.7	0.2	0.4	0.1	27.8	2.8	39.0	10.7	3,849	3,841
Spain	1.2	0.2	1.0	0.2	0.3	0.1	30.9	4.9	47.1	7.8	5,473	5,472
Spain (Murcia)	1.6	0.4	1.4	0.3	0.2	0.1	27.0	5.0	28.2	14.3	2,621	2,617
Netherlands	1.3	0.4	0.7	0.3	0.5	0.2	23.0	7.2	43.2	11.4	2,372	2,370
United States	3.3	0.2	2.2	0.2	1.0	0.1	28.0	1.9	38.1	4.6	9,282	9,275

Table 7A.2 (*cont.*)

Country	Among the total population										Part 1 sample sizes	Sample size used[a]
	30-day PA		30-day PA without lifetime PD cases		30-day PD		30-day PA among 12-month PA cases without lifetime PD		30-day PD among 12-month PD			
	%	SE	%	SE	%	SE	%	SE	%	SE		
All countries combined	**1.6**	**0.0**	**1.2**	**0.0**	**0.4**	**0.0**	**29.2**	**0.7**	**40.6**	**1.7**	**147,264**	**142,714**
WHO regions[b]												
Region of the Americas	1.9	0.1	1.4	0.1	0.5	0.1	27.8	1.3	37.4	3.4	31,718	31,690
African region	0.3	0.1	0.3	0.1	0.0	0.0	24.6	7.2	17.2	14.0	11,067	6,713
Western Pacific region	1.6	0.1	1.2	0.1	0.4	0.0	27.7	1.4	38.0	2.9	37,715	37,694
Eastern Mediterranean region	1.6	0.2	1.3	0.1	0.4	0.1	33.3	2.8	53.8	7.9	12,048	11,999
Western European region	1.5	0.1	1.1	0.1	0.4	0.0	28.5	1.5	43.0	3.2	32,235	32,209
Eastern European region	1.3	0.1	1.1	0.1	0.3	0.1	34.9	1.9	47.6	5.2	22,481	22,409
Comparison between countries[c]	$F_{27,v} = 22.7^*$, $P < 0.001$		$F_{27,v} = 15.1^*$, $P < 0.001$		$F_{27,v} = 10.2^*$, $P < 0.001$		$F_{27,v} = 1.4$, $P = 0.095$		$F_{27,v} = 1.0$, $P = 0.537$			
Comparison between low-, middle-, and high-income country groups[c]	$F_{2,v} = 40.9^*$, $P < 0.001$		$F_{2,v} = 29.4^*$, $P < 0.001$		$F_{2,v} = 14.7^*$, $P < 0.001$		$F_{2,v} = 3.6^*$, $P = 0.028$		$F_{2,v} = 2.1$, $P = 0.119$			
Comparison between WHO regions[c]	$F_{5,v} = 37.8^*$, $P < 0.001$		$F_{5,v} = 19.8^*$, $P < 0.001$		$F_{5,v} = 38.3^*$, $P < 0.001$		$F_{5,v} = 2.7^*$, $P = 0.021$		$F_{5,v} = 1.5$, $P = 0.193$			

*Significant at the 0.05 level, two-sided test.

[a]Sample size used after excluding lifetime panic attack cases with missing age-of-onset.

[b]**Region of the Americas** (Colombia, Mexico, Brazil, Peru, United States, Colombia (Medellin)); **African region** (Nigeria); **Western Pacific region** (PRC (Shenzhen), PRC Beijing and Shanghai, Japan, Australia, New Zealand); **Eastern Mediterranean region** (Israel, Iraq, Lebanon); **Western European region** (Belgium, France, Germany, Italy, Netherlands, Spain, Northern Ireland, Portugal, Spain (Murcia)); **Eastern European region** (Romania, Bulgaria, Poland, Ukraine).

[c]Wald design-corrected F-tests were used to determine if there is variation in prevalence estimates across countries. The denominator degree of freedom, v, is 5367.

PRC: People's Republic of China.

Table 7A.3 Age at selected percentiles on the standardized age-of-onset distributions of DSM-IV panic disorder with projected lifetime risk at age 75

Country	Ages at selected percentiles								Lifetime prevalence of panic disorder		Projected risk at age 75	
	5	10	25	50	75	90	95	99	%	SE	%	SE
Low/lower-middle-income countries	**9**	**13**	**18**	**35**	**50**	**61**	**63**	**69**	**0.8**	**0.1**	**1.4**	**0.2**
Colombia[a]	7	11	14	24	37	46	49	49	1.3	0.2	1.7	0.3
Iraq	11	13	18	35	44	50	55	55	1.4	0.3	2.3	0.5
Nigeria	13	13	19	30	69	69	69	69	0.2	0.1	0.4	0.2
Peru[a]	5	9	16	32	55	55	55	55	0.5	0.1	0.8	0.3
PRC (Beijing/Shanghai)	5	13	13	31	44	48	55	55	0.4	0.1	0.6	0.2
PRC (Shenzhen)	5	6	11	18	37	41	44	44	0.3	0.1	0.4	0.1
Ukraine	9	14	19	31	51	61	63	64	2.2	0.3	3.2	0.5
Upper-middle-income countries	**8**	**13**	**20**	**33**	**49**	**61**	**75**	**75**	**1.1**	**0.1**	**2.0**	**0.3**
Brazil	11	14	24	37	43	62	65	65	1.7	0.2	3.0	0.6
Bulgaria	14	17	25	36	51	75	75	75	1.1	0.1	2.0	0.6
Colombia (Medellin)[a]	5	8	13	21	50	58	58	58	1.3	0.3	1.8	0.5
Lebanon	15	17	25	30	36	61	61	61	0.5	0.1	0.8	0.2
Mexico[a]	7	11	21	31	44	57	57	57	1.0	0.2	1.8	0.4
Romania	6	6	9	21	39	64	64	64	0.7	0.2	0.8	0.2
High-income countries	**9**	**13**	**19**	**31**	**46**	**60**	**66**	**71**	**2.2**	**0.1**	**3.3**	**0.1**
Australia	10	13	19	31	43	56	65	73	3.7	0.3	5.2	0.5
Belgium	7	10	19	25	33	48	60	60	1.6	0.3	2.2	0.5
France	10	13	19	26	36	41	51	58	2.1	0.3	2.6	0.4
Germany	11	19	23	33	46	60	71	71	1.6	0.2	2.6	0.4
Israel	13	19	32	51	61	73	73	73	0.9	0.1	2.0	0.4
Italy	5	14	23	39	57	61	70	70	1.5	0.2	2.3	0.4
Japan	13	14	26	37	45	66	69	69	0.8	0.1	1.1	0.2
New Zealand	7	11	17	27	43	59	66	69	2.8	0.2	4.1	0.3
Northern Ireland	13	14	20	33	45	63	68	68	3.3	0.3	5.5	0.8
Poland[b]	15	21	26	46	55	57	57	57	0.3	0.1	0.7	0.2
Portugal	7	13	19	33	57	60	61	64	1.7	0.3	2.5	0.5
Spain	14	17	24	33	47	60	64	65	1.2	0.2	2.1	0.3
Spain (Murcia)	6	11	18	29	39	44	49	55	1.6	0.4	2.2	0.5
Netherlands	13	15	24	33	48	71	71	71	3.0	0.4	5.2	1.0
United States	7	11	17	26	41	54	56	66	4.7	0.2	6.4	0.4
All countries combined	**9**	**13**	**20**	**32**	**47**	**60**	**66**	**73**	**1.7**	**0.0**	**2.7**	**0.1**
WHO regions												
Region of the Americas	8	11	18	31	44	56	65	69	2.2	0.1	3.4	0.2
African region	13	13	19	30	69	69	69	69	0.2	0.1	0.4	0.2
Western Pacific region	9	13	19	31	46	60	67	73	2.0	0.1	3.1	0.2
Eastern Mediterranean region	12	15	26	38	55	64	73	73	1.0	0.1	1.9	0.3
Western European region	10	14	21	32	46	60	64	71	1.9	0.1	3.0	0.2
Eastern European region	12	14	22	36	53	63	75	75	0.9	0.1	1.7	0.3

[a]The projected risk for these countries is at age 65 because the age range of these surveys is between 18 and 65.
[b]The projected risk for this country is at age 64 because the age range of this survey is between 18 and 64.
PRC: People's Republic of China.

Table 8A.1 Prevalence of agoraphobia (AG) without panic disorder (PD) in the World Mental Health surveys

Country	Lifetime prevalence		12-month prevalence		30-day prevalence		12-month prevalence of AG without PD among lifetime cases		30-day prevalence of AG without PD among 12-month cases		Part 1 sample sizes
	%	SE	%	SE	%	SE	%	SE	%	SE	
Low/lower-middle-income countries	**0.7**	**0.1**	**0.5**	**0.1**	**0.2**	**0.0**	**64.7**	**5.2**	**44.4**	**5.3**	**31,297**
Colombia	2.5	0.3	1.6	0.3	0.7	0.1	66.5	8.1	40.2	6.5	4,426
Iraq	0.8	0.2	0.5	0.2	0.4	0.2	63.5	13.5	71.5	16.6	4,332
Nigeria	0.3	0.1	0.1	0.1	0.1	0.0	44.9	15.7	35.3	18.9	6,752
Peru	0.7	0.1	0.5	0.1	0.2	0.1	68.9	10.9	32.2	12.3	3,930
PRC (Shenzhen)	0.1	0.1	0.1	0.1	0.0	0.0	60.1	17.4	3.9	4.4	7,132
Ukraine	0.3	0.1	0.2	0.1	0.2	0.1	75.9	12.4	68.5	13.1	4,725
Upper-middle-income countries	**1.3**	**0.1**	**0.9**	**0.1**	**0.6**	**0.1**	**68.5**	**3.2**	**62.7**	**3.7**	**19,294**
Brazil	2.5	0.3	1.6	0.3	1.0	0.2	63.0	5.1	64.1	5.1	5,037
Colombia (Medellin)	1.2	0.2	1.0	0.2	0.4	0.1	79.8	7.3	43.5	9.9	3,261
Lebanon	0.5	0.1	0.3	0.1	0.3	0.1	72.7	13.0	90.3	9.5	2,857
Mexico	1.0	0.1	0.7	0.1	0.5	0.1	71.1	5.7	64.4	6.1	5,782
Romania	0.5	0.2	0.3	0.2	0.3	0.2	73.7	17.3	82.9	16.7	2,357
High-income countries	**0.9**	**0.0**	**0.5**	**0.0**	**0.3**	**0.0**	**58.8**	**2.0**	**52.9**	**3.1**	**81,839**
Australia	1.5	0.2	0.7	0.2	0.2	0.1	46.7	5.4	32.4	8.2	8,463
Belgium	0.9	0.2	0.5	0.1	0.4	0.2	54.4	16.0	81.6	18.6	2,419
France	1.0	0.2	0.6	0.1	0.4	0.1	56.9	9.8	63.2	13.2	2,894
Germany	0.5	0.1	0.4	0.1	0.2	0.1	72.4	10.7	66.6	17.1	3,555
Israel	0.6	0.1	0.4	0.1	0.2	0.1	61.3	9.8	41.6	12.5	4,859
Italy	0.8	0.2	0.5	0.1	0.3	0.1	58.1	8.4	58.7	12.1	4,712
Japan	0.2	0.1	0.1	0.0	0.1	0.1	64.8	15.0	75.8	30.1	4,129
New Zealand	1.2	0.1	0.7	0.1	0.3	0.1	55.3	4.0	50.8	6.4	12,790
Northern Ireland	1.9	0.2	1.4	0.2	1.0	0.2	72.9	6.4	73.8	8.5	4,340
Poland	0.2	0.1	0.1	0.0	0.0	0.0	39.4	11.8	50.3	18.8	10,081
Portugal	1.0	0.2	0.7	0.1	0.5	0.1	64.7	6.2	76.0	8.7	3,849
Spain	0.6	0.1	0.4	0.1	0.2	0.0	68.7	8.6	36.6	10.4	5,473
Spain (Murcia)	0.5	0.1	0.2	0.1	0.1	0.1	49.8	19.4	55.3	9.4	2,621
Netherlands	0.6	0.2	0.3	0.1	0.1	0.1	47.7	10.9	36.6	18.8	2,372
United States	1.3	0.1	0.9	0.1	0.4	0.1	64.9	4.6	45.1	6.0	9,282

(cont.)

Table 8A.1 (*cont.*)

Country	Lifetime prevalence		12-month prevalence		30-day prevalence		12-month prevalence of AG without PD among lifetime cases		30-day prevalence of AG without PD among 12-month cases		Part 1 sample sizes
	%	SE	%	SE	%	SE	%	SE	%	SE	
All countries combined	**0.9**	**0.0**	**0.6**	**0.0**	**0.3**	**0.0**	**61.9**	**1.7**	**53.5**	**2.2**	**132,430**
WHO regions[a]											
Region of the Americas	1.5	0.1	1.0	0.1	0.5	0.1	67.0	2.8	50.2	2.9	31,718
African region	0.3	0.1	0.1	0.1	0.1	0.0	44.9	15.7	35.3	18.9	6,752
Western Pacific region	0.9	0.1	0.5	0.1	0.2	0.0	52.1	3.1	42.8	5.3	32,514
Eastern Mediterranean region	0.6	0.1	0.4	0.1	0.3	0.1	64.3	7.5	64.3	9.3	12,048
Western European region	0.9	0.1	0.6	0.1	0.4	0.0	64.0	3.3	64.5	4.6	32,235
Eastern European region	0.2	0.1	0.2	0.0	0.1	0.0	62.0	8.3	68.8	9.8	17,163
Comparison between countries[b]	**$F_{25,v} = 17.2^*$, $P < 0.001$**		**$F_{25,v} = 12.0^*$, $P < 0.001$**		**$F_{25,v} = 12.8^*$, $P < 0.001$**		**$F_{25,v} = 1.3$, $P = 0.124$**		**$F_{25,v} = 1.9^*$, $P = 0.005$**		
Comparison between low-, middle-, and high-income country groups[b]	**$F_{2,v} = 12.4^*$, $P < 0.001$**		**$F_{2,v} = 9.2^*$, $P < 0.001$**		**$F_{2,v} = 13.5^*$, $P < 0.001$**		**$F_{2,v} = 3.3^*$, $P = 0.038$**		**$F_{2,v} = 4.1^*$, $P = 0.016$**		
Comparison between WHO regions[b]	**$F_{5,v} = 47.4^*$, $P < 0.001$**		**$F_{5,v} = 31.4^*$, $P < 0.001$**		**$F_{5,v} = 22.7^*$, $P < 0.001$**		**$F_{5,v} = 2.9^*$, $P = 0.013$**		**$F_{5,v} = 2.9^*$, $P = 0.014$**		

[a]**Region of the Americas** (Colombia, Mexico, Brazil, Peru, United States, Colombia (Medellin)); **African region** (Nigeria); **Western Pacific region** (PRC (Shenzhen), Japan, Australia, New Zealand); **Eastern Mediterranean region** (Israel, Iraq, Lebanon); **Western European region** (Belgium, France, Germany, Italy, Netherlands, Spain, Northern Ireland, Portugal, Spain (Murcia)); **Eastern European region** (Romania, Poland, Ukraine).

[b]Wald design-corrected F-tests were used to determine if there is variation in prevalence estimates across countries. The denominator degree of freedom, v, is 5287.

PRC: People's Republic of China.

Table 8A.2 Age at selected percentiles on the standardized age-of-onset distributions of agoraphobia (AG) without panic disorder (PD) with projected lifetime risk at age 75

Country	Ages at selected percentiles								Lifetime prevalence of AG without PD		Projected risk at age 75	
	5	10	25	50	75	90	95	99	%	SE	%	SE
Low/lower-middle-income countries	**5**	**7**	**11**	**16**	**33**	**50**	**59**	**63**	**0.7**	**0.1**	**0.9**	**0.1**
Colombia[a]	5	6	12	19	41	59	63	63	2.5	0.3	3.3	0.5
Iraq	5	8	11	13	14	19	21	23	0.8	0.2	0.8	0.2
Nigeria	5	5	8	13	14	33	33	33	0.3	0.1	0.3	0.1
Peru[a]	7	10	14	26	59	59	59	59	0.7	0.1	1.2	0.5
PRC (Shenzhen)	5	8	13	13	47	47	47	47	0.1	0.1	0.2	0.1
Ukraine	5	5	6	13	18	49	49	49	0.3	0.1	0.4	0.1
Upper-middle-income countries	**5**	**8**	**13**	**18**	**37**	**54**	**61**	**67**	**1.3**	**0.1**	**1.6**	**0.1**
Brazil	5	9	13	19	41	54	67	67	2.5	0.3	3.3	0.4
Colombia (Medellin)[a]	5	5	5	13	15	31	49	49	1.2	0.2	1.3	0.3
Lebanon	13	13	14	18	31	31	41	41	0.5	0.1	0.5	0.2
Mexico[a]	8	9	14	21	52	61	61	61	1.0	0.1	1.5	0.3
Romania	5	5	20	33	35	36	41	41	0.5	0.2	0.6	0.3
High-income countries	**5**	**8**	**13**	**21**	**36**	**48**	**54**	**66**	**0.9**	**0.0**	**1.2**	**0.1**
Australia	6	11	13	18	33	48	60	66	1.5	0.2	1.9	0.3
Belgium	5	5	13	29	66	66	66	66	0.9	0.2	1.4	0.5
France	8	12	19	26	41	53	58	58	1.0	0.2	1.4	0.2
Germany	11	13	19	25	37	51	51	51	0.5	0.1	0.6	0.1
Israel	7	11	14	36	50	65	65	65	0.6	0.1	0.9	0.2
Italy	5	8	14	19	34	39	40	53	0.8	0.2	1.0	0.2
Japan	5	5	13	23	41	41	47	47	0.2	0.1	0.3	0.1
New Zealand	5	6	13	17	26	38	46	51	1.2	0.1	1.4	0.1
Northern Ireland	6	8	13	21	41	49	51	54	1.9	0.2	2.5	0.3
Poland[b]	5	5	7	13	16	30	30	30	0.2	0.1	0.2	0.1
Portugal	5	5	11	20	33	49	49	66	1.0	0.2	1.2	0.2
Spain	11	11	20	39	47	61	73	73	0.6	0.1	1.0	0.3
Spain (Murcia)	10	10	14	23	33	35	35	41	0.5	0.1	0.6	0.1
Netherlands	14	20	31	40	47	48	48	48	0.6	0.2	1.0	0.3
United States	6	7	13	21	33	48	51	54	1.3	0.1	1.7	0.2
All countries combined	**5**	**7**	**13**	**19**	**36**	**50**	**59**	**66**	**0.9**	**0.0**	**1.2**	**0.1**
WHO regions												
Region of the Americas	5	7	13	19	40	53	59	67	1.5	0.1	2.0	0.1
African region	5	5	8	13	14	33	33	33	0.3	0.1	0.3	0.1
Western Pacific region	5	8	13	18	31	46	51	66	0.9	0.1	1.2	0.1
Eastern Mediterranean region	8	11	13	16	36	51	65	65	0.6	0.1	0.8	0.1
Western European region	6	8	14	25	41	51	61	73	0.9	0.1	1.2	0.1
Eastern European region	5	5	7	16	33	39	49	49	02	0.0	0.3	0.1

[a]The projected risk for these countries is at age 65 because the age range of these surveys is between 18 and 65.
[b]The projected risk for this country is at age 64 because the age range of this survey is between 18 and 64.
PRC: People's Republic of China.

Table 8A.3 Severity of role impairment (Sheehan Disability Scale) associated with 12-month agoraphobia without panic disorder, by country

Country	Proportion with severe role impairment (SDS score: 7–10)										Number of 12-month cases
	Home		Work		Relationship		Social		Any[a]		
	%	SE	%	SE	%	SE	%	SE	%	SE	
Low/lower-middle-income countries	**12.7**	**3.3**	**13.0**	**3.4**	**12.0**	**3.4**	**14.3**	**3.7**	**23.1**	**4.6**	**133**
Colombia	15.7	5.1	13.7	4.9	13.9	5.4	18.8	6.1	25.7	7.0	68
Iraq	5.2	3.2	5.2	3.2	11.6	5.9	7.1	4.7	17.6	7.4	21
Nigeria	–	–	–	–	–	–	–	–	–	–	9
Peru	10.7	10.1	20.7	13.2	10.7	10.1	19.8	11.4	29.8	13.0	17
PRC (Shenzhen)	–	–	–	–	–	–	–	–	–	–	7
Ukraine	27.5	15.7	30.8	16.7	18.2	11.5	11.8	10.9	39.3	17.6	11
Upper-middle-income countries	**14.8**	**3.5**	**18.9**	**3.6**	**26.4**	**4.3**	**24.6**	**4.1**	**31.1**	**4.5**	**189**
Brazil	16.5	5.5	20.3	5.5	24.7	5.8	20.7	4.9	29.1	6.0	88
Colombia (Medellin)	11.8	8.2	23.3	9.9	29.4	11.4	29.8	13.0	39.5	12.9	32
Lebanon	6.9	6.9	–	–	23.2	17.5	23.2	17.5	23.2	17.5	9
Mexico	14.6	6.2	18.6	6.8	23.0	7.5	23.7	7.5	27.4	7.9	56
Romania	–	–	–	–	–	–	–	–	–	–	4
High-income countries	**15.5**	**1.8**	**19.9**	**2.3**	**27.2**	**2.5**	**31.9**	**2.5**	**40.6**	**2.9**	**485**
Australia	38.4	7.9	36.3	9.5	37.4	7.5	46.5	7.8	55.2	8.0	68
Belgium	7.5	7.3	43.8	27.0	55.4	25.1	26.8	14.3	63.0	24.3	9
France	13.9	13.0	–	–	22.3	8.0	12.3	6.3	38.1	12.9	19
Germany	5.1	4.3	14.0	11.8	5.1	4.3	31.0	15.7	36.0	18.6	13
Israel	26.0	11.3	38.4	12.4	36.8	12.2	45.9	12.6	50.6	12.6	17
Italy	35.2	14.1	9.3	5.4	33.6	12.3	30.5	11.1	51.0	13.3	18
Japan	–	–	–	–	36.1	29.1	–	–	36.1	29.1	5
New Zealand	6.1	2.4	12.0	3.9	19.6	4.6	22.7	5.0	30.8	5.7	115
Northern Ireland	20.0	4.4	25.1	5.3	36.9	5.3	58.0	6.7	59.9	6.2	67
Poland	51.4	18.8	85.2	11.8	29.8	16.5	48.2	18.8	68.2	17.4	6
Portugal	8.4	4.3	17.4	6.5	15.0	6.1	17.1	6.5	18.8	6.7	33
Spain	8.0	4.4	9.1	5.0	8.9	4.8	10.6	5.4	17.3	7.4	24
Spain (Murcia)	21.8	17.2	27.9	20.4	93.9	6.3	100.0	0.0	100.0	0.0	7
Netherlands	9.2	9.1	9.2	9.1	9.2	9.1	0.0	0.0	9.2	9.1	7
United States	13.9	3.5	22.6	6.3	28.6	6.5	31.5	6.3	37.2	7.2	77

Table 8A.3 *(cont.)*

Country	Proportion with severe role impairment (SDS score: 7–10)										Number of 12-month cases
	Home		Work		Relationship		Social		Any[a]		
	%	SE	%	SE	%	SE	%	SE	%	SE	
All countries combined	**14.8**	**1.5**	**18.3**	**1.7**	**24.1**	**1.9**	**26.8**	**1.9**	**35.0**	**2.2**	**807**
WHO regions											
Region of the Americas	14.8	2.3	19.3	2.8	22.7	3.0	24.1	3.0	30.9	3.4	338
African region	–	–	–	–	–	–	–	–	–	–	9
Western Pacific region	12.0	2.5	15.3	3.3	23.0	4.0	25.4	4.1	34.5	4.7	195
Eastern Mediterranean region	13.0	5.1	16.2	5.9	22.9	6.9	24.2	7.2	30.6	7.7	47
Western European region	15.9	3.0	17.6	3.1	27.5	3.7	33.4	3.8	42.9	4.4	197
Eastern European region	29.5	10.6	36.6	11.9	33.4	11.9	34.7	12.0	51.9	12.6	21
Comparison between countries[b]	**$F_{25,v} = 1.7^*$, $P = 0.015$**		**$F_{25,v} = 2.1^*$, $P = 0.001$**		**$F_{25,v} = 1.7^*$, $P = 0.017$**		**$F_{25,v} = 2.6^*$, $P < 0.001$**		**$F_{25,v} = 2.1^*$, $P = 0.001$**		
Comparison between low-, middle-, and high-income countries[b]	**$F_{2,v} = 0.3$, $P = 0.772$**		**$F_{2,v} = 1.3$, $P = 0.263$**		**$F_{2,v} = 5.4^*$, $P = 0.005$**		**$F_{2,v} = 6.3^*$, $P = 0.002$**		**$F_{2,v} = 4.8^*$, $P = 0.008$**		
Comparison between WHO regions[b]	**$F_{5,v} = 1.4$, $P = 0.206$**		**$F_{5,v} = 1.5$, $P = 0.186$**		**$F_{5,v} = 1.2$, $P = 0.316$**		**$F_{5,v} = 1.8$, $P = 0.117$**		**$F_{5,v} = 2.2$, $P = 0.056$**		

"-": All 12-month cases associated with role impairment were non-severe.
[a]Highest severity category across four SDS role domains.
[b]Wald design-corrected F-tests were used to determine if there is variation in impairment severity across countries. The denominator degree of freedom, v, is 5287.
PRC: People's Republic of China.

Table 9A.1 Bivariate associations between socio-demographic correlates and DSM-IV social anxiety disorder (SAD) (low/lower-middle-income countries)

Correlates	30-day SAD[a]		Lifetime SAD[b]		12-month SAD among lifetime cases[c]		30-day SAD among 12-month cases[c]	
	OR	(95% CI)	OR	(95% CI)	OR	(95% CI)	OR	(95% CI)
Age-cohort								
18–29	**6.7***	(2.9–15.5)	**7.1***	(4.3–11.6)				
30–44	**4.8***	(2.1–11.0)	**4.7***	(2.8–7.7)				
45–59	**3.6***	(1.4–8.9)	**3.2***	(1.9–5.5)				
60+	**1.0**		**1.0**					
Age-cohort difference[d]	$\chi^2_3 = 26.6^*, P < 0.001$		$\chi^2_3 = 74.7^*, P < 0.001$					
Age-of-onset								
Early					**2.7***	(1.3–5.5)	**1.3**	(0.6–2.8)
Early-average					**1.4**	(0.8–2.4)	**1.4**	(0.7–3.2)
Late-average					**1.1**	(0.6–1.9)	**1.4**	(0.7–2.8)
Late					**1.0**		**1.0**	
Age-of-onset difference[d]					$\chi^2_3 = 9.3^*, P = 0.026$		$\chi^2_3 = 1.3, P = 0.721$	
Time since onset (continuous)					**0.98***	(0.96–0.99)	**0.99**	(0.97–1.02)
Gender								
Female	**1.4**	(0.9–2.1)	**1.1**	(0.9–1.4)	**1.5**	(1.0–2.2)	**1.1**	(0.7–1.9)
Male	**1.0**		**1.0**		**1.0**		**1.0**	
Gender difference[d]	$\chi^2_1 = 2.8, P = 0.092$		$\chi^2_1 = 1.3, P = 0.255$		$\chi^2_1 = 3.7, P = 0.055$		$\chi^2_1 = 0.2, P = 0.679$	
Employment status								
Student	**1.4**	(0.6–3.1)	**1.1**	(0.6–1.8)	**1.7**	(0.6–4.8)	**3.7***	(1.3–10.8)
Homemaker	**1.4**	(0.8–2.4)	**1.0**	(0.8–1.4)	**1.7**	(0.9–3.2)	**1.3**	(0.6–3.0)
Retired	**0.7**	(0.3–1.9)	**1.9**	(1.0–3.8)	**0.6**	(0.2–1.5)	**0.7**	(0.3–2.2)
Other	**1.0**	(0.6–1.7)	**1.0**	(0.7–1.3)	**2.4***	(1.2–4.9)	**0.8**	(0.4–1.7)
Employed	**1.0**		**1.0**		**1.0**		**1.0**	
Employment status difference[d]	$\chi^2_4 = 2.7, P = 0.606$		$\chi^2_4 = 4.2, P = 0.387$		$\chi^2_4 = 9.9^*, P = 0.043$		$\chi^2_4 = 7.4, P = 0.115$	
Marital status								
Never married	**1.1**	(0.7–1.7)	**1.4***	(1.1–1.8)	**0.8**	(0.5–1.3)	**1.0**	(0.5–1.8)
Divorced/separated/widowed	**1.3**	(0.8–2.1)	**1.3**	(0.9–1.8)	**1.0**	(0.5–2.1)	**1.2**	(0.5–2.7)
Currently married	**1.0**		**1.0**		**1.0**		**1.0**	

Table 9A.1 *(cont.)*

Correlates	30-day SAD[a]		Lifetime SAD[b]		12-month SAD among lifetime cases[c]		30-day SAD among 12-month cases[c]	
	OR	(95% CI)	OR	(95% CI)	OR	(95% CI)	OR	(95% CI)
Marital status difference[d]	$\chi^2_2 = 0.8, P = 0.664$		$\chi^2_2 = 7.4^*, P = 0.025$		$\chi^2_2 = 1.0, P = 0.613$		$\chi^2_2 = 0.2, P = 0.927$	
Education level								
No education	**1.2**	(0.4–3.1)	**0.9**	(0.5–1.8)	–	–	**1.1**	(0.3–3.6)
Some primary	**1.4**	(0.6–3.2)	**0.9**	(0.5–1.4)	**1.5**	(0.6–4.2)	**2.8**	(0.9–8.9)
Primary finished	**1.9**	(0.8–4.1)	**1.1**	(0.7–1.8)	**1.6**	(0.7–3.7)	**2.0**	(0.7–6.2)
Some secondary	**1.2**	(0.5–2.5)	**0.9**	(0.6–1.3)	**1.5**	(0.7–3.3)	**1.0**	(0.5–2.4)
Secondary finished	**0.9**	(0.5–1.7)	**1.0**	(0.7–1.4)	**1.5**	(0.8–2.9)	**0.8**	(0.4–1.6)
Some college	**0.6**	(0.3–1.0)	**0.8**	(0.6–1.2)	**1.1**	(0.5–2.1)	**0.5**	(0.2–1.3)
College finished	**1.0**		**1.0**		**1.0**		**1.0**	
Education level difference[d]	$\chi^2_3 = 12.2, P = 0.058$		$\chi^2_3 = 2.6, P = 0.856$		$\chi^2_3 = 3.5, P = 0.739$		$\chi^2_3 = 8.9, P = 0.181$	
Household income								
Low	**0.9**	(0.5–1.6)	**0.9**	(0.6–1.2)	**1.2**	(0.6–2.3)	**1.2**	(0.6–2.6)
Low-average	**1.2**	(0.6–2.1)	**0.9**	(0.7–1.3)	**2.0***	(1.0–4.1)	**0.9**	(0.4–2.1)
High-average	**0.9**	(0.5–1.5)	**0.9**	(0.7–1.2)	**1.8**	(0.9–3.6)	**0.7**	(0.4–1.4)
High	**1.0**		**1.0**		**1.0**		**1.0**	
Household income difference[d]	$\chi^2_3 = 1.4, P = 0.709$		$\chi^2_3 = 1.0, P = 0.800$		$\chi^2_3 = 5.9, P = 0.117$		$\chi^2_3 = 2.4, P = 0.498$	
N[e]	**36,498**		**1,426,232**		**564**		**349**	

*Significant at the 0.05 level, two-sided test.
A dash was inserted for low cell counts (<5 cases).
[a]These estimates are based on logistic regression models adjusted for age, gender, and low/lower-middle-income countries.
[b]These estimates are based on survival models adjusted for age-cohorts, gender, person-years, and low/lower-middle-income countries.
[c]These estimates are based on logistic regression models adjusted for time since SAD onset, age of SAD onset, gender, and low/lower-middle-income countries.
[d]Chi-square test exploring significant differences between blocks of socio-demographic variables.
[e]Denominator N: 36,498 = total sample; 1,426,232 = number of person-years in the survival models; 564 = number of lifetime SAD cases; 349 = number of 12-month SAD cases.

Table 9A.2 Bivariate associations between socio-demographic correlates and DSM-IV social anxiety disorder (SAD) (upper-middle-income countries)

Correlates	30-day SAD[a]		Lifetime SAD[b]		12-month SAD among lifetime cases[c]		30-day SAD among 12-month cases[c]	
	OR	(95% CI)	OR	(95% CI)	OR	(95% CI)	OR	(95% CI)
Age-cohort								
18–29	**2.0***	(1.2–3.1)	**3.9***	(2.7–5.5)				
30–44	**2.1***	(1.3–3.3)	**2.9***	(2.1–4.0)				
45–59	**1.9***	(1.2–3.1)	**2.1***	(1.5–3.1)				
60+	**1.0**		**1.0**					
Age-cohort difference[d]	$\chi^2_3 = 9.8^*, P = 0.021$		$\chi^2_3 = 70.3^*, P < 0.001$					
Age-of-onset								
Early					**1.0**	(0.6–2.0)	**0.5***	(0.3–1.0)
Early-average					**0.8**	(0.5–1.4)	**0.6**	(0.3–1.1)
Late-average					**0.9**	(0.5–1.5)	**1.0**	(0.6–1.7)
Late					**1.0**		**1.0**	
Age-of-onset difference[d]					$\chi^2_3 = 1.0, P = 0.810$		$\chi^2_3 = 6.4, P = 0.092$	
Time since onset (continuous)					**0.99**	(0.98–1.01)	**1.02***	(1.00–1.03)
Gender								
Female	**2.0***	(1.6–2.6)	**1.5***	(1.3–1.8)	**1.6***	(1.1–2.4)	**1.6***	(1.0–2.3)
Male	**1.0**		**1.0**		**1.0**		**1.0**	
Gender difference[d]	$\chi^2_1 = 29.5^*, P < 0.001$		$\chi^2_1 = 19.6^*, P < 0.001$		$\chi^2_1 = 4.7^*, P = 0.030$		$\chi^2_1 = 4.5^*, P = 0.034$	
Employment status								
Student	**1.8**	(1.0–3.3)	**1.4**	(0.9–2.1)	**0.6**	(0.3–1.5)	–	–
Homemaker	**1.3**	(1.0–1.8)	**1.1**	(0.8–1.3)	**1.4**	(0.8–2.3)	**1.8***	(1.1–3.1)
Retired	**0.4***	(0.2–0.9)	**0.7**	(0.5–1.0)	**1.0**	(0.4–2.7)	**0.4**	(0.1–1.3)
Other	**1.4**	(1.0–2.0)	**1.3**	(1.0–1.6)	**1.0**	(0.6–1.8)	**1.2**	(0.7–2.1)
Employed	**1.0**		**1.0**		**1.0**		**1.0**	
Employment status difference[d]	$\chi^2_4 = 15.8^*, P = 0.003$		$\chi^2_4 = 7.8, P = 0.101$		$\chi^2_4 = 3.9, P = 0.414$		$\chi^2_4 = 18.7^*, P = 0.001$	
Marital status								
Never married	**1.0**	(0.7–1.3)	**1.3***	(1.0–1.7)	**1.0**	(0.6–1.6)	**0.8**	(0.5–1.2)
Divorced/separated/widowed	**1.1**	(0.8–1.6)	**1.3***	(1.0–1.7)	**1.0**	(0.6–1.7)	**0.8**	(0.4–1.4)
Currently married	**1.0**		**1.0**		**1.0**		**1.0**	

Table 9A.2 (*cont.*)

Correlates	30-day SAD[a]		Lifetime SAD[b]		12-month SAD among lifetime cases[c]		30-day SAD among 12-month cases[c]	
	OR	(95% CI)	OR	(95% CI)	OR	(95% CI)	OR	(95% CI)
Marital status difference[d]	$\chi^2_2 = 0.4, P = 0.815$		$\chi^2_2 = 8.4^*, P = 0.015$		$\chi^2_2 = 0.0, P = 0.996$		$\chi^2_2 = 1.5, P = 0.484$	
Education level								
No education	**1.4**	(0.7–2.9)	**0.7**	(0.4–1.2)	–	–	**2.1**	(0.6–7.4)
Some primary	**1.7***	(1.1–2.8)	**0.9**	(0.7–1.3)	**3.8***	(2.0–7.3)	**2.2**	(0.9–5.3)
Primary finished	**1.6**	(1.0–2.6)	**1.1**	(0.8–1.6)	**2.4***	(1.1–5.1)	**1.3**	(0.5–3.3)
Some secondary	**1.4**	(0.9–2.2)	**1.2**	(0.9–1.6)	**1.3**	(0.7–2.6)	**1.2**	(0.6–2.4)
Secondary finished	**1.0**	(0.6–1.6)	**0.9**	(0.7–1.2)	**1.1**	(0.6–2.0)	**1.4**	(0.7–2.7)
Some college	**1.0**	(0.6–1.7)	**1.1**	(0.8–1.5)	**1.5**	(0.6–3.8)	**0.7**	(0.3–1.6)
College finished	**1.0**		**1.0**		**1.0**		**1.0**	
Education level difference[d]	$\chi^2_3 = 12.9^*, P = 0.044$		$\chi^2_3 = 10.6, P = 0.102$		$\chi^2_3 = 37.1^*, P < 0.001$		$\chi^2_3 = 9.3, P = 0.157$	
Household income								
Low	**1.2**	(0.8–1.7)	**1.0**	(0.8–1.2)	**0.9**	(0.5–1.6)	**1.6**	(0.8–3.1)
Low-average	**1.2**	(0.8–1.8)	**1.0**	(0.8–1.3)	**1.2**	(0.7–2.0)	**1.6**	(0.9–2.8)
High-average	**1.2**	(0.9–1.6)	**0.8**	(0.7–1.1)	**1.3**	(0.7–2.3)	**2.0***	(1.2–3.5)
High	**1.0**		**1.0**		**1.0**		**1.0**	
Household income difference[d]	$\chi^2_3 = 1.7, P = 0.649$		$\chi^2_3 = 3.1, P = 0.384$		$\chi^2_3 = 2.0, P = 0.580$		$\chi^2_3 = 6.7, P = 0.082$	
N[e]	**28,927**		**1,206,689**		**834**		**601**	

*Significant at the 0.05 level, two-sided test.
A dash was inserted for low cell counts (<5 cases).
[a]These estimates are based on logistic regression models adjusted for age, gender, and upper-middle-income countries.
[b]These estimates are based on survival models adjusted for age-cohorts, gender, person-years, and upper-middle-income countries.
[c]These estimates are based on logistic regression models adjusted for time since SAD onset, age of SAD onset, gender, and upper-middle-income countries.
[d]Chi-square test exploring significant differences between blocks of socio-demographic variables.
[e]Denominator N: 28,927 = total sample; 1,206,689 = number of person-years in the survival models; 834 = number of lifetime SAD cases; 601 = number of 12-month SAD cases.

Table 9A.3 Bivariate associations between socio-demographic correlates and DSM-IV social anxiety disorder (SAD) (high-income countries)

Correlates	30-day SAD[a]		Lifetime SAD[b]		12-month SADamong lifetime cases[c]		30-day SAD among 12-month cases[c]	
	OR	(95% CI)	OR	(95% CI)	OR	(95% CI)	OR	(95% CI)
Age-cohort								
18–29	**3.3***	(2.7–4.2)	**3.3***	(3.0–3.8)				
30–44	**2.8***	(2.3–3.5)	**2.8***	(2.5–3.2)				
45–59	**2.5***	(2.0–3.2)	**2.3***	(2.1–2.7)				
60+	**1.0**		**1.0**					
Age-cohort difference[d]	$\chi^2_3 = 119.5^*, P < 0.001$		$\chi^2_3 = 414.6^*, P < 0.001$					
Age-of-onset								
Early					**1.5***	(1.1–1.9)	**1.0**	(0.8–1.4)
Early-average					**1.5***	(1.2–1.9)	**0.9**	(0.7–1.3)
Late-average					**1.2**	(0.9–1.4)	**0.9**	(0.7–1.1)
Late					**1.0**		**1.0**	
Age-of-onset difference[d]					$\chi^2_3 = 13.4^*, P = 0.004$		$\chi^2_3 = 1.8, P = 0.615$	
Time since onset (continuous)					**0.98***	(0.97–0.98)	**1.01**	(1.00–1.01)
Gender								
Female	**1.6***	(1.4–1.8)	**1.3***	(1.2–1.4)	**1.3***	(1.1–1.5)	**1.2**	(1.0–1.4)
Male	**1.0**		**1.0**		**1.0**		**1.0**	
Gender difference[d]	$\chi^2_1 = 38.8^*, P < 0.001$		$\chi^2_1 = 44.7^*, P < 0.001$		$\chi^2_1 = 8.5^*, P = 0.004$		$\chi^2_1 = 2.8, P = 0.097$	
Employment status								
Student	**1.3**	(1.0–1.8)	**1.1**	(0.9–1.4)	**1.2**	(0.8–1.8)	**1.5**	(1.0–2.3)
Homemaker	**1.4***	(1.2–1.8)	**1.2***	(1.1–1.4)	**1.3***	(1.0–1.7)	**1.3**	(0.9–1.8)
Retired	**0.7***	(0.5–1.0)	**0.8***	(0.7–1.0)	**1.1**	(0.8–1.5)	**1.1**	(0.7–1.6)
Other	**2.2***	(1.8–2.7)	**1.6***	(1.5–1.9)	**2.3***	(1.7–3.1)	**1.0**	(0.7–1.4)
Employed	**1.0**		**1.0**		**1.0**		**1.0**	
Employment status difference[d]	$\chi^2_4 = 81.7^*, P < 0.001$		$\chi^2_4 = 84.1^*, P < 0.001$		$\chi^2_4 = 34.4^*, P < 0.001$		$\chi^2_4 = 5.3, P = 0.258$	

Table 9A.3 *(cont.)*

Correlates	30-day SAD[a]		Lifetime SAD[b]		12-month SADamong lifetime cases[c]		30-day SAD among 12-month cases[c]	
	OR	(95% CI)	OR	(95% CI)	OR	(95% CI)	OR	(95% CI)
Marital status								
Never married	**1.3***	(1.1–1.6)	**1.4***	(1.3–1.6)	**1.5***	(1.2–1.8)	**1.0**	(0.8–1.3)
Divorced/separated/widowed	**1.6***	(1.3–2.0)	**1.3***	(1.2–1.5)	**1.5***	(1.2–1.8)	**1.1**	(0.9–1.4)
Currently married	**1.0**		**1.0**		**1.0**		**1.0**	
Marital status difference[d]	$\chi^2_2 = 30.0^*, P < 0.001$		$\chi^2_2 = 63.3^*, P < 0.001$		$\chi^2_2 = 26.0^*, P < 0.001$		$\chi^2_2 = 0.7, P = 0.709$	
Education level								
No education	–	–	–	–	–	–	–	–
Some primary	**1.9***	(1.1–3.1)	**1.2**	(1.0–1.6)	**2.9***	(1.7–5.0)	**1.5**	(0.7–3.1)
Primary finished	**1.3**	(0.8–1.9)	**1.2**	(1.0–1.5)	**1.7***	(1.0–2.9)	**0.9**	(0.5–1.5)
Some secondary	**1.4***	(1.1–1.8)	**1.2***	(1.1–1.4)	**1.7***	(1.3–2.1)	**1.0**	(0.7–1.4)
Secondary finished	**1.0**	(0.8–1.2)	**1.1**	(1.0–1.2)	**1.3***	(1.1–1.6)	**0.8**	(0.6–1.0)
Some college	**1.1**	(0.9–1.4)	**1.2***	(1.0–1.3)	**1.3***	(1.0–1.7)	**0.8**	(0.6–1.1)
College finished	**1.0**		**1.0**		**1.0**		**1.0**	
Education level difference[d]	$\chi^2_3 = 17.2^*, P = 0.009$		$\chi^2_3 = 15.6^*, P = 0.016$		$\chi^2_3 = 29.4^*, P < 0.001$		$\chi^2_3 = 7.6, P = 0.268$	
Household income								
Low	**1.6***	(1.3–2.0)	**1.2***	(1.1–1.4)	**1.8***	(1.4–2.2)	**1.3**	(1.0–1.8)
Low-average	**1.3***	(1.0–1.6)	**1.0**	(0.9–1.2)	**1.4***	(1.1–1.7)	**1.3**	(1.0–1.8)
High-average	**1.1**	(0.9–1.4)	**1.1**	(1.0–1.2)	**1.1**	(0.9–1.4)	**1.0**	(0.8–1.4)
High	**1.0**		**1.0**		**1.0**		**1.0**	
Household income difference[d]	$\chi^2_3 = 25.1^*, P < 0.001$		$\chi^2_3 = 15.9^*, P = 0.001$		$\chi^2_3 = 32.7^*, P < 0.001$		$\chi^2_3 = 5.7, P = 0.126$	
N[e]	**76,980**		**3,448,640**		**4,360**		**2,510**	

*Significant at the 0.05 level, two-sided test.
A dash was inserted for low cell counts (<5 cases).
[a]These estimates are based on logistic regression models adjusted for age, gender, and high-income countries.
[b]These estimates are based on survival models adjusted for age-cohorts, gender, person-years, and high-income countries.
[c]These estimates are based on logistic regression models adjusted for time since SAD onset, age of SAD onset, gender, and high-income countries.
[d]Chi-square test exploring significant differences between blocks of socio-demographic variables.
[e]Denominator N: 76,980 = total sample; 3,448,640 = number of person-years in the survival models; 4,360 = number of lifetime SAD cases; 2,510 = number of 12-month SAD cases.

Table 9A.4 Among those with 12-month social anxiety disorder, percent reporting treatment in the past 12 months by Sheehan impairment severity

Sector of treatment	Sheehan disability scale category[a]											
	Mild impairment (score: 1–3)			Moderate impairment (score: 4–6)			Severe impairment (score: 7–10)			Any impairment		
	%	SE	Comparison between country income groups[b]	%	SE	Comparison between country income groups[b]	%	SE	Comparison between country income groups[b]	%	SE	Comparison between country income groups[b]
Specialty mental health[c]												
Low/lower-middle-income countries	**10.7**	6.0	$F_{2,v} = 1.4$, $P = 0.25$	**5.2**	2.4	$F_{2,v} = 3.4^*$, $P = 0.03$	**6.3**	2.3	$F_{2,v} = 33.4^*$, $P < 0.001$	**7.8**	1.9	$F_{2,v} = 32.6^*$, $P < 0.001$
Upper-middle-income countries	**13.9**	4.2		**12.4**	2.6		**15.3**	3.0		**13.2**	1.7	
High-income countries	**19.2**	2.0		**12.6**	1.4		**34.4**	1.7		**23.3**	0.9	
All countries combined	**17.5**	1.7		**11.7**	1.1		**27.7**	1.4		**19.8**	0.8	
General medical[d]												
Low/lower-middle-income countries	–	–	$F_{2,v} = 14.4^*$, $P < 0.001$	**9.9**	3.7	$F_{2,v} = 5.1^*$, $P = 0.01$	**7.0**	2.4	$F_{2,v} = 44.8^*$, $P < 0.001$	**7.8**	1.7	$F_{2,v} = 65.6^*$, $P < 0.001$
Upper-middle-income countries	**13.8**	3.9		**12.3**	3.1		**15.0**	2.8		**13.7**	1.7	
High-income countries	**28.8**	2.2		**20.9**	1.9		**39.0**	1.9		**30.8**	1.1	
All countries combined	**23.9**	1.8		**17.8**	1.5		**31.0**	1.5		**25.2**	0.9	
Any health care[e]												
Low/lower-middle-income countries	**12.4**	6.0	$F_{2,v} = 8.6^*$, $P < 0.001$	**15.0**	4.1	$F_{2,v} = 3.3^*$, $P = 0.04$	**12.7**	3.2	$F_{2,v} = 43.7^*$, $P < 0.001$	**14.5**	2.6	$F_{2,v} = 54.3^*$, $P < 0.001$
Upper-middle-income countries	**23.6**	4.6		**22.6**	3.4		**26.0**	3.6		**23.7**	1.9	
High-income countries	**36.7**	2.3		**26.7**	2.0		**54.6**	1.9		**40.9**	1.1	
All countries combined	**32.0**	2.0		**24.5**	1.6		**44.6**	1.6		**34.9**	0.9	
Human services[f]												
Low/lower-middle-income countries	–	–	$F_{2,v} = 5.1^*$, $P = 0.01$	–	–	$F_{2,v} = 0.3$, $P = 0.76$	**3.5**	1.7	$F_{2,v} = 5.1^*$, $P = 0.01$	**3.4**	1.3	$F_{2,v} = 2.5$, $P = 0.08$
Upper-middle-income countries	**4.5**	2.4		**4.8**	2.0		**2.3**	1.2		**3.6**	1.1	
High-income countries	**7.7**	1.6		**3.5**	0.8		**7.1**	1.0		**5.7**	0.5	
All countries combined	**6.5**	1.2		**3.9**	0.8		**5.8**	0.7		**5.1**	0.5	

Table 9A.4 *(cont.)*

Sector of treatment	Sheehan disability scale category[a]											
	Mild impairment (score: 1–3)			Moderate impairment (score: 4–6)			Severe impairment (score: 7–10)			Any impairment		
	%	SE	Comparison between country income groups[b]	%	SE	Comparison between country income groups[b]	%	SE	Comparison between country income groups[b]	%	SE	Comparison between country income groups[b]
CAM[g]												
Low/lower-middle-income countries	–	–	–	–	–	$F_{2,v} = 14.3^*$, $P < 0.001$	–	–	$F_{2,v} = 12.5^*$, $P < 0.001$	**1.6**	0.6	$F_{2,v} = 26.9^*$, $P < 0.001$
Upper-middle-income countries	–	–		**2.7**	1.4		**2.5**	1.2		**2.3**	0.7	
High-income countries	**9.1**	1.7		**5.2**	0.9		**8.5**	1.0		**7.8**	0.6	
All countries combined	**7.3**	1.3		**4.0**	0.7		**6.6**	0.8		**6.1**	0.5	
Any non-health care[h]												
Low/lower-middle-income countries	–	–	$F_{2,v} = 6.3^*$, $P < 0.001$	–	–	$F_{2,v} = 0.2$, $P = 0.80$	**4.7**	1.8	$F_{2,v} = 11.9^*$, $P < 0.001$	**4.5**	1.4	$F_{2,v} = 15.1^*$, $P < 0.001$
Upper-middle-income countries	**5.0**	2.4		**7.3**	2.3		**4.7**	1.7		**5.6**	1.3	
High-income countries	**13.7**	1.9		**7.6**	1.1		**13.6**	1.3		**11.7**	0.7	
All countries combined	**11.3**	1.5		**7.2**	1.0		**11.0**	1.0		**9.8**	0.6	
Any treatment[i]												
Low/lower-middle-income countries	**15.9**	6.1	$F_{2,v} = 9.2^*$, $P < 0.001$	**20.2**	4.9	$F_{2,v} = 2.0$, $P = 0.13$	**15.3**	3.4	$F_{2,v} = 44.5^*$, $P < 0.001$	**18.0**	2.7	$F_{2,v} = 52.3^*$, $P < 0.001$
Upper-middle-income countries	**26.6**	4.7		**24.6**	3.5		**27.2**	3.7		**25.7**	2.1	
High-income countries	**41.8**	2.5		**29.5**	2.0		**57.1**	1.9		**44.2**	1.1	
All countries combined	**36.6**	2.1		**27.4**	1.7		**46.9**	1.6		**38.0**	1.0	

A dash was inserted for low cell counts (<5 cases).
[a]Highest severity category across four SDS role domains.
[b]Wald design-corrected F-tests were used to determine if there is variation in treatment estimates across country income groups. The denominator degree of freedom, v, is 1535. Wald test is only generated where there is more than one stable cell (≥5 cases) for each combination of treatment sector and Sheehan impairment.
[c]The mental health specialist sector, which includes psychiatrist and non-psychiatrist mental health specialists (psychiatrist, psychologist, or other non-psychiatrist mental health professional; social worker or counsellor in a mental health specialty setting; use of a mental health helpline; or overnight admissions for a mental health or drug or alcohol problems, with a presumption of daily contact with a psychiatrist).
[d]The general medical sector (general practitioner, other medical doctor, nurse, occupational therapist, or any healthcare professional).
[e]The mental health specialist sector or the general medical sector.
[f]The human services sector (religious or spiritual advisor or social worker or counsellor in any setting other than a specialty mental health setting).
[g]The CAM (complementary and alternative medicine) sector (any other type of healer such as herbalist or homeopath, participation in an internet support group, or participation in a self-help group).
[h]The human services sector or CAM.
[i]Any treatment listed above.

Table 10A.1 Comorbidity of specific phobia with other DSM-IV disorders

	Specific phobia cases with comorbid disorders									
	Mood disorder[a]		Anxiety disorder[b]		Disruptive behaviour/ impulse-control disorder[c]		Substance-use disorder[d]		Any mental disorder[e]	
	%	SE	%	SE	%	SE	%	SE	%	SE
Lifetime comorbidity[f]										
Lifetime	**34.3**	0.7	**41.2**	0.8	**17.4**	0.7	**15.9**	0.6	**60.5**	0.9
12-month	**35.9**	0.9	**42.9**	0.9	**18.1**	0.7	**15.6**	0.6	**62.0**	1.0
12-month comorbidity[g]										
12-month	**21.0**	0.7	**29.6**	0.8	**10.1**	0.6	**5.3**	0.4	**42.2**	1.0
Temporal priority of specific phobia[h]										
Lifetime	**89.3**	0.7	**71.6**	0.9	**72.5**	1.7	**92.2**	0.9	**72.6**	0.8
12-month	**89.7**	0.8	**72.2**	1.1	**71.5**	2.0	**92.8**	1.0	**72.8**	1.0

[a]Respondents with major depressive episode or bipolar spectrum disorder.
[b]Respondents with panic disorder, generalized anxiety disorder, social phobia, agoraphobia, posttraumatic stress disorder, or separation anxiety disorder.
[c]Respondents with intermittent explosive disorder, attention deficit disorder, conduct disorder, oppositional defiant disorder, binge-eating disorder, or bulimia nervosa.
[d]Respondents with alcohol abuse with or without dependence or drug abuse with or without dependence.
[e]Respondents with any disorder listed above.
[f]Percentage of respondents with either lifetime or 12 month specific phobia who also meet lifetime criteria for at least one of the other DSM-IV disorders.
[g]Percentage of respondents with 12-month specific phobia who also meet 12-month criteria for at least one of the other disorders.
[h]Percentage of respondents with either lifetime or 12-month specific phobia and at least one of the other disorders, whose age-of-onset of specific phobia is reported to be younger than the age-of-onset of all comorbid disorders under consideration.

Table 10A.2 Days-out-of-role due to 12-month specific phobia[a] by role impairment

Sheehan disability domain	Days-out-of-role due to 12-month specific phobia						
	Not severe (score: 0–6)			Severe (score: 7–10)			F-test, P-value[b]
	N	Mean	SE	N	Mean	SE	
Home	3,063	7.1	0.7	727	34.6	3.8	57.9*, P < 0.001
Work	3,125	6.0	0.6	659	42.1	4.3	75.0*, P < 0.001
Relationship	3,254	6.4	0.7	547	47.9	5.0	75.5*, P < 0.001
Social	3,174	5.9	0.6	630	45.1	4.5	79.5*, P < 0.001
Any[c]	2,493	3.8	0.5	1,313	29.1	2.6	104.6*, P < 0.001

[a]Mean (SE) days-out-of role due to 12-month specific phobia: 12.2 (0.9) days.
[b]Bivariate linear regression to test for significant differences in severity. No controls were used.
[c]Mean days-out-of role presented for subgroups of respondents defined by their highest severity category across the four Sheehan disability domains (home, work, relationship, and social).

Table 10A.3 Among those with 12-month specific phobia, percent reporting treatment in the past 12 months by Sheehan impairment severity

Sector of treatment	Sheehan Disability Scale category[a]							
	Mild impairment (score: 1–3)		Moderate impairment (score: 4–6)		Severe impairment (score: 7–10)		Any impairment	
	%	SE	%	SE	%	SE	%	SE
Specialty mental health[b]								
Low/lower-middle-income countries	3.0	1.2	5.9	1.9	5.7	1.7	4.4	0.8
Upper-middle-income countries	8.5	1.4	8.4	1.8	10.4	1.8	9.0	0.8
High-income countries	11.2	1.1	11.6	1.3	21.7	1.7	12.9	0.6
All countries combined	8.6	0.7	9.8	0.9	16.6	1.2	10.4	0.4
General medical[c]								
Low/lower-middle-income countries	4.1	1.1	4.2	1.3	7.7	2.6	4.5	0.7
Upper-middle-income countries	5.0	0.9	8.8	1.8	9.7	2.0	6.8	0.7
High-income countries	21.8	1.4	20.7	1.5	28.8	1.8	21.4	0.7
All countries combined	14.0	0.9	15.1	1.1	21.0	1.3	14.9	0.5
Any health care[d]								
Low/lower-middle-income countries	6.6	1.5	10.1	2.3	13.2	2.9	8.4	1.1
Upper-middle-income countries	12.6	1.5	15.9	2.5	17.9	2.4	14.4	0.9
High-income countries	26.9	1.6	25.6	1.6	39.3	2.0	27.6	0.8
All countries combined	19.0	1.0	20.7	1.2	30.1	1.5	21.0	0.6
Human services[e]								
Low/lower-middle-income countries	–	–	1.3	0.7	–	–	0.9	0.3
Upper-middle-income countries	1.7	0.9	–	–	2.5	0.9	1.2	0.3
High-income countries	3.5	0.6	3.3	0.6	5.3	0.8	3.7	0.4
All countries combined	2.4	0.4	2.4	0.4	4.2	0.6	2.6	0.2
CAM[f]								
Low/lower-middle-income countries	1.0	0.5	–	–	2.1	1.1	1.1	0.3
Upper-middle-income countries	2.6	1.3	1.1	0.6	1.3	0.6	1.8	0.5
High-income countries	4.3	0.7	4.2	0.7	5.4	0.9	4.1	0.4
All countries combined	3.1	0.5	3.0	0.5	3.8	0.6	3.0	0.2
Any non-health care[g]								
Low/lower-middle-income countries	1.3	0.6	2.6	1.0	3.6	1.6	1.9	0.4
Upper-middle-income countries	4.3	1.5	1.3	0.7	3.5	1.0	2.9	0.5
High-income countries	6.6	0.9	6.7	0.9	8.9	1.1	6.8	0.5
All countries combined	4.9	0.6	4.8	0.6	6.7	0.7	5.0	0.3
Any treatment[h]								
Low/lower-middle-income countries	7.5	1.6	11.7	2.5	15.0	2.9	9.6	1.1
Upper-middle-income countries	14.9	1.9	17.0	2.6	19.7	2.5	16.0	1.0
High-income countries	29.6	1.7	28.2	1.7	42.0	2.0	30.1	0.8
All countries combined	21.1	1.1	22.8	1.3	32.5	1.5	23.1	0.6

A dash indicates low cell counts (<5).
[a]Highest severity category across four SDS role domains.
[b]The mental health specialist sector which includes psychiatrist and non-psychiatrist mental health specialists (psychiatrist, psychologist, or other non-psychiatrist mental health professional; social worker or counsellor in a mental health specialty setting; use of a mental health helpline; or overnight admissions for a mental health or drug or alcohol problems. with a presumption of daily contact with a psychiatrist).
[c]The general medical sector (general practitioner. other medical doctor. nurse. occupational therapist, or any healthcare professional).
[d]The mental health specialist sector or the general medical sector.
[e]The human services sector (religious or spiritual advisor or social worker or counsellor in any setting other than a specialty mental health setting).
[f]The CAM (complementary and alternative medicine) sector (any other type of healer such as herbalist or homeopath. participation in an internet support group. or participation in a self-help group).
[g]The human services sector or CAM.
[h]Any treatment listed above.

Table 11A.1 Bivariate associations between socio-demographic correlates and DSM-IV posttraumatic stress disorder (PTSD) (low/lower-middle-income countries)

Correlates	Exposure to TE[a,f]		Lifetime PTSD among exposed[a,f]		30-day PTSD[b]		Lifetime PTSD[a]		12-month PTSD among lifetime cases[c]		30-day PTSD among 12-month cases[c]	
	OR	(95% CI)	OR	(95% CI)	OR	(95% CI)	OR	(95% CI)	OR	(95% CI)	OR	(95% CI)
Age-cohort												
18–29	**1.9***	(1.6–2.2)	**0.8**	(0.4–1.6)	**0.2***	(0.1–0.4)	**4.1***	(2.0–8.3)				
30–44	**1.3***	(1.2–1.5)	**0.9**	(0.6–1.5)	**0.4***	(0.2–0.8)	**2.8***	(1.9–4.4)				
45–59	**1.0**	(0.9–1.2)	**0.9**	(0.5–1.7)	**0.5**	(0.2–1.1)	**1.6**	(1.0–2.5)				
60+	**1.0**		**1.0**		**1.0**		**1.0**					
Age-cohort difference[d]	$\chi^2_3 = 139.8^*$, $P < 0.001$		$\chi^2_3 = 0.4$, $P = 0.946$		$\chi^2_3 = 26.3^*$, $P < 0.001$		$\chi^2_3 = 23.0^*$, $P < 0.001$					
Age-of-onset												
Early									**2.3**	(0.7–7.8)	**0.4**	(0.1–1.8)
Early-average									**0.7**	(0.3–1.5)	**0.5**	(0.1–1.9)
Late-average									**0.8**	(0.3–1.8)	**0.5**	(0.2–1.3)
Late									**1.0**		**1.0**	
Age-of-onset difference[d]									$\chi^2_3 = 5.6$, $P = 0.134$		$\chi^2_3 = 2.9$, $P = 0.402$	
Time since onset (continuous)									**0.95***	(0.93–0.98)	**1.03**	(1.00–1.06)
Gender												
Female	**0.9***	(0.8–0.9)	**2.9***	(1.8–4.8)	**2.5***	(1.3–4.7)	**1.7***	(1.2–2.3)	**1.0**	(0.5–1.9)	**1.7**	(0.7–4.2)
Male	**1.0**		**1.0**		**1.0**		**1.0**		**1.0**		**1.0**	
Gender difference[d]	$\chi^2_1 = 20.3^*$, $P < 0.001$		$\chi^2_1 = 17.9^*$, $P < 0.001$		$\chi^2_1 = 7.4^*$, $P = 0.007$		$\chi^2_1 = 10.3^*$, $P < 0.001$		$\chi^2_1 = 0.0$, $P = 0.932$		$\chi^2_1 = 1.3$, $P = 0.264$	
Employment status												
Student	**0.8**	(0.7–1.0)	–	–	–	–	–	–	–	–	–	–
Homemaker	**0.8***	(0.7–0.9)	**1.6**	(0.7–3.3)	**2.2**	(0.9–5.4)	**1.1**	(0.7–1.9)	**0.9**	(0.3–2.1)	**4.4***	(1.1–18.0)
Retired	**1.0**	(0.8–1.2)	**1.9**	(0.9–3.7)	**1.7**	(0.8–3.8)	**1.1**	(0.6–2.0)	**1.4**	(0.5–4.1)	**1.7**	(0.3–10.7)
Other	**1.1**	(1.0–1.2)	**1.4**	(0.8–2.6)	**1.3**	(0.6–2.9)	**1.0**	(0.6–1.8)	**0.9**	(0.4–2.1)	**1.7**	(0.6–4.8)
Employed	**1.0**		**1.0**		**1.0**		**1.0**		**1.0**		**1.0**	
Employment status difference[d]	$\chi^2_4 = 15.0^*$, $P = 0.005$		$\chi^2_4 = 8.0$, $P = 0.093$		$\chi^2_4 = 307.0^*$, $P < 0.001$		$\chi^2_4 = 0.5$, $P = 0.969$		$\chi^2_4 = 4.8$, $P = 0.311$		$\chi^2_4 = 123.0^*$, $P < 0.001$	

Table 11A.1 *(cont.)*

Correlates	Exposure to TE[a,f]		Lifetime PTSD among exposed[a,f]		30-day PTSD[b]		Lifetime PTSD[a]		12-month PTSD among lifetime cases[c]		30-day PTSD among 12-month cases[c]	
	OR	(95% CI)	OR	(95% CI)	OR	(95% CI)	OR	(95% CI)	OR	(95% CI)	OR	(95% CI)
Marital status												
Never married	**1.0**	(0.9–1.1)	**1.9**	(0.7–5.1)	–	–	**1.5**	(0.7–3.1)	**1.5**	(0.6–4.2)	–	–
Divorced/separated/widowed	**1.1***	(1.0–1.3)	**1.7***	(1.1–2.6)	**1.3**	(0.7–2.6)	**1.3**	(0.9–1.9)	**1.7**	(0.8–3.4)	**0.4**	(0.1–1.1)
Currently married	**1.0**		**1.0**		**1.0**		**1.0**		**1.0**		**1.0**	
Marital status difference[d]	$\chi^2_2 = 4.3$, P = 0.117		$\chi^2_2 = 6.7^*$, P = 0.034		$\chi^2_2 = 5.7$, P = 0.058		$\chi^2_2 = 3.3$, P = 0.190		$\chi^2_2 = 2.6$, P = 0.275		$\chi^2_2 = 8.6^*$, P = 0.014	
Education level												
No education	**0.8**	(0.6–1.1)	–	–	**0.7**	(0.2–2.7)	**1.0**	(0.4–2.5)	**0.5**	(0.2–1.6)	**2.0**	(0.4–11.1)
Some primary	**1.0**	(0.9–1.2)	**1.9**	(1.0–3.5)	**3.6***	(1.2–10.4)	**1.5**	(0.9–2.7)	**1.1**	(0.4–3.2)	**13.6***	(2.4–76.5)
Finished primary	**1.1**	(1.0–1.3)	**1.8**	(1.0–3.4)	**1.3**	(0.4–4.4)	**1.4**	(0.8–2.3)	**0.9**	(0.3–2.6)	**2.1**	(0.4–10.0)
Some secondary	**1.0**	(0.9–1.2)	**1.1**	(0.6–2.3)	**1.9**	(0.7–4.8)	**1.5**	(0.9–2.3)	**0.8**	(0.3–2.0)	**2.9**	(0.8–10.6)
Finished secondary	**1.0**	(0.9–1.1)	**1.0**	(0.6–1.7)	**1.0**	(0.4–2.6)	**1.0**	(0.6–1.8)	**0.8**	(0.3–2.4)	**1.3**	(0.4–4.4)
Some college	**1.0**	(0.9–1.2)	**0.8**	(0.5–1.5)	**0.7**	(0.2–1.9)	**1.0**	(0.6–1.6)	**1.2**	(0.3–3.9)	**0.5**	(0.1–1.9)
Finished college	**1.0**		**1.0**		**1.0**		**1.0**		**1.0**		**1.0**	
Education level difference[d]	$\chi^2_6 = 6.4$, P = 0.383		$\chi^2_6 = 13.6^*$, P = 0.034		$\chi^2_6 = 17.1^*$, P = 0.009		$\chi^2_6 = 5.7$, P = 0.459		$\chi^2_6 = 2.3$, P = 0.894		$\chi^2_6 = 12.2$, P = 0.058	
Household income												
Low	**0.9**	(0.8–1.0)	**1.9**	(0.9–4.3)	**2.0**	(0.7–6.2)	**1.1**	(0.6–1.8)	**1.8**	(0.7–4.2)	**1.2**	(0.3–5.9)
Low-average	**0.9***	(0.8–0.9)	**2.5***	(1.4–4.4)	**2.9***	(1.1–7.4)	**1.4**	(0.9–2.3)	**1.6**	(0.7–3.4)	**1.5**	(0.5–5.1)
High-average	**0.9**	(0.9–1.0)	**1.6**	(0.9–2.8)	**1.8**	(0.8–4.1)	**1.1**	(0.7–1.6)	**1.3**	(0.6–2.8)	**1.4**	(0.5–4.0)
High	**1.0**		**1.0**		**1.0**		**1.0**		**1.0**		**1.0**	
Household income difference[d]	$\chi^2_3 = 10.6^*$, P = 0.014		$\chi^2_3 = 10.2^*$, P = 0.017		$\chi^2_3 = 5.1$, P = 0.167		$\chi^2_3 = 2.6$, P = 0.452		$\chi^2_3 = 2.1$, P = 0.549		$\chi^2_3 = 0.6$, P = 0.897	
N[e]	**153,510**		**157,483**		**11,862**		**467,383**		**394**		**198**	

*Significant at the 0.05 level, two-sided test.
A dash was inserted for small cell counts (<5).
[a]These estimates are based on survival models adjusted for age-cohorts, gender, person-years, and low/lower-middle-income countries.
[b]These estimates are based on logistic regression models adjusted for age, gender, and low/lower-middle-income countries.
[c]These estimates are based on logistic regression models adjusted for time since PTSD onset, age of PTSD onset, gender, and low/lower-middle-income countries.
[d]Chi square test of significant differences between blocks of socio-demographic variables.
[e]Denominator N: 11,862 = total sample; 153,510 , 157,483, and 467,383 = number of person-years in the survival models; 394 = number of lifetime PTSD cases; 198 = number of 12-month PTSD cases.
[f]Iraq is not included into the analysis related to exposure to traumatic events (TEs) because the age of first exposure to TEs is not available in Iraq.

Table 11A.2 Bivariate associations between socio-demographic correlates and posttraumatic stress disorder (PTSD) (upper-middle-income countries)

Correlates	Exposure to TE[a]		Lifetime PTSD among exposed[a]		30-day PTSD[b]		Lifetime PTSD[a]		12-month PTSD among lifetime cases[c]		30-day PTSD among 12-month cases[c]	
	OR	(95% CI)	OR	(95% CI)	OR	(95% CI)	OR	(95% CI)	OR	(95% CI)	OR	(95% CI)
Age-cohort												
18–29	**3.3***	(2.9–3.6)	**1.7***	(1.0–3.0)	**0.8**	(0.4–1.8)	**6.3***	(3.6–11.1)				
30–44	**2.3***	(2.1–2.6)	**1.4**	(0.8–2.4)	**0.9**	(0.5–1.5)	**4.1***	(2.4–7.0)				
45–59	**1.7***	(1.6–1.8)	**1.4**	(0.9–2.1)	**0.8**	(0.4–1.4)	**2.5***	(1.6–3.9)				
60+	**1.0**		**1.0**		**1.0**		**1.0**					
Age-cohort difference[d]	$\chi^2_3 = 524.9$*, P < 0.001		$\chi^2_3 = 4.5$, P = 0.208		$\chi^2_3 = 0.8$, P = 0.855		$\chi^2_3 = 43.6$*, P < 0.001					
Age-of-onset												
Early									**0.7**	(0.4–1.5)	**0.7**	(0.2–2.8)
Early-average									**0.7**	(0.4–1.2)	**1.5**	(0.6–3.7)
Late-average									**0.6**	(0.3–1.1)	**0.7**	(0.3–1.7)
Late									**1.0**		**1.0**	
Age-of-onset difference[d]									$\chi^2_3 = 3.3$, P = 0.345		$\chi^2_3 = 3.1$, P = 0.384	
Time since onset (continuous)									**0.96***	(0.93–0.98)	**0.99**	(0.96–1.02)
Gender												
Female	**0.9***	(0.8–0.9)	**2.7***	(1.9–3.6)	**3.4***	(1.7–6.7)	**2.4***	(1.8–3.3)	**0.9**	(0.6–1.5)	**1.1**	(0.5–2.5)
Male	**1.0**		**1.0**		**1.0**		**1.0**		**1.0**		**1.0**	
Gender difference[d]	$\chi^2_1 = 24.3$*, P < 0.001		$\chi^2_3 = 36.8$*, P < 0.001		$\chi^2_1 = 12.4$*, P < 0.001		$\chi^2_1 = 29.1$*, P < 0.001		$\chi^2_1 = 0.1$, P = 0.779		$\chi^2_1 = 0.1$, P = 0.808	
Employment status												
Student	**0.9**	(0.8–1.1)	**0.6**	(0.2–1.6)	–	–	–	–	–	–	–	–
Homemaker	**0.9***	(0.8–1.0)	**1.1**	(0.8–1.5)	**1.0**	(0.4–2.7)	**1.0**	(0.8–1.4)	**1.3**	(0.7–2.3)	**0.8**	(0.3–2.2)
Retired	**1.0**	(0.9–1.1)	**1.3**	(0.8–2.1)	**1.5**	(0.8–3.1)	**1.3**	(0.8–2.0)	**1.1**	(0.4–2.7)	**2.1**	(0.7–5.8)
Other	**1.1**	(1.0–1.1)	**1.4***	(1.0–2.0)	**1.7**	(1.0–3.1)	**1.5***	(1.1–2.1)	**1.3**	(0.8–2.3)	**1.4**	(0.6–3.4)
Employed	**1.0**		**1.0**		**1.0**		**1.0**		**1.0**		**1.0**	

Table 11A.2 *(cont.)*

Correlates	Exposure to TE[a]		Lifetime PTSD among exposed[a]		30-day PTSD[b]		Lifetime PTSD[a]		12-month PTSD among lifetime cases[c]		30-day PTSD among 12-month cases[c]	
	OR	(95% CI)	OR	(95% CI)	OR	(95% CI)	OR	(95% CI)	OR	(95% CI)	OR	(95% CI)
Employment status difference[d]	$\chi^2_4 = 12.4^*$, P = 0.015		$\chi^2_4 = 7.4$, P = 0.115		$\chi^2_4 = 774.8^*$, P < 0.001		$\chi^2_4 = 8.9$, P = 0.065		$\chi^2_4 = 4.8$, P = 0.308		$\chi^2_4 = 280.7^*$, P < 0.001	
Marital status												
Never married	**1.0**	(0.9–1.1)	**0.7**	(0.5–1.0)	**0.9**	(0.4–2.0)	**0.7**	(0.5–1.0)	**1.1**	(0.6–2.2)	**1.2**	(0.4–3.3)
Divorced/separated/widowed	**1.2***	(1.1–1.3)	**1.7***	(1.2–2.4)	**1.5**	(0.5–4.2)	**1.9***	(1.3–2.6)	**0.6**	(0.3–1.2)	**0.7**	(0.3–1.6)
Currently married	**1.0**		**1.0**		**1.0**		**1.0**		**1.0**		**1.0**	
Marital status difference[d]	$\chi^2_2 = 14.0^*$, P = 0.001		$\chi^2_2 = 13.8^*$, P = 0.001		$\chi^2_2 = 0.6$, P = 0.757		$\chi^2_2 = 17.0^*$, P < 0.001		$\chi^2_2 = 2.4$, P = 0.295		$\chi^2_2 = 0.8$, P = 0.688	
Education level												
No education	**0.9**	(0.8–1.1)	**1.4**	(0.8–2.4)	–	–	**1.4**	(0.8–2.4)	**0.6**	(0.2–2.4)	–	–
Some primary	**1.1**	(1.0–1.2)	**1.4**	(0.9–2.3)	**3.4***	(1.3–8.5)	**1.6**	(1.0–2.5)	**2.4**	(0.9–6.8)	**4.2**	(0.9–20.5)
Finished primary	**0.9**	(0.8–1.1)	**1.3**	(0.7–2.3)	**1.2**	(0.4–3.8)	**1.3**	(0.7–2.3)	**3.2**	(0.9–11.1)	**1.5**	(0.3–8.6)
Some secondary	**1.1**	(1.0–1.2)	**1.5**	(0.9–2.4)	**3.0***	(1.2–7.5)	**1.6**	(1.0–2.7)	**2.1**	(0.8–5.4)	**3.4**	(0.8–14.4)
Finished secondary	**1.1**	(1.0–1.2)	**1.4**	(0.9–2.3)	**2.7***	(1.0–7.0)	**1.5**	(1.0–2.5)	**1.4**	(0.5–3.9)	**2.5**	(0.7–10.0)
Some college	**1.2***	(1.0–1.3)	**1.4**	(0.9–2.3)	**1.6**	(0.5–5.4)	**1.7***	(1.1–2.8)	**2.4**	(0.8–7.5)	**1.4**	(0.3–8.2)
Finished college	**1.0**		**1.0**		**1.0**		**1.0**		**1.0**		**1.0**	
Education level difference[d]	$\chi^2_6 = 20.6^*$, P = 0.002		$\chi^2_6 = 3.2$, P = 0.781		$\chi^2_6 = 17.5^*$, P = 0.008		$\chi^2_6 = 6.5$, P = 0.368		$\chi^2_6 = 9.5$, P = 0.147		$\chi^2_6 = 6.6$, P = 0.362	
Household income												
Low	**0.9***	(0.8–1.0)	**1.5***	(1.1–2.0)	**1.2**	(0.6–2.6)	**1.4**	(1.0–1.9)	**0.9**	(0.5–1.6)	**1.1**	(0.4–2.7)
Low-average	**0.9**	(0.9–1.0)	**1.4**	(0.9–2.0)	**1.5**	(0.5–4.3)	**1.3**	(0.9–1.9)	**1.0**	(0.5–2.2)	**1.3**	(0.5–3.6)
High-average	**1.0**	(0.9–1.0)	**1.6***	(1.1–2.1)	**1.1**	(0.5–2.3)	**1.5***	(1.1–2.1)	**0.6**	(0.3–1.2)	**0.7**	(0.2–2.1)
High	**1.0**		**1.0**		**1.0**		**1.0**		**1.0**		**1.0**	
Household income difference[d]	$\chi^2_3 = 9.2^*$, P = 0.027		$\chi^2_3 = 8.2^*$, P = 0.043		$\chi^2_3 = 0.7$, P = 0.883		$\chi^2_3 = 7.2$, P = 0.066		$\chi^2_3 = 2.7$, P = 0.449		$\chi^2_3 = 1.4$, P = 0.709	
N[e]	**461,399**		**254,602**		**16,913**		**705,959**		**602**		**273**	

*Significant at the 0.05 level, two-sided test.
A dash was inserted for small cell counts (<5).
[a]These estimates are based on survival models adjusted for age-cohorts, gender, person-years, and upper-middle-income countries.
[b]These estimates are based on logistic regression models adjusted for age, gender, and upper-middle-income countries.
[c]These estimates are based on logistic regression models adjusted for time since PTSD onset, age of PTSD onset, gender, and upper-middle-income countries.
[d]Chi-square test of significant differences between blocks of socio-demographic variables.
[e]Denominator N: 16,913 = total sample; 461,399, 254,602, and 705,959 = number of person-years in the survival models; 602 = number of lifetime PTSD cases; 273 = number of 12-month PTSD cases.

Table 11A.3 Bivariate associations between socio-demographic correlates and posttraumatic stress disorder (PTSD) (high-income countries)

Correlates	Exposure to TE[a]		Lifetime PTSD among exposed[a]		30-day PTSD[b]		Lifetime PTSD[a]		12-month PTSD among lifetime cases[c]		30-day PTSD among 12-month cases[c]	
	OR	(95% CI)	OR	(95% CI)	OR	(95% CI)	OR	(95% CI)	OR	(95% CI)	OR	(95% CI)
Age-cohort												
18–29	**1.8***	(1.7–1.9)	**3.1***	(2.5–3.7)	**1.7***	(1.2–2.3)	**5.6***	(4.5–6.9)				
30–44	**1.5***	(1.4–1.6)	**2.4***	(2.0–2.8)	**2.1***	(1.5–2.8)	**4.3***	(3.6–5.1)				
45–59	**1.2***	(1.2–1.3)	**2.0***	(1.7–2.4)	**2.3***	(1.7–3.2)	**2.9***	(2.4–3.5)				
60+	**1.0**		**1.0**		**1.0**		**1.0**					
Age-cohort difference[d]	$\chi^2_3 = 621.7^*$, P < 0.001		$\chi^2_3 = 138.3^*$, P < 0.001		$\chi^2_3 = 34.2^*$, P < 0.001		$\chi^2_3 = 302.6^*$, P < 0.001					
Age-of-onset												
Early									**1.1**	(0.8–1.5)	**0.7**	(0.5–1.1)
Early-average									**0.7***	(0.6–1.0)	**0.6***	(0.4–0.9)
Late-average									**0.7***	(0.5–0.9)	**0.8**	(0.5–1.2)
Late									**1.0**		**1.0**	
Age-of-onset difference[d]									$\chi^2_3 = 17.7^*$, P = 0.001		$\chi^2_3 = 6.2$, P = 0.101	
Time since onset (continuous)									**0.98***	(0.97–0.98)	**1.00**	(0.99–1.02)
Gender												
Female	**0.9***	(0.8–0.9)	**2.6***	(2.3–2.9)	**2.2***	(1.7–2.9)	**2.4***	(2.1–2.7)	**1.1**	(0.8–1.3)	**0.9**	(0.6–1.2)
Male	**1.0**		**1.0**		**1.0**		**1.0**		**1.0**		**1.0**	
Gender difference[d]	$\chi^2_1 = 95.9^*$, P < 0.001		$\chi^2_1 = 262.2^*$, P < 0.001		$\chi^2_1 = 38.6^*$, P < 0.001		$\chi^2_1 = 205.4^*$, P < 0.001		$\chi^2_1 = 0.2$, P = 0.672		$\chi^2_1 = 1.0$, P = 0.328	
Employment status												
Student	**1.0**	(0.9–1.1)	**1.0**	(0.7–1.4)	**1.3**	(0.7–2.5)	**1.0**	(0.8–1.4)	**1.4**	(0.8–2.5)	**1.7**	(0.8–3.8)
Homemaker	**0.9**	(0.9–1.0)	**1.3***	(1.1–1.5)	**1.6***	(1.1–2.1)	**1.2***	(1.0–1.4)	**1.4**	(1.0–1.9)	**1.1**	(0.7–1.6)
Retired	**1.0**	(0.9–1.1)	**1.4***	(1.1–1.7)	**1.0**	(0.6–1.5)	**1.2**	(1.0–1.6)	**1.1**	(0.8–1.7)	**1.4**	(0.9–2.4)
Other	**1.2***	(1.1–1.2)	**2.0***	(1.8–2.4)	**3.4***	(2.6–4.4)	**2.4***	(2.0–2.7)	**1.8***	(1.3–2.4)	**1.4**	(0.9–2.1)
Employed	**1.0**		**1.0**		**1.0**		**1.0**		**1.0**		**1.0**	
Employment status difference[d]	$\chi^2_4 = 29.4^*$, P < 0.001		$\chi^2_4 = 98.2^*$, P < 0.001		$\chi^2_4 = 88.8^*$, P < 0.001		$\chi^2_4 = 143.4^*$, P < 0.001		$\chi^2_4 = 15.5^*$, P = 0.004		$\chi^2_4 = 5.2$, P = 0.271	

Table 11A.3 *(cont.)*

Correlates	Exposure to TE[a]		Lifetime PTSD among exposed[a]		30-day PTSD[b]		Lifetime PTSD[a]		12-month PTSD among lifetime cases[c]		30-day PTSD among 12-month cases[c]	
	OR	(95% CI)	OR	(95% CI)	OR	(95% CI)	OR	(95% CI)	OR	(95% CI)	OR	(95% CI)
Marital status												
Never married	**1.0**	(1.0–1.1)	**1.4***	(1.2–1.6)	**1.0**	(0.8–1.3)	**1.4***	(1.2–1.7)	**1.1**	(0.8–1.4)	**0.9**	(0.6–1.3)
Divorced/separated/widowed	**1.2***	(1.1–1.2)	**1.6***	(1.4–1.8)	**2.1***	(1.6–2.8)	**1.8***	(1.6–2.1)	**1.4***	(1.1–1.7)	**1.0**	(0.7–1.4)
Currently married	**1.0**		**1.0**		**1.0**		**1.0**		**1.0**		**1.0**	
Marital status difference[d]	$\chi^2_2 = 35.1$, P < 0.001		$\chi^2_2 = 54.2$*, P < 0.001		$\chi^2_2 = 29.0$*, P < 0.001		$\chi^2_2 = 80.1$*, P < 0.001		$\chi^2_2 = 5.8$, P = 0.055		$\chi^2_2 = 0.6$, P = 0.756	
Education level												
No education	**0.7***	(0.6–0.9)	**1.4**	(0.7–2.9)	–	–	**1.4**	(0.7–2.6)	–	–	–	–
Some primary	**0.8***	(0.8–0.9)	**1.7***	(1.3–2.2)	**1.2**	(0.7–2.0)	**1.5***	(1.2–2.0)	**1.0**	(0.5–1.7)	**0.8**	(0.4–1.5)
Finished primary	**0.9***	(0.8–0.9)	**2.0***	(1.5–2.7)	**1.4**	(0.8–2.5)	**1.8***	(1.3–2.5)	**1.3**	(0.8–2.2)	**0.7**	(0.3–1.5)
Some secondary	**1.0**	(0.9–1.0)	**1.5***	(1.3–1.8)	**1.3**	(0.9–1.8)	**1.5***	(1.2–1.8)	**0.9**	(0.7–1.3)	**1.0**	(0.6–1.6)
Finished secondary	**1.0**	(0.9–1.0)	**1.1**	(0.9–1.2)	**1.1**	(0.8–1.5)	**1.1**	(0.9–1.2)	**1.2**	(0.9–1.7)	**1.0**	(0.6–1.6)
Some college	**1.0**	(1.0–1.1)	**1.1**	(0.9–1.3)	**1.1**	(0.8–1.6)	**1.1**	(0.9–1.3)	**1.1**	(0.8–1.6)	**1.1**	(0.7–1.6)
Finished college	**1.0**		**1.0**		**1.0**		**1.0**		**1.0**		**1.0**	
Education level difference[d]	$\chi^2_6 = 40.4$*, P < 0.001		$\chi^2_6 = 47.9$*, P < 0.001		$\chi^2_6 = 6.5$, P = 0.374		$\chi^2_6 = 36.4$*, P < 0.001		$\chi^2_6 = 5.3$, P = 0.507		$\chi^2_6 = 5.8$, P = 0.444	
Household income												
Low	**1.0**	(0.9–1.0)	**1.7***	(1.5–2.0)	**2.2***	(1.6–2.8)	**1.7***	(1.5–2.0)	**1.6***	(1.2–2.1)	**1.2**	(0.8–1.8)
Low-average	**1.0**	(0.9–1.0)	**1.4***	(1.2–1.7)	**1.8***	(1.3–2.5)	**1.4***	(1.2–1.7)	**1.3**	(0.9–1.7)	**1.5**	(1.0–2.2)
High-average	**1.0**	(0.9–1.0)	**1.4***	(1.2–1.6)	**1.4**	(1.0–1.9)	**1.4***	(1.2–1.6)	**1.0**	(0.8–1.4)	**1.0**	(0.7–1.5)
High	**1.0**		**1.0**		**1.0**		**1.0**		**1.0**		**1.0**	
Household income difference[d]	$\chi^2_3 = 2.3$, P = 0.507		$\chi^2_3 = 48.2$*, P < 0.001		$\chi^2_3 = 34.4$*, P < 0.001		$\chi^2_3 = 49.6$, P < 0.001		$\chi^2_3 = 14.6$*, P = 0.002		$\chi^2_3 = 4.7$, P = 0.196	
N[e]	**1,031,399**		**897,923**		**42,280**		**1,897,969**		**3,078**		**1,600**	

*Significant at the 0.05 level, two-sided test.
A dash was inserted for small cell counts (<5).
[a]These estimates are based on survival models adjusted for age-cohorts, gender, person-years, and high-income countries.
[b]These estimates are based on logistic regression models adjusted for age, gender, and high-income countries.
[c]These estimates are based on logistic regression models adjusted for time since PTSD onset, age of PTSD onset, gender, and high-income countries.
[d]Chi-square test of significant differences between blocks of socio-demographic variables.
[e]Denominator N: 42,280 = total sample; 1,031,399, 897,923, and 1,897,969 = number of person-years in the survival models; 3,078 = number of lifetime PTSD cases; 1,600 = number of 12-month PTSD cases.

Table 12A.1 Among those with 12-month adult separation anxiety disorder, percent reporting treatment in the past 12 months by Sheehan impairment severity

Sector of treatment	Sheehan Disability Scale category[a]														
	No impairment (score: 0)			Mild impairment (score: 1–3)			Moderate impairment (score: 4–6)			Severe impairment (score: 7–10)			Any impairment		
	%	SE	Comparison between country income groups[b]	%	SE	Comparison between country income groups[b]	%	SE	Comparison between country income groups[b]	%	SE	Comparison between country income groups[b]	%	SE	Comparison between country income groups[b]
Specialty mental health[c]															
Low/lower-middle-income countries	–	–	$F_{2,v} = 3.6^*$, $P = 0.03$	–	–	–	**18.7**	9.3	$F_{2,v} = 0.7$, $P = 0.48$	–	–	$F_{2,v} = 6.2^*$, $P < 0.001$	**7.5**	3.2	$F_{2,v} = 8.1^*$, $P < 0.001$
Upper-middle-income countries	**7.2**	3.6		–	–		**18.7**	5.2		**17.0**	5.8		**14.3**	3.4	
High-income countries	**10.8**	4.9		**33.2**	12.9		**27.9**	6.3		**33.6**	5.6		**26.6**	3.3	
All countries combined	**6.3**	2.2		**18.1**	6.4		**22.0**	3.9		**23.8**	3.7		**17.9**	2.0	
General medical[d]															
Low/lower-middle-income countries	–	–	–	–	–	–	–	–	$F_{2,v} = 4.0^*$, $P = 0.02$	–	–	$F_{2,v} = 5.2^*$, $P = 0.01$	**4.1**	1.7	$F_{2,v} = 13.8^*$, $P < 0.001$
Upper-middle-income countries	–	–		–	–		**14.9**	6.8		**20.7**	5.4		**12.5**	2.8	
High-income countries	**18.8**	6.4		**27.6**	11.6		**22.4**	6.1		**26.8**	4.8		**24.2**	3.0	
All countries combined	**7.5**	2.3		**15.0**	5.8		**14.3**	3.6		**21.9**	3.2		**15.5**	1.7	
Any health care[e]															
Low/lower-middle-income countries	–	–	$F_{2,v} = 2.7$, $P = 0.07$	–	–	–	**20.1**	9.5	$F_{2,v} = 1.2$, $P = 0.32$	–	–	$F_{2,v} = 7.5^*$, $P < 0.001$	**11.7**	3.4	$F_{2,v} = 12.6^*$, $P < 0.001$
Upper-middle-income countries	**9.8**	4.4		–	–		**27.4**	6.7		**31.4**	6.4		**22.5**	3.7	
High-income countries	**21.5**	7.3		**40.7**	14.1		**39.8**	8.4		**49.2**	6.0		**40.8**	4.0	
All countries combined	**11.5**	3.0		**21.5**	6.8		**30.1**	4.9		**37.7**	4.0		**27.7**	2.4	
Human services[f]															
Low/lower-middle-income countries	–	–	–	–	–	–	–	–	–	–	–	–	–	–	–
Upper-middle-income countries	–	–		–	–		–	–		–	–		–	–	
High-income countries	–	–		–	–		**9.4**	4.2		**10.0**	3.4		**7.9**	1.8	
All countries combined	–	–		–	–		**7.7**	2.7		**5.7**	1.8		**4.8**	1.0	
CAM[g]															
Low/lower-middle-income countries	–	–	–	–	–	–	–	–	–	–	–	–	**3.9**	1.1	$F_{2,v} = 2.2$, $P = 0.12$
Upper-middle-income countries	–	–		–	–		–	–		–	–		**2.4**	1.4	
High-income countries	–	–		–	–		–	–		**10.1**	3.3		**6.5**	1.5	
All countries combined	–	–		–	–		**3.3**	1.1		**7.9**	2.3		**4.3**	0.8	

Table 12A.1 *(cont.)*

Sector of treatment	Sheehan Disability Scale category[a]														
	No impairment (score: 0)			Mild impairment (score: 1–3)			Moderate impairment (score: 4–6)			Severe impairment (score: 7–10)			Any impairment		
	%	SE	Comparison between country income groups[b]	%	SE	Comparison between country income groups[b]	%	SE	Comparison between country income groups[b]	%	SE	Comparison between country income groups[b]	%	SE	Comparison between country income groups[b]
Any non-health care[h]															
Low/lower-middle-income countries	–	–	–	–	–	–	**20.1**	10.2	$F_{2,v} = 3.1^*$, $P = 0.05$	–	–	–	**9.2**	3.7	$F_{2,v} = 5.0^*$, $P = 0.01$
Upper-middle-income countries	–	–		–	–		–	–		–	–		**3.6**	1.6	
High-income countries	–	–		–	–		**11.6**	4.6		**15.8**	3.8		**12.1**	2.2	
All countries combined	–	–		–	–		**10.1**	3.0		**11.6**	2.5		**8.0**	1.3	
Any treatment[i]															
Low/lower-middle-income countries	–	–	$F_{2,v} = 2.7$, $P = 0.07$	–	–	–	**32.0**	12.8	$F_{2,v} = 11.1$, $P = 0.34$	**15.8**	5.7	$F_{2,v} = 6.8^*$, $P < 0.001$	**17.6**	4.3	$F_{2,v} = 10.3^*$, $P < 0.001$
Upper-middle-income countries	**9.8**	4.4		–	–		**28.8**	6.7		**33.5**	6.6		**23.8**	3.8	
High-income countries	**21.5**	7.3		**40.7**	14.1		**45.1**	8.8		**54.6**	6.1		**44.5**	4.1	
All countries combined	**11.5**	3.0		**23.1**	7.0		**35.5**	5.4		**41.9**	4.1		**30.9**	2.5	

*Significant at the 0.05 level, two-sided test.
A dash indicates low cell counts (<5 cases).
[a]Highest severity category across four SDS role domains.
[b]Wald design-corrected F-tests were used to determine if there is variation in treatment estimates across country income groups. The denominator degree of freedom, v, is 887. Wald test is only generated where there is more than one stable cell (≥5 cases) for each combination of treatment sector and Sheehan impairment.
[c]The mental health specialist sector, which includes psychiatrist and non-psychiatrist mental health specialists (psychiatrist, psychologist, or other non-psychiatrist mental health professional; social worker or counsellor in a mental health specialty setting; use of a mental health helpline; or overnight admissions for a mental health or drug or alcohol problems, with a presumption of daily contact with a psychiatrist).
[d]The general medical sector (general practitioner, other medical doctor, nurse, occupational therapist, or any healthcare professional).
[e]The mental health specialist sector or the general medical sector.
[f]The human services sector (religious or spiritual advisor or social worker or counsellor in any setting other than a specialty mental health setting).
[g]The CAM (complementary and alternative medicine) sector (any other type of healer such as herbalist or homeopath, participation in an internet support group, or participation in a self-help group).
[h]The human services sector or CAM.
[i]Any treatment listed above..

Table 13A.1 Age at selected percentiles on the standardized age-of-onset distributions of DSM-IV intermittent explosive disorder (IED) with projected lifetime risk at age 75

Country	Ages at selected percentiles								Lifetime prevalence of IED		Projected risk at age 75	
	5	10	25	50	75	90	95	99	%	SE	%	SE
Low/lower-middle-income countries	**7**	**9**	**14**	**18**	**31**	**51**	**61**	**61**	**0.6**	**0.1**	**0.8**	**0.1**
Colombia[a]	7	10	16	21	51	61	61	61	1.2	0.2	1.7	0.4
Iraq	13	13	13	14	23	26	30	31	0.4	0.2	0.4	0.2
Nigeria	5	5	16	19	19	19	19	19	0.0	0.0	0.0	0.0
Peru[a]	6	10	17	27	38	48	48	48	0.6	0.2	0.9	0.3
PRC (Beijing/Shanghai)	8	8	13	14	19	31	41	41	0.5	0.1	0.5	0.1
PRC (Shenzhen)	5	6	9	14	19	29	34	36	0.7	0.1	0.8	0.2
Ukraine	10	12	14	18	27	51	61	61	1.1	0.2	1.3	0.2
Upper-middle-income countries	**9**	**10**	**16**	**19**	**26**	**40**	**47**	**56**	**0.7**	**0.1**	**0.8**	**0.1**
Brazil	8	13	16	19	24	43	47	47	0.7	0.1	0.8	0.1
Bulgaria	6	6	9	13	28	36	36	55	0.2	0.1	0.3	0.1
Lebanon	14	14	17	19	21	23	31	31	0.6	0.1	0.7	0.2
Romania	11	11	14	24	31	45	46	46	0.5	0.2	0.6	0.2
South Africa	10	10	18	22	40	56	56	57	1.2	0.3	1.7	0.5
High-income countries	**6**	**8**	**11**	**16**	**20**	**29**	**37**	**53**	**1.1**	**0.1**	**1.2**	**0.1**
Japan	10	14	15	18	27	41	54	54	0.4	0.1	0.5	0.1
Northern Ireland	6	8	12	17	26	31	35	41	1.1	0.2	1.3	0.2
Poland[b]	13	15	16	21	26	31	36	36	0.2	0.0	0.2	0.1
Portugal	7	14	14	18	37	49	53	53	0.5	0.1	0.7	0.2
United States	6	8	11	14	18	23	28	40	2.7	0.2	3.0	0.2
All countries combined	**7**	**9**	**13**	**17**	**23**	**38**	**49**	**61**	**0.8**	**0.0**	**0.9**	**0.0**
WHO regions												
Region of the Americas	6	8	12	16	21	33	43	61	1.6	0.1	1.8	0.1
African region	10	10	18	21	40	56	56	57	0.5	0.1	0.7	0.2
Western Pacific region	6	8	13	15	19	37	41	54	0.6	0.1	0.6	0.1
Eastern Mediterranean region	13	13	14	17	23	26	30	31	0.5	0.1	0.5	0.1
Western European region	6	8	13	18	29	37	41	53	0.9	0.1	1.0	0.1
Eastern European region	9	11	14	19	28	50	55	61	0.4	0.0	0.5	0.1

[a]The projected risk for these countries is at age 65 because the age range of these surveys is between 18 and 65.
[b]The projected risk for this country is at age 64 because the age range of this survey is between 18 and 64.
PRC: People's Republic of China.

Table 13A.2 Severity of role impairment (Sheehan Disability Scale) associated with 12-month intermittent explosive disorder (IED), by country

Country	Proportion with severe role impairment (SDS score: 7–10)										Number of 12-month IED cases
	Home		Work		Relationship		Social		Any[a]		
	%	SE	%	SE	%	SE	%	SE	%	SE	
Low/lower-middle-income countries	**20.5**	**3.9**	**15.7**	**3.6**	**22.8**	**4.2**	**24.6**	**4.4**	**36.5**	**4.9**	**131**
Colombia	7.3	4.3	19.0	10.4	32.2	11.0	44.0	12.7	46.1	12.9	23
Iraq	28.4	15.8	20.7	12.5	22.6	14.0	29.0	15.3	31.7	15.9	16
Nigeria	–	–	–	–	–	–	–	–	–	–	2
Peru	35.9	11.9	40.8	14.0	23.7	12.5	27.7	14.3	49.6	12.5	9
PRC (Beijing/Shanghai)	–	–	–	–	–	–	–	–	–	–	14
PRC (Shenzhen)	13.6	6.9	1.7	1.7	10.0	6.0	18.9	7.7	23.9	8.1	41
Ukraine	36.6	9.0	30.2	9.3	45.5	10.3	20.9	9.1	56.6	11.0	26
Upper-middle-income countries	**10.4**	**4.1**	**19.0**	**7.1**	**15.4**	**5.1**	**18.9**	**6.0**	**26.7**	**7.8**	**55**
Brazil	9.0	6.4	36.1	15.2	19.4	10.1	19.4	10.1	44.1	15.8	17
Bulgaria	–	–	–	–	–	–	–	–	–	–	7
Lebanon	–	–	–	–	–	–	–	–	–	–	9
Romania	–	–	–	–	–	–	–	–	–	–	6
South Africa	13.8	8.4	17.7	9.6	17.1	9.2	27.8	14.1	29.2	14.4	16
High-income countries	**19.2**	**3.4**	**13.5**	**2.8**	**30.2**	**4.8**	**27.6**	**4.0**	**44.7**	**3.8**	**171**
Japan	–	–	–	–	–	–	–	–	–	–	11
Northern Ireland	19.1	13.4	9.3	6.7	15.1	8.3	8.0	5.8	26.4	12.7	13
Poland	–	–	–	–	–	–	–	–	–	–	9
Portugal	8.1	7.7	8.1	7.7	26.4	15.6	36.5	15.9	36.5	15.9	10
United States	21.8	4.0	14.9	3.5	33.7	6.1	30.9	4.9	50.1	4.4	128

(cont.)

Table 13A.2 (*cont.*)

Country	Proportion with severe role impairment (SDS score: 7–10)										Number of 12-month IED cases
	Home		Work		Relationship		Social		Any[a]		
	%	SE	%	SE	%	SE	%	SE	%	SE	
All countries combined	**18.3**	**2.3**	**15.1**	**2.2**	**25.1**	**2.9**	**25.1**	**2.7**	**38.9**	**2.9**	**357**
WHO regions											
Region of the Americas	19.5	3.2	18.6	3.5	31.6	4.8	31.1	4.1	49.0	3.9	177
African region	13.4	8.1	17.1	9.2	19.5	9.7	30.0	14.3	31.3	14.5	18
Western Pacific region	12.0	5.1	3.4	2.0	9.4	4.5	14.9	5.6	23.9	6.2	66
Eastern Mediterranean region	24.8	11.9	15.5	9.0	23.3	11.5	27.7	12.1	29.5	12.4	25
Western European region	14.3	8.4	8.8	5.0	19.4	8.3	19.4	8.6	30.2	10.2	23
Eastern European region	23.7	6.4	19.9	6.1	27.5	7.5	13.4	5.4	32.8	8.0	48
Comparison between countries[b]	**$F_{16,v} = 1.3$, P = 0.157**		**$F_{16,v} = 1.4$, P = 0.131**		**$F_{16,v} = 1.6$, P = 0.070**		**$F_{16,v} = 1.3$, P = 0.210**		**$F_{16,v} = 1.8$*, P = 0.022**		
Comparison between low-, middle-, and high-income countries[b]	**$F_{2,v} = 1.6$, P = 0.207**		**$F_{2,v} = 0.3$, P = 0.734**		**$F_{2,v} = 1.9$, P = 0.149**		**$F_{2,v} = 0.6$, P = 0.530**		**$F_{2,v} = 2.2$, P = 0.114**		
Comparison between WHO regions[b]	**$F_{5,v} = 0.7$, P = 0.657**		**$F_{5,v} = 2.9$*, P = 0.013**		**$F_{5,v} = 2.5$*, P = 0.028**		**$F_{5,v} = 1.9$, P = 0.098**		**$F_{5,v} = 2.8$*, P = 0.016**		

*Significant at the 0.05 level, two-sided test.
[a]Highest severity category across four SDS role domains.
[b]Wald design-corrected F-tests were used to determine if there is variation in impairment severity across countries. The denominator degree of freedom, v, is 770.

Table 13A.3 Among those with 12-month intermittent explosive disorder, percent reporting treatment in the past 12 months by Sheehan impairment severity

Sector of treatment	Sheehan Disability Scale category[a]											
	Mild impairment (score: 1–3)			Moderate impairment (score: 4–6)			Severe impairment (score: 7–10)			Any impairment		
	%	SE	Comparison between country income groups[b]	%	SE	Comparison between country income groups[b]	%	SE	Comparison between country income groups[b]	%	SE	Comparison between country income groups[b]
Specialty mental health[c]												
Low/lower-middle-income countries	6.1	3.6	$F_{2,v} = 6.5^*$, $P < 0.001$	6.0	2.6	$F_{2,v} = 3.4^*$, $P = 0.03$	6.9	3.1	$F_{2,v} = 2.5$, $P = 0.08$	4.5	1.3	$F_{2,v} = 13.6^*$, $P < 0.001$
Upper-middle-income countries	–	–		–	–		14.8	5.9		10.7	3.3	
High-income countries	18.1	4.2		19.2	4.0		17.4	3.6		17.1	1.9	
All countries combined	10.3	2.5		11.9	2.4		13.7	2.3		10.6	1.1	
General medical[d]												
Low/lower-middle-income countries	–	–	–	–	–	$F_{2,v} = 7.1^*$, $P < 0.001$	10.0	4.0	$F_{2,v} = 3.4^*$, $P = 0.03$	5.7	1.5	$F_{2,v} = 9.0^*$, $P < 0.001$
Upper-middle-income countries	–	–		13.0	4.9		13.5	4.9		11.1	2.3	
High-income countries	15.6	4.7		14.8	3.9		25.1	4.5		17.5	2.4	
All countries combined	11.3	2.9		8.9	1.8		18.3	2.7		11.3	1.2	
Any health care[e]												
Low/lower-middle-income countries	10.4	4.7	$F_{2,v} = 2.6$, $P = 0.08$	6.5	2.7	$F_{2,v} = 6.8^*$, $P < 0.001$	15.8	5.0	$F_{2,v} = 3.9^*$, $P = 0.02$	9.0	1.8	$F_{2,v} = 17.5^*$, $P < 0.001$
Upper-middle-income countries	–	–		21.1	7.3		22.3	6.8		19.7	3.6	
High-income countries	24.3	4.8		25.6	4.3		35.1	4.9		27.4	2.4	
All countries combined	16.2	3.1		16.6	2.6		26.9	3.2		18.2	1.4	
Human services[f]												
Low/lower-middle-income countries	–	–	–	–	–	–	–	–	–	2.5	1.2	$F_{2,v} = 2.5$, $P = 0.08$
Upper-middle-income countries	–	–		–	–		–	–		–	–	
High-income countries	–	–		3.7	1.8		9.6	3.7		5.9	1.7	
All countries combined	3.0	1.5		3.0	1.0		5.9	2.0		3.7	0.9	
CAM[g]												
Low/lower-middle-income countries	–	–	–	–	–	–	–	–	–	1.0	0.5	$F_{2,v} = 3.7^*$, $P = 0.03$
Upper-middle-income countries	–	–		–	–		–	–		–	–	
High-income countries	–	–		–	–		6.0	2.3		4.5	1.2	
All countries combined	3.6	1.6		2.4	0.9		3.6	1.2		2.5	0.6	

Table 13A.3 (*cont.*)

Sector of treatment	Sheehan Disability Scale category[a]											
	Mild impairment (score: 1–3)			Moderate impairment (score: 4–6)			Severe impairment (score: 7–10)			Any impairment		
	%	SE	Comparison between country income groups[b]	%	SE	Comparison between country income groups[b]	%	SE	Comparison between country income groups[b]	%	SE	Comparison between country income groups[b]
Any non-health care[h]												
Low/lower-middle-income countries	–	–	–	–	–	–	–	–	–	**3.0**	1.2	$F_{2,v}=5.1^*$, $P=0.01$
Upper-middle-income countries	–	–		–	–	–	–	–	–			
High-income countries	**7.4**	3.3		**6.6**	2.3		**15.1**	4.2		**9.4**	2.1	
All countries combined	**4.2**	1.6		**4.4**	1.2		**9.2**	2.3		**5.4**	1.0	
Any treatment[i]												
Low/lower-middle-income countries	**12.7**	4.9	$F_{2,v}=2.6$, $P=0.08$	**7.6**	2.8	$F_{2,v}=8.4^*$, $P<0.001$	**17.4**	5.2	$F_{2,v}=5.1^*$, $P=0.01$	**11.3**	2.1	$F_{2,v}=16.3^*$, $P<0.001$
Upper-middle-income countries	–	–		**21.1**	7.3		**22.3**	6.8		**19.7**	3.6	
High-income countries	**25.8**	4.7		**29.3**	4.1		**41.4**	5.7		**31.2**	2.8	
All countries combined	**17.9**	3.1		**18.6**	2.5		**30.5**	3.5		**20.7**	1.6	

*Significant at the 0.05 level, two-sided test.
A dash was inserted for low cell counts (<5 cases).
[a]Highest severity category across four SDS role domains.
[b]Wald design-corrected F-tests were used to determine if there is variation in treatment estimates across country income groups. The denominator degree of freedom, v, is 770. Wald test is only generated where there is more than one stable cell (≥5 cases) for each combination of treatment sector and Sheehan impairment.
[c]The mental health specialist sector, which includes psychiatrist and non-psychiatrist mental health specialists (psychiatrist, psychologist, or other non-psychiatrist mental health professional; social worker or counsellor in a mental health specialty setting; use of a mental health helpline; or overnight admissions for a mental health or drug or alcohol problems, with a presumption of daily contact with a psychiatrist).
[d]The general medical sector (general practitioner, other medical doctor, nurse, occupational therapist or any healthcare professional).
[e]The mental health specialist sector or the general medical sector.
[f]The human services sector (religious or spiritual advisor or social worker or counsellor in any setting other than a specialty mental health setting).
[g]The CAM (complementary and alternative medicine) sector (any other type of healer such as herbalist or homeopath, participation in an internet support group, or participation in a self-help group).
[h]The human services sector or CAM.
[i]Any treatment listed above.

Table 15A.1 Bivariate associations between socio-demographic correlates and DSM-IV oppositional defiant disorder (ODD) (low/lower-middle-income countries)

Correlates	Lifetime ODD[a]		12-month ODD among lifetime cases[b]	
	OR	(95% CI)	OR	(95% CI)
Age-cohort				
18–24	**2.3***	(1.3–4.3)		
25–34	**1.1**	(0.6–2.0)		
35+	**1.0**			
Age-cohort difference[c]	$\chi^2_3 = 11.2^*, P = 0.004$			
Age-of-onset				
Early			–	–
Early-average			–	–
Late-average			–	–
Late			–	
Age-of-onset difference[c]				
Time since onset (continuous)			**0.91***	(0.84–0.98)
Gender				
Female	**0.5***	(0.3–0.8)	**1.5**	(0.5–4.8)
Male	**1.0**		**1.0**	
Gender difference[c]	$\chi^2_1 = 9.0^*, P = 0.003$		$\chi^2_1 = 0.4, P = 0.509$	
Employment status				
Student	**0.8**	(0.4–1.6)	–	–
Homemaker	**1.0**	(0.6–1.9)	–	–
Retired	–	–	–	–
Other	**1.9***	(1.1–3.5)	**3.3**	(0.7–15.3)
Employed	**1.0**		**1.0**	
Employment status difference[c]	$\chi^2_4 = 647.8^*, P < 0.001$		–	
Marital status				
Never married	**1.3**	(0.7–2.5)	**4.4***	(1.3–14.8)
Divorced/separated/widowed	**0.8**	(0.3–2.1)	–	–
Currently married	**1.0**		**1.0**	
Marital status difference[d]	$\chi^2_2 = 1.2, P = 0.555$		–	
Education level				
No education	–	–	–	–
Some primary	**1.2**	(0.4–4.1)	–	–
Finished primary	**1.8**	(0.6–5.4)	–	–
Some secondary	**1.9**	(0.8–4.4)	–	–
Finished secondary	**1.4**	(0.6–3.3)	–	–
Some college	**1.0**	(0.4–2.5)	–	–
Finished college	**1.0**		–	
Education level difference[c]	$\chi^2_6 = 1045.7^*, P < 0.001$		–	
Household income				
Low	**0.6***	(0.3–1.0)	–	–
Low-average	**0.8**	(0.5–1.4)	–	–
High-average	**1.0**	(0.6–1.7)	–	–
High	**1.0**		–	
Household income difference[c]	$\chi^2_3 = 5.3, P = 0.150$		–	
N[d]	**89,254**		**133**	

*Significant at the 0.05 level, two-sided test.
[a]These estimates are based on survival models adjusted for age-cohorts, gender, person-years, and low/lower-middle-income countries.
[b]These estimates are based on logistic regression models adjusted for time since ODD onset, age of ODD onset, gender, and low/lower-middle-income countries.
[c]Chi-square test of significant differences between blocks of socio-demographic variables.
[d]Denominator N: 89,254 = number of person-years in the survival models; 133 = number of lifetime ODD.

Table 15A.2 Bivariate associations between socio-demographic correlates and DSM-IV oppositional defiant disorder (ODD) (upper-middle-income countries)

Correlates	Lifetime ODD[a]		12-month ODD among lifetime cases[b]	
	OR	(95% CI)	OR	(95% CI)
Age-cohort				
18–24	**2.6***	(1.7–4.1)		
25–34	**1.6***	(1.1–2.2)		
35+	**1.0**			
Age-cohort difference[c]	$\chi^2_3 = 17.3^*, P < 0.001$			
Age-of-onset				
Early			**5.8***	(1.3–26.5)
Early-average			**1.9**	(0.5–6.9)
Late-average			**1.5**	(0.4–5.5)
Late			**1.0**	
Age-of-onset difference[c]			$\chi^2_3 = 8.3^*, P = 0.040$	
Time since onset (continuous)			**0.98**	(0.96–1.01)
Gender				
Female	**0.7**	(0.5–1.0)	**0.9**	(0.5–1.8)
Male	**1.0**		**1.0**	
Gender difference[c]	$\chi^2_1 = 3.8, P = 0.052$		$\chi^2_1 = 0.1, P = 0.788$	
Employment status				
Student	**1.7**	(0.8–3.8)	**2.0**	(0.4–9.2)
Homemaker	**1.5**	(0.9–2.6)	**1.1**	(0.4–3.4)
Retired	**1.8**	(0.5–6.1)	–	–
Other	**1.2**	(0.8–1.9)	**2.5***	(1.1–6.1)
Employed	**1.0**		**1.0**	
Employment status difference[c]	$\chi^2_4 = 4.5, P = 0.348$		$\chi^2_4 = 316.9^*, P < 0.001$	
Marital status				
Never married	**1.3**	(0.8–1.8)	**1.3**	(0.7–2.4)
Divorced/separated/widowed	**1.9**	(1.0–3.7)	**1.2**	(0.4–3.7)
Currently married	**1.0**		**1.0**	
Marital status difference[c]	$\chi^2_2 = 4.3, P = 0.117$		$\chi^2_2 = 0.6, P = 0.740$	
Education level				
Some primary	**2.0**	(0.8–5.0)	**2.0**	(0.8–5.2)
Finished primary	**1.9**	(0.8–4.7)	**4.0***	(1.1–15.6)
Some secondary	**2.4***	(1.0–5.9)	**0.8**	(0.2–3.3)
Finished secondary	**1.2**	(0.5–2.5)	**1.5**	(0.3–7.4)
Some college	**2.4***	(1.1–5.6)	**1.7**	(0.4–7.9)
Finished college	**1.0**		**1.0**	
Education level difference[c]	$\chi^2_6 = 10.8, P = 0.094$		$\chi^2_6 = 12.7^*, P = 0.049$	
Household income				
Low	**0.9**	(0.6–1.4)	**1.7**	(0.6–4.6)
Low-average	**1.0**	(0.6–1.6)	**0.8**	(0.3–2.5)
High-average	**1.0**	(0.6–1.6)	**1.7**	(0.5–5.5)
High	**1.0**		**1.0**	
Household income difference[c]	$\chi^2_3 = 0.3, P = 0.956$		$\chi^2_3 = 2.1, P = 0.559$	
N[d]	**322,917**		**259**	

*Significant at the 0.05 level, two-sided test.

[a]These estimates are based on survival models adjusted for age-cohorts, gender, person-years, and upper-middle-income countries.

[b]These estimates are based on logistic regression models adjusted for time since ODD onset, age of ODD onset, gender, and upper-middle-income countries.

[c]Chi-square test of significant differences between blocks of socio-demographic variables.

[d]Denominator N: 322,917 = number of person-years in the survival models; 259 = number of lifetime ODD.

Table 15A.3 Bivariate associations between socio-demographic correlates and DSM-IV oppositional defiant disorder (ODD) (high-income countries)

Correlates	Lifetime ODD[a]		12-month ODD among lifetime cases[b]	
	OR	(95% CI)	OR	(95% CI)
Age-cohort				
18–24	**2.1***	(1.6–2.7)		
25–34	**1.2**	(0.9–1.6)		
35+	**1.0**			
Age-cohort difference[c]	$\chi^2_3 = 39.4^*, P < 0.001$			
Age-of-onset				
Early			**4.0***	(1.7–9.6)
Early-average			**1.5**	(0.6–3.9)
Late-average			**2.0**	(0.9–4.6)
Late			**1.0**	
Age-of-onset difference[c]			$\chi^2_3 = 12.6^*, P = 0.006$	
Time since onset (continuous)			**1.02**	(0.99–1.06)
Gender				
Female	**0.8**	(0.7–1.0)	**1.6**	(0.9–2.6)
Male	**1.0**		**1.0**	
Gender difference[c]	$\chi^2_1 = 3.5, P = 0.060$		$\chi^2_1 = 3.0, P = 0.085$	
Employment status				
Student	**1.0**	(0.6–1.5)	–	–
Homemaker	**0.7**	(0.4–1.1)	**2.0**	(0.8–5.1)
Retired	**0.2***	(0.1–0.6)	–	–
Other	**1.9***	(1.5–2.4)	**1.7**	(0.9–3.4)
Employed	**1.0**		**1.0**	
Employment status difference[c]	$\chi^2_4 = 37.7^*, P < 0.001$		$\chi^2_4 = 4.6, P = 0.331$	
Marital status				
Never married	**0.9**	(0.7–1.2)	**1.3**	(0.7–2.6)
Divorced/separated/widowed	**1.5***	(1.0–2.1)	**1.7**	(0.7–3.7)
Currently married	**1.0**		**1.0**	
Marital status difference[c]	$\chi^2_2 = 4.9, P = 0.086$		$\chi^2_2 = 1.7, P = 0.435$	
Education level				
Some primary	**1.6**	(0.8–3.1)	–	–
Finished primary	**1.9***	(1.1–3.3)	**2.5**	(0.7–9.6)
Some secondary	**2.1***	(1.4–3.2)	**4.4***	(1.6–11.9)
Finished secondary	**1.7***	(1.3–2.3)	**2.2**	(1.0–4.7)
Some college	**1.4**	(1.0–1.9)	**1.7**	(0.6–5.4)
Finished college	**1.0**		**1.0**	
Education level difference[c]	$\chi^2_6 = 349.1^*, P < 0.001$		$\chi^2_6 = 11.4^*, P = 0.045$	
Household income				
Low	**1.2**	(0.9–1.6)	**2.3***	(1.1–4.9)
Low-average	**1.0**	(0.7–1.4)	**3.0***	(1.2–7.6)
High-average	**1.0**	(0.7–1.5)	**1.0**	(0.4–2.5)
High	**1.0**		**1.0**	
Household income difference[c]	$\chi^2_3 = 1.8, P = 0.606$		$\chi^2_3 = 11.8^*, P = 0.008$	
N[d]	**490,671**		**721**	

*Significant at the 0.05 level, two-sided test.
[a]These estimates are based on survival models adjusted for age-cohorts, gender, person-years, and high-income countries.
[b]These estimates are based on logistic regression models adjusted for time since ODD onset, age of ODD onset, gender, and high-income countries.
[c]Chi-square test of significant differences between blocks of socio-demographic variables.
[d]Denominator N: 490,671 = number of person-years in the survival models; 721 = number of lifetime ODD cases.

Index

For EU product safety concerns, contact us at Calle de José Abascal, 56–1°, 28003 Madrid, Spain or eugpsr@cambridge.org.

www.ingramcontent.com/pod-product-compliance
Lightning Source LLC
LaVergne TN
LVHW062126200926
848484LV00007B/1774